Antibiotics

Volume IV

Biosynthesis

Edited by
John W. Corcoran

With 164 Figures

Springer-Verlag
Berlin Heidelberg New York 1981

Professor John W. Corcoran, Ph.D.
Department of Biochemistry
The Medical and Dental Schools
Northwestern University
Chicago, IL 60611, USA

ISBN-13: 978-3-642-67726-7 e-ISBN-13: 978-3-642-67724-3
DOI: 10.1007/978-3-642-67724-3

Library of Congress Cataloging in Publication Data. Main entry under title: Biosynthesis. (Antibiotics; v. 4). Bibliography: v. 1, p. 1. Antibiotics Synthesis. I. Corcoran, John W. II. Series. QD375.B56 615'.329 80-20092.

Softcover reprint of the hardcover 1st edition 1981

Typesetting, printing, and bookbinding: Universitätsdruckerei H. Stürtz AG, Würzburg
2131/3130-543210

Preface

The Series on Antibiotics produced by Springer-Verlag began more than a decade ago with the nearly simultaneous appearance of two volumes, one dealing with the mode of action of antibiotics and the other concerning the biosynthesis of them. The standards set by the original Editors were high, and these books have proved useful to many. The rapid advances in our knowledge of the mode of action of antibiotics and other antitumor agents has stimulated two further works in the same series (Volume III, 1975; and Volumes V/1 and V/2, 1979). For some time it had appeared to Dr. Konrad Springer that the time might 'be ripe' for bringing the subject of the biosynthesis of antibiotics up-to-date. This Editor agreed to survey the literature and discuss this possibility with his colleagues who are active in research on antibiotics. In spite of the appearance of numerous review articles, both of a highly specialized and general nature, on the biosynthesis of antibiotics, it was agreed generally that it would be extremely useful to add a new volume on biosynthesis to the Series. Such a work should focus on collecting a group of contributions dealing with those antibiotics whose biosynthesis is understood in much greater detail now than it was in the middle 1960's. Since Volume II on biosynthesis continues to be available, this addition to the series has not dealt with each and every antibiotic whose biosynthesis was studied long ago. Neither does it attempt to be encyclopedic, and cover all the numerous substances whose biosynthesis has been touched on during the intervening years. In the end, the Editor decided to aim for a volume which would describe the current state of knowledge of the major antibiotics, but which would not attempt to cover the many antibiotics and related natural products whose biosynthesis is either similar 'in principle' to these or has not been studied yet in any great detail. The contributors were asked to organize their chapters around central themes or patterns wherever possible.

It is sincerely hoped that this volume will be useful to research workers interested in antibiotics and the subject of their biosynthesis. The detail aimed at in the collection should make the book useful as a reference for those in this category, but it is hoped that it will be useful also to present and future students who lack much understanding of how nature plays the role of synthetic organic chemist in assembling the complex and fascinating molecules that antibiotics are. The biosynthesis of antibiotics reflects all the metabolic activities of nature, in particular the non-mammalian ones, and thus this volume represents a summary of the intermediary metabolism of those biological systems that provide most of our useful drugs.

Obviously, not all the important antibiotic substances have been included in the present volume, but it is believed that the goal set has been met and that the major examples are presented. It was originally intended to include general sections on the use of genetic techniques in the study (and manipulation) of biosynthetic pathways, and to have other general sections dealing with methodology – in particular the tremendous effect of new developments in chromatography and spectrometry on our ability to work out biosynthetic mechanisms. However, as the plans for the book developed, it became obvious that the individual chapters themselves would offer the most powerful testimony to the utility of these approaches and methods. One area exists, however, where there has been far less development during the past years than one would have expected. This is the study by classical biochemical techniques of the enzymatic steps in a whole biosynthetic pathway for an antibiotic. It is true that there are exceptions (6-methylsalicylate and the patulin pathway, transmethylases that form ethers and esters, etc.) but a detailed attempt to characterize all of the enzymes of a complex pathway has hardly been started. For this reason, and hopefully as a model for this approach, the Editor himself has hesitantly included one chapter (erythromycin) that is constructed along this line.

The Editor was fortunate in being able to enlist the major primary contributors to the literature on the biosynthesis of antibiotics, and he has enjoyed supurb cooperation in the delivery of manuscripts. For this he thanks his colleagues.

With the rapid strides currently being made in the study of the biosynthesis of antibiotics, this present volume will be 'past history' before its appearance. However, this is as it should be, and those whose scientific lives have been devoted to this fascinating subject will look forward to the next volume in the Series on Antibiotics with the subject of the biosynthesis of antibiotics.

In addition to the many colleagues who have helped in so many ways to make this volume a reality, the Editor wishes to give special thanks to several who provided him with stimulating discussion during certain phases of its preparation. They are: E.P. Abraham (Oxford), E.F. Gale (Cambridge); C. Hassall (Welwyn Garden City); D. Hopwood (Norwich); W.B. Whalley (London); D. Arigoni, H. Gerlach, W. Keller-Schierlein and V. Prelog (Zürich); P. Sensi and G. Lancini (Milan); and J.R. Martin (North Chicago).

The Editor acknowledges with gratitude the encouragement and support of Dr. Konrad Springer and Ms. Conny Fourneé in the planning and preparation of this volume. Thanks are given also to Northwestern University for a leave of absence that facilitated the Editor's role, and the courtesy of the School of Pharmacy (University of London) in providing the Editor with a temporary home during part of his leave is acknowledged with deepest appreciation.

Chicago, Autumn 1980

JOHN W. CORCORAN

Acknowledgments

The Editor thanks his teachers, especially Hans and Frieda, and his colleagues at Western Reserve and Columbia Universities (1949–1968) for his devotion to 'Nature' as a synthetic organic chemist.

This volume is dedicated to Alena with deepest appreciation for her loyal and loving support.

Contents

Contributors

ABRAHAM, E.P., Sir William Dunn School of Pathology, University of Oxford, Oxford OX1 3RE, Great Britain

CHANG, CHING-JER, Department of Medicinal Chemistry and Pharmacognosy, Purdue University, West Lafayette, IN 47907, USA

CORCORAN, JOHN W., Department of Biochemistry, The Medical and Dental Schools, Northwestern University, Chicago, IL 60611, USA

FLOSS, HEINZ G., Department of Medicinal Chemistry and Pharmacognosy, Purdue University, West Lafayette, IN 47907, USA

GRANDI, MARIA, Gruppo Lepetit, via Durando, 38, 20158 Milano, Italy

HOPWOOD, DAVID A., John Innes Institute, Norwich, NR4 7UH, Great Britain

HORNEMANN, ULFERT, Department of Medicinal Chemistry and Pharmacognosy, Purdue University, West Lafayette, IN, 47907, USA

HURLEY, LAURENCE H., College of Pharmacy, University of Kentucky, Lexington, KY 40506, USA

HUTCHINSON, C. RICHARD, School of Pharmacy, University of Wisconsin, Madison, WI 53706, USA

KURAHASHI, KIYOSHI, Institute for Protein Research, Osaka University, 5311, Yamada-Kami, Suita, Osaka, Japan

LANCINI, GIANCARLO, Gruppo Lepetit, via Durando, 38, 20158 Milano, Italy

NAKAGAWA, AKIRA, School of Pharmaceutical Sciences, Kitasato University, Tokyo 108, Japan

ŌMURA, SATOSHI, Microbial Chemistry, School of Pharmaceutical Sciences, Kitasato University, 5-9-1 Shirokane, Minato-ku, Tokyo 108, Japan

O'SULLIVAN, J., Sir William Dunn School of Pathology, University of Oxford, Oxford OX1 3RE, Great Britain

PEARCE, CEDRIC J., Department of Chemistry, University of Illinois, Champaign-Urbana, IL 61801, USA

RINEHART, KENNETH L., JR., Department of Chemistry, University of Illinois, Champaign-Urbana, IL 61801, USA

SPEEDIE, MARILYN, K., College of Pharmacy, University of Maryland, Baltimore, MD 21201, USA

SUHADOLNIK, ROBERT, J., Department of Biochemistry, Temple University, School of Medicine, Philadelphia, PA, 19140, USA

WESTLEY, JOHN W., Hoffmann-La Roche Inc., Nutley, NJ 07110, USA

The Biosynthesis of Tetracycline and Anthracycline Antibiotics

C. RICHARD HUTCHINSON

I. Introduction

The tetracycline antibiotics (1–5), which are produced by fermentation of various *Streptomyces* species, "are a group of natural products having notable antibacterial activity toward a broad range of pathogenic microorganisms and characterized [clinically] by very low toxicity to the mammalian hosts of these pathogens." MCCORMICK introduced his definitive review of the biosynthesis of the tetracycline antibiotics twelve years ago with this statement (MCCORMICK, 1967). Despite the continued interest in the chemistry of these 2-naphthacenecarboxamide-4-(dimethylamino)-1,4,4a,5,6,11,12a-octahydro-3,6,10,12,12a-pentahydroxy-6-methyl-1,11-dioxo antibiotics (HLAVKA and BOOTHE, 1973; DURCKHEIMER, 1975), the literature contains only a few reports about their biosynthesis since the pioneering studies of the LEDERLE group (MCCORMICK, 1967; MITSCHER, 1968). As most additions to the knowledge of the tetracycline's biosynthetic pathway were reviewed in 1973 by VANĚK et al., the present account highlights only the important experimental results obtained in the period 1968–1978. This review also covers the biosynthesis of the anthracycline antibiotics, typified by daunomycin and adriamycin, because they have a close structural and biogenetic relationship to the tetracyclines. I also summarize the available data about the microbial genetics of the tetracycline antibiotics to show that

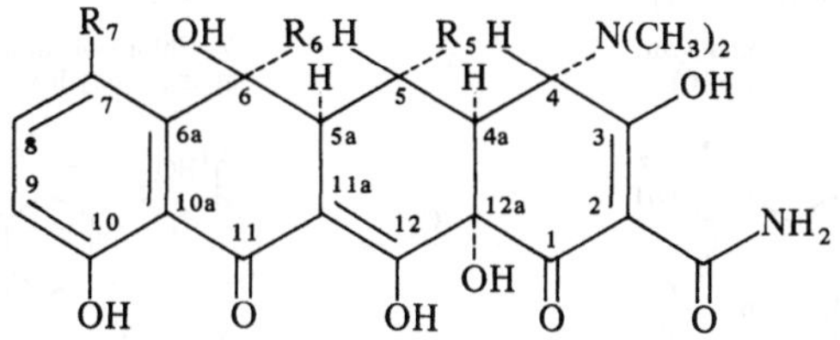

	R_5	R_6	R_7	
6-Demethyltetracycline	H	H	H	(1)
7-Chloro-6-demethyl tetracycline	H	H	Cl	(2)
Tetracycline	H	CH_3	H	(3)
5-Hydroxytetracycline	OH	CH_3	H	(4)
7-Chlorotetracycline	H	CH_3	Cl	(5)

Fig. 1. Structures of tetracycline antibiotics

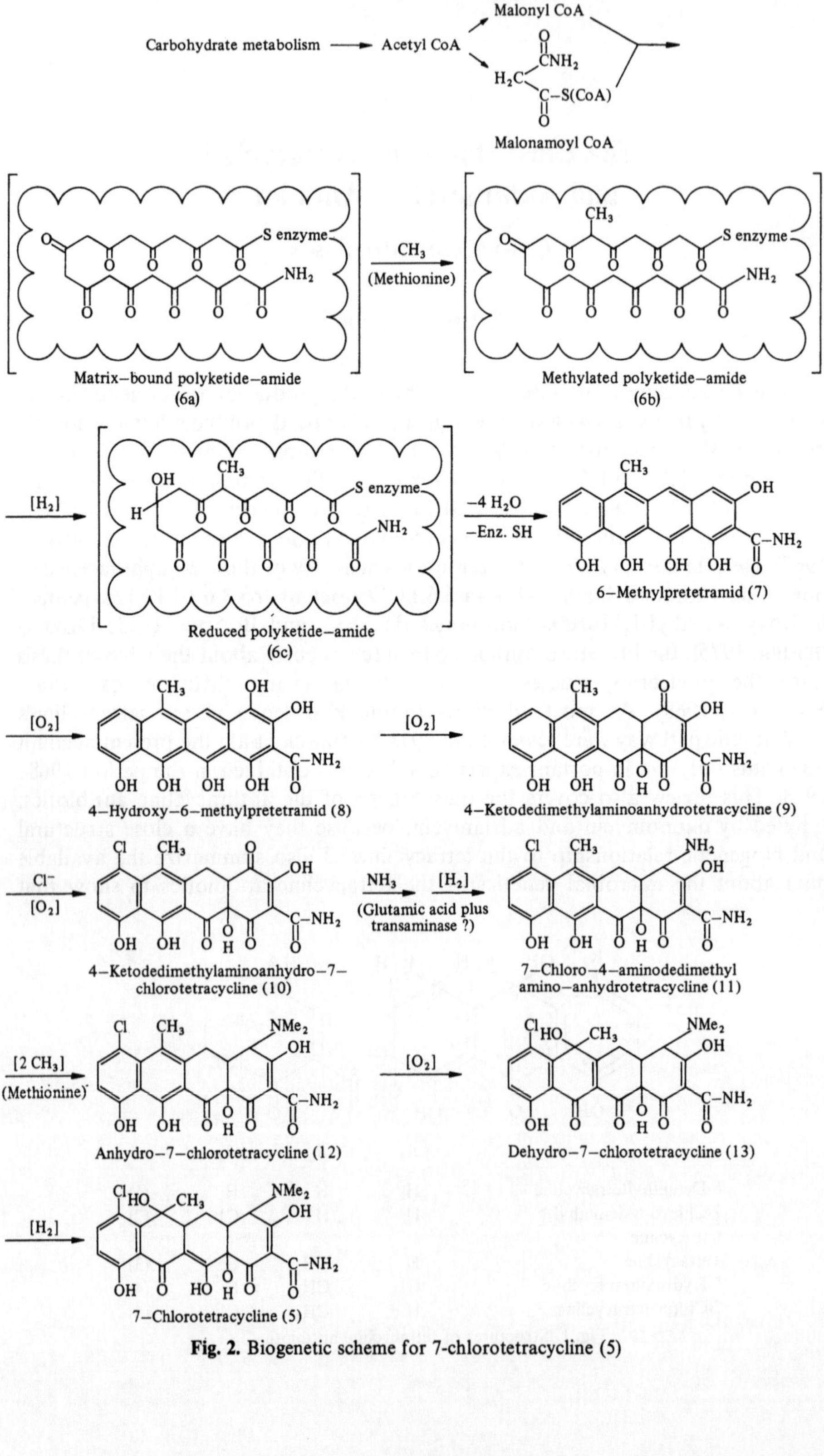

Fig. 2. Biogenetic scheme for 7-chlorotetracycline (5)

such studies may soon lead to important advances in the understanding of the biosynthesis of such antibiotics at the molecular level.

II. Tetracycline Biosynthesis

The results of experimental studies carried out by the LEDERLE group and others (McCORMICK, 1967; MITSCHER, 1968) are consistent with the biogenetic scheme for the tetracyclines (Fig. 2). It has not been directly proven that decapolyketides (6a–6c) are enzyme-bound intermediates between the primary metabolic precursor, acetate, and 6-methylpretetramid (7). Yet this is a reasonable mechanistic concept by analogy to the biogenesis of other acetate-derived aromatic polyketides (LYNEN and TADA, 1961; DIMROTH et al., 1970), since acetate is the precursor of all of the tetracyclines' hydronaphthacene ring carbons (MILLER et al., 1956; SNELL et al., 1960; GATENBECK, 1961; CATLIN et al., 1969). Although C(6) methylation (6a→6b) and C(8) deoxygenation (6c→7) presumably occur at the decapolyketide level, the introduction of the other non-acetate derived atoms [C(7) chlorine, C(4) dimethylamino, C(4), (4a), (5) and (5a) hydrogens, and C(4), (6) and (12a) oxygens] occurs after 7 by discrete reactions. Cell-free systems derived from *S. aureofaciens* can achieve some of these transformations [11→5, 7-deschloro-11→1, 13→4 and 5], but the use of 'point-blocked' mutants of *S. aureofaciens* provides most of the support for the intermediates of the biosynthetic pathway past 7 (McCORMICK, 1965, 1967). Mutant strains were isolated, following treatment of the wild-type organism with UV irradiation or chemical mutagens, that converted 7 to 1 or to 5, and 9 to 1 and 5. Other mutants converted 12 or 13 to 5. In fact, the observation that 7, 8, 12, and 13 accumulated during fermentations of certain of the point-blocked mutants was the initial signal that these substances are intermediates of the biosynthetic pathway to tetracycline (3) and 7-chlorotetracycline (5). Such experiments represent a milestone in biosynthetic investigations for they were the first successful use of mutants to map an antibiotic's biosynthetic pathway.

The carboxamide functionality at C(2) of 1–5 is unique among aromatic polyketides because it implicates malonamoyl CoA (Fig. 2), or an equivalent thioester, as the starter unit in the decapolyketide's formation. This was unprecedented at the most active time of experimental studies of tetracycline biosynthesis, since investigators believed that acetate, not malonate, was the principal starter unit for aromatic polyketide biosynthesis (BIRCH, 1957). Moreover, *S. rimosus* mutants were known that produced the 2-acetyl-2-decarboxamido tetracycline antibiotics, 14–16 (HOCHSTEIN et al., 1960; MILLER and HOCHSTEIN, 1962). GATENBECK found that both [1-^{14}C] malonate and [^{14}C] bicarbonate labeled the C(2) carboxamido carbon of oxytetracycline (4). This result and the isolation of protetrone (17) and the 6-methyl analog of protetrone (18) from fermentation of a *S. aureofaciens* mutant (McCORMICK and JENSEN, 1968a; McCORMICK et al., 1968b) are consistent with a malonate or malonamide starter unit for tetracycline biosynthesis. Nevertheless, the appropriate double-labeling experiments to confirm the involvement of an *intact* malonamide starter unit (McCORMICK, 1965; MITSCHER, 1968) were not successful, or have not been done.

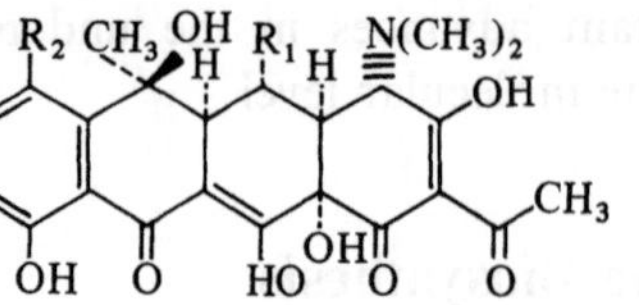

R_1	R_2	
H	H	(14)
H	Cl	(15)
OH	H	(16)

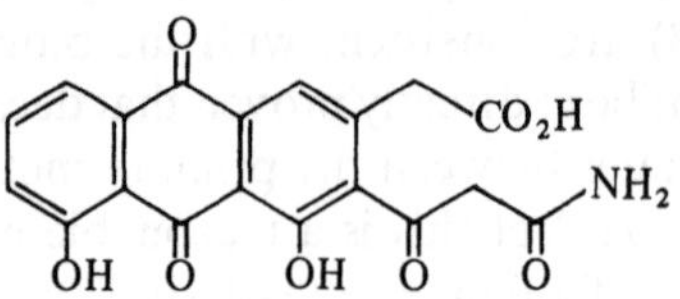

(17)

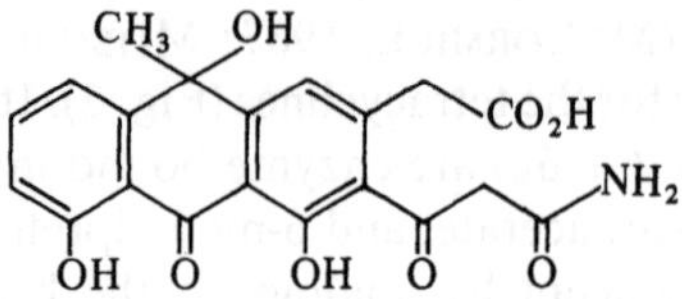

(18)

VANĚK and co-workers have recently re-examined this problem. PODOJIL et al. (1973) found that [U-^{14}C] asparagine labeled the C(2) carboxamido carbon of tetracycline (3) in fermentations of *S. aureofaciens* ten times more efficiently than it labeled C(6) or the D ring carbons. Subsequent feeding experiments showed that [1,3-^{14}C]-malonic acid semiamide, or its methyl ester, were apparently hydrolyzed to [1,3-^{14}C] malonate before their incorporation into 3, and that several ^{14}C-labeled substances known to be rather direct precursors of malonate in vivo (e.g., uracil and propionate) labeled 3 only by apparent conversion to C_2 units (BEHAL et al., 1974). The Czechoslovakian group proposed that asparagine could be converted to malonamic acid in vivo by pathways that conserved either its α or γ carboxamido group, from which malonamoyl CoA could result by adenylation and reaction with CoASH (PODOJIL, 1973). Their hypothesis awaits confirmation by a double-labeling experiment, which is absolutely necessary since the available data suggest that the introduction of the C(2) carboxamide unit occurs *after* the C(1) and C(2) carbons of the starter unit are loaded onto the enzyme that catalyzes the formation of the decapolyketide.

The route by which acetate serves as the precursor of the tetracyclines' hydronaphthacenecarboxamide ring is more complex than a simple acetate-to-malonate (plus malonamide) polymerization. Two research groups discovered that although [1-^{14}C] acetate labeled oxytetracycline (4) in the expected alternate positions [C(1), (3), (4a), (5a), (6a), (8), (10), (11) and (12)], [2-^{14}C] acetate labeled 4 somewhat randomly in fermentations of *S. rimosus* (TURLEY and SNELL, 1966; GATENBECK, 1961). CATLIN et al. (1969) confirmed the latter results, demonstrating that about 14% of the ^{14}C at C(2) of acetate entered the 'carbonyl carbon' positions of 4, normally labeled only by C(1) of acetate, after 72 h of metabolism in the presence of [2-^{14}C] acetate. Although these workers could not directly determine the relative molar ^{14}C-labeling of all carbons of 4, it was clear that [2-^{14}C] acetate did not label only C(2), (4) to (7), (9), (10a), (11a) and (12a) of 4.

TURLEY and SNELL (1966) reported that the relative molar ^{14}C-labeling of ring A *vs* rings BCD of 4 was unequal and markedly varied depending on the length of time [2-^{14}C] acetate was metabolized by fermentations of *S. rimosus*. This is a curious observation for it seems to imply that either the tetracycline carbon ring system was biosynthesized from more than a single polyketide chain, or that portions of the carbon ring system underwent independent and differential metabolic turnover *via* synthesis-resynthesis pathways. The conclusion SNELL and TURLEY drew from their data may be invalid, however. These authors used the specific radioactivity of a degradation product of 4, terracinoic acid (rings BCD), to calculate by difference the contribution ring A made to the specific radioactivity of 4, which had been isolated from feeding experiments of 18-, 24-, and 50-h duration. The percentage contribution that terracinoic acid and ring A made to the specific radioactivity of 4 was normalized to the number of C_2 units in each of these two subunits of the antibiotic. This normalized value showed that ring A contained about 1.2 times the relative ^{14}C-labeling of rings BCD after 18 h metabolism, about 1.05 times after 24 h, and about 0.8 times after 50 h. However, although ring A of 4 contains three acetate-derived C_2 units, C(2) of ring A is part of the starter unit, the carboxamido portion of which has often been found to have a specific radioactivity larger than the expected value of one-tenth the specific radioactivity of a [^{14}C] acetate-labeled tetracycline (GATENBECK, 1961; BEHAL, 1974). Since TURLEY and SNELL could not correct their data for the amount that the C(2)-$CONH_2$ subunit contributed to the ring A labeling, it is possible that the ^{14}C-labeling of this subunit only was changing as a function of time. This would be consistent with the results of BEHAL et al. (1974) discussed above.

Some of the Czechoslovakian group's recent observations permit a deeper appreciation of the complex pathway traversed by acetate during its incorporation into the tetracycline antibiotics (VANĚK et al., 1973; HOŠŤÁLEK and VANĚK, 1973). A comparative analysis of low (wild-type) and high-producing strains of *S. aureofaciens* showed that chlorotetracycline (5) biosynthesis occurred only after 12 h fermentation, becoming most active between 45 and 120 h of cultivation. The initial fermentation period ('anabolic phase') was characterized by a high primary metabolic activity as reflected in mycelial RNA content, the rate of protein and lipid synthesis, the activity of oxidative processes and tricarboxylic cycle enzymes, and the intracellular level of ATP. This phase was followed by the 'catabolic phase' during which 5 appeared in the medium and the rate of protein and lipid synthesis declined then ceased; the latter appeared to be associated with aggregation of the ribosomes in the cytoplasm. The latter process may have been the result of a ribosome-chlorotetracycline interaction. The presence and activities of several enzymes that might have provided acetyl and malonyl CoA for antibiotic biosynthesis were maximal in the anabolic phase, then declined rapidly during the onset and development of antibiotic biosynthesis. Interestingly, the intracellular ATP content (necessary for activation of exogenous acetate) and the incorporation of [1-^{14}C] acetate into the fatty acids markedly decreased during the time of rapid increase in chlorotetracycline formation. The authors concluded that these observations and others indicated that the carboxylation of acetyl Co A to malonyl Co A was not the sole source of the C_2 units used for antibiotic biosynthesis. Some of the available (exogenous) acetate must have been withdrawn, part into the dicarboxylic acid pool and part elsewhere, from which malonyl Co A was provided indirectly for chlorotetracycline biosynthesis. The exact sequence of biochemical events must be rather efficient since the LEDERLE group and SNELL et al. reported 10% yields in conversion of acetate to tetracyclines (MCCORMICK, 1967).

In view of the extensive studies of precursor-product relationships among the known tetracycline antibiotics, it seems unlikely that significant new information will result from further research of this type. And it is, therefore, interesting that the Czechoslovakian group at Prague has directed its investigations of tetracycline biosynthesis towards the microbial genetics of *S. aureofaciens*. Several definitive reviews are available: VANĚK et al., 1970; HOŠŤÁLEK and VANĚK, 1973; HOŠŤÁLEK et al., 1976.

These investigators are seeking an answer to the fundamental question of the molecular basis of polygenic inheritance in the biosynthesis of chlorotetracycline (5). An early paper (VANĚK et al., 1970) analyzed the problem of the number of genes required for the biosynthesis of 5. A biogenetic scheme containing 72 possible intermediates was devised to account for the full capacity of the 11 enzymatic systems necessary for the formation of 5. Only 27 of these intermediates were known; the other 45 were hypothetical. This fact and others was said to require an operon *ctc*-cluster of structural (biosynthetic) genes controlled by a single operator gene. Later papers (HOŠŤÁLEK and VANĚK, 1973; HOŠŤÁLEK et al., 1976) dealt with the primary and secondary metabolic changes found in *S. aureofaciens* mutant strains, which were obtained by treatment with UV irradiation and/or N-methyl-N′-nitro-N-nitrosoguanidine. The authors reported detailed observations of many qualitative (morphological, metabolite production) and quantitative (enzyme activities) differences among eight standard and mutant strains. They concluded that high antibiotic-producing strains had several changes in the primary metabolic pathways, particularly their control systems, which permitted expression of that part of the genome which usually remains repressed in the wild strain. Thus in high production strains, "an amphibolic type of metabolism ensues and intermediates formed during dissimilation of the [fermentation carbon source] sugar are not drawn into energy-producing metabolism but rather are exploited for secondary biosynthesis" (HOŠŤÁLEK et al., 1976).

Despite the enormous amount of effort which has been devoted to studying tetracycline biosynthesis, no information is available about the antibiotic production at the molecular level. The results of the few cell-free experiments (*inter alia*) have not been used to provide purified biosynthetic enzymes. However, UMEZAWA's laboratory has recently reported that treatment of *Streptomyces* strains with acriflavine eliminated the chlorotetracycline biosynthetic capacity in more than 1% of the cultures (H. UMEZAWA, 1977). A Czechoslovakian group has reported similar results upon acridine orange treatment (ZELINKOVA et al., 1976). These are exciting findings because they suggest that tetracycline biosynthesis is controlled by plasmid DNA. If this is verified, it should enable a detailed study of the molecular mechanisms of tetracycline biosynthesis analogous to studies of biosynthesis of other microbial antibiotics mediated by plasmid DNA (UMEZAWA, 1977; HORNEMANN and HOPWOOD, 1978; YAGISAWA et al., 1978).

III. Anthracycline Biosynthesis

The anthracycline antibiotics also are produced by species of the genus, *Streptomyces*. Representative structures are shown in Figure 3; the microbial sources are given in parentheses below each structural formula. The great utility of adriamycin (20) in cancer chemotherapy (CARTER, 1975) has stimulated interest in anthracycline chemistry, synthesis, metabolism, and biosynthesis. Several definitive reviews are available on these topics, excluding synthesis (BROCKMANN, 1963; OKI, 1977; VANĚK et al., 1977).

The anthracycline aglycones (anthracyclinones) are formally derived from a decapolyketide as are the tetracyclines. OLLIS and co-workers demonstrated

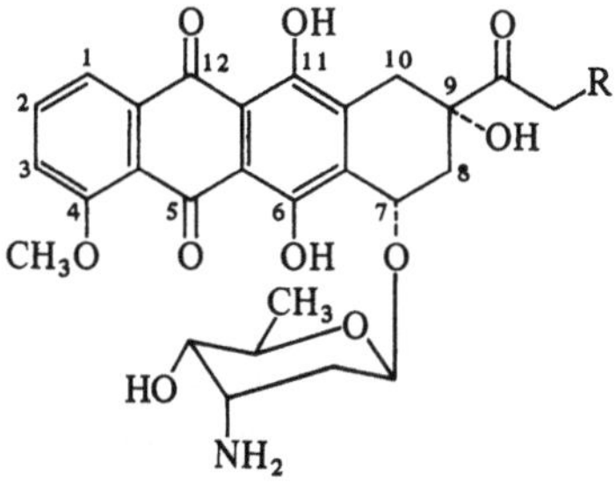

(19) R = H

(20) R = OH

(*S. peucetius*)

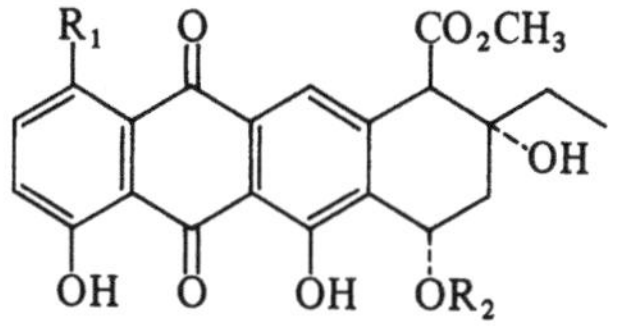

(21) R_1 = H; R_2 = H

(22) R_1 = OH; R_2 = H

(23) R_1 = H; R_2 =

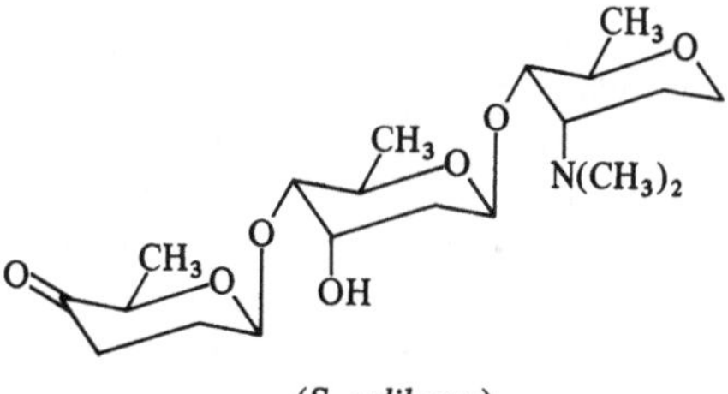

(*S. galilaeus*)

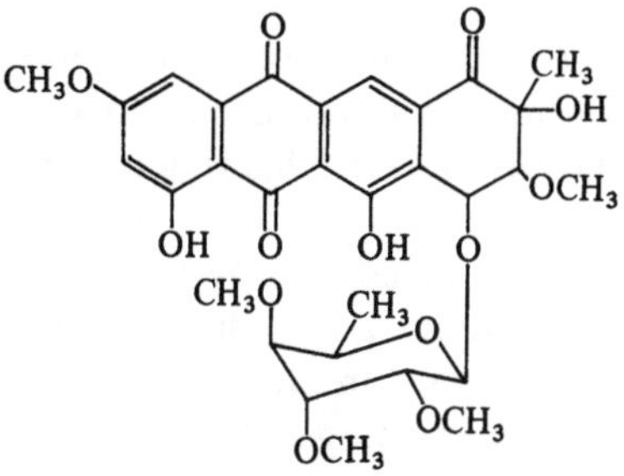

(24)

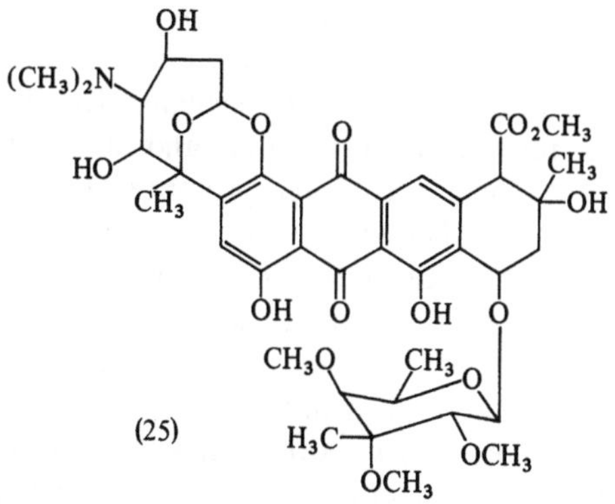

(25)

(*S. nogalater, S. elgreteus*)

Fig. 3. Representative structures of anthracycline antibiotics of *Streptomyces*

in 1960 that [^{14}C] propionate and acetate labeled ε-pyrromycinone (rutilantinone, 22) at the expected positions for its biosynthesis by way of the hypothetical decapolyketide, 26, and the naphthacene, 27:

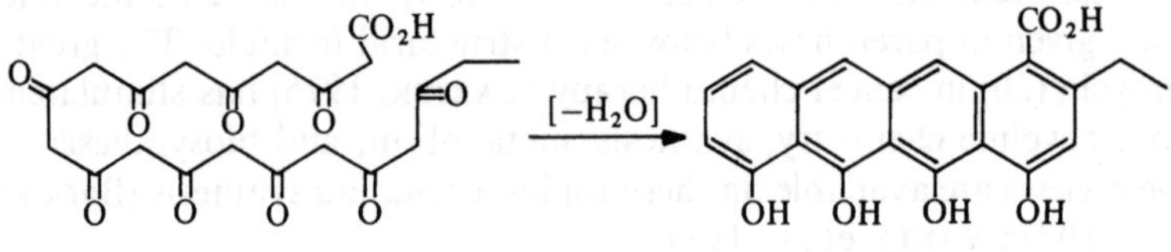

(26) (27)

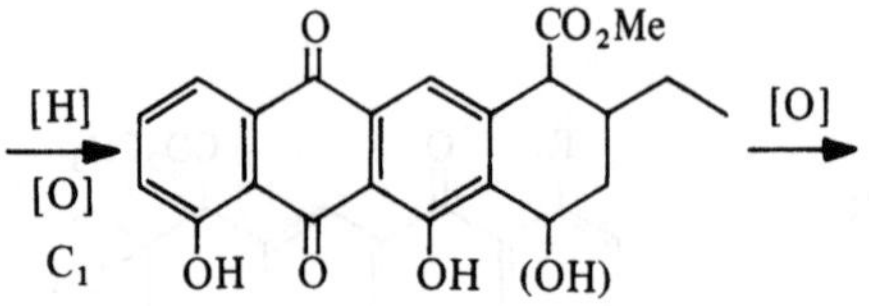

(28) (22)

Although an aklavinone (28) is also a likely intermediate in the biogenesis of 22, no information is available about the sequential events leading to ring A reductions, and the oxidations at C(4), C(7), and C(9). The recent results on incorporation of [^{13}C] acetate into daunomycin (19) (CASEY et al., 1978) and into steffimycin B (24) and nogalamycin (25) (WILEY et al., 1978) confirmed the polyketide origin of these anthracycline antibiotics by direct analysis of the ^{13}C-labeling patterns of 19, 24, and 25 using ^{13}C NMR spectroscopy. This technique permitted the authors to ascertain the three antibiotics' complete ^{13}C-labeling pattern, thereby obviating the difficulties that had arisen using radioisotope labels, which required tedious and incomplete chemical degradation for label localization (OLLIS et al., 1960). The C_2 units of 19, 24, and 25 appeared to be equally ^{13}C-enriched within the limits of the sensitivity of the spectroscopic technique, which indicates that they are derived from a single decapolyketide chain. Propionate is the starter unit of this decapolyketide (CASEY et al., 1978; PARANOSENKOVA and KARPOV, 1976).

Both BROCKMANN (1963) and VANĚK et al. (1977) have proposed reasonable and detailed biogenetic schemes for the anthracycline antibiotics, but no one has reported experimental validation of their proposals to date. This is necessary since, for example, the presence of 7-deoxyaklavinones in *S. galileus* indicates that the C(7) hydroxyl of the anthracyclinones could be introduced by oxidation of a C(7) methylene, or by reduction of a C(7) ketone. Also, the presence of both ring A aromatic and saturated anthracyclines in Nature does not enable us to know whether one precedes the other in a given biogenetic pathway, or whether both result from a common branch-point intermediate. For example, we have shown recently that the cyclization of A to B can be achieved in vitro (VEDEJS et al., unpublished results), which indicates that the A ring of anthracyclines could be formed from a tricyclic intermediate, rather than from a naphthacene. The inability of tetracycline-producing microorganisms to incorporate protetrone or its 6-methyl analogue into the tetracycline antibiotics does not support such an hypothesis, however.

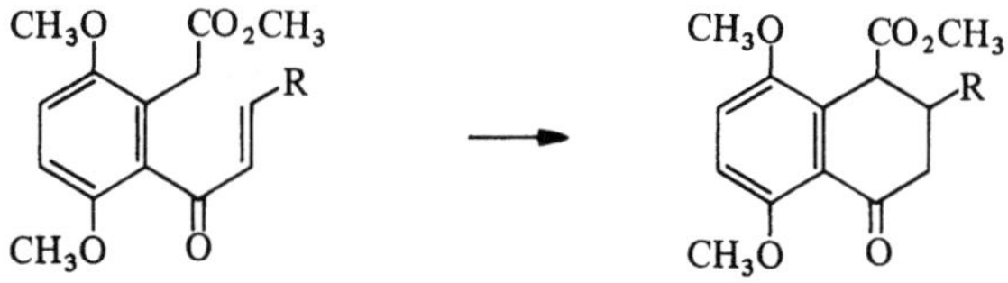

(A) (B)

It is interesting to note that both the tetracyclines and anthracycline aglycones lack the D ring hydroxy – at C(8) in 3 and at C(3) in 19 – corresponding to the same decapolyketide carbonyl position. Presumably this hydroxyl is lost by reduction followed by dehydration at the putative enzyme-bound stage preceding the cyclization that results in the primary naphthacene which serves as the precursor of the two types of antibiotics. This 'dehydrated' decapolyketide must have a *cis* double bond at the position originally held by the carbonyl to permit the reduced polyketide chain to adopt a favorable conformation for closure to 7 or 27. The same holds for the analogous reduction-dehydration steps involved in the biosynthesis of 6-methylsalicylic acid (LYNEN and TADA, 1961). Investigations of the solution chemistry of poly-β-carbonyl compounds by T.M. HARRIS and others (T.M. HARRIS and C.M. HARRIS, 1977; T.M. HARRIS et al., 1974) have confirmed that it also is important in vitro. For example, HARRIS' group carried out efficient syntheses of the heptaketides, chrysophanol (30), and eleutherin (31) from the formally reduced heptaketide intermediate, 29.

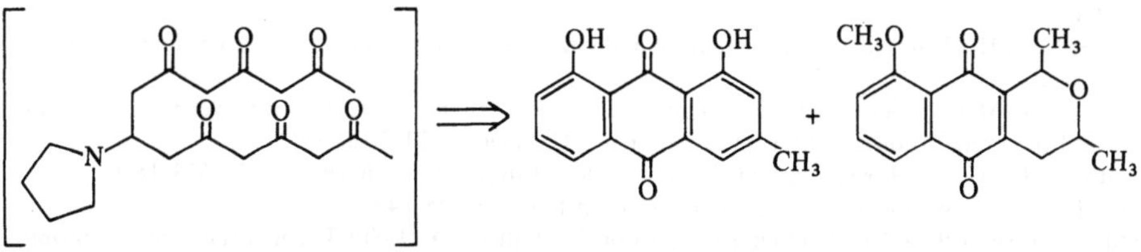

(29) (30) (31)

Acknowledgments. The preparation of this chapter was facilitated by a Research Career Development Award from the National Institutes of Health (CA 00253). I am indebted to Dr. J.R.D. MCCORMICK and Mrs. S.B. HASSAM for critical reading of the manuscript.

References

Běhal V, Podojil M, Hošťálek Z, Vaněk Z, Lynen F (1974) Regulation of the biosynthesis of excessive metabolites. XVI. Origin of the terminal group of tetracyclines. Folia Microbiol 19:146–150

Birch AJ (1957) Biosynthetic relations of some natural phenolic and enolic compounds. Fortschr Chem Org Naturst 14:186–216

Brockmann H (1963) Anthracyclinone und anthracycline. Fortschr Chem Org Naturst 21:122–182
Carter SK (1975) Adriamycin – a review. J Natl Cancer Inst 55:1265–1274
Casey ML, Paulick RC, Whitlock HC (1978) Carbon-13 Nuclear Magnetic Resonance study of the biosynthesis of daunomycin and islandicin. J Org Chem 43:1627–1634
Catlin ER, Hassall CH, Parry DR (1969) The biosynthesis of phenols. Part XVIII. Carbon-14 labelling in rings C and D of oxytetracycline incorporating [2-^{14}C] acetic acid. J Chem Soc C:1363–1366
Dimroth P, Walter H, Lynen F (1970) Biosynthese von 6-Methylsalicylsaure. Eur J Biochem 13:98–110
Durckheimer W (1975) Tetracyclines: chemistry, biochemistry, and structure-activity relationships. Angew Chem Int Edn 14:721–734
Gatenbeck S (1961) The biosynthesis of oxytetracycline. Biochem Biophys Res Commun 6:422–426
Harris TM, Harris CM (1977) Tetrahedron 33:2159–2185
Harris TM, Harris CM, Hindley KB (1974) Fortschritte Org Naturstoffe 31:218–282
Hlavka JJ, Boothe JH (1973) The tetracyclines. Fortschr Arzneimittel 17:210–240
Hochstein FA, Schach von Wittenau M, Tanner FW, Maurai K (1960) 2-Acetyl-2-decarboxamido-oxytetracycline. J Am Chem Soc 82:5934–5937
Hornemann U, Hopwood D (1978) Isolation and characterization of desepoxy-4,5-didehydro-methylenomycin A. A precursor of the antibiotic methylenomycin A in SCPl+ strains of *Streptomyces coelicolor* A3(2). Tetrahedron Lett 2977–2979
Hošťálek Z, Blumauerová M, Ludvik J, Jechová, Běhal V, Čaślavská J, Čurdová E (1976) The role of the genome in secondary biosynthesis in *Streptomyces aureofaciens*. In: MacDonald KD (ed) 2nd Int Symp Genet Indust Microorg, pp 155–177. Academic Press, London New York
Lynen F, Tada M (1961) Die Biochemischen Grundlagen der "Polyacetat-Regel." Angew Chem 73:513–519
McCormick JRD (1965) Biosynthesis of the tetracyclines. In: Vaněk Z, Hošťálek Z (eds) Biogenesis of antibiotic substances, pp 73–92. Academic Press, London New York
McCormick JRD (1967) Tetracyclines. In: Gottlieb D, Shaw PD (eds) The antibiotics. Biosynthesis, vol II, pp 113–122. Springer, Berlin Heidelberg New York
McCormick JRD, Jensen ER (1968) Biosynthesis of tetracyclines. X. Protetrone. J Am Chem Soc 90:7126–7127
McCormick JRD, Jensen ER, Arnold NH, Corey HS, Joachim UH, Johnson S, Miller PA, Sjolander ND (1968) Biosynthesis of tetracyclines. XI. The methylanthrone analog of protetrone. J Am Chem Soc 90:7127–7129
Miller MW, Hochstein FA (1962) Isolation and characterization of two new tetracycline antibiotics. J Org Chem 27:2525–2528
Miller PA, McCormick JRD, Doerschuk AP (1956) Studies of Chlorotetracycline biosynthesis and the preparation of Chlorotetracycline – ^{14}C. Science 123:1030–1031
Mitscher LA (1968) Biosynthesis of the tetracycline antibiotics. J Pharm Sci 57:1633–1649
Oki T (1977) New anthracycline antibiotics. J Antibiot 30:705–845
Ollis WD, Sutherland TO, Codner RC, Gordon JJ, Miller DA (1960) The incorporation of propionate in the biosynthesis of ε-pyrromycinone (rutilantinone). Proc Chem Soc London 347–349
Paranosenkova VI, Karpov VL (1976) The study of rubomycin biosynthesis. Bioorg Khim 1:1755–1758
Podojil M, Vaněk Z, Běhal V, Blumauerová M (1973) Regulation of biosynthesis of excessive metabolites. XIV. Incorporation of [U-^{14}C] asparagine into the molecule of tetracycline. Folia Microbiol 18:415–417
Snell JF, Birch AJ, Thomson PL (1960) The biosynthesis of tetracycline antibiotics. J Am Chem Soc 82:2402
Turley RH, Snell JF (1966) Biosynthesis of tetracycline antibiotics. In: Snell JF (ed) Biosynthesis of antibiotics, vol I, pp 95–120. Academic Press, London New York
Umezawa H (1977) Recent advances in bioactive microbial secondary metabolites. J Antibiot 30:138–163
Vaněk Z, Hošťálek Z (1973) Molecular basis of polygenic inheritance in the biosynthesis of chlorotetracycline. In: Vaněk Z, Hošťálek Z, Cudlín J (eds) Genetics of industrial microorganisms, vol II, pp 353–371. Elsevier, Amsterdam London New York

Vaněk Z, Cudlín J, Blumauerová M, Hošťálek Z (1970) How many genes are required for the synthesis of chlorotetracycline? Folia Microbiol 16:225–240
Vaněk Z, Hošťálek Z, Blumauerová M, Mikulík K, Podojil M, Běhal V, Jechová V (1973) The biosynthesis of tetracycline. Pure Appl Chem 34:463–486
Vaněk Z, Tax J, Komersová I, Sedmera P, Vokoun J (1977) Anthracyclines. Folia Microbiol 22:139–159
Wiley PF, Elrod DW, Marshall VP (1978) Biosynthesis of the anthracycline antibiotics nogalamycin and steffimycin B. J Org Chem 43:3457–3461
Yagisawa M, Rossana HTS, Davies JE (1978) Possible involvement of plasmids in biosynthesis of neomycin. J Antibiot 31:809–813
Zelinkova E, Čajkovská C, Zelinka J (1976) Acridine orange inhibits mycelial growth and chlorotetracycline production. Biologia (Bratislava) 31:727–730 [Chem Abstr 85:156184d]

Biosynthesis of Ansamycins

GIANCARLO LANCINI and MARIA GRANDI

I. Introduction

The term ansamycin designates a class of natural compounds produced by different organisms and characterized by a cyclic structure consisting of an aromatic group and an aliphatic chain that forms a bridge between two non-adjacent positions of the aromatic moiety. This typical handle shape (lat.: ansa) led PRELOG and OPPOLZER (1973) to propose the name ansamycin. According to the aromatic group we distinguish naphthalene ansamycins and the benzene ansamycins. This is not merely a chemical subdivision, since the structural differences correspond with different biological properties. Reviews on ansamycins have been published by PRELOG and OPPOLZER (1973), RINEHART, Jr., et al. (1976), WEHRLI (1977), and BRUFANI (1977). Rifamycin biosynthesis has been reviewed by LANCINI and WHITE (1976) and LANCINI and PARENTI (1978).

II. Natural Ansamycins with a Naphthalene Ring

To this group belong the following compounds:

A. Rifamycins,
B. Halomycins,
C. Tolypomycin Y,
D. Streptovaricins,
E. Naphthomycin.

All these products have antibacterial activity, especially against gram-positive bacteria and *Mycobacterium tuberculosis*. The first four compounds act through inhibition of RNA synthesis by formation of a complex with bacterial RNA polymerase. Naphthomycin inhibits bacterial growth by an as yet unknown mechanism of action.

A. Rifamycins

Rifamycins were first isolated by SENSI et al. (1959) from culture filtrates of an actinomycetes classified as *Streptomyces mediterranei* by MARGALITH and BERETTA (1960) as a complex of at least five different antibiotics. Later, the

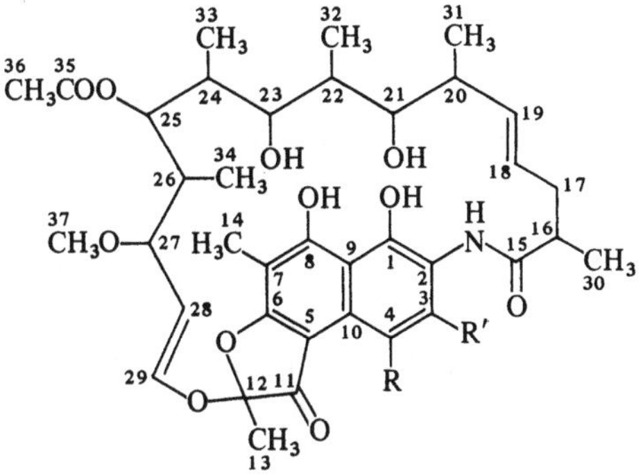

Name	R	R'
Rifamycin SV	OH	H
Rifamycin B	OCH_2COOH	H
Rifamycin L	$OCOCH_2OH$	H
3–Methylthiori-famycin SV	OH	SCH_3
Halomycin B	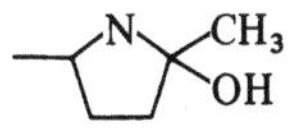	H

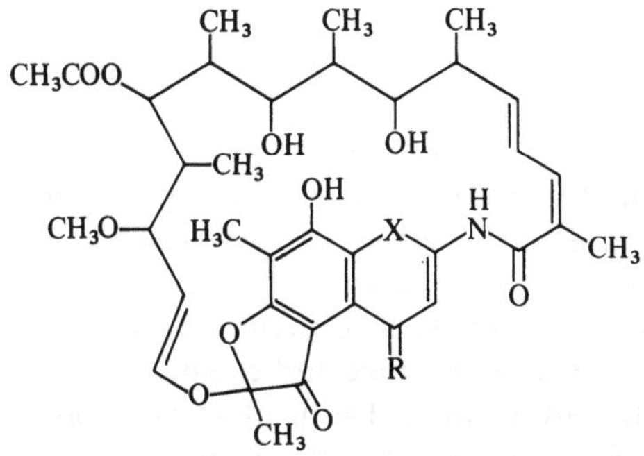

Name	R	X
Rifamycin S	=O	C=O
Rifamycin O	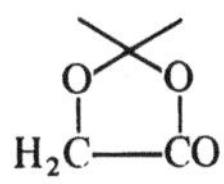	C=O
Rifamycin G	O	O

Fig. 1. Natural rifamycins and halomycin B

taxonomic position of this microorganism was revised by THIEMANN et al. (1969), who proposed its transfer from *Streptomyces* to *Nocardia* on the basis of the presence of meso-diaminopimelic acid in its cell wall.

Conditions of fermentation and rifamycin production have been reviewed by SENSI and THIEMANN (1967). It is noteworthy that diethyl barbituric acid added to fermentation media causes drastic changes so that instead of the complex of five or more products rifamycin B is almost exclusively produced.

Among the products of the original strain of *N. mediterranea,* only three have been obtained in a pure state and their structures determined. These are rifamycin B (OPPOLZER et al., 1964), rifamycin Y (LEITICH et al., 1967), (LANCINI et al., 1967), and rifamycin G (LANCINI and SARTORI, 1976) (Fig. 1).

Of these compounds, rifamycin G and rifamycin Y are inactive, whereas rifamycin B appears to be moderately active against gram-positive organisms only because it is transformed spontaneously into the active rifamycin S (FURESZ and TIMBAL, 1963). They are mentioned here because they were produced with other components of the rifamycin complex that are more active, but have never been thoroughly studied because of their instability. Several other rifamycins obtained from mutant *N. mediterranea* strains will be discussed later.

Other microbial strains that produce members of the rifamycin family were subsequently isolated: (Fig. 1) rifamycin O was obtained from *Streptomyces*

4107A by SUGAWARA et al. (1964), rifamycin SV was obtained from an Australian isolate of *N. mediterranea,* strain NT 19, by BIRNER et al. (1972), and rifamycins B and O from *Streptomyces tolipophorus,* as minor components by KISHI et al. (1972). From a new species of *Micromonospora,* later named *M. lacustris,* CELMER et al. (1975) isolated 3-methylthio-rifamycin SV and rifamycin S.

Both rifamycin SV and rifamycin O had been previously obtained chemically from rifamycin B by SENSI et al. (1960) and their structure was elucidated with that of rifamycin B by OPPOLZER and PRELOG (1973). Rifamycin SV and a semisynthetic derivative, rifampicin, are widely used in clinical medicine; rifampicin is the most effective antibiotic known for the cure of tuberculosis.

B. Halomycins

These were isolated by WEINSTEIN et al. (1967) as a complex of at least four components, active in the inhibition of gram-positive bacteria. The producing organisms were identified as belonging to the genus *Micromonospora* and were named *M. halophytica* and *M. halophytica* var. *nigra.*

The structure of one component of the complex, halomycin B (see Fig. 1) was elucidated by GANGULY et al. (1974) by spectroscopic and chemical means. The antibiotic differs from rifamycin B only in the substituent at position 4; it is easily transformed into rifamycin S on treatment with nitrous acid, and can be prepared by synthesis from rifamycin O. There are no data on the other components of the complex to indicate whether these are ansamycins also.

C. Tolypomycin Y

This was isolated by SHIBATA et al. (1971) in the course of a screening program for new broad spectra antibiotics. The producing strain, judged to be a new species, was named *Streptomyces tolypophorus.* It is a mesophilic streptomycete, characterized by the formation of sclerotic granules. The strain produces several antibiotics, among which tolypomycin Y was noticed because it is produced earlier in the course of the fermentation, and because it has different activity and stability (HASEGAWA et al., 1971). The same authors reported that the addition of iron salts increases the production of tolypomycin Y by two to five times. When more then 0.05% of ferrous sulfate was present, rifamycin B and O were also produced in the culture. The other components of the fermentation broth, named tolypomycins A to F, are not described. The structure of tolypomycin Y (Fig. 2) has been elucidated by KISHI et al. (1969). It differs from rifamycin S in the ansa chain, where C-19, C-20, and C-31 form a cyclopropane ring. At C-18 a keto group is found. Cross resistance is observed between tolypomycin Y and rifamycins.

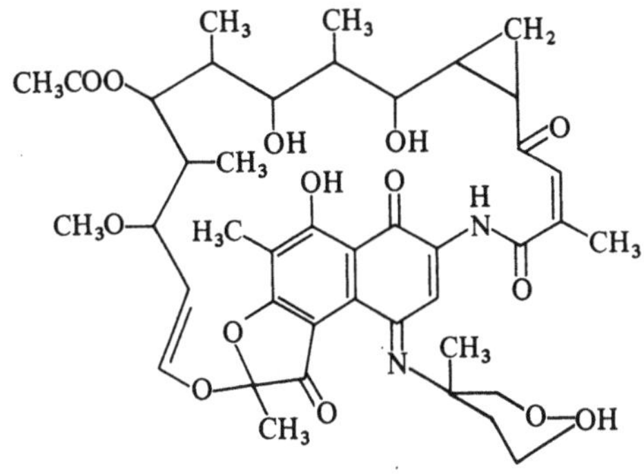

Fig. 2. Tolypomycin Y

D. Streptovaricins

These were isolated from *Streptomyces spectabilis* by SIMINOFF et al. (1957) as a complex of antibiotics active against gram-positive bacteria and *M. tuberculosis*. The characteristics of the producing strain have been described by WAKSMAN (1961). The structures of the various components of the complex were elucidated by RINEHART and ANTOSZ (1972), who described streptovaricin C, and RINEHART et al. (1971), who described other members of the complex, streptovaricins A, B, D, E, G, and J (Fig. 3). The main characteristic by which streptovaricins differ from rifamycins is that the ansa is a continuous carbon-carbon chain, whereas in rifamycins it also contains an oxygen atom.

During the separation of the components of the complex, two classes of precursors have been isolated from the same fermentation broth, protostreptovaricins I to V by DESHMUKH et al. (1976) and damavaricins by RINEHART et al. (1976). Their role in biosynthesis will be discussed in section IV. Compounds analogous to streptovaricin have been isolated by YAMAZAKI (1968), as a complex from fermentation broths of *Streptomyces* B-44PI, a strain differing from *Streptomyces spectabilis* only in some nutritional requirements. Three members of this complex were found to be identical to streptovaricins.

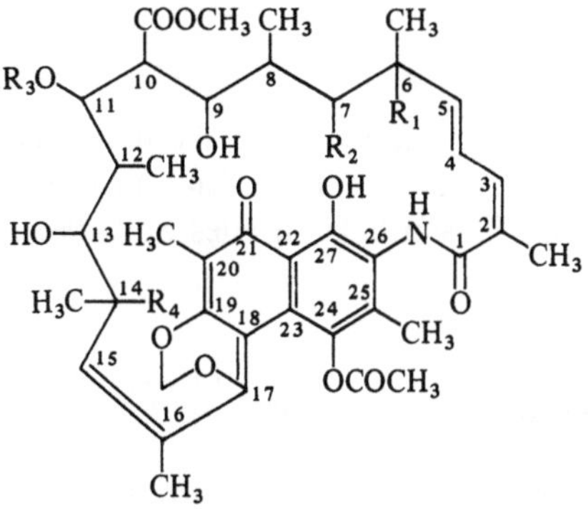

	R_1	R_2	R_3	R_4
A	OH	OH	$COCH_3$	OH
B	H	OH	$COCH_3$	OH
C	H	OH	H	OH
D	H	OH	H	H
E	H	=O	H	OH
G	OH	OH	H	OH
J	H	$OCOCH_3$	H	OH

Streptovaricins A–E, G and J

Fig. 3. Natural streptovaricins

Some years ago interest in streptovaricins was renewed because these compounds were found to be active in inhibiting the reverse transcriptase of some oncogenic RNA viruses (CARTER et al., 1971; RINEHART, et al., 1974).

E. Naphthomycin

Isolated by BALERNA et al. (1969) from *Streptomyces collinus* Lindenbein Tu. 105, naphthomycin is active against gram-positive bacteria. It differs from other naphthalene ansamycins in that it does not inhibit bacterial RNA polymerase. It is antagonized by Vitamin K and by cysteine or other sulfhydryl compounds. The structure of an antibiotic isolated from *Streptomyces* Sp. X-I2384 identical to the compound isolated by BALERNA was elucidated by WILLIAMS (1975) (Fig. 4). It differs from the other naphthalene ansamycins in that the skeleton of the ansa chain contains six additional carbon atoms, and there is a halogen at C-3 of the chromophore.

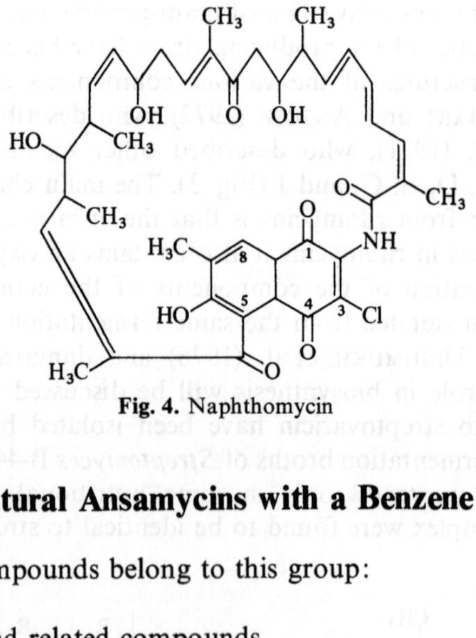

Fig. 4. Naphthomycin

III. Natural Ansamycins with a Benzene Ring

The following compounds belong to this group:

A. Geldanamycin
B. Maytansine and related compounds
C. Ansamitocin

These compounds have been isolated from *Streptomyces* or from higher plants. They are mainly active in eukaryotes, with a mechanism of action probably not related to RNA polymerase inhibition. Biosynthetic studies have been carried out only on geldanamycin.

A. Geldanamycin

This was isolated from *Streptomyces hygroscopicus* var. *geldanus* by DEBOER et al. (1970) while screening for substances inhibiting the growth and multiplica-

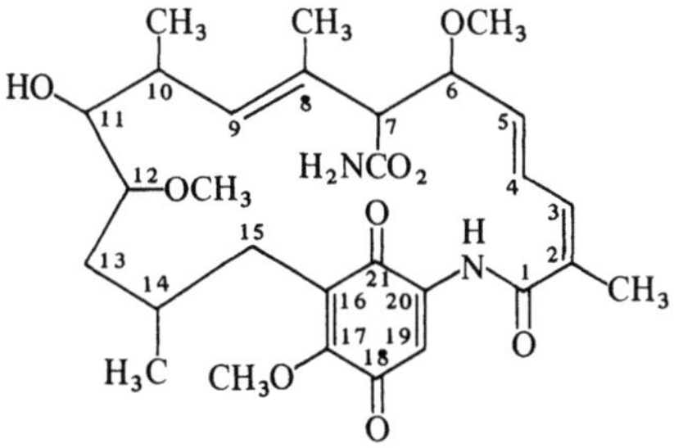

Fig. 5. Geldanamycin

tion of protozoa. The antibiotic was separated from other metabolites by extraction with n-butanol and the structure was elucidated by SASAKI et al. (1970) (Fig. 5). Besides having a benzoquinone instead of a naphthoquinone derivative as the aromatic moiety, geldanamycin possesses a shorter ansa chain than the naphthalene ansamycins (15 carbons instead of the 17 of the streptovaricins). As in the streptovaricins, the ansa is a continuous carbon chain linked directly by a C-C bond to one side of the aromatic ring and by an amide bond to the other side. The pattern of hydroxylation and methylation of the aliphatic ansa has some similarity to that of naphthalene ansamycins but there are also differences, such as the presence of a carbamate substituent at C-7.

B. Maytansine and Related Compounds

In the course of a search for tumor inhibitors from plant sources maytansine was first isolated from an alcoholic extract of the fruits of *Maytenus ovatus* by KUPCHAN et al. (1972), who also determined its structure (Fig. 6). The same authors have isolated analogous compounds from *Maytenus buchananii,* named maytanprine and maytanbutine (KUPCHAN et al., 1972b) and from *Putterlika verrucosa,* named maytanacine and maytansinol (KUPCHAN et al., 1975). Colubrinol acetate and colubrinol are products structurally related to the maytansines that have been isolated from alcoholic extracts of *Colubrina texensis* by WANI et al. (1973), along with maytanbutine. These antibiotics have the benzene chromophore of geldanamycin and the same number of carbon atoms in the skeleton of the ansa chain (Fig. 6).

The isolation of similar complex secondary metabolites from organisms taxonomically so different as plants and *Streptomyces* was a great surprise. It was even suggested that the producer was a *Streptomyces* contaminant of the plant fruits. However, there are differences from geldanamycin in the pattern of ansa substitution which appears to be more complex, and in the aromatic nucleus which has a chlorine at position 19 (corresponding to position 3 of rifamycins).

C. Ansamitocin

This group of maytansinoid compounds has been recently isolated from a new species of the genus *Nocardia,* named strain C-15003 by HIGASHIDE

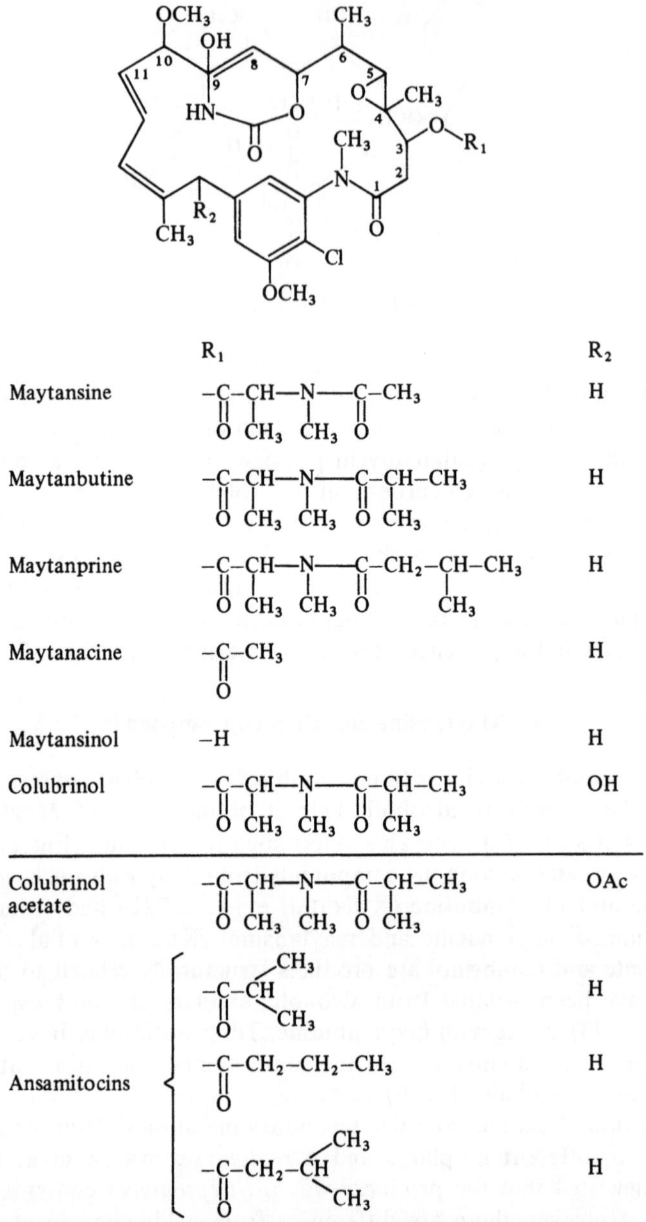

Fig. 6. Maytansine and related compounds, colubrinol and ansamitocin

et al. (1977). The strain forms many coraemia-like bodies and mobile heteromorphic cells. Two components of the complex were found to be identical to maytansine and maytansinol propionate. The other three are unknown maytansinoids (Fig. 6). The discovery of compounds identical to maytansine but produced by *Streptomyces* reinforces the suspicion that a contaminating microorganism may be the true source of maytansine and colubrinol.

Table 1. Origin and main characteristics of natural ansamycins

Family	Origin	Products	Chromophore	Extra substituent on chromophore	Ansa	Biological activity
Rifamycins	*Nocardia mediterranea* *Streptomyces tolypophorus* *Micromonospora lacustris*	Rifamycin complex (A,B,C,D,E) Rifamycin B, Y, G Rifamycin O, B	Naphthalenic		17-Carbon interrupted by oxygen	Antibacterial
	Streptomyces str. 4107 A_2	3-Methylthio rifamycin SV		Methylthio at C-3		
	Nocardia mediterranea str. NT 19	Rifamycin S Rifamycin O Rifamycin SV				
Halomycins	*Micromonospora halophytica*	Halomycin B				
Tolypomycin	*Streptomyces tolypophorus*	Tolypomycin Y				
Streptovaricins	*Streptomyces spectabilis*	Protostreptovaricins Damavaricins Streptovaricins		Methyl at C-25	17-Carbon continuous chain	
	Streptomyces B44P	Streptovaricins				
Naphthomycin	*Streptomyces collinus* *Streptomyces str X12384*	Naphthomycin		Cl at C-3	23-Carbon continuous chain	Antibacterial Antifungal
Geldanamycin	*Streptomyces hygroscopicus*	Geldanamycin	Benzenic		15-Carbon continuous chain	Antiprotozoal
Maytansines	Celastraceae Rhamnaceae	Maytansines		Cl at C-19		Antitumor
Colubrinol	Rhamnaceae	Colubrinol		Cl at C-19		Antitumor
Ansamitocins	*Nocardia* sp. C-1003	Ansamitocins		Cl at C-19		Antitumor

IV. Origin of the Ansamycin Carbon Skeleton

A. Acetate-propionate Incorporation into Rifamycins

1. Preliminary Experiments

Once the structure of rifamycins (and, later, that of streptovaricins) had been established, it became evident that the carbon skeleton of the ansa closely resembles that of macrolide antibiotics of the erythromycin type (CORCORAN and CHICK, 1966). In fact, in the ansa chain the methyl groups alternate with hydroxyl groups and this suggests that, as has been shown for the macrolides, it originates from a polyketide chain formed by condensation of *methylmalonate* units, with the insertion of one or two *malonate* units.

The aromatic nucleus could originate by cyclization of a polyketide chain, as was demonstrated for tetracyclines, or from an intermediate of aromatic amino acid synthesis. Preliminary experiments in our laboratories support the hypothesis of a macrolide-type of biosynthesis. Addition to the fermentation broth of ^{14}C methionine labeled in the methyl group (Brufani et al., 1973) gave rise to rifamycin B exclusively labeled in the methoxyl carbon on C-27. This strongly suggested that all the other methyls, including those of the chromophore, were derived from methylmalonate. ^{14}C-labeled propionate added to fermentation broths was efficiently incorporated into rifamycin B. This was also considered to be evidence for the above-mentioned biosynthetic scheme, since *propionate* is easily converted into *methylmalonate* by microbial cells. Acetate, the normal precursor of malonate, was also incorporated, although with lesser efficiency.

2. Studies with ^{3}H- and ^{14}C-labeled Propionate

The distribution of radioactivity in rifamycin molecules after addition to fermentation broths of propionate labeled in various positions was examined in cooperative studies by Prelog and the Lepetit Laboratories (Brufani et al., 1973).

The rifamycin B obtained after the fermentations was converted to rifamycin S which was then split by appropriate reactions into the fragments indicated

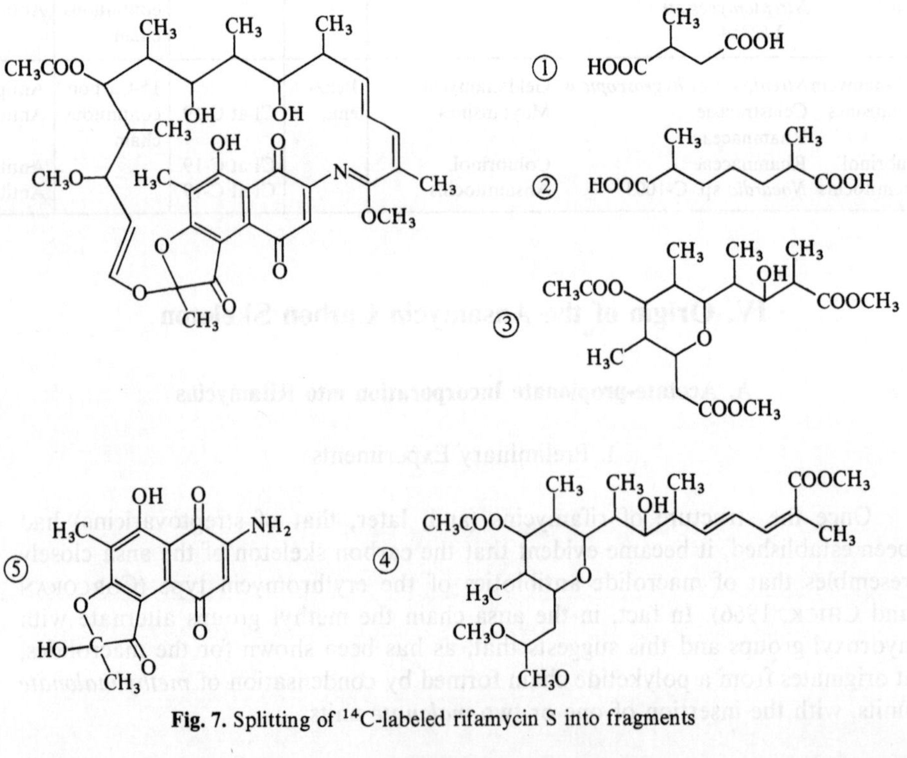

Fig. 7. Splitting of ^{14}C-labeled rifamycin S into fragments

Table 2. Radioactivity distribution after ^{14}C-propionate incorporation

	$^{14}CH_3$-CH_2-COOH		CH_3-CH_2-$^{14}COOH$		CH_3-$^{14}CH_2$-COOH	
	Percent	Ratio	Percent	Ratio	Percent	Ratio
Rif S	100%	7	100%	8	100%	8
Frag 1	13.24	0.93	–		11.64	0.93
Frag 2	29.94	2.09	36.23	2.89	28.48	2.27
Frag 3	57.81	4.04	–		62.25	4.98
Frag 4	74.51	5.21	85.21	6.81	72.2	5.77
Frag 5	28.67	2.00	12.32	0.98	24.54	1.96

in Figure 7. When methyl-labeled propionate was used as the precursor, the radioactivity of the fragments (see Table 2) was proportional to the number of methyl groups they included. Five propionate units appear to be incorporated into the ansa chain and two into the aromatic moiety. However, when carboxyl-labeled propionate was added different results were obtained (see Table 2). The ratio of the radioactivity of the ansa chain to that in the aromatic moiety appeared to be 7:1. When propionate labeled in the methylene carbon was used ansa: chromophore was 6:2. Repetition of the experiment with propionate labeled with ^{3}H in the methyl and ^{14}C in the carboxyl group confirmed the results.

These findings were interpreted to support the assumption that the rifamycin ansa and part of the chromophore originates by condensation of methylmalonate units. Also the stereochemistry of the chain is surprisingly similar to that of erythromycin, suggesting synthesis by a similar enzyme system. However, the differences in incorporation observed with propionate labeled in different positions were difficult to interpret and the data were considered to be insufficient to allow a detailed hypothesis about chain formation.

3. Incorporation of ^{13}C-acetate and ^{13}C-propionate

The use of ^{13}C-enriched precursors made it possible to identify unambiguously the carbon atoms derived from acetate and propionate (White et al., 1973). ^{13}C-Propionate and ^{13}C-acetate were pulse-fed twice a day for 96 h to *N. mediterranea* cultures to increase the incorporation. The rifamycin B obtained was chemically converted to rifamycin S and examined by CMR spectroscopy. The spectrum was compared to the natural abundance proton-decoupled CMR spectrum of rifamycins, in which each peak has been assigned to its corresponding C-atom. The addition of $^{13}CH_3$-CH_2-COOH confirmed that the 5 methyl group on the ansa chain (C-30, C-31, C-32, C-33, C-34) and the 2 on the chromophore (C-13, C-14) were derived from the methyl groups of propionate. No other carbon was enriched by this precursor.

When CH_3-CH_2 $^{13}COOH$ was used, the ansa chain carbon atoms C-15, C-19, C-21, C-23, C-25, which were in the appropriate positions with respect to methyls, were enriched; but, to our surprise C-29 and C-27 were also labeled. In the aromatic moiety, only C-6 was enriched.

When CH_3-$^{13}CH_2$-COOH was used, the expected C-7, C-16, C-20, C-22, C-24, C-26, and C-28, adjacent to those derived from the carboxyl propionate were labeled, but C-12 was also found to be ^{13}C enriched.

The interpretation of acetate incorporation was complicated by its metabolic conversion, through the Krebs cycle, into succinate and then to methylmalonate. For this reason, the carbons enriched by 2-^{13}C propionate and 3-^{13}C-propionate were also enriched by 2-^{13}C-acetate. In addition to this indirect incorporation, when $^{13}CH_3$-COOH was used, C-17 and C-11 were enriched; when CH_3-$^{13}COOH$ was used, the enrichment was in C-18 and C-5. The carbons of the acetoxyl group (C-35 and C-36) were also, as expected, enriched by ^{13}C-acetate.

In conclusion, in the rifamycin carbon skeleton, 23 atoms appear to be derived from propionate, through incorporation of eight 'propionate' units, one methyl group of which must be subsequently lost. This loss and the distribution of the units are in agreement and explain the results obtained with radioactive labels. Four atoms besides those of the acetoxy groups are derived from 'acetate' units. The remaining seven atoms, all part of the aromatic moiety, can not originate from the acetate-propionate pathway.

4. Formation of the Rifamycin Carbon Skeleton

Assuming that, as in macrolide biosynthesis, the incorporation of acetate-propionate units is evidence for a malonate-methylmalonate pathway of chain construction, the results obtained can be interpreted as showing that the rifamycin molecule is synthesized by a regular, clockwise condensation of 'propionate' and 'acetate' units, initiated by a seven-carbon aromatic moiety (Fig. 8a). This hypothesis requires that after chain completion the molecule undergoes two major modifications: 1. oxidation, resulting in insertion of oxygen between the carboxyl and the methylene of one propionate unit; 2. loss of a methyl group.

The existence of a precursor that is modified in this way was postulated, and a product with the expected characteristics was identified in *N. mediterranea* metabolites (see rifamycin W), thus confirming the validity of the postulation.

B. Acetate-propionate Incorporation into Streptovaricins

The structural resemblance between the streptovaricins and the rifamycins makes it probable that their biosyntheses are closely similar. Also, the ansa chains of both streptovaricin and the rifamycin precursor, rifamycin W, are continuous carbon atom chains.

Incorporation studies with ^{13}C-enriched precursors were carried out in streptovaricin D and streptovaricin C by MILAVETZ et al. (1973) and by KAKINUMA et al. (1976).

Comparison by the CMR technique of the compounds obtained after incorporation of ^{13}C-precursors with the spectrum of natural abundance indicated that, as in rifamycin, the molecule is formed by amide-head condensation starting

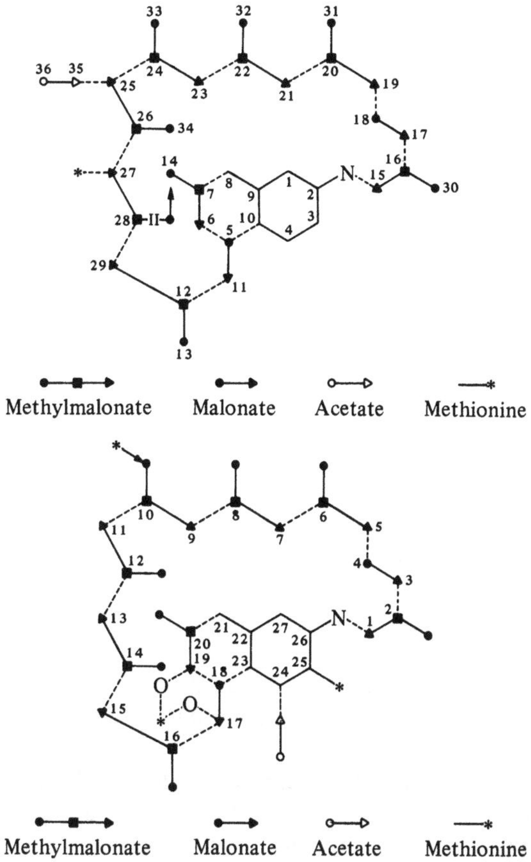

Fig. 8. a Scheme of biosynthesis of rifamycin ansa chain after condensation of malonate-methylmalonate. **b** Scheme of biosynthesis of streptovaricin ansa chain after condensation of malonate-methylmalonate

from the aromatic nucleus, of eight methylmalonate and two malonate units (Fig. 8b). In fact, 1-^{13}C-propionate labels carbon atoms C-1, C-5, C-7, C-9, C-13, C-15, and C-19 whereas 2-^{13}C malonate enriches equally C-4 and C-18. (Note that the numbering of streptovaricins differs from that commonly used for rifamycins.) Incorporation of methionine ^{14}C-labeled in the methyl group indicates that the 'extra' methyl at C-25 (corresponding to C-3 in rifamycins) as well as the methylene atom and the methoxy carbon are derived from methionine. No studies have been made of the origin of the aromatic moiety, but the lack of any significant labeling after acetate-propionate incorporation suggests that it originates from the aromatic amino acid pathway.

C. Origin of the Aromatic Ring

Only seven atoms of the rifamycin S carbon skeleton do not arise from propionate or acetate, namely, the six atoms of the quinone ring (C-1, C-2,

C-3, C-4, C-10, and C-9) plus the adjacent C-8. ^{14}C-Incorporation studies by KARLSSON et al. (1974) demonstrated that two precursors preferentially labeled the chromophore: 3,4-^{14}C-glucose and 1-^{14}C-glycerate. Glycerate presumably enters the glycolytic pathway as 3-phosphoglycerate: this intermediate would also be labeled in its carboxyl group when formed from 3,4-^{14}C-glucose. The labeling of the chromophore by these two precursors presumably occurs via the same intermediate, i.e., a three-carbon glycolytic pathway molecule. This could be phosphoenolpyruvate, which is also a building unit in the biosynthesis of aromatic amino acids.

^{13}C-Incorporation studies by WHITE and MARTINELLI (1974) gave further information on the origin of the aromatic nucleus. They found that after 1-^{13}C-glucose incorporation two carbon atoms were enriched: C-10 and C-1 with enrichment factors of 1.9 and 2.4 respectively. After 1-^{13}C-glycerate incorporation, the two carbons enriched were C-8 and C-3, with enrichment factors of 4.4 and 2.0. These data are consistent with a shikimate-type origin of the chromophore, by way of the sequence of reactions shown in Figure 9. However, it was found that labeled shikimate added to fermentation broths does not label the aromatic ring in a specific way. This result could indicate that the precursor is an intermediate on the aromatic pathway, before shikimate, that is dehydroquinate or dehydroshikimate, or as suggested by BRUGISSER (1975), that intact shikimate cannot enter cells of *N. mediterranea*. A recent genetic approach by GHISALBA and NÜESCH (1978a, b) provides further evidence that the aromatic moiety is synthesized by the shikimate pathway. Two *N. mediterranea* mutants were isolated by these authors:

1. Mutant A8, auxotrophic for aromatic amino acids, producing very low amounts of rifamycin B. Sugar analysis indicated that the mutant accumulated a mixture of aldopentose and ketopentose, but no sedoheptulose. Crude extracts of this mutant were analyzed and shown to be lacking in a transketolase. Therefore the mutant is unable to synthesize 3-deoxyheptulosonic acid, an essential precursor of shikimate.

2. Mutant A10, auxotrophic for aromatic amino acids, but producing about the same amount of rifamycin B as the parent strain. The mutant accumulated shikimic acid and 3-hydroshikimic acid, but no shikimate-3-phosphate. It seems very likely that the mutant lacks shikimate kinase.

Therefore, the authors postulated that the precursor of the aromatic ring is a compound intermediate between 3-deoxy-sedoheptulosonic acid and shikimate, which agrees with the incorporation found by WHITE and MARTINELLI (1974).

D. Hypothesis about the Precursors of the Building Units

The origin of the carbon skeleton of the rifamycins by condensation of 'acetate' and 'propionate' units has been well established, as described above. Further studies by KARLSSON et al. (1974) indicated that, as in the biosynthesis of macrolide antibiotics, malonate and methylmalonate are the actual activated forms in which the acetate and propionate precursors are incorporated. They

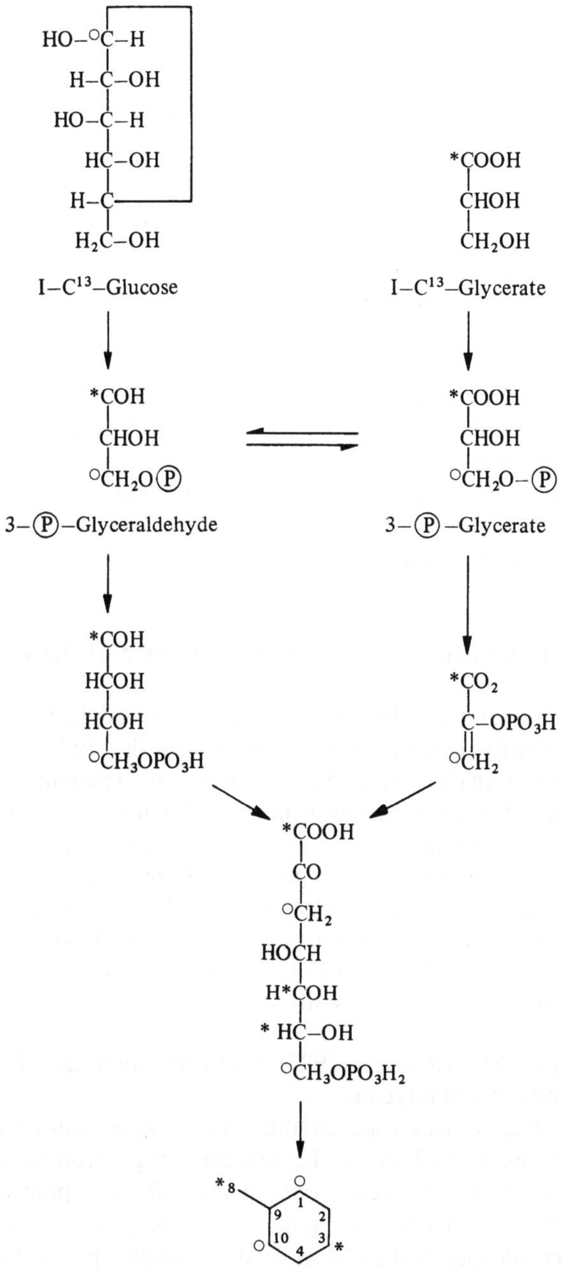

Fig. 9. Formation of the aromatic ring from 1-^{13}C glucose and 1-^{13}C glycerate

have observed that the rifamycin S ansa and chromophore have the same ratio of isotope labeling when either methyl-labeled propionate or methyl-labeled methylmalonate were used as precursors. Moreover, unlabeled propionate efficiently dilutes the incorporation of radioactive methylmalonate.

Comparison of ^{13}C-acetate and ^{13}C-malonate incorporation shows that these precursors label the same atoms in the carbon skeleton, while the acetoxy at C-25 is preferentially labeled by acetate.

Preliminary experiments carried out in our laboratories indicate that among the possible metabolic pathways from glucose to methylmalonate, the ones most likely involved in rifamycin biosynthesis are:

1. glucose → pyruvate → acetyl CoA $\xrightarrow{\text{Krebs cycle}}$ succinyl CoA → methylmalonyl CoA
2. glucose → pyruvate → acetyl CoA $\xrightarrow{\text{glyoxylate cycle}}$ succinate → methylmalonyl CoA.

In fact, when 1-^{13}C-glucose is used as a precursor, the ansa carbon atoms known to be derived from the methyl or the methylene carbon of propionate are about equally enriched, the methylene ones perhaps slightly more. Carbons derived from the propionate carboxyl are less enriched. This is consistent with the above-reported pathway and different labeling ratios would have been given by other biosynthetic pathways.

E. Origin of the Geldanamycin Carbon Skeleton

The assumption that similar pathways are followed in the biosynthesis of all ansamycins recently received strong support from the studies of geldanamycin precursors by RINEHART's group. Nuclear magnetic resonance spectra of the antibiotic obtained from fermentation in the presence of ^{13}C-propionate once again indicated that the ansa chain is built starting from a C_7N_1 initiating unit and grows in the direction of the amide linkage (Fig. 10).

Unlike the rifamycins and streptovaricins, which possess a longer chain, only four 'propionate' units are present in geldanamycin. The label from 1-^{13}C propionate was found as expected in C-1, C-7, C-9, and C-13. The three methoxy methyls were shown to come from the methyl of methionine (JOHNSON et al., 1974).

Further studies (HABER et al., 1977) confirmed that the the origin of the C_7H_1 unit is similar to rifamycins.

When 6-^{13}C-glucose was used as the precursor, a strong enrichment was observed in carbons 17 and 21 of the benzene ring, strongly suggesting that this moiety derived from an intermediate of the shikimate pathway of aromatic aminoacid synthesis. Carbon 6 of glucose, in fact, is the source of C-3 in phosphoenolpyruvate and of the C-4 in erythrose-4-phosphate, the two building units of the aromatic ring in this pathway. Since shikimate is not incorporated into geldanamycin, 3-dehydroquinate or 3-dehydroshikimate were again suggested to be the most likely intermediates.

Also, enrichments from C-6 of glucose in the ansa carbons which are derived from the methyl or the methylene of propionate units are about the same or greater than that observed for carbons derived from the propionate carboxyl group. These results agree with the above-reported finding of 1-^{13}C-glucose

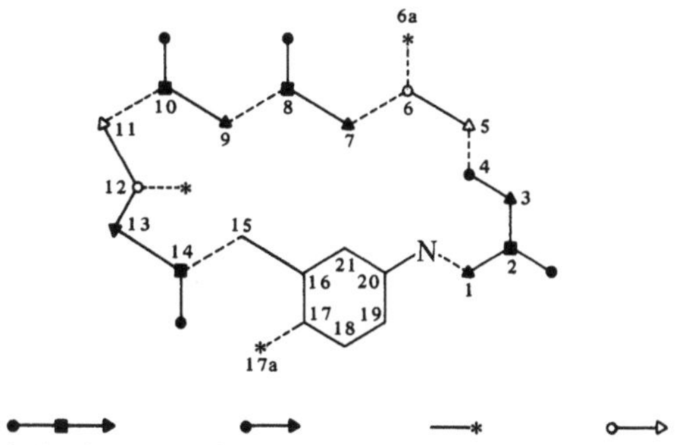

Fig. 10. Scheme of biosynthesis of geldanamycin ansa chain after condensation of malonate-methylmalonate

incorporation into rifamycins. Since after glycolysis C-1 and C-6 of glucose are interchangeable, similar patterns of methylmalonate formation and incorporation must be assumed to exist for both the antibiotics. A difference from other ansamycins has been found in the origin of the two-carbon units in the geldanamycin ansa. Both in streptovaricins and in rifamycins, two acetate-malonate units participate in ansa chain formation. In the geldanamycin ansa there are three two-carbon units, none of which was labeled by propionate. Only one of these (the C-3, C-4 unit) appears to be labeled by ^{13}C-malonate. 1-^{13}C-glycolate added to the fermentation yielded geldanamycins labeled at C-5 and C-11. Moreover, C-12 and C-6 both have hydroxyl substituents. An unusual incorporation of glycolate can thus be surmised to be responsible for the remaining two-carbon units C-5, C-6 and C-11, C-12.

The carbamate residue of geldanamycin is derived from the guanidino group of arginine, since the latter, double-labeled with ^{15}N and ^{13}C appeared to be incorporated as an intact unit into position 7 of the antibiotic.

V. Intermediate and Late Steps in Ansamycin Biosynthesis

A. Biosynthetic Relationship among Rifamycins

Two classical approaches have been extensively used to determine the biosynthetic relationships among natural rifamycins: 1. examination of the microorganism's ability to convert one product into another and 2. the isolation of mutant strains blocked in the biosynthetic pathways. Several products have been obtained by the last method and now, between intermediates and final products, about twenty rifamycins are known, either produced by microorganisms isolated from the soil or by mutant strains of *N. mediterranea*. The complex picture of the biosynthetic relationships can be simplified by grouping the rifamycins into families according to their structural and biogenetic similarities. A graphical representation of these families and their connections is given in Figure 11. The central role of rifamycin S (or its hydroquinone form, rifamycin SV) can

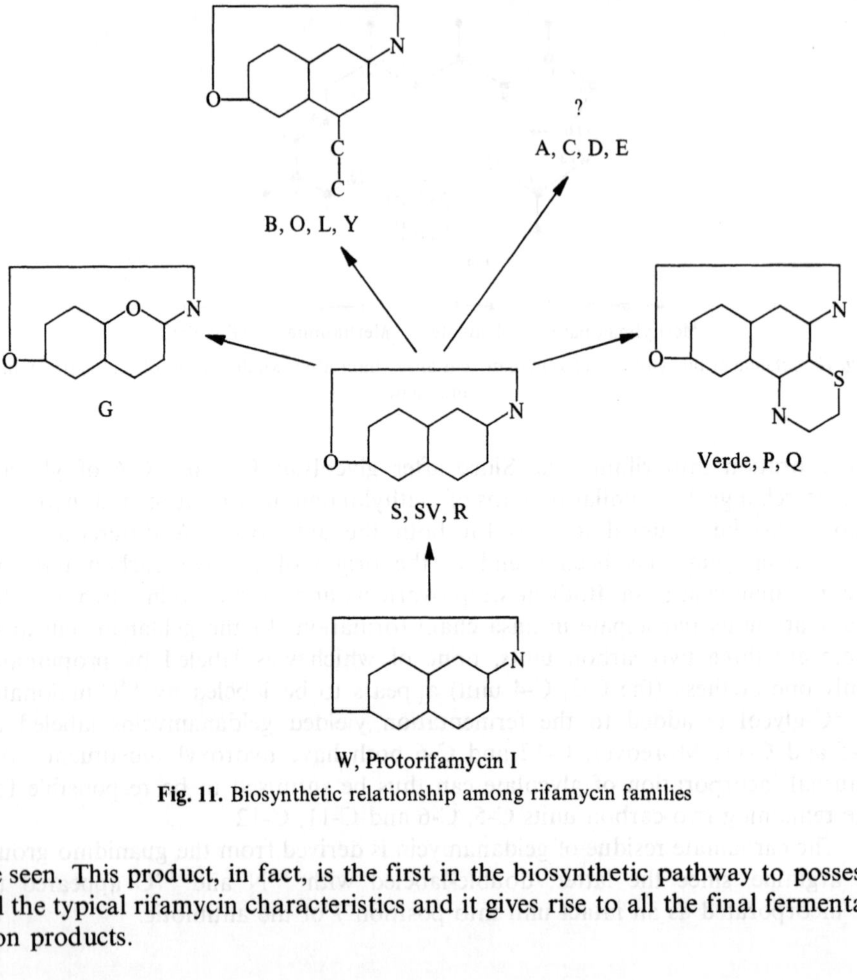

Fig. 11. Biosynthetic relationship among rifamycin families

be seen. This product, in fact, is the first in the biosynthetic pathway to possess all the typical rifamycin characteristics and it gives rise to all the final fermentation products.

1. Rifamycin W Family

This family includes the early precursors of the rifamycins, soon after the assembling of the carbon skeleton and is characterized by an as yet unmodified, all-carbon, ansa chain (Fig. 12).

The recently isolated protorifamycin I (GHISALBA et al., 1979) appears to be the earliest intermediate, since it is converted into rifamycin W (from which it differs only in lacking the hydroxyl group at position 8) by *N. mediterranea* blocked mutants 126 and W 2800, both producers of rifamycin W. Rifamycin W was first isolated by WHITE et al. (1974) from a morphologic variant of *N. mediterranea*. Its discovery confirmed that rifamycins were made from one chain of 'acetate' and 'propionate' units. In addition to the continuous carbon ansa, it still retains the propionate-derived methyl group that is missing in rifamycin S (MARTINELLI et al., 1974). This methyl group is hydroxylated, an indication that its subsequent loss is by way of an oxidative sequence of reactions.

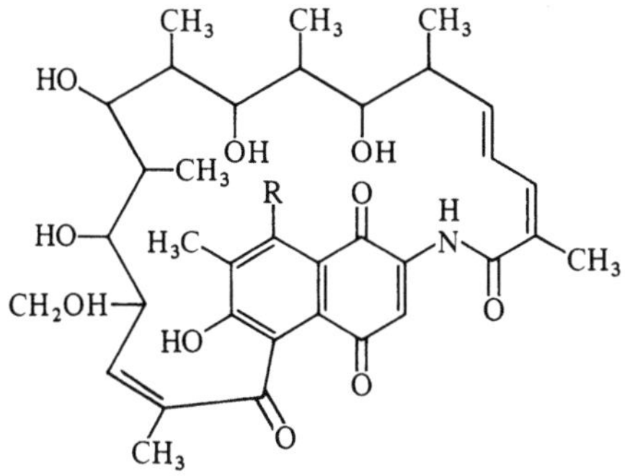

Protorifamycin I R = H
Rifamycin W R = OH

Fig. 12. Structure of protorifamycin 1 and rifamycin W

^{14}C-Labeled rifamycin W is converted into labeled rifamycin B by the mycelium of *N. mediterranea,* good evidence that it is a true intermediate in the biosynthesis of rifamycin B. Protorifamycin I and rifamycin W have only minor structural differences from protostreptovaricins, the early streptovaricin precursors, thus supporting the assumption that both these families of antibiotics are derived from a common precursor.

2. Rifamycin S Family

This family includes the first products in the biosynthetic pattern that possess the typical rifamycin structural features, that is, the ether linkage in the ansa and the naphthoquinone-furanone moiety. The aromatic nucleus does not have any extra substituents (Fig. 13).

In addition to rifamycin S (the quinone form) and rifamycin SV (the hydroquinone form), which are easily interchangeable, rifamycin R (or 30-hydroxy-rifamycin S) and 27-demethyl-rifamycin SV (or 27-demethoxy-27-hydroxy-rifamycin SV) belong to this family.

Rifamycin S and SV were first obtained by chemical degradation of rifamycin B by SENSI and co-workers (1961). They were recognized by LANCINI and SENSI (1967) to be intermediates in rifamycin biosynthesis because they were converted to rifamycin B in the *N. mediterranea* fermentation, and by LANCINI and HENGELLER (1969) who, after a target-oriented screening, isolated a blocked mutant able to accumulate substantial amounts of rifamycin S (or SV) in fermentation broth.

As mentioned before BIRNER et al. (1972) later isolated from soil a strain producing rifamycin SV. 27-Demethyl-rifamycin SV and rifamycin R were isolated from other *N. mediterranea* mutants (LANCINI and WHITE, 1973, WHITE et al., 1975). Their biogenetic relationships to rifamycin S have not been demonstrated experimentally. The 27-demethyl-rifamycin SV is thought to be an intermediate in rifamycin SV biosynthesis, although the order in which the different modifications between rifamycin W and rifamycin S take place is unknown.

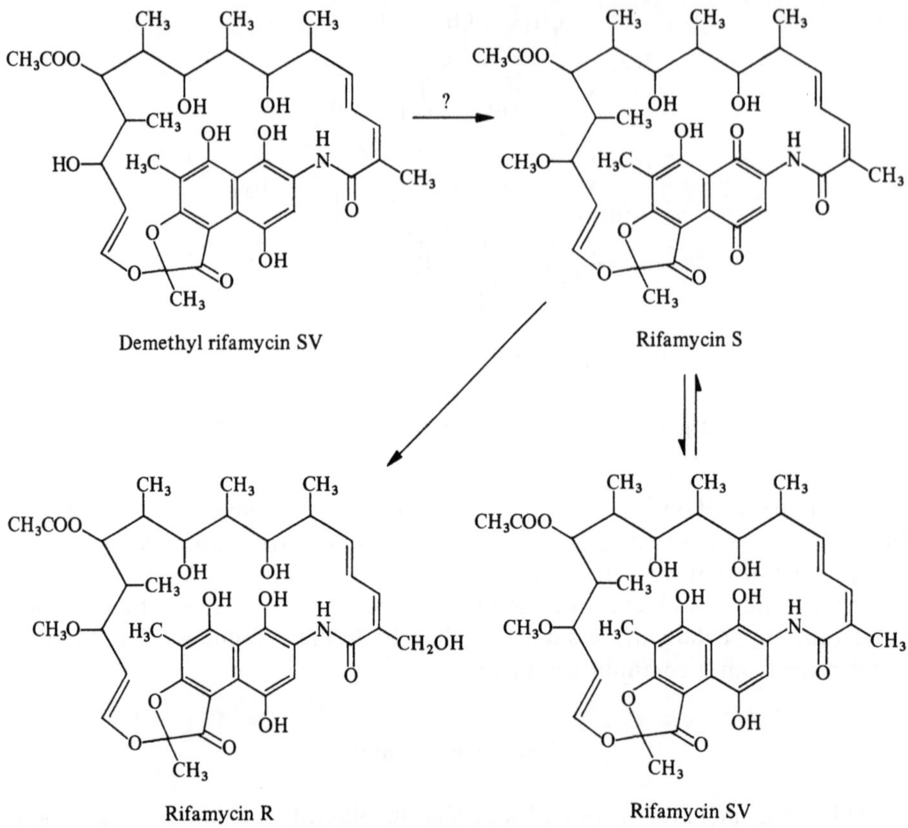

Fig. 13. Rifamycin S family

The conditions under which rifamycin R is produced indicate that it originates by oxidation of rifamycin S (MARTINELLI et al., 1978).

3. Rifamycin B Family

This includes the compounds that have a two-carbon unit of the type -O-CH_2-CO- at position 4 of rifamycin SV or S (Fig. 14). In rifamycin B, the main product of *N. mediterranea* when grown in the presence of barbital, the chain has the acidic form -OCH_2COOH. Its origin from rifamycin SV has been demonstrated as mentioned before, by the conversion of labeled SV into ^{14}C-labeled rifamycin B, both in *N. mediterranea* fermentations and by washed mycelium. The origin of the glycolic moiety has been studied, but no firm conclusion could be drawn (LANCINI et al., 1969). It is possible that a three-carbon intermediate of glycolysis (such as 3-phosphoglyceric acid or 3-phosphohydroxypyruvate) is first attached to position 4 of rifamycin and then degraded by decarboxylation. In the experiments on the conversion of rifamycin S to rifamycin B, the formation of a novel product was observed. This was rifamycin L in which the glycolic moiety is linked to oxygen 4 of rifamycin SV by an ester bond

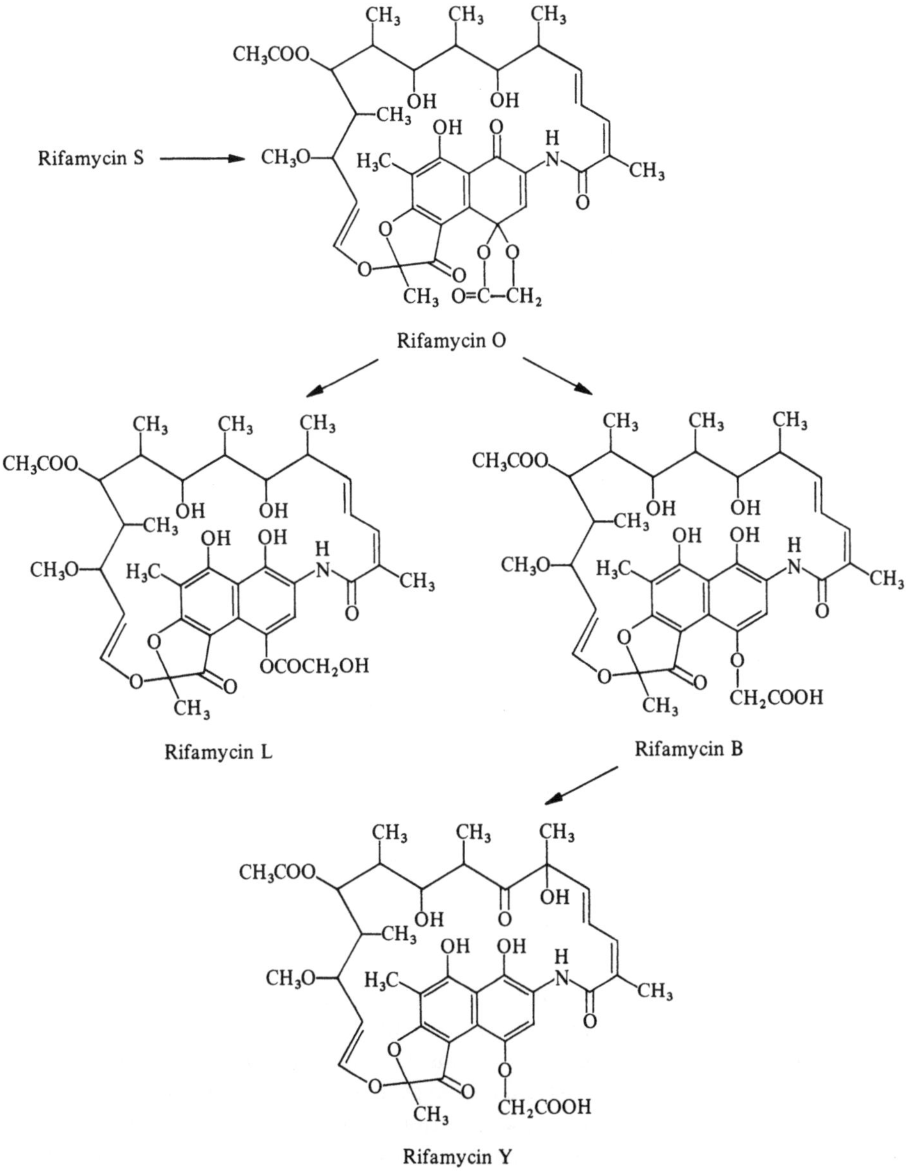

Fig. 14. Rifamycin B family

(LANCINI et al., 1969). This led to the suggestion that rifamycin O, in which the glycolic chain is cyclized at position 4 of rifamycin S, might be a common precursor of both rifamycin B and L. The former could be derived by hydrolysis (chemical or enzymatic) of the ester bond, the latter by opening of the ether linkage. No direct evidence in support of this assumption is available, but rifamycin O has been isolated from the fermentation broth of a streptomycete (SUGAWARA et al., 1964).

Rifamycin Y is found as a minor component in rifamycin B fermentations (LEITICH et al., 1967). Its origin from rifamycin B, from which it differs in the degree of ansa oxygenation, has been demonstrated by LANCINI and co-workers (1967) using ^{14}C-labeled compounds.

4. Rifamycin G

In this compound, one of the end products of *N. mediterranea* fermentation in the absence of barbiturate, the carbon 1 of rifamycin S is replaced by an oxygen atom (Fig. 15). Its origin from rifamycin SV has been demonstrated by its high yield when rifamycin SV is converted into rifamycin G by *N. mediterranea* mycelium and by experiments using ^{14}C-labeled compounds (LANCINI and SARTORI, 1976).

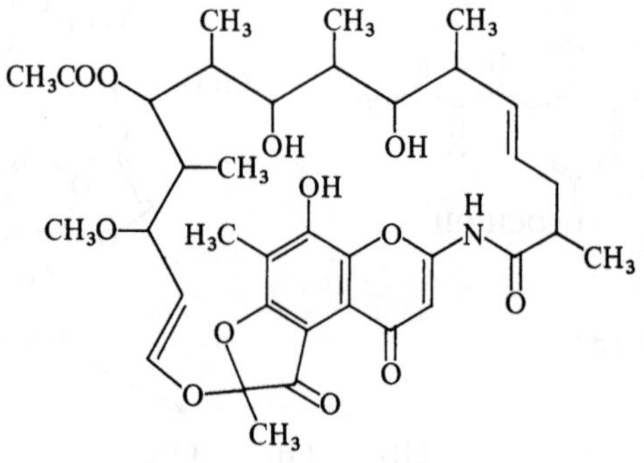

Fig. 15. Rifamycin G

5. Rifamycin complex

The structure of rifamycins A, C, D, and E, produced along with rifamycin B and G by the original *N. mediterranea* strain, are still unknown. The origins of the two main compounds, rifamycins C and D, from rifamycin SV are suggested by the results of co-synthesis experiments in which a non-producing *N. mediterranea* mutant was grown with a rifamycin SV producer. In the presence of barbital the production of rifamycin B was observed, when barbital was omitted rifamycins C and D were produced (WHITE, unpublished results).

6. Sulphur-substituted Rifamycins

From a mutant strain (strain D-2) blocked in the conversion of rifamycin SV into rifamycin B a novel series of rifamycins with a heterocyclic ring attached to positions 3 and 4 were obtained (CRICCHIO et al., 1979, CRICCHIO and LANCINI, 1978). These have been named rifamycin Verde (or green), Q and P (Fig. 16). In all cases the ring contains a sulphur atom, linked to position 3 of rifamycin

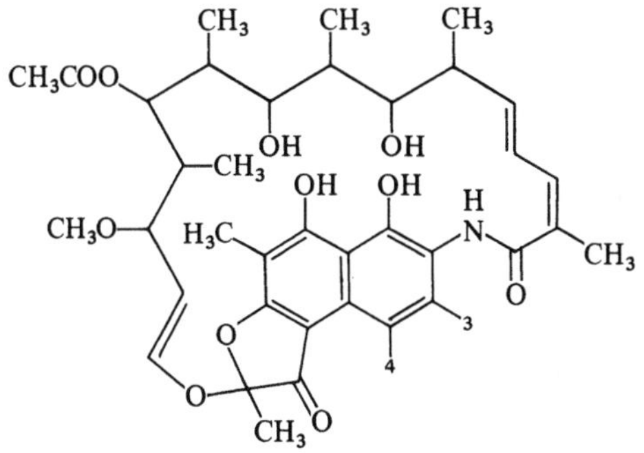

Name

Rifamycin Verde

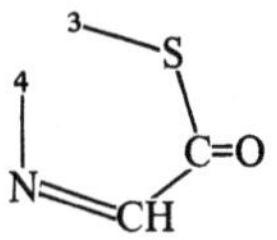

Rifamycin P

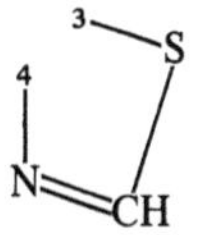

Rifamycin Q

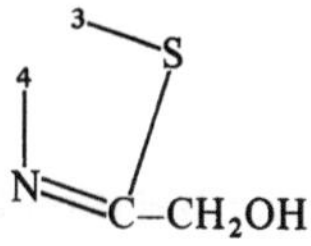

Fig. 16. Sulphur-substituted rifamycins

SV, and a nitrogen substitutes for the oxygen at position 4. All these derivatives are derived from rifamycin S, as shown by the isolation of labeled compounds when ^{14}C-labeled rifamycin S was added to strain D-2 cultures. The origin of the heterocyclic ring from cysteine was demonstrated by addition to the fermentation medium of this amino acid labeled either with ^{35}S or with ^{14}C.

Recent results, however, demonstrate that probably only rifamycin Q is the direct result of enzymatic activity in the microorganisms. Rifamycin Verde and P are formed in the fermentation broth by chemical reactions, even after the enzymes have been inactivated (CRICCHIO et al., 1979).

A sulphur-substituted rifamycin (3-methylrifamycin SV) has been isolated by CELMER et al. (1975) from a micromonospora strain. Its origin from rifamycin SV may be surmised.

Summary of the rifamycin biosynthetic pattern.

1. a. Glucose → erythrose-4-phosphate + phosphoenolpyruvate
→ shikimic type intermediate → benzene ring

b. Glucose → TCA cycle or glyoxylate cycle → succinyl-CoA → methylmalonyl-CoA
c. Glucose → acetyl-CoA → malonyl-CoA
2. Benzene ring + 2-malonyl-CoA + 8-methylmalonyl-CoA → polyketide type chain → protorifamycin I (or earlier unknown intermediate)
3. Protorifamycin I → rifamycin W
4. Rifamycin W $\xrightarrow{a,\,b,\,c}$ rifamycin S and SV $\xrightarrow{ox.}$ rifamycin R
   a. Insertion of oxygen in the ansa chain
   b. Closure of the furanone ring
   c. Oxidation and cleavage of methyl on the ansa
5. Modification of rifamycin SV (or S), leading to different groups of final products.
   a. Introduction of a two-carbon substituent at position 4. Rifamycin S → rifamycins Q, L, B → rifamycin Y
   b. Replacement of C-1 with oxygen. Rifamycin S → rifamycin G
   c. Unknown alterations. Rifamycin S → rifamycin C, D
   d. Introduction of cysteine at C-3 and C-4.

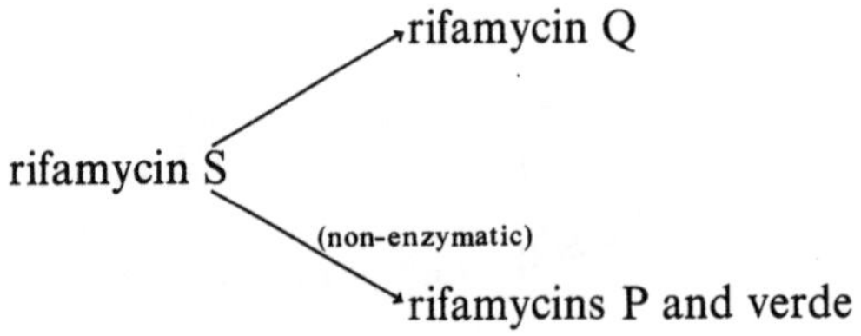

B. Biosynthetic Relationships among Streptovaricins

As with the other ansamycins and macrolide antibiotics, no intermediate between the building units of the chain and an assembled molecule containing all of the skeletal carbon atoms of the antibiotic has been observed so far for the streptovaricins. Some evidence is available about the sequence of events following assembly of the carbon skeleton. This evidence includes: a. the identification of metabolites produced in small amounts by *S. spectabilis* and b. transformation of labeled streptovaricins by *S. spectabilis* cultures or cell-free preparations.

1. Protostreptovaricins

The earliest identified precursors of streptovaricins are protostreptovaricins I→V, described by DESHMUCK et al. (1976) (Fig. 17). Their biogenetic positions can be inferred from the absence of the hydroxyl group at C-21 (note that protorifamycin I lacks the corresponding hydroxyl group at C-8) and from the presence in protostreptovaricins I→IV of an intact methyl at C-10 (which appears to have been oxidized to a carboxyl group in streptovaricins).

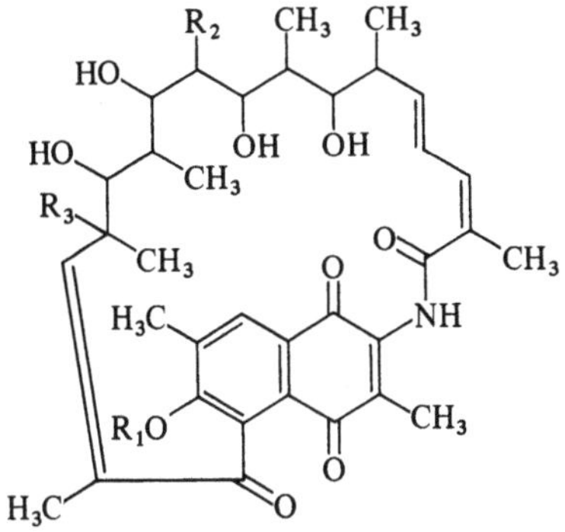

Protostreptovaricins I–V

	R_1	R_2	R_3
I	H	CH_3	H
II	CH_3	CH_3	H
III	H	CH_3	OH
IV	CH_3	CH_3	OH
V	H	H	H

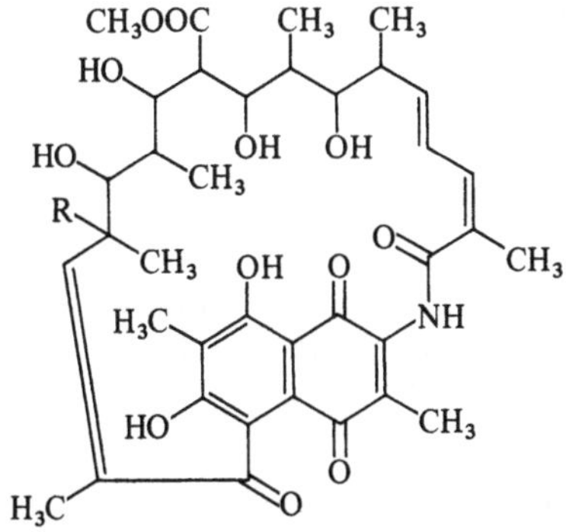

Damavaricins C and D

	R
C	H
D	OH

Fig. 17. Protostreptovaricins and damavaricins

Protostreptovaricin V has one methyl group fewer, but, since it is not certain which of the aliphatic methyls is missing, the position of this compound in the biosynthetic pathway is not clear.

Protostreptovaricin I appears to be the simplest metabolite and thus is reputed to be the earliest intermediate. Protostreptovaricins II, III, and IV appear to be derived from it by methylation and hydroxylation.

2. Damavaricins

Damavaricin D (Fig. 17) was isolated by RINEHART et al. (1976) as a minor product of *S. spectabilis* fermentation. It can also be obtained from streptovaricin D by chemical conversion. Similarly, damavaricin C was obtained from streptovaricin C. It differs from damavaricin D in the presence of a hydroxyl group at C-14. Damavaricins C and D appear to be intermediates between the protostreptovaricins and the streptovaricins, since they possess the methyl-derived carboxyl group at C-10 and the hydroxyl at C-21, but still lack the methylenedioxy group, with the concurrent enolization at C-17, and the acetyl at C-24.

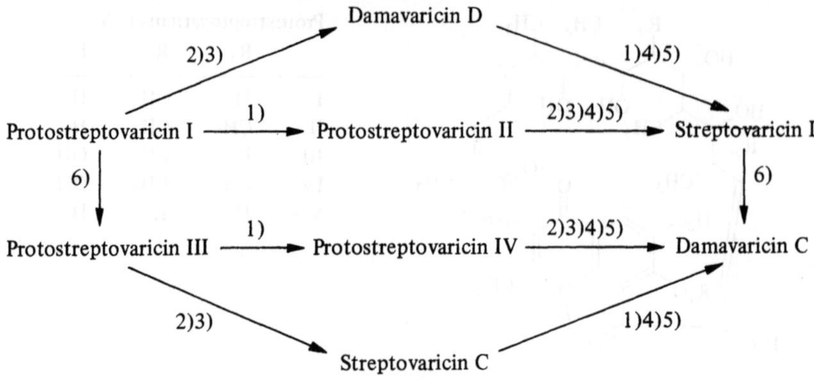

Fig. 18. Proposed routes from protostreptovaricins to streptovaricins. Numbered steps are: 1. methylation of 19-hydroxyl; 2. conversion of 10-methyl to 10-carbomethoxyl group; 3. hydroxylation at C-21; 4. enolization at C-17, oxidation of 17-hydroxyl and 19-methoxyl to methylenedioxy group; 5. reduction at C-24 and C-27 to hydroquinone, acetylation of 24-hydroxyl; 6. hydroxylation at C-14

The biosynthetic routes from protostreptovaricins to damavaricins and to streptovaricins proposed by RINEHART and SHIELD (1976) are shown in Figure 18.

3. Late Steps in Streptovaricin Biosynthesis

The relationships among the streptovaricins have been studied by MILAVETZ et al. (1973) (see RINEHART and SHIELD, 1976). ^{14}C-labeled streptovaricin D was added to a culture of *S. spectabilis* and after a 2-h incubation labeled streptovaricin C could be recovered.

In a separate experiment, tritium-labeled streptovaricin C was added to a cell-free enzyme preparation. Streptovaricins B and A were found to be labeled after incubation. On the basis of these findings and of structural considerations,

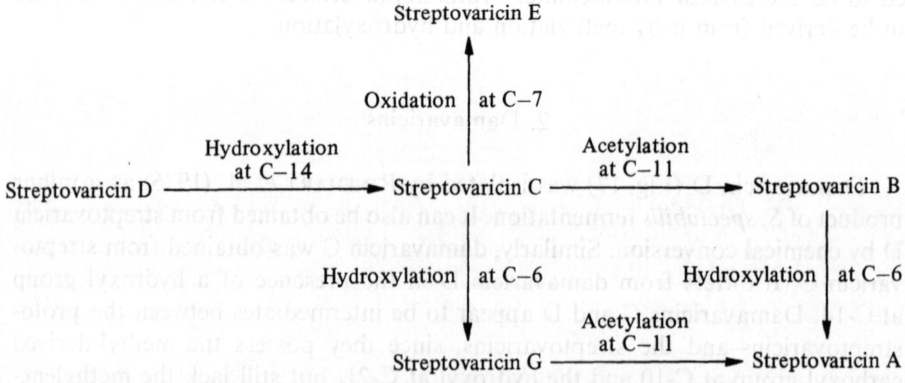

Fig. 19. Probable biosynthetic relationship of the streptovaricins

Rinehart and Shield (1976) proposed the scheme in Figure 19 for the biosynthetic relationships of the streptovaricins.

VI. Discussion

From the evidence available it is possible to conclude that the ansamycins are a large family of secondary metabolites, produced by a variety of organisms, with a common biogenetic pattern. Their carbon structures originate from a chain of a number of two- or three-carbon units joined together by a head-to-tail type of condensation as in the synthesis of the macrolide antibiotics. A unique feature of the ansamycins is that the chain is always initiated from a seven-carbon cyclic unit which is the origin of part or all of the molecule aromatic nucleus. Methylmalonate and malonate appear to be, as usual, the building units of the chain; it is, however, noteworthy that in geldanamycin a different two-carbon unit, possibly glycollate, is also incorporated. The chain invariably forms a macrocycle closed by an amide bond to the aromatic nucleus, rather than by a lactone as in the macrolides. In naphthalene ansamycins, in which it is longer, the ansa chain folds to form the second aromatic ring. The source of the seven-carbon cyclic initiator of the chain is an interesting problem. Its structure is basically that of a benzoic acid derivative meta-substituted with an amino group. This is most unusual because in primary metabolism substitutions of this type occur only in the ortho position, as in anthranilic acid, or in the para position, as in p-aminobenzoic acid. Its origin from one of the intermediates of the aromatic amino acid pathway has been established, but this intermediate has not been identified with certainty and nothing is known of the subsequent steps leading to the final compound. The biosynthesis of rifamycins, streptovaricins, and geldanamycin has been studied. Extension of the results to other ansamycins is based only on structural considerations. There is obviously a need for confirmatory experiments, especially for compounds apparently produced by such very different organisms as plants.

Of the three classical methods for study of biosynthesis, only two have been applied: incorporation of precursors and isolation of intermediates either from blocked mutant strains or as minor components of the fermentation mixture containing the product. No attempts have been made to identify the enzymes involved in the reactions and very few cell-free experiments have been performed. On the other hand, the elucidation of the ansamycin biosynthesis pattern has demonstrated that ^{13}C labeling coupled with carbon magnetic resonance spectroscopy is a powerful tool that provides a relatively simple, precise method for identification of the individual carbons into which precursors are incorporated, permitting the solution of what appeared, at least in the case of rifamycin, to be a very complex puzzle. Moreover, even when the precursor of a moiety, as in the case of the aromatic ring, has not been identified, the semiquantitative determination of incorporation of the carbons of glucose by means of ^{13}C labeling gave precise indications of the metabolic pathway by which the molecules originated. The understanding of the relationships between primary and secondary metabolism will certainly be increased by extensive use of this method.

References

Balerna M, Keller-Schierlein W, Martius C, Wolf H, Zähner H (1969) A Naphthomycin, ein Antimetabolit von Vitamin K. Arch Mikrobiol 65:303–317

Birner J, Hodgson PR, Lane WR, Baxter EH (1972) An australian isolate of *Nocardia mediterranea* producing rifamycin SV. J Antibiot 25:356–359

Brufani M (1977) The ansamycins. In: Sammes PG (ed) Topics in antibiotic chemistry, vol I, pp 93–217. London

Brufani M, Kluepfel D, Lancini GC, Leitich J, Mesentsev AS, Prelog V, Schmook FP, Sensi P (1973) Über die Biogenese des Rifamycins S. Helv Chim Acta 56:2315–2323

Brugisser S (1975) Zur Biosynthese des Rifamycin Chromophores. Dissertation Nr 5435. Federal School of Technology, Switzerland

Carter WA, Brockman WW, Li L, Reusser F (1971) Selective inhibition of RNA tumor virus "Reverse transcriptase" by the streptovaricins. Clin Res 19:No 2, 490

Celmer WD, Cullen WP, English AR, Jefferson MT, Oscarson JR, Routien JB, Sciavolino FC (1975) 3-Methyl-thiorifamycin SV and CP-32.650, novel sulphur containing ansamycins from a new species of Micromonospora. In: 15th Intersci Conference Antimicrob Agents Chemother 260

Corcoran JW, Chick M (1966) Biochemistry of the macrolide antibiotics In: Snell JF (ed) Biosynthesis of antibiotics, Vol I, pp 159–201. Academic Press, London New York

Cricchio R, Lancini GC (1978) Structure determination and synthesis of rifamycins P.Q. and Verde, novel metabolites from mutants of *Nocardia mediterranea*. Proc IIth IUPAC Int Symp Chem Nat Prod, vol I. Varna, Bulgaria

Cricchio R, Antonini P, Lancini GC, Tamborini G, White RJ, Martinelli E (1980) Thiazo rifamycins, Part I. Structure and synthesis of rifamycins P, Q and Verde, novel metabolites from mutants of *Nocardia mediterranea*. Tetrahedron 36:1415–1421

DeBoer C, Meulman PA, Wnuk RJ, Peterson DH (1970) Geldanamycin, a new antibiotic. J Antibiot 23:442–447

Deshmukh PV, Kakinuma K, Ameel JJ, Rinehart KL Jr, Wiley PF, Li LH (1976) Protostreptovaricins I-V. J Am Chem Soc 98:870–872

Füresz S, Timbal MT (1963) Antibacterial activity of rifamycins. Chemotherapia 7:200–208

Ganguly AK, Szmulewicz S, Sarre OZ, Greeves D, Morton J, McGlotten J (1974) Structure of Halomycin B. JCS Chem Commun 395–396

Ghisalba O, Nüesch J (1978a) A genetic approach to the biosynthesis of the rifamycin-chromophore in *Nocardia mediterranea*, I. Isolation and characterization of a pentose-excreting auxotrophic mutant of *Nocardia mediterranea* with drastically reduced rifamycin production. J Antibiot 31:202–214

Ghisalba O, Nüesch J (1978b) A genetic approach to the biosynthesis of the rifamycin-chromophore in *Nocardia mediterranei*. II. Isolation and characterization of a shikimate excreting auxotrophic mutant of *Nocardia mediterranea* with normal rifamycin-production. J Antibiot 31:215–225

Ghisalba O, Traxler P, Nüesch J (1979) Early intermediated in the biosynthesis of ansamycins. I. Isolation and identification of protorifamycin I. in press

Haber A, Johnson RD, Rinehart KL Jr (1977) Biosynthetic origin of the C_2 units of geldanamycin and distribution of label from D-[6-^{13}C]glucose. J Am Chem Soc 99:3541–3544

Hasegawa T, Higashide E, Shibata M (1971) Tolypomycin, a new antibiotic. II. Production and preliminary identification of tolypomycin Y. J Antibiot 24:817–822

Higashide E, Asai M, Ootsu K, Tanida S, Kozai Y, Hasegawa T, Kishi T, Sugino Y, Yoneda M (1977) Ansamitocin, a group of novel maytansinoid antibiotics with antitumor properties from *Nocardia*. Nature (London) 270:721–722

Johnson RD, Haber A, Rinehart KL Jr (1974) Geldanamycin biosynthesis and carbon magnetic resonance. J Am Chem Soc 96:3316–3317

Kakinuma K, Milavetz BI, Rinehart KL Jr (1976) Carbon-13 nuclear magnetic resonance spectra of the streptovaricins and related compounds. J Org Chem 41:1358–1364

Karlsson A, Sartori G, White RJ (1974) Rifamycin biosynthesis: further studies on origin of the ansa chain and chromophore. Eur J Biochem 47:251–256

Kishi T, Harada S, Asai M, Muroi M, Mizuno K (1969) Tolypomycin. II; Structures of tolyposamine and tolypomycin Y. Tetrahedron Lett 7:97–100

Kishi T, Yamana H, Muroi M, Harada S, Arai M, Hasegawa T, Mizuno K (1972) Tolypomycin, a new antibiotic. III Isolation and characterization of Tolypomycin Y. J Antibiot 25:11–15

Kupchan SM, Komoda Y, Court WA, Thomas GJ, Smith RM, Karim A, Gilmore CJ, Haltiwanger RC, Bryan RF (1972a) Maytansine, a novel antileukemic ansa macrolide from *Maytenus ovatus*. J Am Chem Soc 94:1354–1356

Kupchan SM, Komoda Y, Thomas GJ, Hintz HP (1972b) Maytanprine and Maytanbutine, new antileukaemic ansa macrolides from *Maytenus buchananii*. JCS Chem Commun 1065

Kupchan SM, Branfman AR, Sneden AT, Verma AK, Dailey RC, Jr, Komoda Y, Nagao Y (1975) Novel Maytansinoids. Naturally occurring and synthetic antileukemic esters of maytansinol. J Am Chem Soc 97:5294–5295

Lancini GC, Hengeller C (1969) Isolation of rifamycin SV from a mutant *Streptomyces mediterranei* strain. J Antibiot 22:637–638

Lancini GC, Parenti F (1978) Rifamycin biogenesis. In: Wherli W (ed) Acta 5th FEMS Symp, pp 129–139. Academic Press, London New York

Lancini GC, Sartori G (1976) Rifamycin G, a further product of *Nocardia mediterranea* metabolism. J Antibiot 29:466–468

Lancini GC, Sensi P (1967) Studies on the final steps in rifamycins biosynthesis. In: Spitzy KH, Haschek H (eds) Proc 5th Int Congr Chemother, vol I, pp 41–47. Verlag der Wiener Medizinischen Akademie

Lancini GC, White RJ (1973) Rifamycin fermentation studies. Process Biochem 8:July 14–16

Lancini GC, White RJ (1976) Rifamycin biosynthesis. In: MacDonald KD (ed) 2nd Int Symp Genet Indust Microorg, pp 139–153. Academic Press, London New York

Lancini GC, Thiemann JE, Sartori G, Sensi P (1967) Biogenesis of rifamycins. The conversion of rifamycin B into rifamycin Y. Experientia 23:899–900

Lancini GC, Gallo GG, Sartori G, Sensi P (1969) Isolation and structure of rifamycin L and its biogenetic relationship with other rifamycins. J Antibiot 22:369–377

Leitich J, Prelog V, Sensi P (1967) Rifamycin Y und seine Umwandlungsprodukte. Experientia 23:505–507

Margalith P, Beretta G (1960) Rifomycin XI. Taxonomic study on *Streptomyces mediterranei* Nov. sp. Mycopathol Mycol Appl 8:321–330

Martinelli E, Gallo GG, Antonini P, White RJ (1974) Structure of rifamycin W. A novel ansamycin from a mutant of *Nocardia mediterranea*. Tetrahedron 30:3087–3091

Martinelli E, Antonini P, Cricchio R, Lancini GC, White RJ (1978) Rifamycin R, a novel metabolite from a mutant of *Nocardia mediterranea*. J Antibiot 31:949–951

Milavetz B, Kakinuma K, Rinehart KL Jr, Rolls JP, Haak WJ (1973) Carbon-13 magnetic resonance spectroscopy and the biosynthesis of streptovaricin. J Am Chem Soc 95:5793–5795

Oppolzer W, Prelog V (1973) Über die Konstitution und die Konfiguration der Rifamycine B, O, S und SV. Helv Chim Acta 56:2287–2314

Oppolzer W, Prelog V, Sensi P (1964) Konstitution des Rifamycins B und verwandter Rifamycine. Experientia 20:336–339

Prelog V, Oppolzer W (1973) Ansamycine, eine neuartige Klasse von mikrobiellen Stoffwechselprodukten. Helv Chim Acta 56:2279–2287

Rinehart KL Jr, Antosz FJ (1972) Chemistry of the streptovaricins. VII Revised structures for streptovarone and streptovaricin C. J Antibiot 25:71–73

Rinehart KL Jr, Shield LS (1976) Chemistry of ansamycin antibiotics. Fortschr Chem Org Naturst 33:231–307

Rinehart KL Jr, Maheshwari ML, Antosz FJ, Mathur HH, Sasaki K, Schacht RJ (1971) Chemistry of the streptovaricins. VIII. Structures of streptovaricins A, B, D, E, F, and G. J Am Chem Soc 93:6273–6274

Rinehart KL Jr, Antosz FJ, Sasaki K, Martin PK, Maheshwari ML, Reusser F, Li LH, Moran D, Wiley PF (1974) Relative biological activities of individual streptovaricins and streptovaricin acetates. Biochemistry 13:861–867

Rinehart KL Jr, Antosz FJ, Deshmukh PV, Kakinuma K, Martin PK, Milavetz BI, Sasaki K, Witty TR, Li LH, Reusser F (1976) Identification and preparation of damavaricins, biologically active precursors of streptovaricins. J Antibiot 29:201–203

Sasaki K, Rinehart KL Jr, Slomp G, Grostic MF, Olson EC (1970) Geldanamycin. I. Structure assignment. J Am Chem Soc 92:7591–7593

Sensi P, Thiemann JE (1967) Production of rifamycins. Prog Indust Microbiol 6:21–60
Sensi P, Margalith P, Timbal MT (1959) Rifomycin, a new antibiotic. Preliminary report. Farmaco Ed Sci 14:146–147
Sensi P, Ballotta R, Greco AM (1960) Rifomycin, V-Rifomycin O, a new antibiotic of the rifomycin family. Farmaco Ed Sci 15:228–234
Sensi P, Ballotta R, Greco AM, Gallo GG (1961) Rifomycin, XV – Activation of rifomycin B and rifomycin O. – Production and properties of rifomycin S and rifomycin SV. Farmaco Ed Sci 16:165–180
Shibata M, Hasegawa T, Higashide E (1971) Tolypomycin, a new antibiotic. I. *Streptomyces tolypophorus* nov. sp., a new antibiotic, tolypomycin-producer. J Antibiot 24:810–816
Siminoff P, Smith RM, Sokolski WT, Savage GM (1957) Streptovaricin. I. Discovery and biologic activity. Am Rev Tuberc Pulm Dis 75:576–583
Sugawara S, Karasawa K, Watanabe M, Hidaka T (1964) Production of rifamycin O by Streptomyces 4107 A_2. J Antibiot Ser A 17:29–32
Thiemann JE, Zucco G, Pelizza G (1969) A proposal for the transfer of *Streptomyces mediterranei* Margalith and Beretta 1960 to the genus Nocardia as Nocardia mediterranea (Margalith and Beretta) Comb. Nov Arch Mikrobiol 67:147–155
Waksman SA (1961) The actinomycetes, vol II, p 276. Williams and Wilkins Co, Baltimore
Wani MC, Taylor HL, Wall ME (1973) Plant antitumor agents: Colubrinol acetate and colubrinol, antileukaemic ansa macrolide from *Colubrina texensis*. JCS Chem Commun 390
Weinstein MJ, Luedemann GM, Oden EM, Wagman GH (1967) Halomycin, a new *Micromonospora*-produced antibiotic. Antimicrob Agents Chemother 435–441
Wherli W (1977) Ansamycins. Chemistry, biosynthesis and biological activity. In: Topics in current chemistry, vol 72, pp 21–49. Springer, Berlin Heidelberg New York
White RJ, Martinelli E (1974) Ansamycin biogenesis: incorporation of [I-^{13}C]glucose and [I-^{13}C]glycerate into the chromophore of rifamycin S. FEBS Lett 49:233–236
White RJ, Martinelli E, Gallo GG, Lancini GC, Beynon P (1973) Rifamycin biosynthesis studied with ^{13}C enriched precursors and carbon magnetic resonance. Nature (London) 243:273–277
White RJ, Martinelli E, Lancini GC (1974) Ansamycin biogenesis: Studies on a novel rifamycin isolated from a mutant strain of *Nocardia mediterranea*. Proc Natl Acad Sci USA 71:3260–3264
White RJ, Lancini GC, Sensi P (1975) New natural rifamycins. In: Proc 1th Int Congr IAMS Symp, vol III, pp 483–492. T Hasegawa Science Council of Japan
Williams TH (1975) Naphthomycin, a novel ansa macrocyclic antimetabolite. Proton NMR spectra and structure elucidation using lanthanide shift reagent. J Antibiot 28:85–86
Yamazaki H (1968) Studies on antimicrobial substance B44P (streptovaricin) produced by a strain of actinomycetes. I. J Antibiot 21:204–208

Polyether Antibiotics – Biosynthesis

J.W. WESTLEY

The increasing interest in both synthetic and natural ionophores, particularly the polyether antibiotics, has generated a number of reviews including a book by OVCHINNIKOV et al. (1974) and journal reviews by HODGSON (1974), TRUTER (1976) and one devoted to the biological activities of polyether antibiotics by PRESSMAN (1976). The isolation, separation, and purification of some commercially important polyether antibiotics such as lasalocid and monensin were the subject of a very detailed and comprehensive review by HAMILL and CRANDALL (1978). A broader review deals with many aspects of research into polyether antibiotics (WESTLEY, 1977). The review that follows is restricted to studies on the *biosynthesis* of five polyether antibiotics: lasalocid, monensin, narasin, salinomycin, and lysocellin.

Almost 30 years have elapsed since the isolation of the first polyether antibiotics by HARNED et al. (1951) who isolated nigericin and BERGER et al. (1951) who reported on three antibiotics, which were subsequently found to range in size from a C_{24} up to a C_{36} backbone. The first, X-537A was the smallest and is now known as lasalocid; the second, X-464 was later found to be identical to HARNED's nigericin; and the third, X-206, with one of the longest carbon skeletons (C_{36}) of the polyethers, was structurally elucidated many years later (BLOUNT and WESTLEY, 1975). The fourth polyether antibiotic, dianemycin, was first mentioned in the literature in 1958 by LARDY and after another 9 years, the fifth, monensin, was reported by AGTARAP et al. (1967). AGTARAP et al. included in this paper the structure of monensin, which was the first polyether structure to be elucidated. This marked a turning point for the polyether antibiotics. In the following decade, 1968–1978, the number of these antibiotics increased from 5 to 46 (Table 1). The catalyst for this upsurge of interest was a report in 1968 by SHUMARD and CALLENDER that four of the five known polyethers, monensin, nigericin, dianemycin, and X-206 were potent *coccidiostats,* that is, these antibiotics are able to control coccidial infections in poultry when added at approximately 100 ppm to the feed. Coccidia are parasitic protozoa of the subphylum Sporozoa, which exhibit a particular affinity for the epithelial cells in the digestive tracts of birds and mammals; the genus found most often in poultry is *Eimeria.* The extent of the disease can be estimated by the current world market for coccidiostats, recently estimated at U.S. $ 100 million by WHEN-CHI LIU et al. (1978).

Monensin was the first polyether antibiotic to be patented as a coccidiostat (HANEY and HOEHN, 1968) and within a few years after release (in 1971) monensin

Table 1. Polyether Antibiotics (1951–1978)

Antibiotic[a]	Producing organism	References
Class 1a		
Alborixin	*Streptomyces albus*	ALLEAUME et al. (1975) GACHON et al. (1976)
Antibiotic X-206	*Streptomyces* X-206	BERGER et al. (1951) BLOUNT and WESTLEY (1975)
CP 38,986	*Streptomyces flaveolus* ATCC 31100	CELMER et al. (1977)
CP 44,161	*Dactylosporangium salmoneum* ATCC 31222, 31223, 31224	TONE et al. (1978)
Deoxy(0-8)-salinomycin (SY-1)	*Streptomyces albus* ATCC 21838	WESTLEY et al. (1977) SHIBATA et al. (1976)
Deoxy(0-8)-*epi*-17-salinomycin	*Streptomyces albus* ATCC 21838	WESTLEY et al. (1977)
Grisorixin (K358)	*Streptomyces griseus*	GACHON et al. (1970)
Laidlomycin	*Streptomyces eurocidus* var. *asterocidius*	KITAME et al. (1974)
Lonomycin A	*Streptomyces ribosidificus* ATCC 31051	OMURA et al. (1976)
Emericid, RP31559	*Streptomyces hygroscopicus* NRRL 5787	NINET et al. (1976)
A218	*Streptomyces hygroscopicus* FERM-P928	TSUJI et al. (1976)
DE 3936	*Streptomyces hygroscopicus* 9735-1 (FERM-P3159)	OHSHIMA et al. (1976)
Lonomycin B, C	*Streptomyces ribosidificus*	SETO et al. (1978b)
Monensin A, B, C, and D	*Streptomyces cinnamonensis* ATCC 15413 and NRRL B1588	HANEY et al. (1968) AGTARAP et al. (1967)
Mutalomycin (S11743)	*Streptomyces mutabilis* NRRL 8088	FEHR et al. (1977)
Narasin A (A28086A; 4-methyl-salinomycin), B and D	*Streptomyces aureofaciens* NRRL 5758, NRRL 8092	OCCOLOWITZ et al. (1976) KINASHI and OTAKE (1976)
Nigericin	*Streptomyces violaceoniger* NRRL B1356	HARNED et al. (1951)
X-464	*Streptomyces* X-464	BERGER et al. (1951)
Polyetherin A	*Streptomyces hygroscopicus* E-749 (ATCC 21368)	KUBOTA et al. (1968)
Helixin C	*Streptomyces* sp.	SMEBY et al. (1952)
K-178	*Streptomyces albus* K-178	HORVATH et al. (1964)
Azalomycin M	*Streptomyces hygroscopicus* ATCC 13810	OKAZAKI and ARAI (1966)
Duamycin	*Streptomyces hygroscopicus duamyceticus*	MISATO et al. (1970)
Noboritomycin A and B	*Streptomyces noboritoensis* NRRL 8123	KELLER-JUSLEN et al. (1978)
RP 30504	*Streptomyces gallinarius* DS 25881, NRRL 5785	FLORENT et al. (1976)
Salinomycin	*Streptomyces albus* ATCC 21838	KINASHI et al. (1973)
Salinomycin AII	*Streptomyces albus* ATCC 21838	YONEHARA et al. (1975)

Table 1 (continued)

Antibiotic[a]	Producing organism	References
Antibiotic X-14766A	*Streptomyces malachitofuscus* subsp. *downeyi*	WESTLEY et al. (1980)
Class 1b		
A204 A and B	*Streptomyces albus* NRRL 3384	HAMILL and HOEHN (1972) JONES et al. (1973)
Antibiotic 6016	*Streptomyces* sp. 6016	SETO et al. (1978c) OTAKE et al. (1978a)
Carriomycin (T42082)	*Streptomyces hygroscopicus* T42082	OTAKE et al. (1977) IMADA et al. (1978)
Dianemycin	*Streptomyces hygroscopicus* NRRL 3444	HAMILL et al. (1969) CZERWINSKI and STEINRAUF (1971)
Etheromycin	*Streptomyces hygroscopicus*	MITANI et al. (1977)
CP-38295	*Streptomyces hygroscopicus* ATCC 31050	CELMER et al. (1976)
Lenoremycin (Ro 21-6150)	*Streptomyces hygroscopicus* X-14563	BLOUNT et al. (1975) LIU et al. (1976)
(A130A)	*Streptomyces hygroscopicus* A130 ATCC 21840	KUBOTA et al. (1975)
K-41	*Streptomyces hygroscopicus* K41	SHIRO et al. (1978)
(A 32887)	*Streptomyces albus* NRRL 11109	OCCOLOWITZ et al. (1978)
Septamycin (BL-580α)	*Streptomyces hygroscopicus* NRRL 5678	KELLER-JUSLEN et al. (1975)
(A28695A)	*Streptomyces albus* NRRL 3883	HAMILL and HOEHN (1974)
BL-580β (A28695B)	*Streptomyces hygroscopicus* NRRL 5647	MARTIN and KANTOR (1974)
BL-580Δ	*Streptomyces hygroscopicus* NRRL 8180	MARTIN et al. (1977)
Class 2a		
Lasalocids A (X-537A), B, C, D and E	*Streptomyces lasaliensis* NRRL 3382 and ATCC 31180	BERGER et al. (1951) WESTLEY et al. (1970a) JOHNSON et al. (1970)
iso-Lasalocid A		WESTLEY et al. (1974b, c)
Lysocellin	*Streptomyces cacaoi* var. *asoensis* K-9 Met	EBATA et al. (1975) OTAKE et al. (1975)
(X-14537)	*Streptomyces longwoodensis* ATCC 29251	PROSSER and PALLERONI (1976)
Ionomycin	*Streptomyces conglobatus* ATCC 31005	MEYERS et al. (1975)
Class 2b		
A23187	*Streptomyces chartreusis* NRRL 3882	CHANEY et al. (1974) GALE et al. (1975)
X-14547A	*Streptomyces antibioticus* NRRL 8167	WESTLEY et al. (1978) LIU et al. (1978)

[a] Classification of polyethers in this table is according to the system proposed by WESTLEY (1977)

accounted for about 80% of the American market. The American patent for lasalocid as a coccidiostat was issued to BERGER in 1973 and the antibiotic was finally released in late 1976 to compete with monensin both in the United States and worldwide. The trade names of the two preparations are Coban® (monensin) and Avatec® (lasalocid).

I. Biosynthesis of Polyether Antibiotics

All the polyether antibiotics described up to mid-1978 were isolated from the genus *Streptomyces*. The first exception was announced by TONE et al. in 1978 when they reported the isolation of CP 44,161 from *Dactylosporangium salmoneum*, which although belonging to the order Actinomycetales is in a different family (Actinoplanaceae) than the *Streptomyces* which belong to the Streptomycetaceae. The name is derived from *daktylos* (finger, Greek) from the finger-like sporangium which contain their motile spores. A more specific biochemical difference between *Dactylosporangium* and *Streptomyces* is found in the 2,6-diaminopimelic acid present in the cell walls. In the former, this acid has the *meso* configuration whereas *Streptomyces* contain the *LL* form (Fig. 1).The most fruitful sources have been *S. albus* and *S. hygroscopicus* which account for half of the polyether antibiotics listed in Table 1.

Of the nearly fifty polyether antibiotics known, the biosynthesis of only five has been investigated, but results from these studies, on lasalocid (WESTLEY et al. 1970b, 1972, 1974a, b, and c), monensin (DAY, et al., 1973), narasin

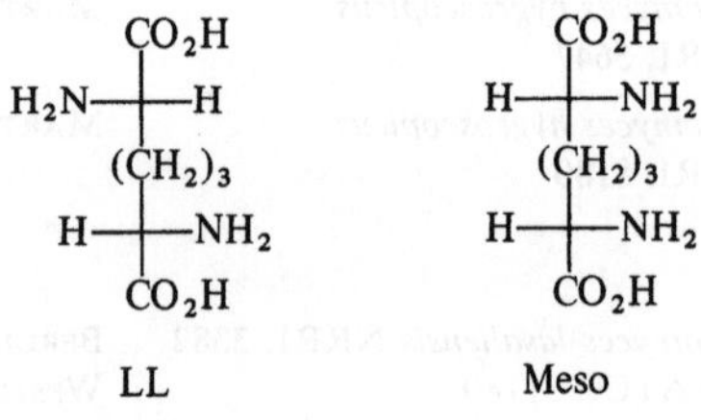

Fig. 1. 2,6-Diaminopimelic acid

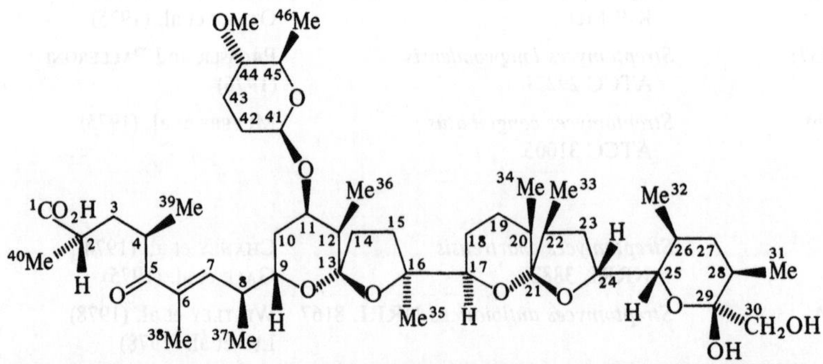

Fig. 2. Numbering system for polyether antibiotics. The example illustrated is lenoremycin

(DORMAN, et al., 1976), salinomycin (SETO, et al., 1977b), and lysocellin (OTAKE, et al., 1978b) have been very consistent, suggesting a general route which can be applied to predict the biosynthesis of other polyether antibiotics. One result of the biosynthetic studies has been the formulation and general acceptance of a universal numbering system for polyether antibiotics (WESTLEY, 1976) exemplified by lenoremycin (Fig. 2).

A. Lasalocid

Although not recognized as a polyether antibiotic at the time, one of the first three antibiotics of this class to be reported was X-537A since renamed lasalocid (BERGER et al., 1951). The structure of the antibiotic (JOHNSON et al., 1970; WESTLEY et al., 1970a) and absolute configuration were shown by a combination of X-ray and chemical degradation to be I. The anticoccidial activity of lasalocid against pathogenic species of *Eimeria* in broiler chickens has been described in detail by MITROVIC and SCHILDKNECHT (1974).

In the same year that the structure of lasalocid was reported, the first of five reports on the biosynthesis of the antiotic appeared (WESTLEY et al., 1970b).

1. ^{14}C Incorporation into Lasalocid

Negative results with [^{14}C]formate, [Me-^{14}C]methionine, [Me-^{14}C]ethionine, and [2-^{14}C]mevalonate ruled out transmethylation, transethylation, or the introduction of terpenoid units as possible mechanisms leading to the branched alkyl groups in lasalocid A. The other two ^{14}C-labeled acids *not* incorporated into (I) were salicylic and shikimic acid (Table 2).

The effective utilization of sodium (1-^{14}C]acetate, sodium [1-, 2-, or 3-^{14}C]propionate, and sodium [1-, 2-, or 3,4-^{14}C] butyrate showed that the antibi-

Table 2. Incorporation of ^{14}C-Labeled substrates into lasalocid

Substrate for lasalocid	Percentage incorporation
[1-^{14}C]Acetate	0.2
[1-^{14}C]Propionate	1–4
[2-^{14}C]Propionate	0.2
[3-^{14}C]Propionate	3.7
[1-^{14}C]Butyrate	2–10
[2-^{14}C]Butyrate	1.6
[3,4-^{14}C]Butyrate	8.5
[2-^{14}C]Malonate	0.4
[Me-^{14}C]2-Methylmalonate	0.5
[2-^{14}C]2-Ethylmalonate	1.8
[1-^{14}C]3-Hydroxybutyrate	11.1
[1-^{14}C]Stearate	0.8

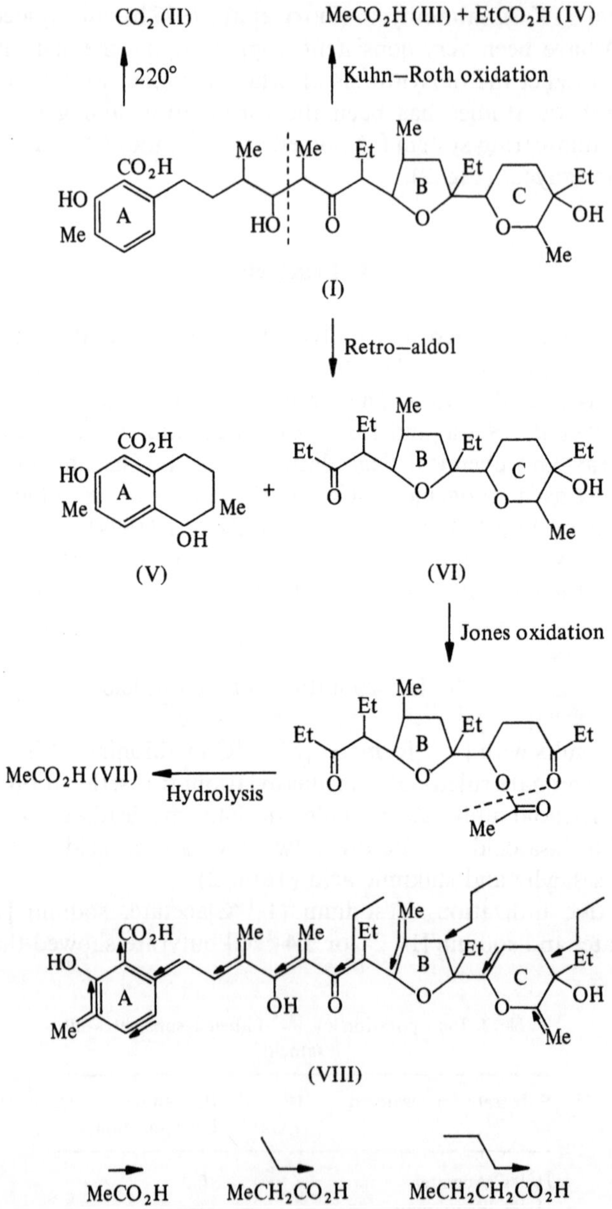

Scheme 1. Reactions used to determine the labeling pattern in ^{14}C-derived lasalocid A (VIII)

otic was derived from these three units probably after conversion to malonate, 2-methylmalonate, and 2-ethylmalonate, respectively. This mechanism is well established in the case of acetate and propionate (Birch, 1957; Lynen, 1967; Kaneda et al., 1962), but the involvement of *butyrate* and 2-*ethylmalonate* had no precedent in the literature.

Degradation experiments and ^{13}C nmr (next two sections) showed the incorporation pattern to be as indicated by VIII in Scheme 1.

2. Chemical Degradation of ^{14}C-Labeled Lasalocid A (Scheme 1)

Pyrolytic decarboxylation of lasalocid A at 220° C gave radioactive CO_2 (II) only in the case of [1-^{14}C]acetate-derived antibiotic, showing that C-1 in (I) is derived from an acetate carboxyl. Retro-aldol cleavage of (I) followed by oxidation of (VI) and hydrolysis gave acetic acid (VII) from the C-methyl group at C-23 in (I). This C-methyl was shown to originate as an acetate unit by obtaining radioactive (VII) from [1-^{14}C]acetate-derived (I) (Table 3). The relative molar activity of fragments II and VII (8.9 and 10.5% respectively) suggest that 10 or 11 acetate units are involved in lasalocid biosynthesis. However, as later results indicate (see below) only five acetates are *directly* incorporated into the antibiotic. This implies that in the [1-^{14}C]acetate labeling experiment, in addition to the five molecules of acetate involved directly in lasalocid biosynthesis, a further six were incorporated *indirectly* after prior conversion to butyrate.

Kuhn-Roth oxidation of (I) produced acetic acid (III) from the eight C-methyls and propionic acid (IV) from the three C-ethyls in the molecule. These acids were separated by silica gel chromatography as their p-bromophenacyl esters. If all the ^{14}C atoms in a labeled (I) preparation are situated in the C-methyl groups, the theoretical relative molar activity of (IV) would be 12.5%. Similarly, if all the ^{14}C atoms are in C-ethyl groups, the theoretical activity of (IV) would be 33.3%. When this reaction was carried out on [2- or 3-^{14}C] propionate-derived (I), the resulting acetic acid had activity of 11.2% and 10.5%, respectively, whereas [1-^{14}C]propionate-derived (I) gave inactive acetic acid. The propionic acid (IV) produced in the oxidation was virtually inactive in all three cases. These results show clearly that the propionate units incorporated into (I) are only at C-methyl positions in the antibiotic. Retro-aldol cleavage of the three [^{14}C]propionate-derived samples of (I) demonstrated that there are four propionate units in the molecule and that one is situated at the C-11,

Table 3. Results of chemical degradation of lasalocid from different substrates[a]

Lasalocid derived from following substrates	Percentage relative molar activity of					
	(II)	(III)	(IV)	(V)	(VI)	(VII)
[1-^{14}C]Acetate	8.9	3.4	4.1	45.7	56.4	10.5
[1-^{14}C]Propionate	0	0	0.8	75.3	25.1	–
[2-^{14}C]Propionate	–	11.2	0.7	47.1	50.7	–
[3-^{14}C]Propionate	–	10.5	1.0	45.3	50.8	–
[1-^{14}C]Butyrate	0	0.1	0.2	2.6	97.4	–
[2-^{14}C]Butyrate	–	0.3	26.6	9.5	91.2	–
[3,4-^{14}C]Butyrate	–	9.3	27.3	3.5	96.5	–
[2-^{14}C]Malonate	–	–	–	48.0	52.0	–
[Me-^{14}C]Methylmalonate	–	–	–	50.4	49.5	–
[2-^{14}C]2-Ethylmalonate	–	–	–	1.6	98.4	–
[1-^{14}C]3-Hydroxybutyrate	–	–	–	12.6	87.4	–
[1-^{14}C]Stearate	–	–	–	40.7	57.9	–

[a] The degradation reactions and products are shown in Scheme 1

C-12 bond, the site of this cleavage. This results in a (V):(VI) ratio of 1:1 (or 2:2) in the [2- and 3-^{14}C]propionate experiments, but 3:1 in the [1-^{14}C]propionate case. The four propionate-derived C-methyls must be at C-4, C-10, C-12, and C-16 since the C-23 methyl is acetate-derived.

Kuhn-Roth oxidation of the three [^{14}C]butyrate-derived samples established that the butyrate units incorporated into (I) are only at the C-ethyl positions. Thus, [1-^{14}C]butyrate-derived (I) gave virtually inactive acetic and propionic acid, [2-^{14}C]butyrate-derived (I) gave inactive acetic, but active propionic acid (26.6%, theoretical 33.3%) and [3,4-^{14}C]butyrate-derived (I) gave active acetic (9.3%, theoretical 12.5%) and active propionic acid (27.3%). The results from retro-aldol cleavage showed that all butyrate incorporation was taking place in the ketone (VI) part of the molecule, but could not be used to determine whether one, two, or all three of the C-ethyls were butyrate-derived. This question was subsequently answered by ^{13}C incorporation experiments described in the next section.

The high level of incorporation observed for antibiotic derived from [1-^{14}C]3-hydroxybutyrate and the label distribution (Table 3) suggests that this precursor is either transported, or converted to 2-ethylmalonate, more efficiently than butyrate itself. The even distribution of label indicated for [1-^{14}C]stearate-derived antibiotic suggests that the C_{18} acid is utilized primarily as a source for malonyl Co A.

3. ^{13}C Incorporation into Lasalocid A

The assignment of the ^{13}C spectrum of lasalocid A (I) was completed by SETO et al. (1978a) using model compounds like the lasalocid retro-aldol ketone VI (Scheme 1) together with the biosynthetic results obtained earlier (WESTLEY et al., 1974a). The assignments are listed in Table 4, alongside the abundance of ^{13}C in lasalocid produced by *S. lasaliensis* with [1-^{13}C]acetate, [1-^{13}C]propionate, and [1-^{13}C]butyrate as substrates in three separate experiments. The numbering system for the antibiotic is indicated in Figure 3.

The ^{13}C enrichments considered most significant were those that resulted in at least a doubling of the natural abundance signal as determined by ^{13}nmr (WESTLEY et al., 1972).

In the case of [1-^{13}C]butyrate-derived lasalocid (I), three carbons were enriched consistent with the C-ethyls at C-14, -18, and -22 being butyrate-derived. The results with [1-^{13}C]propionate-derived (I) were consistent with the conclu-

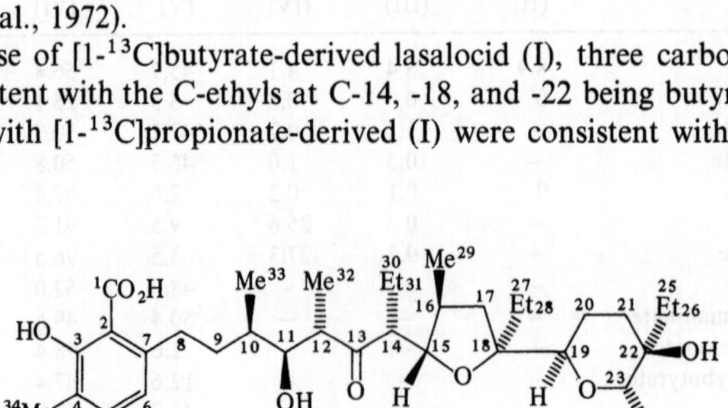

Fig. 3. Numbering system for lasalocid A

Table 4. Incorporation of [1-^{13}C]acetate, [1-^{13}C]propionate and [1-^{13}C]butyrate into lasalocid as determined by ^{13}C nmr[a]

Carbon number	Functional group	^{13}C Shift in ppm[b] for I (in CD_2Cl_2)	% Abundance[c] of ^{13}C in I produced from		
			$CH_3{}^{13}CO_2Na$	$CH_3CH_2{}^{13}CO_2Na$	$CH_2CH_2CH_2{}^{13}CO_2Na$
1	$-CO_2H$	173.6	2	1	1
2	=C–	111.2	1	1	1
3	=C–OH	161.6	1	4.5	1
4	=C̲–CH_3	124.1	1	1	1
5	=CH	135.1	3	1	1.5
6	=CH	121.6	1	1	1
7	=C̲–CH_2	144.4	2.5	1	1
8	$-CH_2$	34.8	1	4	1
9	$-CH_2$	37.0	1	1	1
10	–C̲H(CH_3)	34.9	1	1	1
11	–CH(OH)	72.8	1.5	4	1.5
12	–C̲H(CH_3)	48.9	1	1	1
13	–C=O	214.1	1	1	4
14	–C̲H(C_2H_5)	55.4	1	1	1
15	–CH–O	84.2	1.5	4	1.5
16	–C̲H(CH_3)	34.8	1	1	1
17	$-CH_2$	38.7	1	1	5
18	–C(O)	86.7	1	1	1
19	–CH(O)	70.9	3	1	1
20	$-CH_2$	20.0	1	1	1
21	$-CH_2$	30.2	1	1	4
22	–C(O)	72.4	1	1	1
23	–CH(O)	76.6	3	1	1.5
24	$-CH_3$	14.0	1	1	1
25	$-CH_2$	30.7	1	1	1
26	$-CH_3$	6.6	1	1	1
27	$-CH_2$	30.6	1	1	1
28	$-CH_3$	9.2	1	1	1
29	$-CH_3$	15.9	1	1	1
30	$-CH_2$	16.7	1	1	1
31	$-CH_3$	12.9	1	1	1
32	$-CH_3$	13.2	1	1	1
33	$-CH_3$	13.4	1	1	1
34	$-CH_3$	15.7	1	1	1

[a] Concentration of natural abundance and ^{13}C-enriched lasalocid A was 0.76 M. The 1 H decoupled ^{13}C nmr FOURIER transform spectra were recorded in 10 mm spinning sample tubes on a Bruker HFX-90/6 spectrometer at 22.63 MHz, using an internal ^{19}F lock of C_6F_6 at 84.66 MHz. A Fabritek FT-1083 Computer was used for accumulation of free induction decays and Fourier Transformation

[b] Downfield from internal Me_4Si

[c] Corrected to nearest 0.5%

sion from the earlier ^{14}C experiments that the four C-methyl groups at C-4, -10, -12, and -16 were propionate-derived (Scheme 1).

Sodium [1-^{13}C]acetate at 0.5 gm/l in *S. lasaliensis* fermentations gave antibiotic in which five carbons were enriched (Table 4). The enrichments at C-1 and C-23 confirmed earlier results with [^{14}C]acetate and the other three enrichments at C-5, -7, and -19 accounted for the biosynthetic origin of the remaining six carbon atoms in the molecule [(VIII) in Scheme 1].

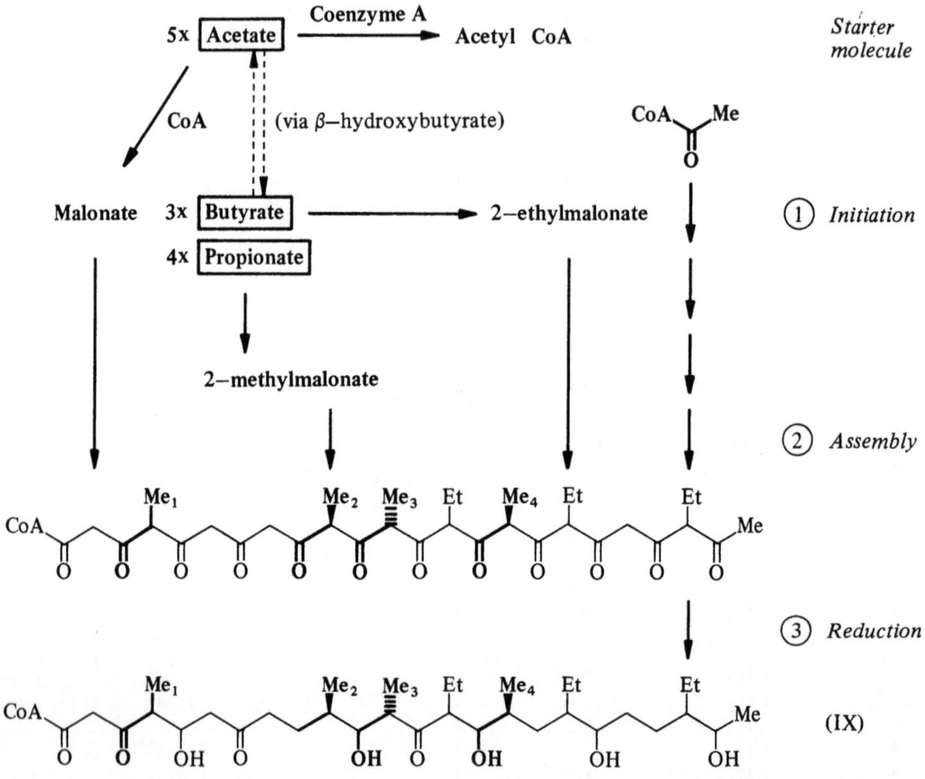

(IX)

Scheme 2. Proposed outline for assembly of the carbon skeleton (IX) of lasalocid A. Propionate-derived C-methyl groups (in bold face) are replaced between 1–4 times/100 molecules of (IX) by butyrate-derived *C-ethyls*, resulting in the production of four homologs (XV)

Summarizing the results from the ^{14}C and ^{13}C incorporation studies, the carbon skeleton (IX) of the antibiotic appears to be assembled via an enzyme complex (*lasalocid synthetase*) in a manner similar to that proposed in Scheme 2. The initiation of the polyketide chain involves acetyl Co A as a starter unit followed by extension steps involving 2-ethylmalonyl Co A, malonyl Co A, and 2-methylmalonyl Co A and continues until the twelfth and final biosynthetic unit, a malonyl Co A, has been added.

During this extension of the carbon skeleton, reduction of selected carbonyls to either secondary alcohol or methylene functions probably occurs to form

(IX) or an equivalent type of linear precursor which then undergoes cyclization to form the three rings A, B, and C present in (I).

4. Biosynthetic Cyclization of Lasalocid A

In an attempt to find partially cyclized intermediates between the linear precusor (IX) and the antibiotic (I), crude extracts of *S. lasaliensis* from which (I) had been crystallized, were subjected to close scrutiny. The first compounds isolated and characterized from these mother liquors were two novel C-17 metabolites (WILLIAMS et al., 1973) unrelated to lasalocid. From the fourth crop of a large scale crystallization of lasalocid A sodium salt, a new crystalline salt with identical ultraviolet, infrared, and microanalysis to the parent antibiotic was isolated as *iso*-lasalocid (XIV). Bromination of (XIV) followed by X-ray analysis revealed the nature of the isomer. The difference between (I) and (XIV) resides entirely in the C ring (Fig. 4).

The absolute configuration of the ten asymmetric centers in (XIV) and (I) are identical except for the two terminal carbons C-22 and C-23. In the case of XIV, C-22 is *S* and C-23 *R*, whereas in (I), the absolute configuration of these asymmetric centers is reversed. These differences together with the size of ring C suggest a common precusor for (I) and (XIV), such as the epoxide (XIII) (WESTLEY et al., 1974b) with the configuration 22(R), 23(R). Microorganisms such as *Pseudomonas oleovorans* are known to epoxidize alkenes (MAY and ABBOTT, 1972) and such an olefinic precursor is the proposed structure XI which could arise from the linear precursor (IX) by dehydration either before or after cyclization of the aromatic ring (in X). The final cyclization after formation of the B ring by the mechanism proposed in Scheme 3 (XII→XIII), can apparently proceed by two routes. Acid-catalyzed cyclization of (XII) would be expected to proceed to *iso*-lasalocid A (XIV) by selective cleavage (KIRK, 1973) of the C-O bond to the more substituted carbon (C-22) according to the Markonikoff rule. Going back one step to the diepoxide (XII), a concerted mechanism is possible (Scheme 4) in which the all *R* intermediate is converted directly into *iso*-lasalocid (WESTLEY et al., 1974b). Support for the all *R* configuration proposed for intermediates (XII) and (XIII) in Scheme 3 has been provided recently by OHTA and TETSUKAWA (1978) who demonstrated that *Corynebacterium equi* transforms terminal olefins exclusively to the *optically pure (R)-epoxide*.

In terms of the biosynthesis of lasalocid, the isolation of (XIV) indicates strongly that the cyclization to ring C is the last step in the formation of the antibiotic. As this cyclization follows a non-Markonikoff route, the proposal was made that, like many *polyether antibiotics*, the epoxide, (XIII), assumes the cyclic conformation indicated in Scheme 3. The subsequent cyclization is then subject to conformational rather than the electronic (Markonikoff) effects.

In addition to lasalocid A and *iso*-lasalocid A, four isomeric homologs B, C, D, and E (XV, Fig. 4) have also been isolated and characterized. The separation of the four isomers was achieved by multiple counter current distributions and the structures were assigned primarily on the results of mass spectro-

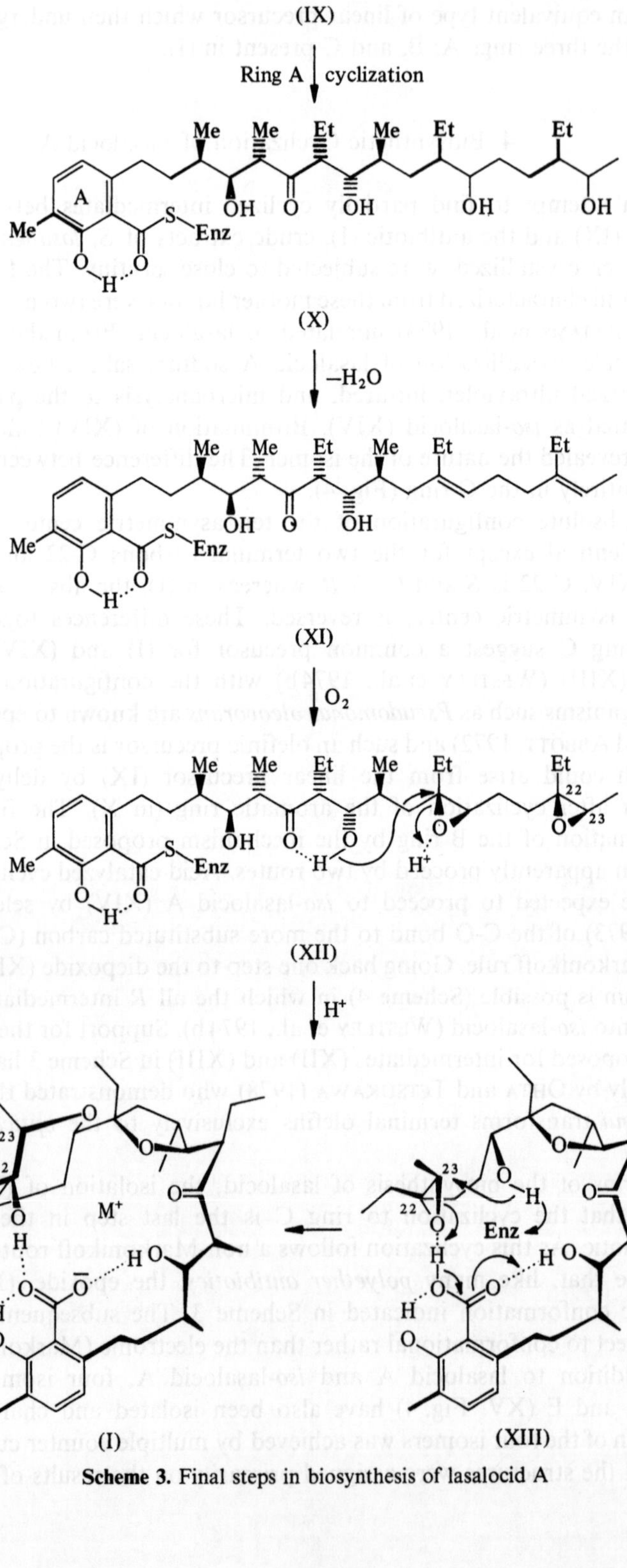

Scheme 3. Final steps in biosynthesis of lasalocid A

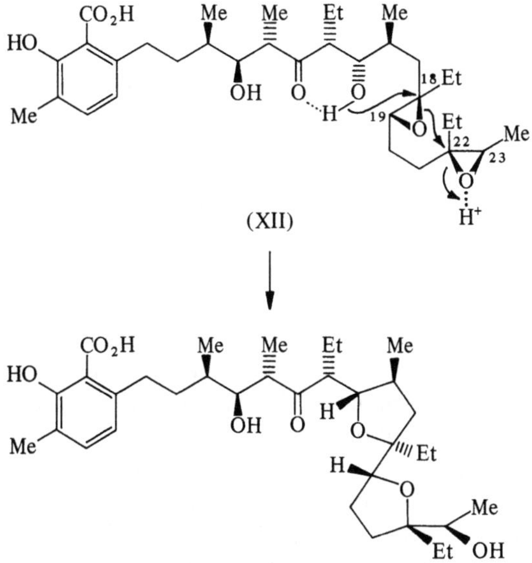

(XII)

(XIV)

Scheme 4. Mechanism proposed for the formation of *iso*-lasalocid (XIV) from the hypothetical diepoxide precursor (XII) of lasalocid

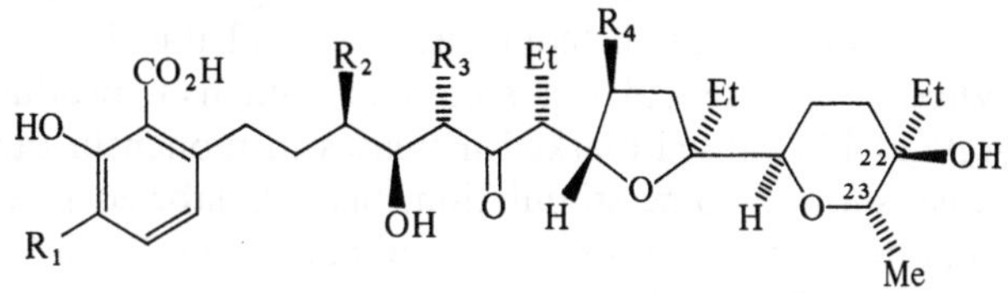

I Lasalocid A — $R_1 = R_2 = R_3 = R_4 = Me$

XV { Lasalocid B — $R_1 = Et, R_2 = R_3 = R_4 = Me$
C — $R_2 = Et, R_1 = R_3 = R_4 = Me$
D — $R_3 = Et, R_1 = R_2 = R_4 = Me$
E — $R_4 = Et, R_1 = R_2 = R_3 = Me$ }

XIV Iso–lasalocid A

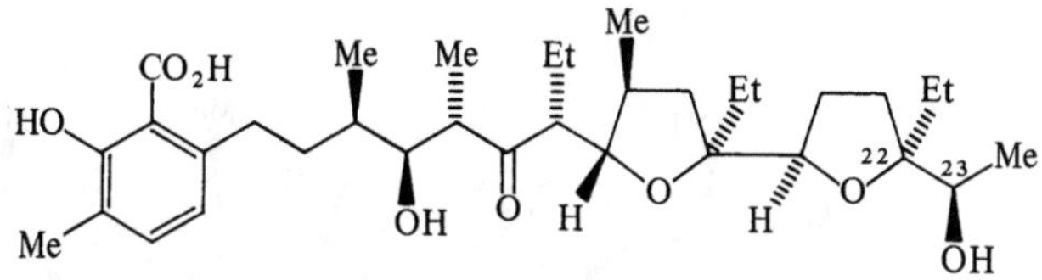

Fig. 4

metric analysis (WESTLEY et al., 1974c). The four homologs probably arise by the replacement of each propionate in the antibiotic precursor molecule (Scheme 2) by a fourth butyrate unit. This replacement results in the formation of the four distinct isomeric homologs of lasalocid, each of which contain an unprecedented *four* C-*ethyl* groups (Fig. 4).

As the total homolog content in lasalocid fermentations varies from 4% up to 16%, it appears that the replacement of each propionate by butyrate can occur from 1–4 times/100 molecules of lasalocid generated by *S. lasaliensis*.

We found no evidence of an ethyl homolog at C-23, which supports the thesis that this particular C-methyl arises from acetate in contrast to the other four propionate-derived methyls at C-4, 10, 12, and 16.

B. Monensin

Monensin is the first polyether antibiotic to become a commercial success. Both as a poultry coccidiostat (Coban®) and as a ruminant growth promotant (Rumensin®), monensin dominates the American markets which, together amount to about U.S. $70 million.

As was noted for *S. lasaliensis, S. cinnamonensis* also produces homologs and three have been described by GORMAN et al. (1968). In factor B, the ethyl group on ring C of monensin is replaced by a methyl; in C, the methyl at the carboxyl terminal asymmetric center is replaced by ethyl and in D, the methyl on ring B is replaced by ethyl (Fig. 5).

The biosynthetic study of DAY et al. (1973) was restricted to monensin, but the homologs are probably formed in a similar way to the lasalocid homologs discussed earlier. The authors first investigated the stimulation of monensin synthesis using potential, 'cold' precursors (Table 5).

Whereas acetate did not stimulate monensin production, propionate and butyrate at 1% caused marked increases in monensin titers and 2-methylmalonate also showed some stimulation. Six ^{14}C-labeled precursors were tested for incorporation and the results are summarized in Table 6. The monensin labeled from these different ^{14}C precursors was then subjected to degradation experiments summarized in Scheme 5.

The periodate oxidation of monensin gave two isolable products, a lactone (XVIIa) missing one of monensin's carbons and formaldehyde (XVIIb) isolated as a dimedone derivative. Chromic acid oxidation cleaved the molecule into a C_{11} acid (XIX) and a C_{23} neutral fragment (XVIII). The same carbon

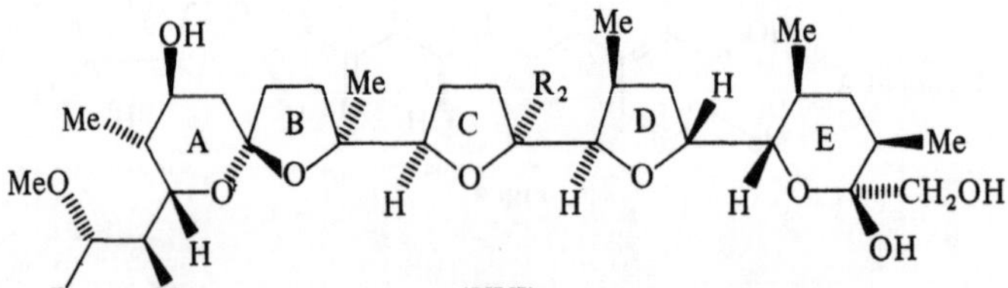

(XVI)

Monensin $R_1 = CH(Me)CO_2H$, $R_2 = Et$ $C_{36}H_{62}O_{11}$
Factor B $R_1 = CH(Me)CO_2H$, $R_2 = Me$ $C_{35}H_{60}O_{11}$
Factor C $R_1 = (CH_2)_3CO_2H$, $R_2 = Me$ $C_{37}H_{64}O_{11}$

Fig. 5

Table 5. Stimulation of monensin synthesis in synthetic medium by unlabeled precursors

Addition	Level tested	Monensin (mcg/ml) produced at 7 days	Percentage increase
0		630	
Sodium propionate	0.1%[a]	1365	+*117*
	0.1%	700	+ 11
	0.2%	265	− 60
	0.3%	50	−100
Sodium acetate	0.1%	640	0
	0.5%	25	−100
Sodium butyrate	0.05%	830	+ 31
	0.1%	1165	+ *85*
	0.2%	140	−100
2-Methyl malonic acid	0.1%	715	+ 14
	0.5%	115	− 82

[a] Addition in this case was made after 42 h. In the other ten experiments addition was made at 0 h

Table 6. Incorporation of ^{14}C-precursors into monensin

Precursor	Percentage incorporation
Glucose-U-^{14}C	0.70
Sodium acetate-1-^{14}C	1.11
Sodium acetate-2-^{14}C	1.86
Sodium propionate-2-^{14}C	19.80
Sodium butyrate-2-^{14}C	3.18
L-Methionine-methyl-^{14}C	6.40

($-CH_2OH$ attached to ring E) is lost as in the periodate reaction and another carbon lost is the C-8 carbon in ring A. Finally, the antibiotic was subjected to Kuhn-Roth oxidation and the resulting acetic and propionic acid separated.

Incorporation experiments showed that while acetate and glucose were incorporated at 0–2% level, butyrate, methionine, and in particular propionate (19.8%) were more efficiently incorporated into the monensin molecule.

When the periodate oxidation was performed on [1-^{14}C] acetate-derived monensin, the resulting formaldehyde (XVII b) had an RMA of 0.5% whereas [2-^{14}C]acetate-derived antibiotic gave XVII b with a relative molar activity (RMA) of 8.1%, which is consistent with carbons C-25, 26 being acetate derived with C-25 corresponding to carboxyl and C-26 to methyl of acetic acid. This is the same as for lasalocid except that in monensin, the terminal methyl group is subsequently oxidized (biosynthetically) to $-CH_2OH$. The results of the chromic acid oxidation (Table 7) reveal that the ratio of RMA values for XVIII:XIX is 4:3 for propionate-derived antibiotic, consistent with the incor-

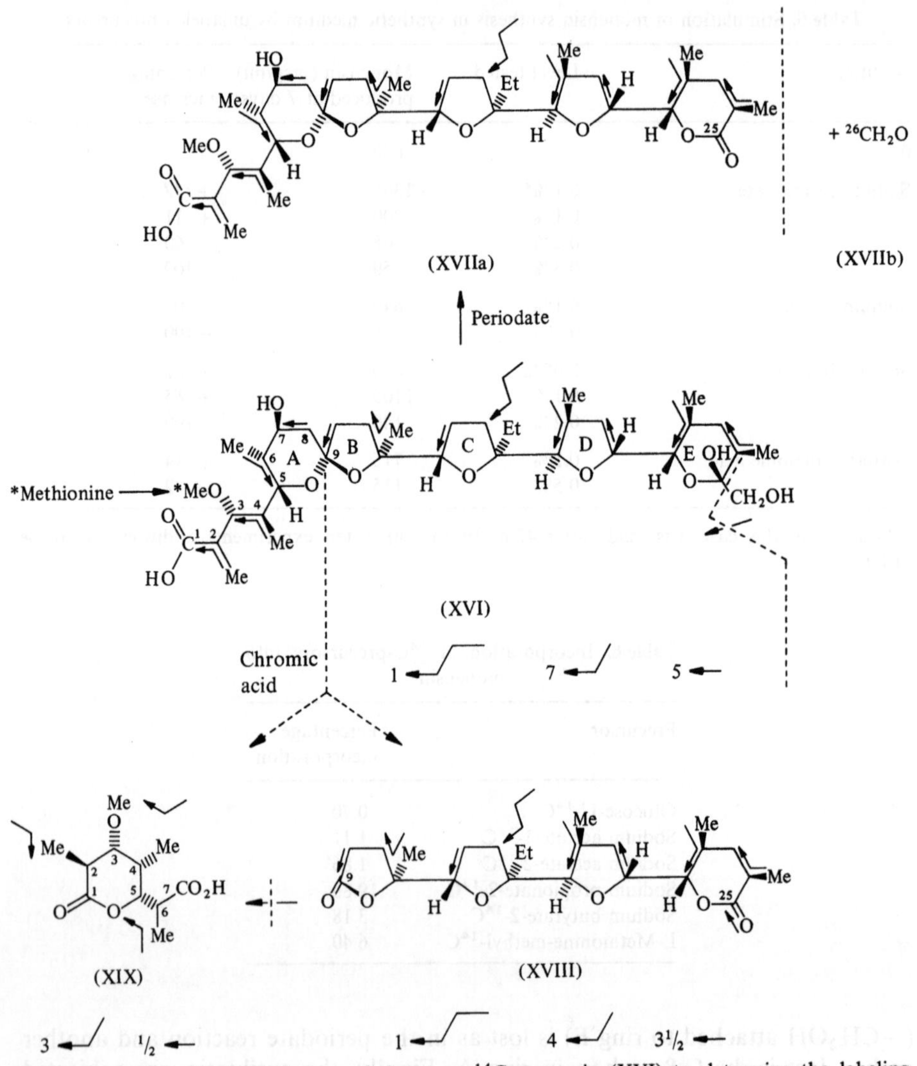

Scheme 5. Chemical degradations carried out on ^{14}C-monensin (XVI) to determine the labeling pattern. Results are given in Table 7

poration of seven of these C_3 units into XVI as proposed in Scheme 5. The ratio for [1-^{14}C]acetate-derived antibiotic was 4.5:1 compared to the theoretical ratio of 4:1 based on Scheme 5, and for butyrate 5:1 (theory > 100:1), suggesting that, although there is a considerable amount of randomization between acetate and butyrate due to β-oxidation, the proposed route to XVI (Scheme 5) is probably correct.

In conclusion, this study of DAY et al. (1973), although hampered by considerably greater randomization than that encountered in the earlier lasalocid work, clearly indicated that the antibiotic is formed from a butyrate, five acetates,

Table 7. Relative molar activity (RMA)[a] of degradation products from ^{14}C-Monensin

^{14}C-Monensin derived	XVIIb	XIX	XVIII
from [1-^{14}C]Acetate	0.3 (0)	18.7 (20)	83.6 (80)
from [2-^{14}C]Acetate	8.1 (20)		
from [2-^{14}C]Propionate	0.2 (0)	44.8 (43)	57.6 (57)
from [1-^{14}C]Butyrate			
from [2-^{14}C]Butyrate	3.1 (0)	17.3 (0)	83 (100)
from [3-^{14}C]Butyrate			
from [Me-^{14}C]Methionine	0.1 (0)	96.2 (100)	3.9 (0)

[a] Values in parentheses are calculated, based on labeling pattern proposed in Scheme 5

and seven propionates. For the first time it was demonstrated unequivocally that the methoxyl group in monensin (and probably other polyethers) is derived from methionine. Using [1-^{13}C] and [2-^{13}C]acetate, attempts were made to confirm the ^{14}C results, but too low enrichment made it impossible to solve the labeling pattern by ^{13}C nmr.

C. Salinomycin and Narasin

Since the structure and therefore biosynthesis of salinomycin (XX) and narasin (4-methylsalinomycin, XXI) are so similar they are considered together in this section (Fig. 6.).

The structure of salinomycin was established by X-ray crystallographic analysis of the *p*-iodophenacyl ester (KINASHI et al., 1973). Some three years later comparing the mass spectral fragmentation patterns of XX and narasin (XXI), OCCOLOWITZ et al. (1976) found them extremely similar. In fact, the only difference was due to the addition of a methyl group in XXI substituted at the C-4 position of XX. This same conclusion was arrived at independently by KINASHI and OTAKE (1976). From the mass spectra of XXI the absolute stereochemistry at C-4 could not be deduced. This problem was finally solved by ^{13}C-nmr spectroscopy (SETO et al., 1977a) which was able to establish the 4-methyl substituent as equatorial, with the absolute S configuration.

The investigations into the biosynthesis of the two antibiotics in both cases involved ^{13}C-nmr spectroscopy, but the two independent groups working on salinomycin (SETO et al., 1977b) and narasin (DORMAN et al., 1976) used somewhat different approaches.

In the case of salinomycin, model compounds were studied such as the retro-aldol ketone (VI, Scheme 1) from lasalocid and the α-lactone (XXII) produced by base cleavage of XX. The assignment of XXII in turn was determined by selective proton decoupling. Solving the ^{13}C-nmr of XXII assisted in the assignment of carbons C_{24}-C_{33} in XX. SETO et al. also used double-labeling methods with [1,2-^{13}C]acetate and [1,2-^{13}C]propionate-derived salinomycin

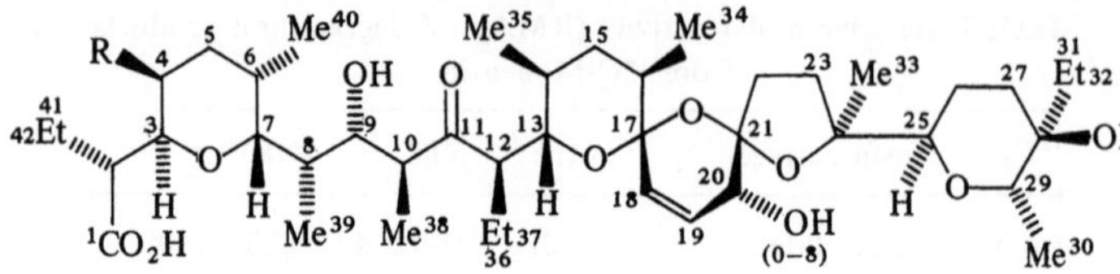

Salinomycin, R = H (XX)
Narasin, R = Me (XXI)

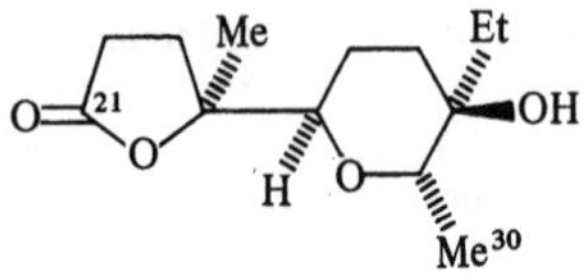

Salinomycin, α–lactone (XXII)

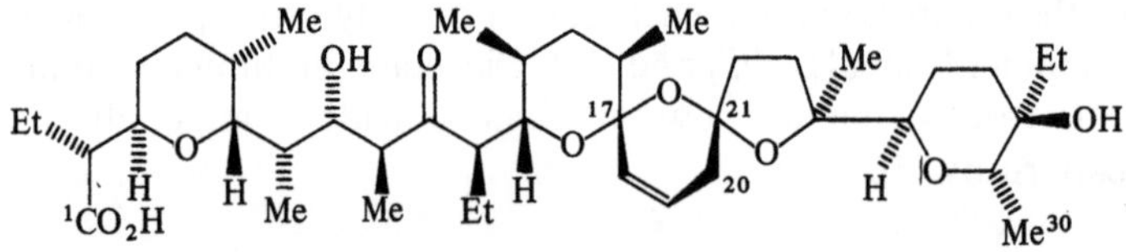

Deoxy–(0–8)–salinomycin (XXV)

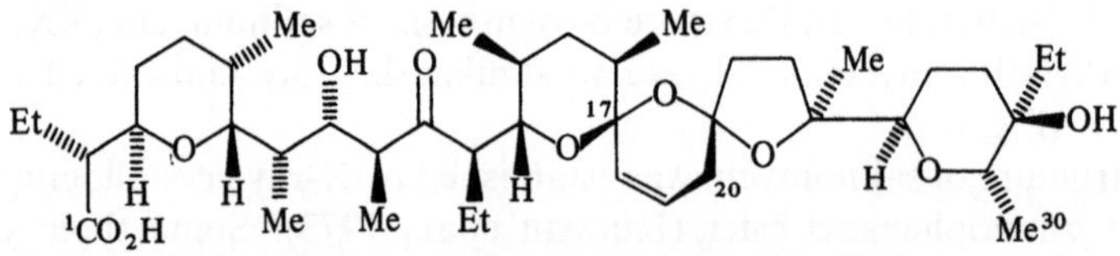

Epi–17–deoxy–(0–8)–salinomycin (XXIV)

Fig. 6

(XX) to help solve more of the 42 assigments in XX. The complete assignments of both salinomycin (XX) and narasin (XXI) are presented in Table 8.

The biosynthesis of narasin was studied (DORMAN et al., 1976) using six ^{13}C-labeled substrates and comparing the resulting ^{13}C-narasin samples with natural abundance antibiotic for enrichments, using ^{13}C-nmr. The results are summarized in Table 9.

From the results in Table 9, the following conclusions can be drawn:

1. *Three butyrate units* are involved in the biosynthesis of narasin (XXI).
2. *Seven propionate units* are also involved.
3. By difference only, *five acetates* must also be involved, but the attempt to confirm this using [2-^{13}C]acetate as substrate for the fermentation yielded narasin with no ^{13}C enrichments greater than 2, which is probably due

Table 8. ^{13}C nmr assignments of salinomycin by SETO et al. (1977b) and narasin by DORMAN et al. (1976)

Carbon number[a]	δ (XX)	δ (XXI)
1	177.2 A[b]	178.4
2	48.9 A	49.3 B2[c]
3	74.9 A	73.9
4	20.1 A	28.0 P2
5	26.4 P	36.2
6	28.0 P	29.0 P2
7	75.2 P	75.1
8	32.6 P	41.1 P2
9	68.7 P	72.0
10	49.2 P	49.9 P2
11	214.5 A	216.5
12	56.5 A	56.1 B2
13	71.7 P	78.4
14	36.5 P	32.9 P2
15	38.6 P	35.5
16	40.7 P	36.6 P2
17	99.2 A	99.6
18	121.6 A	122.0
19	132.4 A	132.0
20	67.2 A	67.6
21	106.4 A	106.5
22	36.2 A	38.7
23	30.2 P	30.5
24	88.5 P	88.5 P2
25	73.7 A	68.5
26	21.9 A	21.8
27	29.3 A	29.4
28	70.9 A	70.8 B2
29	77.2 A	71.1
30	14.5 A	14.3
31	30.6 A	30.9 B3
32	6.3 A	6.3 B4
33	25.8	26.1 P3
34	17.9	13.0 P3
35	15.6	12.1 P3
36	22.7 A	12.1 B4
37	11.9 A	16.4 B3
38	12.8	7.0 P3
39	7.0	15.7 P3
40	11.2	18.0 P3
41	16.6 A	24.0 B3
42	13.2 A	13.2 B4

[a] Carbons italicized are those which are assigned the same chemical shift (within 2 ppm) by both SETO and DORMAN

[b] Assignment by (A) [1,2-^{13}C]acetate or (P) [1,2-^{13}C]propionate labeling

[c] Assignment by enrichment studies with B2, B3, B4 [(2-^{13}C, 3-^{13}C and 4-^{13}C)butyrate] or P2, P3[(2-^{13}C and 3-^{13}C) propionate]

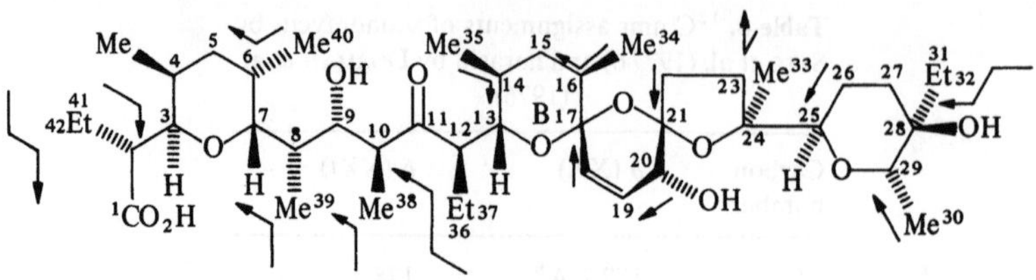

(XXIII)

Fig. 7

Table 9. ^{13}C Enrichment in narasin from six different substrates

Substrate used in the biosynthesis of ^{13}C-narasin	Total carbons enriched	Chemical shifts (ppm) of the enriched resonances							Degree of enrichment
[2-^{13}C]Propionate	7	28	29 [a]	32.9	36.6	41.1	49.9	88.5	>2
[3-^{13}C]Propionate	7	7	12.1	13	15.7	18	19	26.1	>5
	4 [b]	6.3	13.2	49.3	56.1				2–3.5
[2-^{13}C]Butyrate	3	49.3	56.1	70.8					>17
	3 [b]	38.7	67.6	122					2–2.6
[3-^{13}C]Butyrate	3	10.4	24	30.9					>16
	7 [b]	28	29	32.9	36.6	41.1	49.9	88.5	> 7.5–9.5
[4-^{13}C]Butyrate	3	6.3	12.1	13.2					>14
	6 [b]	7	12.1	13	15.7	18	19	26.1	10.8–12.6
[2-^{13}C]Acetate	0	No enrichments greater than 2							

[a] Enrichment = 1.9, but in this case, is probably significant

[b] Secondary, or lower enrichments

to the many sources of ^{12}C-acetate available in the fermentation diluting out the added ^{13}C-acetate.

4. From these first three conclusions, the labeling pattern of narasin appears to be as illustrated for XXIII (Fig. 7).
5. As noted in the case of macrocyclic antibiotics by OMURA et al. (1975), metabolic interconversions of substrates (particularly ^{13}C-butyrate) cause complications in the interpretation of biogenetic results. Three examples from the study of narasin follow:
   a. Inspection of the results from Table 9 reveals that the secondary enrichments in [3 and 4-^{13}C]butyrate-derived narasin are identical to major enrichments from the [2 and 3-^{13}C]propionate experiments. The most likely interpretation is that the secondary labeling in the butyrate-derived sample arose from *α-oxidation* of butyrate to propionate prior to incorporation.
   b. By α-oxidation, the secondary enrichments in [2-^{13}C]butyrate-derived narasin should correspond to the major enrichments in [1-^{13}C]propionate-

derived antibiotic, but, unfortunately, [1-^{13}C]propionate was not tested. However, there were three indirectly derived carbon atoms in the [2-^{13}C]butyrate spectrum at δ 38.7, 67.6, and 122 ppm, which have been assigned to carbons C-18, C-20 and C-22 in Table 8. Assuming these assignments are correct, the proposed labeling pattern (Fig. 7., XXIII) for narasin would mean that the indirectly derived carbons from [2-^{13}C]-butyrate are going into [2-^{13}C]acetate-derived positions by *β-oxidation,* as has been noted earlier (WESTLEY et al., 1972) for lasalocid (Fig. 8).

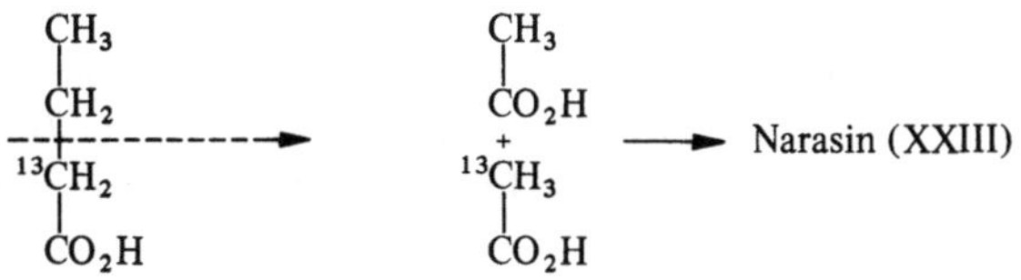

Fig. 8

Considering the relative levels of the secondary enrichments in *Streptomyces aureofaciens,* α- rather β- oxidation is the primary cause of randomization in narasin biosynthesis.

c. The set of lower enrichments observed in the case of [3-^{13}C]propionate corresponded to two [4-^{13}C] and two [2-^{13}C]butyrate carbons suggesting that propionate can be converted to butyrate by *Streptomyces aureofaciens,* which, if true, represents the first documented example known (DORMAN et al., 1976) (Fig. 9).

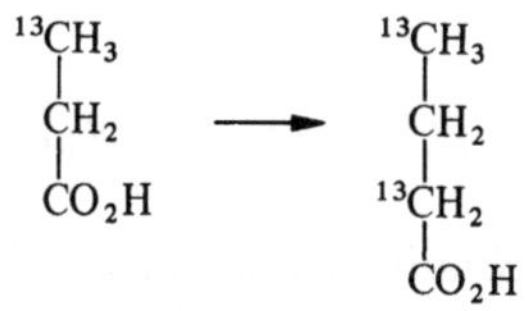

Fig. 9

However, as there appears to be a high level of enzymatic activity capable of α-oxidation (see above), a more likely explanation might be the α-oxidation of propionate to acetate which is then converted to butyrate (Fig. 10).

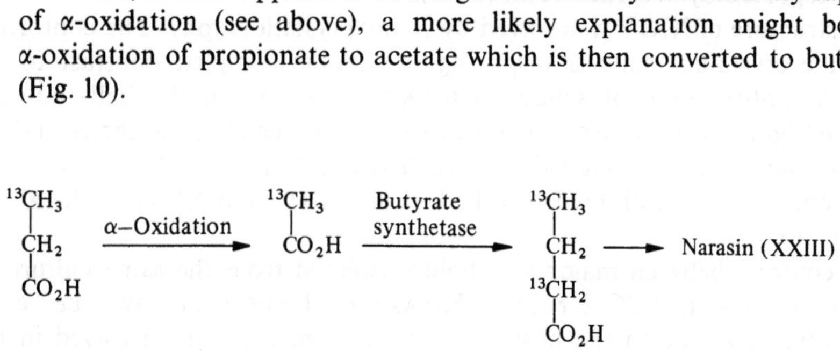

Fig. 10

Comparing the lists of assignments presented in Table 8 for the two antibiotics, reveals that 23 out of 42 signals are in good agreement (chemical shift difference <2 ppm) between the two studies. The difference in structure between XX and XXI (4-methyl substitution) accounts for the difference in chemical shift for C-4 and C-5, but this structural change is not great enough to account for differences in assignment of from 3–10 ppm reported for: C-8, 9, 13, 14, 15, 16, 22, 25, and C-34 to C-42.

Most of these seventeen carbons, in the case of salinomycin (XX) were assigned by the double-labeling technique employing [1,2-^{13}]acetate and propionate as precursors for ^{13}C-(XX) (SETO et al., 1977b). AB-type coupling of ^{13}C-^{13}C were observed for CH_2-CH arising from C-5, 6 and C-15, 16, and for $CO-CH_2$ due to C-23, 24. Three pairs of the AB-type ($CH-CHO$) were noted that fit C-8, 9, C-10, 11 (confirmed by ^{13}C-homo nuclear spin decoupling) and C-13, 14.

From the [1,2-^{13}C]acetate experiment, as from the propionate one, the following pairs were assigned: C-1, 2; C-3, 4; C-11, 12; C-17, 18; C-19, 20; C-21, 22; C-25, 26; C-27, 28; C-29, 30; C-31, 32; C-36, 37; and C-41, 42. The remaining methyls were assigned by analogy with model compounds (SETO et al., 1977b). This combination of double-labeling experiments with very closely related model compounds would seem to insure that the assignments of XX made by SETO are essentially correct. For narasin, although the enrichment results clearly indicate the labeling pattern proposed in XXIII, some of the individual assignments for the carbons listed in Table 8 might be worth checking using [1,2-^{13}C]acetate, propionate, or butyrate. Whatever the outcome of such a study, the important role that α-oxidation plays in *Streptomyces aurefaciens* fermentation will not be effected and would only have been revealed by the enrichments described by DORMAN et al. (1976).

1. Biosynthetic Cyclization of Salinomycin

From deposited cultures of *Streptomyces albus* (ATCC 21838) and employing a different fermentation medium, a new antibiotic, deoxy-(0-8)-*epi*-17-salinomycin (XXIV) was isolated as the major product, with an approximately *tenfold higher yield* than its epimer, deoxy-(0-8)-salinomycin (XXV) and salinomycin (XX) as reported by WESTLEY et al. (1977).

The structure of XXIV was solved by X-ray crystallography. The conformation in the crystalline state is surprisingly linear, in complete contrast to the U-shaped conformation of salinomycin (XX) as shown in the ball-and-stick models in Figure 11. In spite of the quite distinct conformations in the crystalline state, the only *configurational* difference between XX and XXIV is at C-17 and the only structural difference is the lack in XXIV (and XXV) of the allylic hydroxyl at C-20.

The contrast between major metabolites isolated from the same culture of *Streptomyces albus* (ATCC 21838) by KINASHI et al. (1973) and WESTLEY et al. (1977) provides a clue to the possible cyclization mechanisms involved in the biosynthesis of salinomycin. In the initial studies, salinomycin (XX) was the

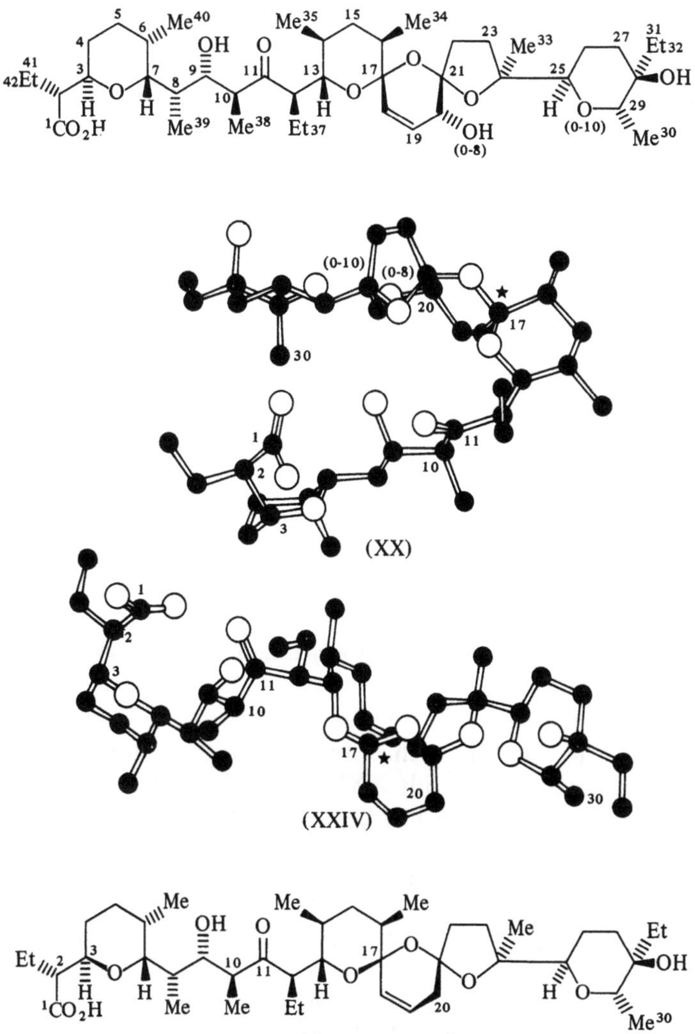

Fig. 11

major activity isolated, whereas in the 1977 report, the epimer at C-17 of deoxy(0-8)-salinomycin (XXIV) was found to be produced at ten times the level of both XX and the simple deoxy-(0-8) derivative (XXV). If the allylic alcohol, 0-8 is assumed to be present in a hypothetical *linear precursor* (diene-diepoxide in Scheme 6) to XX then the foregoing results implicate this hydroxyl as the key to the stereochemistry at C-17. To help explain the kind of role that 0-8 might play in the biosynthesis of salinomycin, a highly speculative mechanism is proposed (Scheme 6). Presumably, 0-8 is hydrogen-bonded to an oxygen earlier in the carbon backbone, such as the carbonyl at C-11. This would force the linear precursor to assume a U-shaped conformation similar to XX in Figure 11. Cyclization to the hemiketal (step a in the scheme) would then be comformationally restricted to a single epimer. The non-hydroxylated precursor, however, would be expected to assume the conformation with least

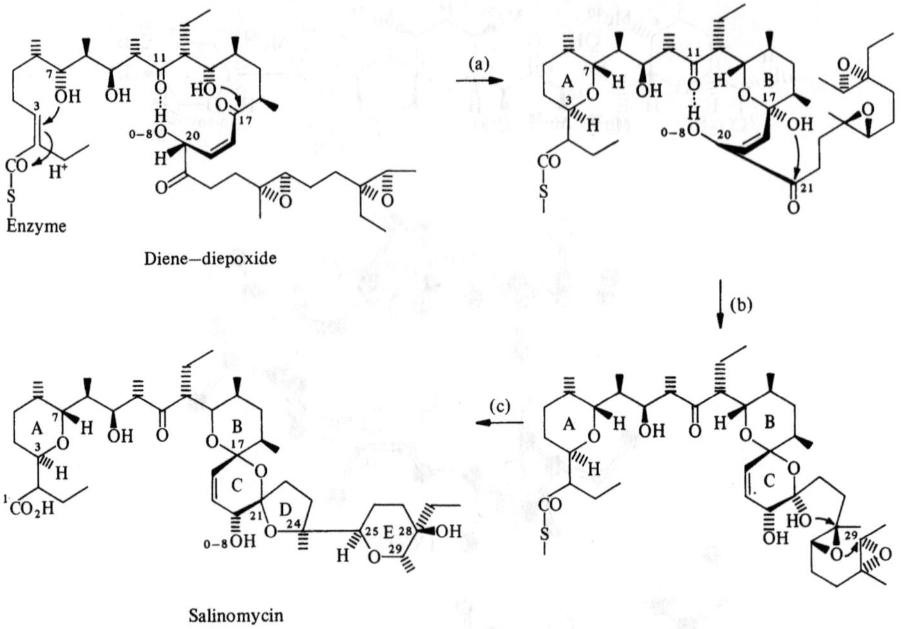

Scheme 6. Speculative cyclization mechanisms involved in the final steps of salinomycin biosynthesis

steric hindrance, which in turn cyclizes to ring B with the opposite stereochemistry at C-17 and eventually yields XXIV (Fig. 11). The formation of ring C of salinomycin (step b) is followed by the same type of epoxide-opening cyclizations (step c) to form rings D and E as those implicated in the formation of the identical rings (B and C in Scheme 3) present in lasalocid. Whatever the actual mechanism, the formation of the last three rings of both XX and XXIV must proceed similarly as carbons C-21, 24, 25, 28, and 29 all have the same configuration in both molecules. The basis of these speculations is sure to be tested in the chemical syntheses of tri-spiroketal polyether antibiotics, which are now under way in several laboratories.

D. Lysocellin

Lysocellin is a relatively small (C_{23} backbone) polyether antibiotic produced by *Streptomyces cacaoi* var. *asoensis* K-9 Met$^-$, the structure of which was established by X-ray analysis (Otake et al., 1975). The section of the lysocellin (XXVI) molecule that encompasses C-8 to C-16 is identical to the C-10 to C-18 fragment of lasalocid (I), which was useful to Otake et al. (1978b) in their assignment of the ^{13}C-nmr spectrum of XXVI, because of the earlier assignment of I by Seto et al. (1978a). In addition to lasalocid as a model, the retro-aldol ketone (VI) from lasalocid and the analogous ketone (XXVII) from lysocellin also proved useful (Fig. 12), particularly in assigning the ten methyl groups present in XXVI.

Lysocellin

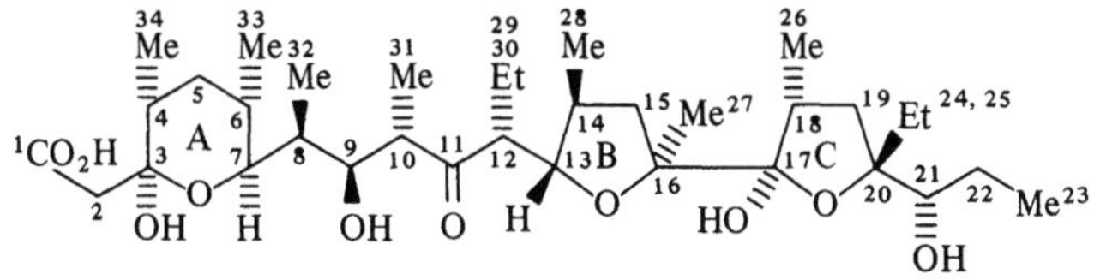

(XXVI)

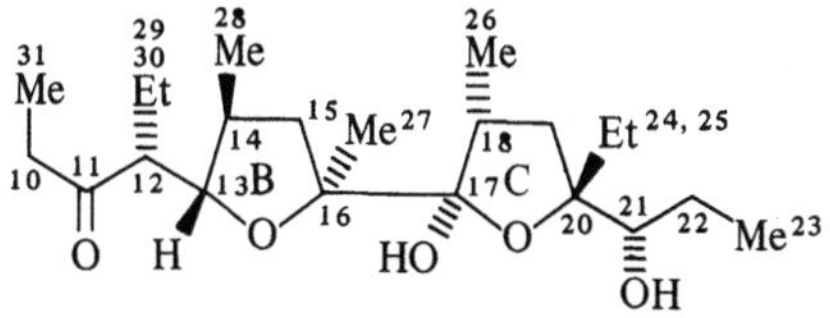

(XXVII)

Lasalocid A

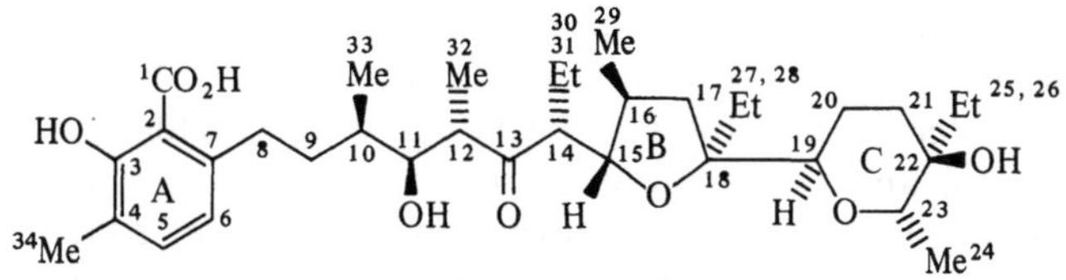

(I)

Iso–lasalocid A (XIV)

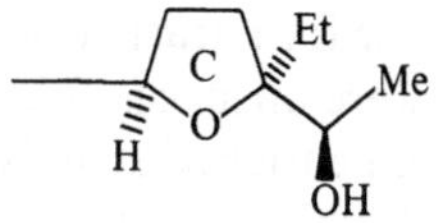

Fig. 12

In a series of reports on the use of high resolution proton nmr spectra (300 MHz) to study the solution conformation of ionophores, M. ANTEUNIS (Ghent, Belgium) has assigned the ^{1}H spectra of inter alia, lasalocid (1976), A23187 (1977a), A204A (1977b), monensin (1977c), dianemycin, lenoremycin (1977d), and *lysocellin* (1977e) in a number of different solvents. From the lysocellin study, the chemical shifts of the oxymethine protons attached to carbons C-7, 9, 13, and 21 were used by OTAKE to assign the four oxymethine *carbons* in the ^{13}C-nmr spectrum by selective decoupling experiments.

A third approach utilized in this attempt to assign the ^{13}C-nmr of XXVI, was the double-labeling technique. The antibiotic (XXVI) was produced by *Streptomyces cacaoi* var. *asoensis* K-9 Met^{-}, on a medium containing (1,2-^{13}C] propionate. By detecting coupled AB-type systems in the enriched spectrum, the carbons, C-8, 10, 14, and 22, attached to the four oxymethine carbons (C-7, 9, 13, and 21) were assigned. There were altogether eight AB-type ^{13}C-^{13}C coupled carbons in the spectrum of [1,2-^{13}C]propionate-derived XXVI (Table 10).

By using the three approaches exemplified by the oxymethine and neighboring carbon systems discussed above, the complete assignment of the ^{13}C-nmr

Table 10. ^{13}C-^{13}C coupling observed in the ^{13}C-nmr spectrum of XXVI derived from [1,2-^{13}C]propionate

Carbons	Chemical shifts	Coupling constants (Hz)
C-3, 4	98.1, 39.3	45.7[a]
C-17, 18	108.1, 38.3	39.3
C-7, 8	79, 32.3	40.0
C-9, 10	75.7, 47.5	41.5
C-13, 14	83.5, 34.6	34.9
C-15, 16	42.7, 86.0	36.9
C-21, 22	71.6, 25.4	38.4
C-5, 6	36.6, 32.3	33.3

[a] Average value from the published data

spectrum of XXVI was achieved (Table 11). With this information in hand, OTAKE et al. proceeded to investigate the biosynthesis of XXVI.

As noted earlier, the C_{23} backbone of lysocellin indicated propionic acid as initiator and eleven sub-units involved in the biosynthesis of the antibiotic (WESTLEY 1976). This was confirmed by enrichment studies using [1,2-^{13}C]propionate, mentioned earlier, together with [1-^{13}C]propionate and [1-^{13}C]butyrate as substrates for *S. cacaoi* var. *asoensis* K-9 Met$^-$ and then examining the ^{13}C spectrum of the resulting labeled XXVI (OTAKE et al., 1978b). As was the case for narasin (DORMAN et al., 1976), all attempts to incorporate [1-^{13}C]acetate were unsuccessful. The [1-^{13}C]propionate experiment gave XXVI with *eight* 30-fold enriched signals due to carbons C-3, 5, 7, 9, 13, 15, 17, and 21, whereas the [1-^{13}C]butyrate yielded XXVI with *two* tenfold enriched peaks C-11 and C-19 together with approximately eight-fold enrichment of the same eight carbons that were enriched in the [1-^{13}C]propionate labeling experiment. This result constitutes another example of butyrate to propionate conversion prior to incorporation into a polyether antibiotic. However, the mechanism is *different* to that observed earlier for *Streptomyces aureofaciens* by DORMAN et al. (1976) where *α-oxidation* appeared to be the predominant route (Fig. 13):

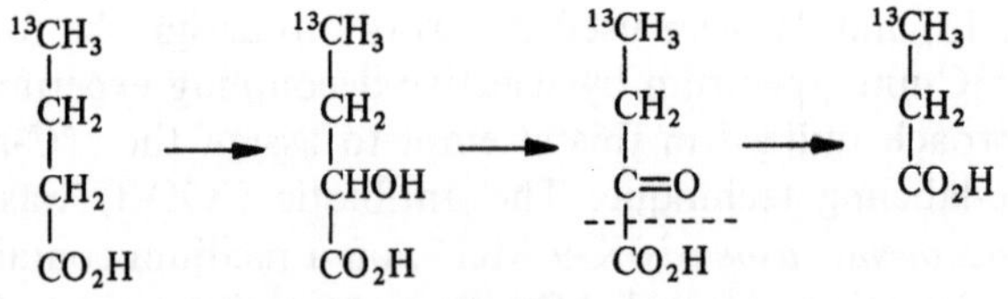

Fig. 13

First demonstrated by MEAD and LEWIS (1963), α-oxidation is consistent with DORMAN's results from labeling narasin with 3- and 4-^{13}C-butyrate and 2- and 3-^{13}C-propionate and might also play a role in lysocellin biosynthesis (α-oxidation of [1-^{13}C]butyrate would give unlabeled, and therefore undetected

Table 11. Assignment of ^{13}C resonances of lysocellin sodium salt

Carbon number	Functional group	Chemical shift (ppm)
1	CO_2^-	177.7
2	CH_2	45.9
3	OC(O)	98.1
4	CH	39.3
5	CH_2	36.6
6	CH	32.3
7	CH(O)	79.3
8	CH	32.3
9	CH(O)	75.7
10	CH	47.5
11	C=O	214.6
12	CH	55.0
13	CHO	83.5
14	CH	34.6
15	CH_2	42.7
16	C(O)	86.0
17	OC(O)	108.1
18	CH	38.3
19	CH_2	37.6
20	C(O)	87.1
21	CH(O)	71.6
22	CH_2	25.4
23	CH_3	11.3
24	CH_2	31.4
25	CH_3	7.5
26	CH_3	14.7
27	CH_3	23.8
28	CH_3	16.6
29	CH_2	14.9
30	CH_3	12.6
31	CH_3	12.8
32	CH_3	5.4
33	CH_3	16.6
34	CH_3	15.5

propionate). OTAKE's results using [1-^{13}C]butyrate and propionate, however, indicate that another mechanism may be predominant in *S. cacaoi* var. *asoensis* for butyrate/propionate conversion, in which the carboxyl group is retained. OMURA et al. (1975, 1976b) observed similar results in macrolide biosynthesis and the most likely intermediates in this second type of conversion are succinate and 2-methylmalonate (Fig. 14):

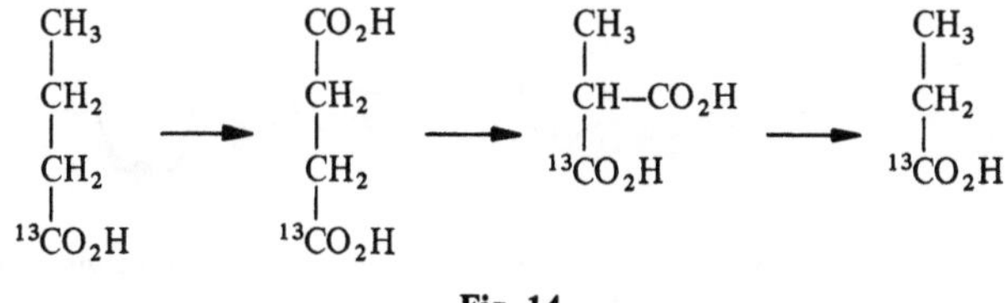

Fig. 14

II. Summary

The polyether antibiotics, with the exception of CP-44,161 (see Table 1) are all products of *Streptomyces*. From the evidence presented here, they appear to be assembled via the polyketide route discovered and refined by BIRCH (1957), KANEDA et al. (1962), TANNENBAUM (1967) and LYNEN (1967) inter alia for the biosynthesis of fatty acids and other natural products such as orsellinic acid. From this earlier work, the activation of acetate by transformation to its co-enzyme A ester, the role of malonyl Co A and the nature of the reductive enzymes utilized in the biosynthesis of the so-called *acetogenins* have all been thoroughly documented. In a similar fashion, the roles of propionyl and 2-methyl-malonylCo A have also been well defined.

One of the first novel results arising from the biosynthetic studies of the polyether antibiotics was that aromatic methyl groups (in this case, the one substituted on the chromophore of lasalocid) could be derived from propionate. All the examples known at the time were derived from C_1 donors such as methionine (see reference to THOMAS, 1978). Another discovery from the same study, came in the first unequivocal demonstration of the formation of a *C-ethyl group from a complete butyric acid molecule*. This novel observation was subsequently demonstrated for the other four polyether antibiotics reviewed here.

An aspect of the biosynthesis of polyether antibiotics that could be most significant to synthetic chemists attempting to make these antibiotics is the nature of the cyclization mechanisms involved in formation of the many reduced furans and pyrans, which characterize this class of natural products. Four possibilities are outlined in Fig. 15.

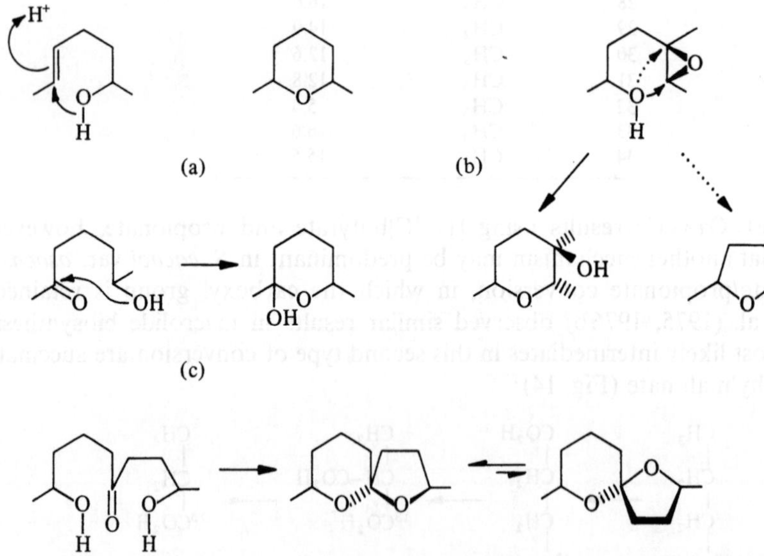

Fig. 15. Possible cyclization mechanisms leading to the many tetrahydro-furans and pyrans found in polyether antibiotics

Mechanisms equivalent to (a) in Figure 15 are probably responsible for the majority of cyclizations involved in the formation of the cyclic ethers, and the common occurrence of *lactols* in the class suggest that at least in some cases they might be intermediates (derived in turn from γ- or δ-hydroxyketones) in the cyclization process (WESTLEY et al., 1974b). The evidence for mechanism (b) was discussed in some detail in the section on lasalocid and recently, Y. KISHI's group at Harvard have employed synthetic routes similar to (b) and (c) in their elegant syntheses of *iso*-lasalocid, lasalocid, and monensin (FUKUYAMA et al., 1979; NAKATA et al., 1978).

One commonly occurring moiety which has not been investigated biosynthetically is the 2,3,6-trideoxy-4-*O*-methyl-D-*erythro*hexapyranose present in the eleven monovalent glycoside polyethers (Class 1b, Table 1) including lenoremycin (Fig. 1). The same sugar, lacking the methoxyl group, 2,3,6-trideoxy-D-*erythro*-hexapyranose(amicetose) is present in the antibiotic amicetin (HANESSIAN and HASKELL, 1964).

Acknowledgment. The author wishes to thank Dr. R. Thomas for his many useful comments and suggestions.

References

Agtarap A, Chamberlin JW, Pinkerton M, Steinrauf L (1967) The structure of monensic acid. J Am Chem Soc 89:5737

Alleaume M, Busetta B, Farges C, Gachon P, Kergomard A, Staron T (1975) X-Ray structure of alborixin, a new antibiotic ionophore. Chem Commun 1975:411

Anteunis MJO (1976) Solution conformation of lasalocid and lasalocid-Na^+ (X-537A). Bioorg Chem 5:327

Anteunis MJO (1977a) Solution conformation of ionophore A23187 and its magnesium salt. Bioorg Chem 6:1

Anteunis MJO, Verhegge C (1977b) Solution conformation of the ionophore A204A, Na^+-salt. Bull Soc Chim Belge 86:353

Anteunis MJO (1977c) Solution conformation of antibiotic (monensin)-sodium salt. Bull Soc Chim Belge 86:367

Anteunis MJO, Rodios N-A, Verhegge G (1977d) Solution conformation of dianemycin, its sodium salt and of lenoremycin-Na. Bull Soc Chim Belge 86:609

Anteunis MJO (1977e) Solution conformation of lysocellin, Na^+, more than a simple structural analog of lasalocid, Na^+. Bull Soc Chim Belge 86:187

Berger J (1973) Coccidiostats. U S Patent 3, 719, 753

Berger J, Rachlin AI, Scott WE, Sternbach LH, Goldberg MW (1951) The isolation of three new crystalline antibiotics from *Streptomyces*. J Am Chem Soc 73:5295

Birch AJ (1957) Biosynthetic relations of some phenolic and enolic compounds In: Fortschritte der Chemie Organischer Naturstoffe, vol XIV, p 186. Springer, Berlin Heidelberg New York

Blount JF, Westley JW (1975) X-ray crystal and molecular structure of antibiotic X-206. Chem Commun 1975:533

Blount JF, Evans RH, Liu C-M, Hermann T, Westley JW (1975) X-ray crystal structure of Ro 21-6150 (lenoremycin), a polyether antibiotic related to dianemycin. Chem Commun 1975:853

Celmer WD, Cullen WP, Jefferson MT, Routien JB, Sciavolino FC, Moppet CE (1976) CP 38295, a new polycyclic ether antibiotic. Belg Patent 831947

Celmer WD, Cullen WP, Moppett CE, Oscarson JR, Routien JB (1977) CP 38,986, new polycyclic ether antibiotic. US Patent 4,022,885

Chaney MO, Demarco PV, Jones ND, Occolowitz JL (1974) The structure of A23187, a divalent cation ionophore. J Am Chem Soc 96:1932

Czerwinski EW, Steinrauf LK (1971) Structure of the antibiotic dianemycin. Biochem Biophys Res Commun 45:1284

Day LE, Chamberlin JW, Gordee EZ, Chen S, Gorman M, Hamill RL, Ness T, Weeks RE, Stroshane S (1973) Biosynthesis of monensin. Antimicrob Agents Chemother 4:410

Dorman DE, Paschal JW, Nakatsukasa WM, Huckstep LL, Neuss N (1976) The use of ^{13}C-NMR. Spectroscopy in biosynthetic studies. II. Biosynthesis of narasin, a new polyether ionophore from fermentation of *Streptomyces aureofaciens*. Helv Chim Acta 59:2025

Ebata E, Kasahara H, Sekine K, Inoue Y (1975) Lysocellin, a new polyether antibiotic. I. Isolation, purification, physico chemical and biological properties. J Antibiot 28:118

Fehr T, King HD, Kuhn M (1977) Mutalomycin, a new polyether antibiotic. Taxonomy, fermentation, isolation and characterization. J Antibiot 30:903

Florent J, Lunel J, Mancy D (1976) Anticoccididial substance (RP 30504). U S Patent 3,989,820

Fukuyama T, Akasaka K, Karanewsky DS, Wang C-LJ, Schmid G, Kishi Y (1979) Total synthesis of monensin, III. Stereocontrolled total synthesis of monensin. J Am Chem Soc 101:262

Gachon P, Kergomard A, Veschambre H, Esteve C, Staron T (1970) Grisorixin, a new antibiotic related to nigericin. Chem Commun 1970:1421

Gachon P, Farges C, Kergomard A (1976) Alborixin, a new antibiotic ionophore: Isolation, structure, physical and chemical properties. J Antibiot 29:603

Gale RM, Higgins CE, Hoehn MM (1975) Antibiotic A23187 and process for preparation thereof. U S Patent 3,923,823

Gorman M, Chamberlin JW, Hamill RL (1968) Monensin, a new biologicallyactive compound. V. Compounds related to monensin. Antimicrob. Agents & chemotherapy. 1967. p 363–368

Hamill RL, Crandall LW (1978) "Polyether Antibiotics" In: Weinstein MJ, Wagman GH (eds) Journal of Chromatography Library, vol V, p 479. entitled *Antibiotics*. Elsevier, Amsterdam

Hamill RL, Hoehn MM (1972) Antibiotics A204I and A204II and method for the production thereof. U S Patent 3,705,238

Hamill RL, Hoehn MM (1974) Antibiotics A28695A and A28695B and a process for production thereof. U S Patent 3,839,558

Hamill RL, Hoehn MM, Pittenger GE, Chamberlin J, Gorman M (1969) Dianemycin, an antibiotic of the group affecting ion transport. J Antibiot 22:161

Hanessian S, Haskell TH (1964) Configuration of the anomeric linkages in amicetin. Tetrahendon Lett 2451

Haney ME, Hoehn MM (1968) Monensin, a new biologically active compound. I. Discovery and isolation. Antimicrob Agents Chemother 1967:349

Harned RL, Hioy PH, Corum CJ, Jones KL (1951) Nigericin, a new crystalline antibiotic from an unidentified streptomyces. Antibiot Chemother 1:594

Hodgson KO (1974) The ionophoric antibiotics: Structural chemistry and interaction with the alkali-metal cations. Intra Sci Chem Rep 8:27

Horvath L, Lorekovich L, Varga JM (1964) Antibiotics produced by streptomyces. III. A new antibiotic K178; biological studies. Z Allf Mikrobiol 4:236

Imada A, Nozaki Y, Hasegawa T, Igarashi S, Yoneda M (1978) Carriomycin, a new polyether antibiotic produced by *Streptomyces hygroscopicus*. J Antibiot 31:7

Johnson SM, Herrin J, Liu SJ, Paul IC (1970) The crystal and molecular structure of an antibiotic containing a high proportion of oxygen. J Am Chem Soc 92:4428

Jones ND, Chaney MO, Chamberlin JW, Hamill RL, Chen S (1973) Structure of A204A, a new polyether antibiotic. J Am Chem Soc 95:3399

Kaneda T, Butte JC, Tauman SB, Corcoran JW (1962) Actinomycete antibiotics III. The biogenesis of erythronolide, the C_{21} branched chain lactone in erythromycin. J Biol Chem 237:322

Keller-Juslen C, King HD, Kis ZL, von Wartburg A (1975) Septamycin, a polyether antibiotic. Taxonomy, fermentation, isolation and characterization. J Antibiot 28:854

Keller-Juslen C, King HD, Kuhn M, Loosli HR, von Wartburg A (1978) Norboribomycins A and B, new polyether antibiotics. J Antibiot 31:820

Kinashi H, Otake N (1976) An interpretation of the mass spectra of salinomycin and its derivatives. Agric Biol Chem 40:1625

Kinashi H, Otake N, Yonehara H, Sato S, Saito Y (1973) The structure of salinomycin, a new member of the polyether antibiotics. Tetrahedron Lett 1973:4955

Kirk DN (1973) Selectivity in reactions of epoxides. Chem Ind 1973:109

Kitame F, Ishida N (1976) The constitution of laidlomycin, a new antimycoplasmal antibiotic J Antibiot 29:759

Kitame F, Utsuhikawa K, Kohama T, Saito T, Kikuchi M, Ishida N (1974) Laidlomycin, a new antimycoplasmal polyether antibiotic. J Antibiot 27:884

Kubota T, Matsutani S, Shiro M, Koyama H (1968) The structure of polyetherin A. Chem Commun 1968:1541

Kubota T, Hinoh H, Mayama M, Motokawa K, Yasuda Y (1975) Antibiotic A-130, Isolation and Characterization. J Antibiot 28:931

Lardy HA, Johnson D, McMurray NC (1958) Antibiotics as tools for metabolic studies. I. A Survey of toxic antibiotics in Respiratory, Phosphorylative and Glycolytic Systems. Arch Biochem Biophys 78:587

Liu C-M, Evans RH, Jr, Fern L, Hermann T, Jenkins E, Liu M, Palleroni NJ, Prosser BLat, Sello LH, Stempel A, Tabenkin B, Westley JW, Miller PA (1976) Studies on a new polyether antibiotic, Ro 21-6150. J Antibiot 29:21

Liu C-M, Westley JW, Hermann TE, Liu M, Evans RH Jr, Blount JF, Bull DN, Palleroni NJ, Prosser BLat, Miller PA (1978) Antibiotic X-14547A, a novel ionophorous antibiotic produced by *Streptomyces antibioticus* NRRL 8167. Presented at the 18th Intersci. Conf. Antimicrob Agents Chemother. October 2–4, Atlanta, Georgia

Liu W-C, Slusarchyk D, Astle G, Trejo WH, Brown WE, Meyers E (1978) Ionomycin, a new polyether antibiotic. J Antibiot 31:815

Lynen F (1967) Biosynthetic pathways from acetate to natural products. In: The chemistry of natural products, vol IV, p 137. Butterworth, London

Martin JHEJ, Hertz MR (1977) Anticoccidial Antibiotic BL 580Δ. Preparation by fermentation of *Streptomyces hygroscopicus*. Belg Patent 856, 314

Martin JHEJ, Kantor S (1974) Antibiotic BL 580. U S Patent 3,812,249

May SW, Abbott BJ (1972) Enzymatic epoxidation. I. Alkene epoxidation by the ω-hydroxylation system of *Pseudomonas oleovorans*. Biochem Biophys Res Commun 48:1230

Mead JF, Lewis GM (1963) A one carbon degradation of the long chain fatty acids of brain sphingo-lipids. J Biol Chem 238:1634

Meyers E, Slusarchyk D, Kund W-C Liu (1975) Ionomycin. U S Patent 3,873,693

Misato T, Huang KT, Shirato S, Seino A, Shibuya M, Miki K (1970) Jpn Patent 70-26719

Mitani M, Umetsu T, Yamanish T, Otake N (1977) Effects of Monovalent and divalent cation ionophores on blood platelets. J Antibiot 30:239

Mitrovic M, Schildknecht EG (1974) Anticoccidial activity of lasalocid in chicks. Poult Sci 53:1448

Nakata T, Kishi Y (1978) Synthetic studies on polyether antibiotics. III. A stereocontrolled synthesis of isolasalocid ketone from acyclic precursors. Tetrahedron Lett 2745

Nakata T, Schmid G, Vranesic B, Okayawa M, Smithpalmer T, Kishi Y (1978) A total synthesis of lasalocid A. J Am Chem Soc 100:2933

Ninet L, Benazet F, Depaire H, Florent J, Lunel J, Mancy D, Abraham A, Cartier JR, De Chezelles N, Godard C, Moreau M, Tissier R, Lallemand JY (1976) Emericid, a new polyether antibiotic from *Streptomyces hygroscopicus* (DS 24307). Experientia 15:319

Occolowitz JL, Berg DH, Dobono M, Hamill RL (1976) The structure of narasin and a related ionophore. Biomed Mass Spectrosc 3:272

Occolowitz JL, Dorman DE, Hamill RL (1978) Structure of the polyether antibiotic K-41 by mass spectrometry and nuclear magnetic resonance spectrometry. Chem Commun 1978:683

Ohshima N, Ishizaki N, Abe K, Ukawa M, Marumoto Y, Nakatsuka K, Horiuchi T, Yonooka Y, Yoshino S, Kanda N (1976) Antibiotic DE-3936, a polyether antibiotic identical with lonomycin. J Antibiot 29:354

Ohta H, Tetsukawa H (1978) Microbial epoxidation of long-chain terminal olefins. Chem Commun 1978:849

Okazaki H, Arai M (1966) Azalomycin M. Jpn Patent 13,791 (66)

Omura S, Nakagawa A, Takeshima H, Atusmi K, Miyazawa J, Piriou F, Lukacs G (1975) Biosynthetic studies using ^{13}C enriched precursors on the 16-membered macrolide antibiotic, Leucomycin A_3. J Am Chem Soc 97:6600

Omura S, Shibata M, Machida S, Sawada J (1976a) Isolation of a new polyether antibiotic, lonomycin. J Antibiot 29:15

Omura S, Takeshima H, Nakagawa A, Kanemoto N, Lukacs G (1976b) Studies on carboxylic

acid metabolism in macrolide – producing microorganisms using carbon-^{13}C magnetic resonance. Bioorg Chem 5:451
Otake N, Koenuma M, Kinashi H, Sato S, Saito Y (1975) The crystal and molecular structure of the silver salt of lysocellin, a new polyether antibiotic. Chem Commun 1975:92
Otake N, Nakayama H, Miyamae H, Sato S, Saito Y (1977) X-ray crystal structure of the thallium salt of carriomycin, a new polyether antibiotic. Chem Commun 1977:590
Otake N, Ogita T, Nakayama H, Miyamae H, Sato S, Saito Y (1978a) X-ray crystal structure of the thallium salt of antibiotic-6016, a new polyether ionophore. Chem Commun 1978:875
Otake N, Seto H, Koenuma M (1978b) The assignment of the ^{13}C-NMR spectrum of lysocellin and its biosynthesis. Agric Biol Chem 42:1879
Ovchinnikov Y, Ivanov VT, Shkrob AM (1974) Membrane-active complexones. Elsevier Scientific, New York
Pressman BC (1976) Biological Applications of Ionophores. Annu Rev Biochem 45:501
Prosser B, Lat, Palleroni N (1976) *Streptomyces longwoodensis* sp. Nov. Int J Syst Bacterol 26:319
Seto H, Yahagi T, Miyazaki Y, Otake N (1977a) Studies on the ionophorous antibiotics. IX. The structure of 4-methylsalinomycins (Narasin). J Antibiot 30:530
Seto H, Miyazaki Y, Fujita KI, Otake N (1977b) The assignment of ^{13}C-nmr spectrum of salinomycin. Tetrahedron Lett 2417
Seto H, Westley JW, Pitcher RG (1978a) The complete assignment of the ^{13}C spectra of lasalocid and the sodium salt-complex of the antibiotic. J Antibiot 31:289
Seto H, Mizoue K, Otake N, Yamagishi M, Mitzutani T (1978b) Studies on the ionophorous antibiotics. XVII. The structures of lonomycins B and C. J Antibiot 31:929
Seto H, Otake N, Yonehara H (1978c) structural studies on polyether antibiotics by ^{13}C-nmr spectroscopy. Presented at the 18th Int Conf Antimicrob Agents Chemother. October 2–4. Atlanta Georgia
Shibata A, Miyazaki Y, Tsuda K, Otake N, Kinashi H (1976) Antibiotic SY-1. Jpn Patent 76–86, 191
Shiro M, Nakai H, Nagashima K, Tsuji N (1978) X-ray Determination of the structure of polyether antibiotic K-41. Chem Commun 1978:682
Shumard RF, Callender ME (1968) Monensin, a new biologically active compound. VI. Anticoccidial activity. Antimicrob Agents Chemother 1967:369
Smeby RR, Leben C, Keit GW, Strong FM (1952) Phytopathology 42:506
Tanenbaum SW (1967) Some acetate derived antibiotics. In: Gottlieb, Shaw (eds) Antibiotics, vol II. Springer, Berlin Heidelberg New York
Thomas R, of the University of Surrey, Dept. of Chemistry pointed out this fact to me after delivering a lecture at Rutgers in May, 1978
Tone J, Shibakawa R, Maeda H, Inoue K, Nishyama S, Ishiguro M, Cullen WP, Routien JB, Chappell LR, Moppett CE, Jefferson MJ, Celmer WD (1978) CP 44,161, a new polyether produced by a new species of *Dactylosporangium*. Presented at the 18th Intersci Conf Antimicrob Agents Chemother. October 2–4, Atlanta Georgia
Truter M (1976) Calcium in biological systems. Symp Soc Exp Biol 30:19
Tsuji N, Nagashima K, Kobayashi M, Wakisaka Y, Kawamura Y, Kozuki S, Mayama M (1976) Two new antibiotics, A-218 and K-41. J Antibiot 29:10
Westley JW (1976) A proposed numbering system for polyether antibiotics. J Antibiot 29:584
Westley JW (1977) Polyether antibiotics: versatile carboxylic acid ionophores produced by Streptomyces. Adv. Appl. Microbiol 22:177
Westley JW, Evans RH, Williams T, Stempel A (1970a) Structure of antibiotic X-537A (lasalocid) Chem Commun 1970:71
Westley JW, Evans RH, Pruess DL, Stempel A (1970b) Biosynthesis of antibiotic X-537A (lasalocid). Chem Commun 1970:71
Westley JW, Pruess DL, Pitcher RG (1972) Incorporation of [1-^{13}C]-butyrate into X-537A (lasalocid). Chem Commun 1972:162
Westley JW, Evans RH Jr, Harvey G, Pitcher RG, Pruess DL, Stempel A, Berger J (1974a) The Biosynthesis of Lasalocid I: incorporation of ^{13}C and ^{14}C labelled substrates into lasalocid A. J Antibiot 27:288–297
Westley JW, Blount JF, Evans RH Jr, Stempel A, Berger J (1974b) The Biosynthesis of Lasalocid II: X-ray analysis of a naturally occurring isomer of lasalocid A. J Antibiot 27:597–604

Westley JW, Benz W, Donahue J Evans RH Jr, Scott CG, Stempel A, Berger J (1974c) The biosynthesis of lasalocid III: isolation and structure determination of four homologs of lasalocid A. J Antibiot 27:744–753

Westley JW, Blount JF, Evans RH, Liu C-M (1977) C-17 Epimers of deoxy-(0-8)-salinomycin from *Streptomyces albus.* J Antibiot 30:610

Westley JW, Evans RH, Liu C-M, Hermann T, Blount JF (1978) Structure of antibiotic X-14547A, a carboxylic acid ionophore produced by *Streptomyces antibioticus.* NRRL 8167. J Am Chem Soc 100:6784

Westley JW, Evans RH, Liu C-M, Hermann T, Blount JF and Miller PA (1980) Structure and activity of antibiotic X-14766A a novel polyether antibiotic produced by *Streptomyces malachitofuscus* subsp. *downeyi.* ACS Meeting August 25–28, Las Vegas

Williams TH, Stempel A, Evans RH, Jacoby A, Westley JW (1973) The structure determination of a novel C_{17} meabolite from *Streptomyces* X-537 using Eu $(DPM)_3$. Experientia 29:257

Yonehara H, Otake N, Kinashi H, Miyazaki Y (1975) A new antibiotic salinomycin AII and process for producing the same. Jpn Patent 50-132190

Biosynthesis of Aminocyclitol Antibiotics

CEDRIC J. PEARCE and KENNETH L. RINEHART, JR.

I. Introduction

The history of the aminocyclitol antibiotics dates from the discovery in 1943 of streptomycin by Waksman's group at Rutgers (SCHATZ et al., 1946). This was followed by the discovery of neomycin, paromomycin, kanamycin, gentamicin, sisomicin, butirosin, ribostamycin, spectinomycin, fortimicin, validamycin, minosaminomycin, and hygromycin, to name but some of the naturally occurring members of this class of compounds. The number of antimicrobial

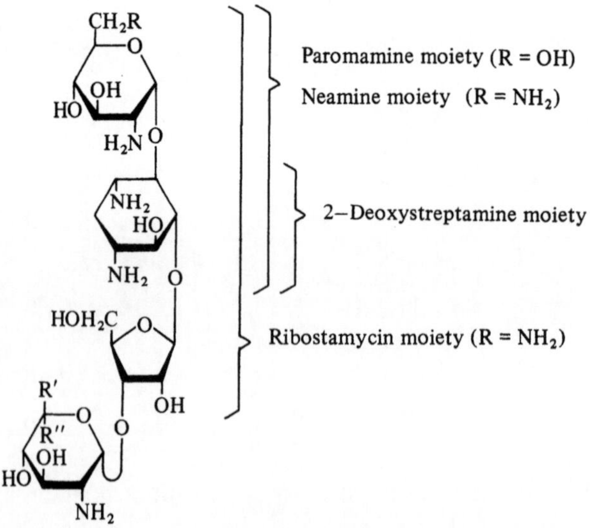

	R	R′	R″
Neomycin B	NH_2	H	CH_2NH
Neomycin C	NH_2	CH_2NH_2	H
Paromomycin I	OH	H	CH_2NH_2
Paromomycin II	OH	CH_2NH_2	H

Fig. 1

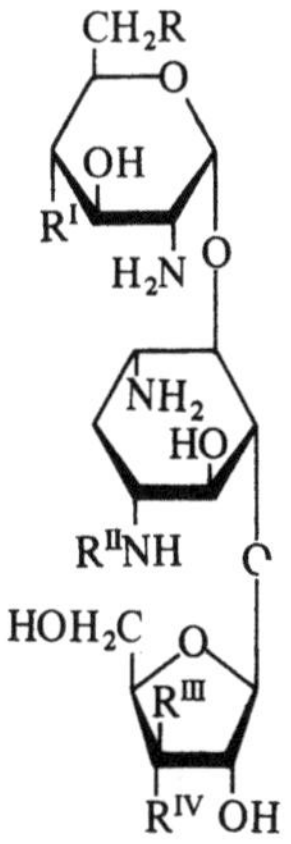

	R	RI	RII	RIII	RIV
Ribostamycin	NH_2	OH	H	H	OH
Xylostasin	NH_2	OH	H	OH	H
Butirosin A	NH_2	OH	*	OH	H
Butirosin B	NH_2	OH	*	H	OH
4′–Deoxybutirosin A	NH_2	H	*	OH	H
4′–Deoxybutirosin B	NH_2	H	*	H	OH
LL BM408α	OH	OH	H	H	OH
DAH–Butirosin A	OH	OH	*	OH	H
DAH–Butirosin B	OH	OH	*	H	OH

$*R^{II} = -COCHOHCH_2CH_2NH_2$

Fig. 2

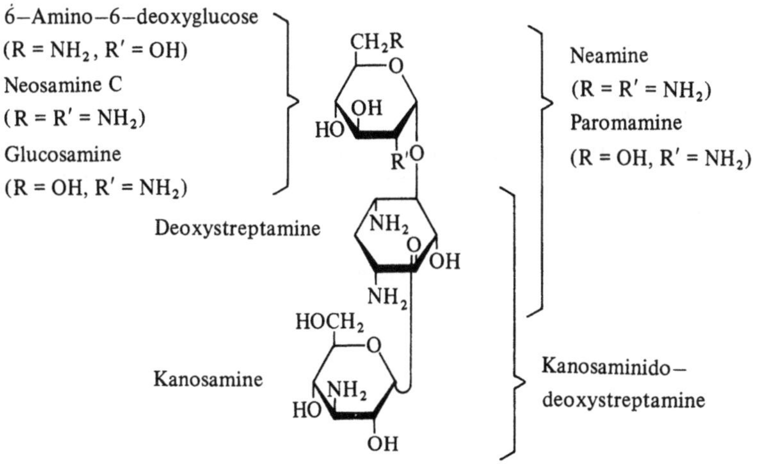

	R	R′
Kanamycin A	NH_2	OH
Kanamycin B	NH_2	NH_2
Kanamycin C	OH	NH_2

Fig. 3

agents belonging to this group is increased further by the addition of many synthetic and semisynthetic aminocyclitol-containing compounds which have biological activity. Many of the aminocyclitol antibiotics have been used successfully as clinical agents.

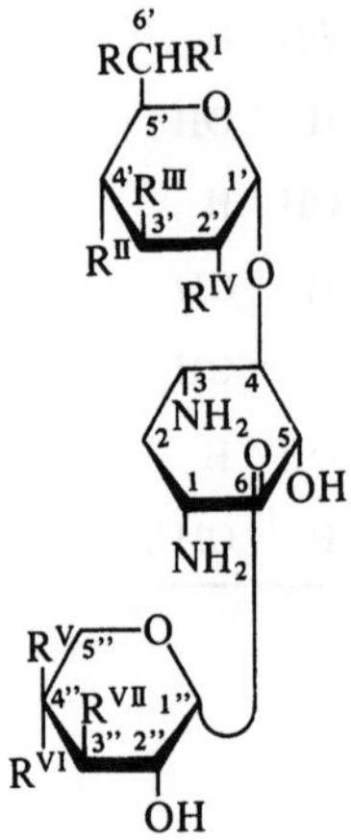

	R	R^I	R^{II}	R^{III}	R^{IV}	R^V	R^{VI}	R^{VII}
Gentamicin A	H	OH	OH	OH	NH_2	H	OH	$NHCH_3$
A_1	H	OH	OH	OH	NH_2	OH	H	$NHCH_3$
A_2	H	OH	OH	OH	NH_2	H	OH	OH
A_3	H	NH_2	OH	OH	OH	OH	H	$NHCH_3$
A_4	H	OH	OH	OH	NH_2	H	OH	$N(CHO)CH_3$
X_2	H	OH	OH	OH	NH_2	OH	CH_3	$NHCH_3$
B	H	NH_2	OH	OH	OH	OH	CH_3	$NHCH_3$
B_1	CH_3	NH_2	OH	OH	NH_2	OH	CH_3	$NHCH_3$
C_1	CH_3	$NHCH_3$	H	H	NH_2	OH	CH_3	$NHCH_3$
C_{1a}	H	NH_2	H	H	NH_2	OH	CH_3	$NHCH_3$
C_2	CH_3	NH_2	H	H	NH_2	OH	CH_3	$NHCH_3$
C_{2a}*	CH_3	NH_2	H	H	NH_2	OH	CH_3	$NHCH_3$
C_{2b}‡ ("C_{2a}")	H	$NHCH_3$	H	H	NH_2	OH	CH_3	$NHCH_3$
G–418	CH_3	OH	OH	OH	NH_2	OH	CH_3	$NHCH_3$
JI–20A (Gentamicin X_5)	H	NH_2	OH	OH	NH_2	OH	CH_3	$NHCH_3$
JI–20B	CH_3	NH_2	OH	OH	NH_2	OH	CH_3	$NHCH_3$

*Stereoisomer of C_2 at C–6′

‡Sagamicin

Fig. 4

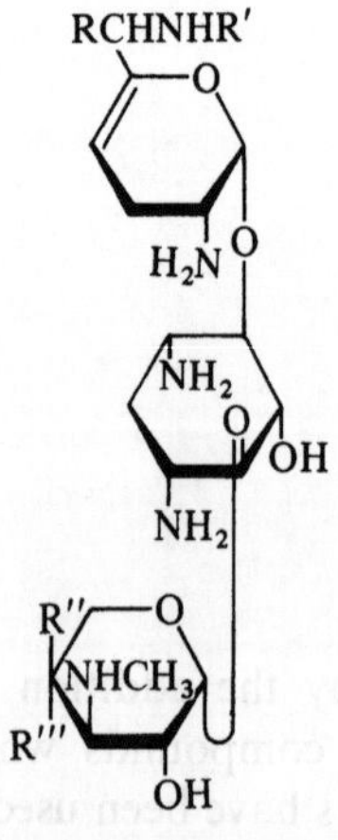

	R	R′	R″	R‴
Sisomicin	H	H	OH	CH_3
Verdamicin	CH_3	H	OH	CH_3
G–52 (Sch 17726)	H	CH_3	OH	CH_3
66–40B	H	H	H	OH
66–40D	H	H	OH	H

Fig. 5

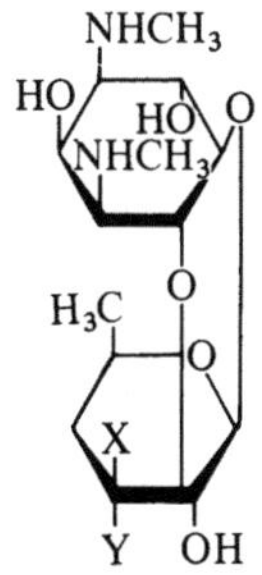

Spectinomycin (hydrate form): X = Y = OH

Dihydrospectinomycin: X = H, Y = OH

Fig. 6

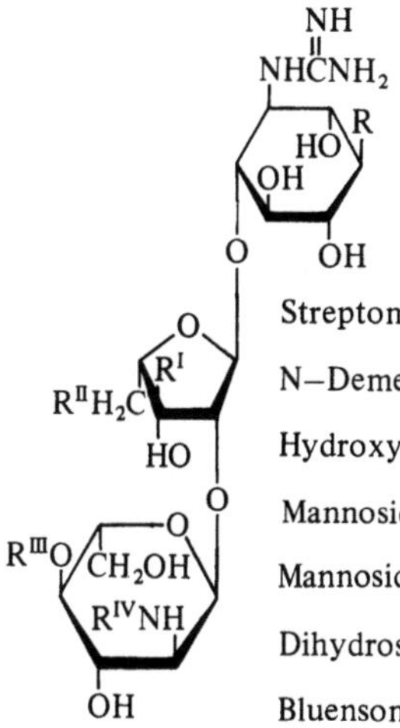

	R	R^I	R^{II}	R^{III}	R^{IV}
Streptomycin	–NHC(=NH)NH_2	CHO	H	H	CH_3
N–Demethylstreptomycin	–NHC(=NH)NH_2	CHO	H	H	H
Hydroxystreptomycin	–NHC(=NH)NH_2	CHO	OH	H	CH_3
Mannosidostreptomycin	–NHC(=NH)NH_2	CHO	H	*	CH_3
Mannosidohydroxystreptomycin	–NHC(=NH)NH_2	CHO	OH	*	CH_3
Dihydrostreptomycin	–NHC(=NH)NH_2	CH_2OH	H	H	CH_3
Bluensomycin	–OCONH_2	CH_2OH	H	H	CH_3

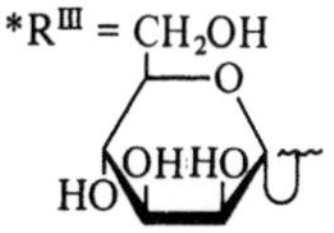

Fig. 7

The naturally occurring aminocyclitol antibiotics can be classified according to their aminocyclitol unit. The 2-deoxystreptamine-containing class of antibiotics includes the neomycins (Fig. 1), paromomycins (Fig. 1), ribostamycins (Fig. 2), butirosins (Fig. 2), kanamycins (Fig. 3), gentamicins (Fig. 4), and sisomicins (Fig. 5). The actinamine-containing antibiotics, spectinomycin and dihydrospectinomycin (Fig. 6), are in a group by themselves. A third class of compounds contains streptidine or bluensidine, and includes streptomycin and bluensomycin (Fig. 7). Finally, there are the fortimicins, which contain the aminocyclitol fortamine (Fig. 8). Another class of antibiotics contains monoaminocyclitols, of which validamycin (Fig. 9) is an example.

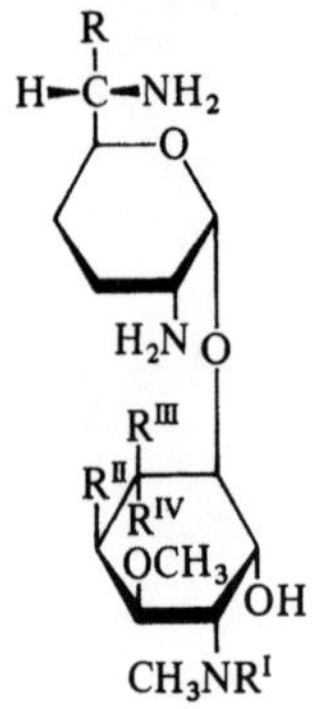

		R	R^{I}	R^{II}	R^{III}	R^{IV}
Fortimicin	A	CH_3	$COCH_2NH_2$	OH	H	NH_2
	B	CH_3	H	OH	H	NH_2
	C	CH_3	$COCH_2NHCONH_2$	OH	H	NH_2
	D	H	$COCH_2NH_2$	OH	H	NH_2
	KE	H	H	OH	H	NH_2
Sporaricin	A	CH_3	$COCH_2NH_2$	H	NH_2	H
	B	CH_3	H	H	NH_2	H

Fig. 8

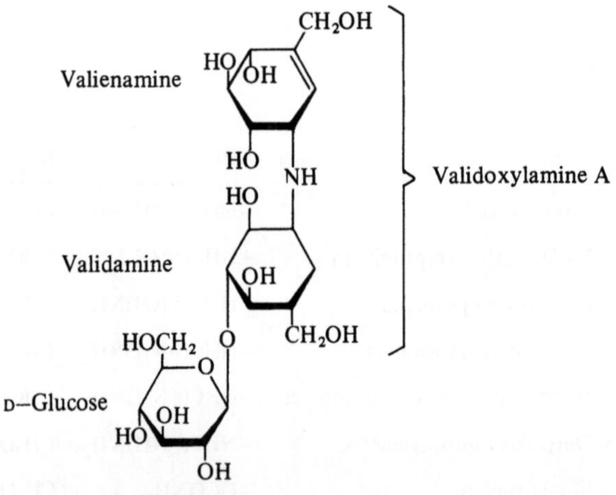

Validamycin A

Fig. 9

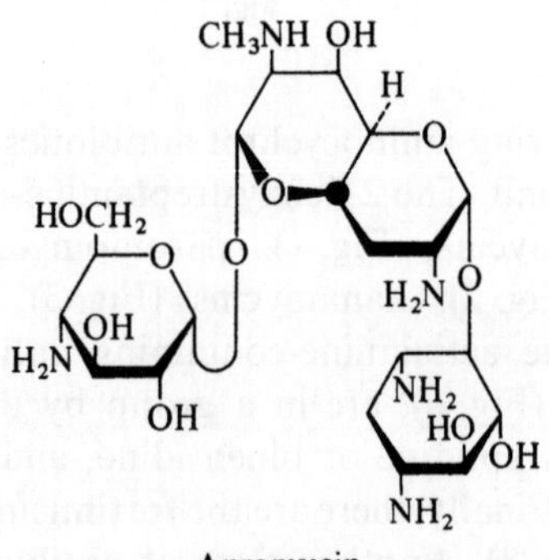

Apramycin

Fig. 10

The deoxystreptamine-containing antibiotics can be further classified according to whether this nucleus is 4-substituted (e.g., apramycin, Fig. 10), 4,5-disubstituted (e.g., neomycin and ribostamycin, Figs. 1 and 2), or 4,6-disubstituted (e.g., kanamycin and gentamicin, Figs. 3 and 4). Usually, the deoxystreptamine-linked substituents are complex amino sugars.

This review will be largely concerned with the 2-deoxystreptamine-containing antibiotics, as knowledge about the biosynthesis of these compounds has greatly increased in the past few years. For comparison with the above class of compounds there is a discussion of streptomycin, validamycin, and spectinomycin biosyntheses and the role of plasmids in the production of this class of antibiotics.

II. Neomycin and Paromomycin

Neomycin was the first deoxystreptamine-containing antibiotic to be discovered and most work on biosynthesis of the deoxystreptamine-containing antibiotics has been on the processes leading to neomycins. The limited amount of work on the biosynthesis of paromomycin is included in this section because the routes leading to these antibiotics are probably similar. Support for this relationship comes from the observations that *Streptomyces fradiae*, an organism which normally produces neomycins, also produces small quantities of paromomycins (HESSLER et al., 1970) and a mutant of *S. rimosus*, which normally produces paromomycin, will synthesize neomycin in the presence of neamine (PEARCE et al., 1976).

The structure of neomycin B is shown in Figure 1. In addition to deoxystreptamine (ring II), there are the two diaminohexoses, 2,6-diamino-2,6-dideoxy-D-glucose (neosamine C, ring I) and 2,6-diamino-2,6-dideoxy-L-idose (neosamine B, ring IV), and ribose (ring III). Paromomycin is similar to neomycin B except that ring I is D-glucosamine rather than neosamine C.

Studies prior to 1967 (FOGHT, 1963; SCHIMBOR, 1966) demonstrated that both [1-^{14}C]glucose and [6-^{14}C]glucose are well incorporated into neomycin and that all subunits are equally well labeled except ribose, which is labeled to a somewhat lesser extent.

The specificity of labeling of the subunits of neomycin by ^{14}C-labeled glucose has also been investigated (FOGHT, 1963; SCHIMBOR, 1966) and it was shown that C-1 of glucose labels C-1 of the neosamines and C-6 of glucose labels C-6 of the neosamines (FALKNER, 1969). A reasonable pathway for the conversion of glucose to neosamines B and C, involving glucosamine as an intermediate, is shown in Figure 11. The labeling pattern in ribose implies that two pathways must be followed since part of the label from [1-^{14}C]glucose is lost and part labels C-1 of ribose, while part of the label from [6-^{14}C]glucose is lost and part labels C-5 of ribose (FOGHT, 1963). Retention of C-6 may be via the hexose monophosphate pathway (MAGASANIK, 1962) and retention of C-1 of glucose via the glucuronate pathway (FEINGOLD et al., 1960). The degradation scheme for deoxystreptamine allowed localization of the label in one or the other half of the molecule and it was demonstrated that label from both [1-^{14}C]-

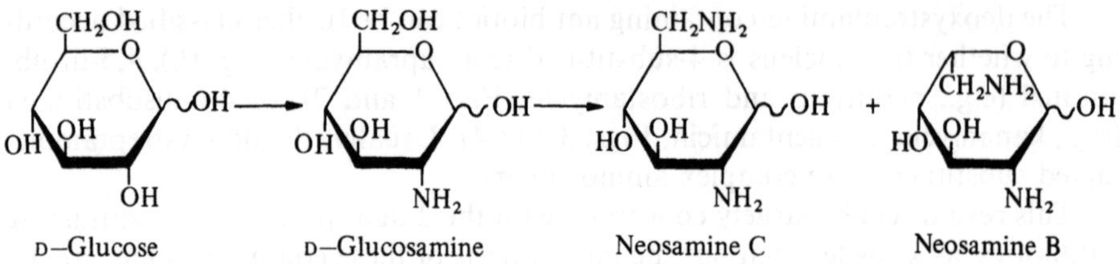

Fig. 11

and [6-^{14}C]glucose was found in that part of deoxystreptamine consisting of C-1 through C-3 (FOGHT, 1963).

In view of the unsatisfactory degradation scheme for ^{14}C-labeled deoxystreptamine, ^{13}C magnetic resonance (^{13}C NMR) spectroscopy was enthusiastically embraced as a tool for studying aminocyclitol biosynthesis. Thus, [6-^{13}C]glucose was incubated with *S. fradiae* (RINEHART et al., 1974a), the neomycin produced was isolated and N-acetylated, and its ^{13}C NMR spectrum was observed. The results demonstrated that C-6 of glucose labels the neosamine subunits at C-6 and labels ribose at C-5, as had been determined earlier in the ^{14}C studies. In addition, it was possible by ^{13}C NMR spectroscopy to locate the label at C-2 of deoxystreptamine. Deoxystreptamine biosynthesis is discussed further below.

A number of potential intermediates between glucose and the subunits of neomycin have been investigated. Early studies showed that [1-^{14}C]glucosamine was better incorporated into neomycin than [1-^{14}C]glucose (FOGHT, 1963). When [1-^{13}C]glucosamine was administered (RINEHART et al., 1974a), the C-1 carbons of the neosamines, ribose, and deoxystreptamine were labeled. The neosamines were labeled at a much higher level by glucosamine than by glucose, which argues that glucosamine is further along the biosynthetic pathway to the neosamines than is glucose. Alternatively, it may indicate a greater uptake of glucosamine and, therefore, a larger pool of labeled material available for neomycin biosynthesis.

On the other hand, ribose, of course, lacks nitrogen and is presumably formed from glucosamine via glucose. A glucosamine-6-phosphate deaminase, which can accomplish this transformation, has been isolated from *Escherichia coli* (COMB and ROSEMAN, 1956; WOLFE et al., 1957), and this enzyme or a similar one could convert glucosamine to glucose in *S. fradiae*.

Both ribose and deoxystreptamine are less labeled (relative to the neosamines) by glucosamine than by glucose. This and the similar level of ^{13}C label in ribose and deoxystreptamine from both [1-^{13}C]glucosamine and [6-^{13}C]glucose suggest that deoxystreptamine, like ribose, arises from glucose directly and from glucosamine via glucose. That the nitrogen of glucosamine is indeed lost in its conversion to deoxystreptamine has been confirmed using [^{15}N]glucosamine (RINEHART et al., 1974b; ROLLS et al., 1975). The neomycin produced when *S. fradiae* was incubated with this substrate was degraded and the results showed that the labeled nitrogen atoms are found only in the neosamine subunits, i.e., that the deoxystreptamine nitrogen atoms are unlabeled.

In addition to labeled glucose and glucosamine, the labeled subunits themselves (except neosamine B) have been administered to *S. fradiae* to determine whether they are biosynthetic intermediates. [1-^{14}C]Ribose labeled all the subunits, presumably via glucose, but it labeled the ribose subunit most heavily and it was directly incorporated, since the label remained at the C-1 position of ribose in neomycin (SCHIMBOR, 1966). [1-^{14}C]Deoxystreptamine (isolated from neomycin derived from a [1-^{14}C]glucose feeding) was only incorporated into the deoxystreptamine moiety of neomycin (FOGHT, 1963). On the other hand, [1-^{14}C]neosamine C was found to be not incorporated into neomycin (FALKNER, 1969), possibly because the intermediates between glucosamine and the neosamine moieties of neomycin are nucleotide- or enzyme-bound.

In a repetition of earlier work on neomycin it has recently been reported that ^{14}C-labeled *D*-glucose, *D*-glucosamine, deoxystreptamine, and ribose are also incorporated into the neomycin-related antibiotic paromomycin (Fig. 1) by *Streptomyces albus* var. *metamycinus* nov. var. (REUTER et al., 1977). Degradation studies showed that [^{14}C]glucose labels all subunits equally, [^{14}C]glucosamine is incorporated predominantly into glucosamine and neosamine B, 50% of label from ^{14}C-ribose is found in that pentose and the other 50% is distributed throughout the rest of the molecule, and [^{14}C]deoxystreptamine is incorporated only into that subunit.

Thus, while it is known that deoxystreptamine is biosynthesized from *D*-glucose and that carbons 1 and 6 of this compound label carbons 1 and 2, respectively, of deoxystreptamine, until recently little was known about the steps involved in this interconversion, except that *myo*-inositol, which might be expected to be involved as a product of glucose cyclization, as it is in the biosynthesis of other aminocyclitols (see section on streptomycin and spectinomycin), does not appear to be an intermediate (FALKNER, 1969).

A second technique developed by SHIER and co-workers in this laboratory (SHIER et al., 1969; SHIER, 1970; SHIER et al., 1972) has been used to examine the biosynthesis of deoxystreptamine and its antibiotics. Mutant strains of *S. fradiae* were developed which produce neomycin only in the presence of added deoxystreptamine, thus confirming that it appears underivatized as a biosynthetic intermediate. Although the use of the *S. fradiae* mutants has not as yet shed light on the intermediate involved in the conversion of glucose into deoxystreptamine, studies using a similar mutant of *Micromonospora purpurea* (DAUM et al., 1977; ROSI et al., 1977), unable to synthesize gentamicin in the absence of added deoxystreptamine, have been more successful.

The *M. purpurea* mutant was shown to produce gentamicin from deoxystreptamine and 2,4/3,5-tetrahydroxycyclohexanone, and 2-hydroxygentamicin from streptamine and 2,4,6/3,5-pentahydroxycyclohexanone (Fig. 12). This suggests that 2,4/3,5-tetrahydroxycyclohexanone is an intermediate in the biosynthesis of deoxystreptamine and, therefore, of gentamicin. It also provides indirect evidence that *myo*-inositol is not involved in deoxystreptamine biosynthesis because *myo*-inosose (2,4,6/3,5-pentahydroxycyclohexanone), the oxidation product of *myo*-inositol produced by a ubiquitous pathway, is converted to hydroxygentamicin rather than gentamicin.

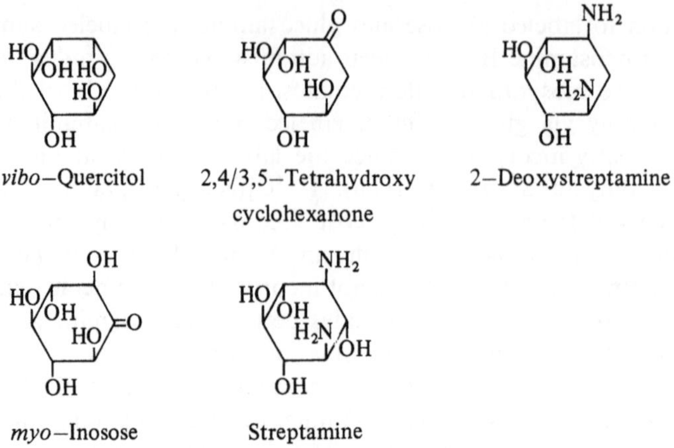

Fig. 12

This work argues that the 2-hydroxy group is lost prior to or during *D*-glucose cyclization. Thus, it may be possible that 6-deoxyglucose or a related compound cyclizes to form a pentahydroxycyclohexane-type intermediate. Of particular interest in this matter is the recent study (BYRNE and RINEHART, 1978), which shows that dTDP-glucose is converted by cell-free extracts of a neomycin-producing strain of *S. fradiae* into dTDP-6-deoxyglucose. However, it was not demonstrated that this nucleotide is involved in neomycin biosynthesis.

dl-Vibo-quercitol (Fig. 12) was also converted to an antibiotic by the mutant of *M. purpurea* (DAUM et al., 1977) and it seems reasonable to speculate that this was a result of vibo-quercitol oxidation to produce 2,4/3,5-tetrahydroxycyclohexanone, which was used for deoxystreptamine biosynthesis followed by incorporation into gentamicin. A reasonable route for the conversion of *vibo*-quercitol and 2,4/3,5-tetrahydroxycyclohexanone into 2-deoxystreptamine is outlined in Figure 13. Although in this figure C-3 is aminated prior to C-1, which contrasts with streptidine biosynthesis where C-1 is aminated prior to C-3, whether this is the actual order of amination is uncertain. A possible solution to this dichotomy would be to repeat the experiments of DAUM et al. (1977) using resolved *D*- and *L*-vibo-quercitol and 2,4/3,5-tetrahydroxycyclohexanone

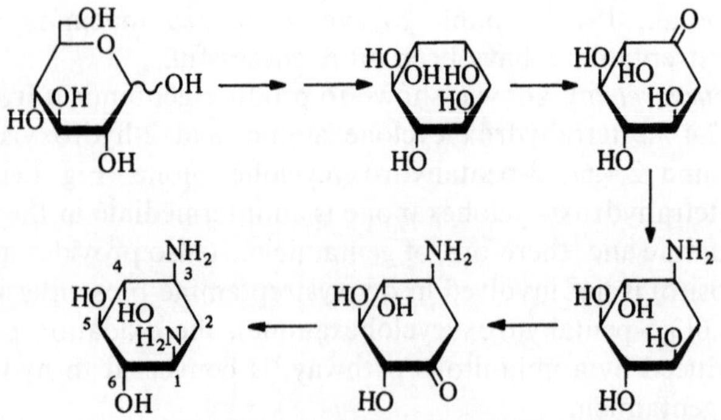

Fig. 13

in order to ascertain which isomer is the precursor for gentamicin biosynthesis and, therefore, 2-deoxystreptamine. Thus, if the *L*-isomers were used for antibiotic biosynthesis this would suggest that the *3*-amino group is added prior to the *1*-amino group. In addition, assuming that the cyclization of glucose, or a glucose-derived cyclization precursor, results in a cyclitol with the same hydroxyl configuration as that of the *myo*-inositol produced by glucose cyclization (EISENBERG et al., 1964), except that the C-6 hydroxyl is missing, then the *L*-isomer of *vibo*-quercitol would be produced, supporting the idea that C-3 is aminated first. From the available evidence it is not possible to decide on the order of amino group addition. The scheme in Figure 13 is, however, in complete agreement with the observed carbon isotope labeling data.

CHEN and WALKER (1977) have demonstrated enzymatic activity in *S. fradiae* and *M. purpurea* resulting in amination of keto-cyclitols by *L*-glutamine as amino-donor, and it seems reasonable that this will be the amino donor for at least one amination involved in deoxystreptamine biosynthesis.

The same type of mutants have also been employed in studying larger subunits as potential intermediates between deoxystreptamine and neomycin. Although the deoxystreptamine idiotroph of *S. fradiae* was unable to convert any of the potential neomycin biosynthesis intermediates of the pseudodi- or trisaccharide type into the antibiotic (SHIER et al., 1974), a similar mutant of *S. rimosus* forma *paromomycinus*, which produces the related antibiotic paromomycin when incubated in the presence of deoxystreptamine, was shown to be able to convert neamine into neomycin (PEARCE et al., 1976). Evidence that neamine was converted directly into the antibiotic, and not hydrolyzed to produce deoxystreptamine which was then incorporated into the antibiotic, was provided by incubating *S. rimosus* in the presence of neamine labeled with ^{3}H and ^{14}C in the diaminohexose moiety but only ^{14}C in the deoxystreptamine subunit and demonstrating that the $^{3}H:^{14}C$ ratio of the neomycin produced was the same as the starting material. It was also demonstrated that the neamine labeled only the neamine moiety of neomycin (PEARCE et al., 1976; PEARCE, 1977).

The observation that neamine is converted into neomycin by D^{-} *S. rimosus* has been confirmed by SEBEK (personal communication) although these investigators found incorporation only when using lower concentrations of neamine in the medium. It was suggested that under their experimental conditions the producing organism was more sensitive to neamine than under the conditions used in the previous experiments of PEARCE et al. (1976).

A number of rationalizations have been provided to explain the apparent inability of the D^{-} mutant of *S. fradiae* to convert neamine into neomycin (SHIER et al., 1974). It seems plausible that this is due to the high sensitivity of *S. fradiae* to neamine. Thus, it is possible that, although neamine is in fact an intermediate of neomycin biosynthesis in the experiment performed, the neamine concentration used was high enough to impair normal biochemical functions.

There are two possible routes for the assembly of neomycin from preformed subunits. In route i) of Figure 14 neamine (rings I, II) is an intermediate; in route ii) the compound comprising rings II–III or the one comprising rings

2–Deoxystreptamine (Ring I) —i)→ Neamine (Rings I–II)

↓ ii) ↓

5–*O*–(β–Ribosyl)–2–deoxystreptamine (Rings II–III) ——→ Neomycin

Fig. 14

II–III–IV is an intermediate. Although in the past a choice between these two pathways has been difficult, the experiments described above suggest that neamine is probably an intermediate in neomycin biosynthesis. Further support for this pathway comes from the earlier observation that *S. fradiae* produces neamine as well as neomycin and under certain growth conditions this can be the major fermentation product (PERLMAN and O'BRIEN, 1953), but whether it is produced by the major neomycin biosynthesis pathway is not certain.

The operation of such a pathway would suggest that route ii) of Figure 14 is not usually utilized. Negative evidence for the exclusion of this pathway is provided by the observation that, while 6-deoxyneamine does support antibiotic production when added to the growth medium of a D^- mutant of *S. rimosus,* 5-*O*-(β-D-ribosyl)-2,6-dideoxystreptamine (rings II–III of 6-deoxyneomycin) does not (PEARCE et al., 1978). This is exactly what would be predicted, assuming that a pseudodisaccharide of the rings I–II type were an obligatory intermediate, but the usual warnings concerning negative evidence are appropriate.

Neamine could be converted into neomycin by a number of routes, the most obvious one being the addition of rings III–IV as one unit to produce the complete antibiotic or the synthesis of ribostamycin from neamine and its conversion into neomycin.

Although neobiosamines, rings III–IV, have never been isolated from fermentation broths, their involvement in neomycin biosynthesis has been proposed by FALKNER (1969). The evidence for this suggestion is that rings III–IV of neomycin synthesized in the presence of radioactive precursors were labeled less than rings I–II. As the radioactive precursors were added after incubation of the culture had started, it was proposed that a portion of rings III–IV (or rings III and IV) had been synthesized prior to the addition of labeled compound and, therefore, contained less radioactivity than rings I–II, which were suggested to be synthesized subsequent to the addition of the label.

In contrast, a mutant of *S. fradiae* has recently been isolated which was unable to produce neomycin but which did produce ribostamycin (BAUD et al., 1977). The authors of this work were able to isolate revertants that produce neomycin. It could be that the mutant is unable to complete the final step in neomycin assembly, i.e., the addition of ring IV. However, there are alternative explanations: it is possible that the organism cannot synthesize rings III–IV and, although it would normally add rings III–IV to neamine as one unit, it adds ring III alone because that is the only unit available.

An unambiguous choice between these two routes is not possible at this time and details regarding the later stages of neomycin assembly need further examination. Paromamine has been implicated in the biosynthesis of a number of aminocyclitol antibiotics (see the section on butirosins, gentamicins, and sisomicins). The role, if any, that paromamine or any related 6′-deamino-6′-hydroxy intermediate plays in neomycin biosynthesis has not, to our knowledge, been investigated as yet.

Phosphate derivatives have been proposed as intermediates involved in the final steps of neomycin biosynthesis (MAJUMDAR and MAJUMDAR, 1969, 1970, 1971; BANDYOPHADHYAY and MAJUMDAR, 1974) and neomycin derivatives which have been assigned phosphoamide structures have been isolated and reported to enhance antibiotic yields when added to the production medium. In addition, an alkaline phosphatase which can convert these compounds to neomycin has been observed in the producing organism and the de novo synthesis of this enzyme has been directly correlated with neomycin biosynthesis (MAJUMDAR and MAJUMDAR, 1971). Cleavage of a neomycin phosphoamide or phosphate has been postulated to be the last step in the biosynthesis of neomycin. One possible advantage of biosynthesis occurring via this route is that the biologically active neomycin is released from the nontoxic neomycin phosphate derivative at the last possible moment. It is unfortunate that the position of the phosphorylation has not been determined.

As a practical outcome of the neomycin biosynthetic study, the same deoxystreptamine negative mutants used to study neomycin and paromomycin biosynthesis have been employed to prepare antibiotics related to neomycin and paromomycin by the incorporation of related aminocyclitols. This procedure for preparing antibiotics is referred to as mutasynthesis (RINEHART and STROSHANE, 1976), the compounds produced as mutasynthetic antibiotics, and the aminocyclitols introduced as mutasynthons. The principle has also been used to prepare analogues of other aminocyclitol-containing antibiotics (see RINEHART, 1977 for a review). NAGAOKA and DEMAIN (1975) have proposed that the mutant organism be called an idiotroph and defined as a mutant requiring a special nutrient to produce a product peculiar to that organism. They have also been referred to as D^- mutants. The use of these organisms to biosynthesize novel aminocyclitol antibiotics is discussed in depth elsewhere (RINEHART and STROSHANE, 1976; RINEHART, 1977) and only those results which are relevant to the biosynthesis of these antibiotics will be included here.

III. Ribostamycin

Although there have been no reported studies employing labeled precursor incorporation, it is assumed the biosynthesis of ribostamycin (Fig. 2) parallels that of neomycin since it is part of the latter antibiotic.

In the same way that deoxystreptamine idiotrophs were developed for *S. fradiae* and *S. rimosus*, similar mutants have been isolated for the ribostamycin-producing organism *Streptomyces ribosidificus* (KOJIMA and SATOH, 1973). This organism was shown to convert deoxystreptamine and neamine into ribostamycin. Applying the arguments used earlier for the involvement of deoxystreptamine and neamine in neomycin biosynthesis, it seems probable that these two compounds are intermediates in ribostamycin biosynthesis. Although it was not shown whether neamine was converted into ribostamycin as an intact unit, this can be presupposed because 3′,4′-dideoxyneamine is converted into 3′,4′-dideoxyribostamycin and is, therefore, probably converted as an intact pseudodisaccharide.

IV. Butirosins

Butirosins A and B are derivatives of xylostasin and ribostamycin (Fig. 2), respectively, substituted at the amino group of C-1 of deoxystreptamine with an α-hydroxy-γ-aminobutyryl (HABA) group. These two compounds, and the related 6′-deamino-6′-hydroxy butirosins A and B, are produced by *Bacillus circulans*. As with ribostamycin, all knowledge of the biosynthesis of these compounds comes from the use of idiotrophs. Initial reports using a D^- mutant demonstrated that deoxystreptamine was converted into butirosins but that 1-*N*-HABA-deoxystreptamine and neamine were not (CLARIDGE et al., 1974). More recently, however, two neamine idiotrophs of *B. circulans* have been isolated which are able to synthesize butirosins from precursors other than deoxystreptamine (TAKEDA et al., 1978a, b). These workers demonstrated that butirosins A and B were produced in varying ratios from deoxystreptamine, paromamine, neamine, and ribostamycin. Butirosin A was also produced from xylostasin and butirosin B. 6′-Deamino-6′-hydroxybutirosin A was produced from DAH-xylostasin and DAH-butirosin B. Based on these observations it was proposed that the biosynthesis of butirosins occurs via the route outlined in Figure 15.

Note that no proof other than chromatographic data was presented as to the identity of the antibiotics produced in the experiments above, nor was it shown whether or not the pseudodi- and pseudotrisaccharides were incorporated intact or whether they were hydrolyzed to produce neamine or deoxystreptamine which was then incorporated into the antibiotic.

The possibility of HABA-neamine or HABA-deoxystreptamine as biosynthetic intermediates cannot as yet be dismissed. It has been shown that 2,5-dideoxystreptamine is converted into 5-deoxybutirosamine (5-deoxy rings I–II of butirosin) by another strain of *B. circulans* (TAYLOR and SCHMITZ, 1976), requiring that HABA addition be possible at the pseudodisaccharide (or, less likely, the deoxystreptamine) level. It is possible that the D^- mutant is impermeable to HABA-derivatives which would give rise to antibiotic production.

V. Kanamycin

Biosynthetic studies on kanamycin A (Fig. 3) (KOJIMA et al., 1968, 1969), an antibiotic produced by *Streptomyces kanamyceticus*, demonstrated that *D*-glucose is a precursor for all three subunits. Surprisingly, it was also shown

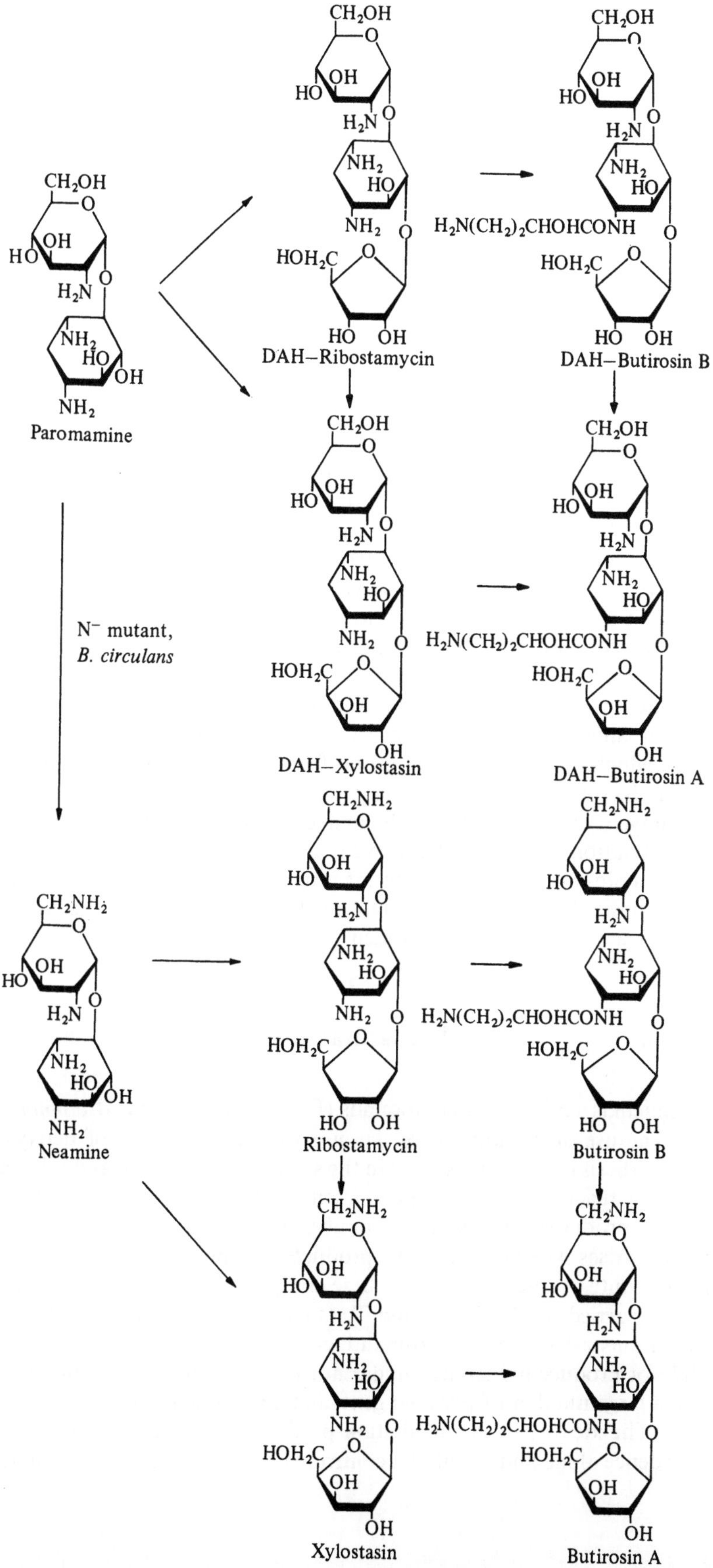
Paromamine
N⁻ mutant,
B. circulans
Neamine
DAH–Ribostamycin
DAH–Xylostasin
Ribostamycin
Xylostasin
$H_2N(CH_2)_2CHOHCONH$
DAH–Butirosin B
DAH–Butirosin A
Butirosin B
Butirosin A

that *D*-[1-^{14}C]glucosamine is a precursor, but only for the 6-amino-6-deoxy-*D*-glucose moiety (ring I), with optimum glucosamine incorporation occurring when the labeled compound is added at a slightly later stage in the fermentation than glucose. Because the conversion of *D*-glucosamine to 6-amino-6-deoxy-*D*-glucose probably involves *D*-glucose as an intermediate, incorporation of *D*-glucosamine into other subunits (II and III) would also be expected. Paromamine (rings I–II of kanamycin C) was isolated in the same experiments and was also shown to be labeled by *D*-glucose and *D*-glucosamine. Again *D*-glucosamine was shown to be incorporated only into ring I of paromamine, but as this is *D*-glucosamine itself, this is not surprising.

Deoxystreptamine-requiring idiotrophs of *S. kanamyceticus* have been isolated (SHIER, 1970; SHIER et al., 1972, 1974; KOJIMA and SATOH, 1973). Although these organisms were able to convert deoxystreptamine into kanamycin, they were unable to incorporate neamine (rings I–II of kanamycin B), paromamine (rings I–II of kanamycin C), or kanosaminidodeoxystreptamine (rings II–III of all kanamycins) into the pseudotrisaccharide antibiotics.

Kanamycin production in *S. kanamyceticus* has been shown to be preceded by the formation of kanamycin acetyltransferase, an enzyme which acetylates the 6′-amino group of kanamycin using acetyl-CoA as the acetyl donor (SATOH et al., 1975a, b). 6′-N-Acetyl-kanamycin A was shown to accumulate both inside the cells and in the culture medium and kanamycin production was shown to be accompanied by the appearance of *N*-acetylkanamycin amidohydrolase, an enzyme which cleaves the acetyl group from *N*-acetylkanamycin to produce kanamycin (SATOH et al., 1976). One conclusion from this study is that *N*-acetylkanamycin is a precursor for kanamycin, the last step in its biosynthesis being deacetylation by *N*-acetylkanamycin amidohydrolase. An obvious advantage of such a biosynthetic sequence to the producing organism is that kanamycin can be synthesized as a non-toxic intermediate, its biological activity being released only at the last possible moment.

VI. Gentamicin

Gentamicin is a mixture of compounds (Fig. 4) produced by *Micromonospora purpurea*. The use of mutants of *M. purpurea* in investigations of deoxystreptamine biosynthesis has been presented in the section on neomycin and this section discusses those reactions unique to gentamicin-type antibiotic biosynthesis. Since *M. purpurea* produces such a large number of related pseudotrisaccharides, the question arises whether these are products of minor modifications of one biosynthetic route or whether some of these compounds are precursors of others. Experiments carried out by TESTA and TILLEY (1976) argue for the latter. These workers demonstrated that a paromamine-producing mutant of *M. purpurea* which did not produce gentamicin under normal fermentation conditions could transform a large number of possible gentamicin precursors into the gentamicin C complex. The identity of the incubation products was indicated by chromatographic evidence alone and should be confirmed by other techniques. The results

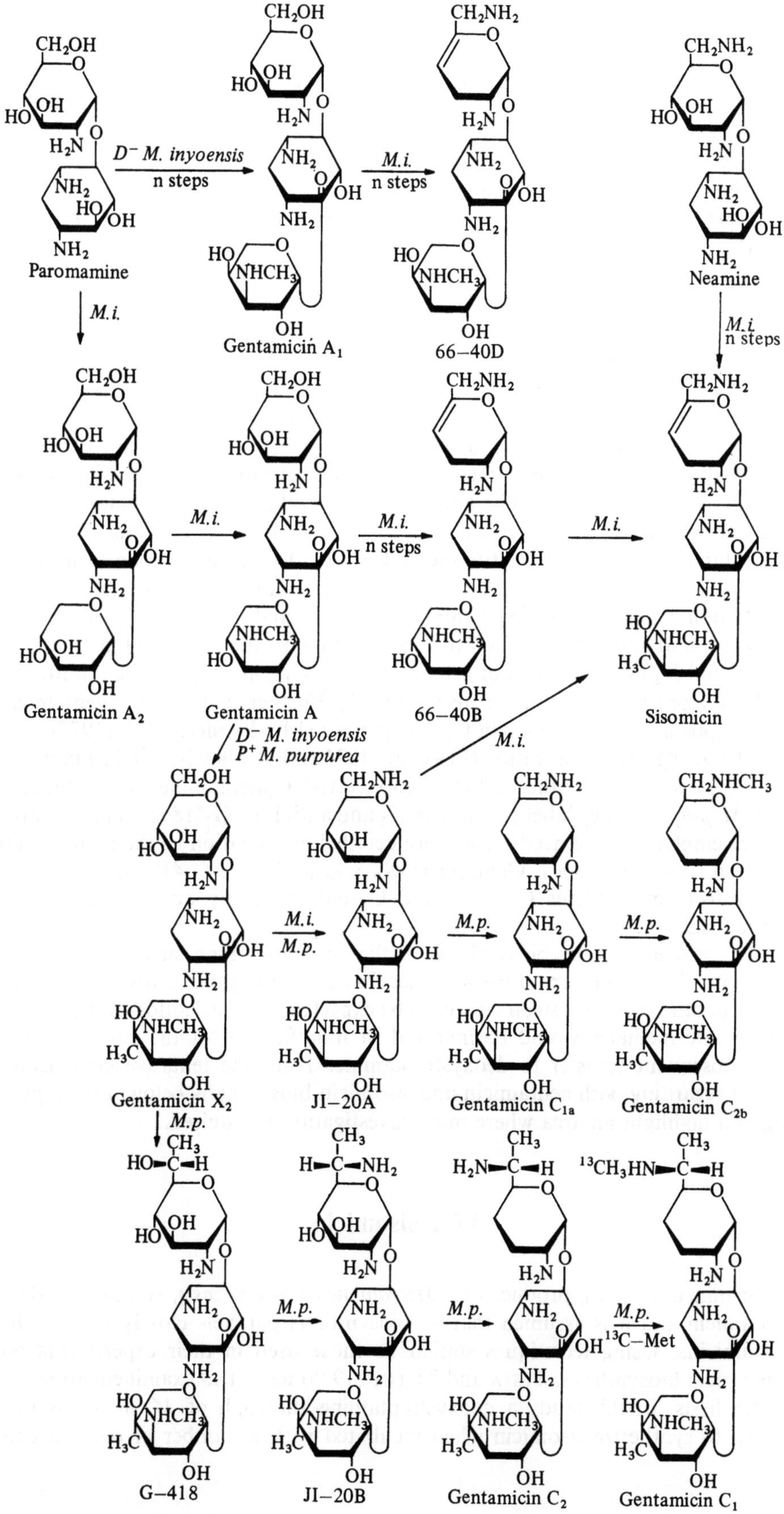

Paromamine
D⁻ M. inyoensis
n steps
Gentamicin A₁
M.i.
n steps
66–40D
Neamine
M.i.
n steps
M.i.
Gentamicin A₂
M.i.
Gentamicin A
M.i.
n steps
66–40B
M.i.
Sisomicin
D⁻ M. inyoensis
P⁺ M. purpurea
M.i.
Gentamicin X₂
M.i.
M.p.
JI–20A
M.p.
Gentamicin C₁a
M.p.
Gentamicin C₂b
M.p.
G–418
M.p.
JI–20B
M.p.
Gentamicin C₂
M.p.
¹³C–Met
Gentamicin C₁

from incubating the mutant with various gentamicin components were used to support the scheme for gentamicin biosynthesis outlined in Figure 16, which involves a branch point at gentamicin X_2 with one branch leading to gentamicins C_{1a} and C_{2b} and the other leading to gentamicins C_1 and C_2. The evidence for the involvement of paromamine as an intermediate was not presented, although this does seem to be a biosynthetic precursor for the related sisomicin, as noted below.

The conversion of gentamicin A to gentamicins C_1 and C_{2b} involves three and two methylation steps, respectively. LEE et al. (1973, 1974) showed that ^{14}C from *L*-[*methyl*-^{14}C]methionine was incorporated into gentamicins C_1, C_{1a}, and C_2. Use of [^{13}C-*methyl*]- and [^{2}H-*methyl*]methionine showed that methionine provides the *C*- and *N*-methyl groups of gentamicins (DANIELS et al., 1976).

Small quantities of gentamicins A, X_2, and antibiotic G-418 (Fig. 4) are produced by *M. purpurea*. The addition of *L*-[*methyl*-^{14}C]methionine to 1-day-old cultures of *M. purpurea* resulted in a small amount of label appearing in gentamicins A, X_2, and antibiotic G-418 after 15-min incubation (LEE et al., 1976a), while gentamicins C_1, C_{1a}, and C_2 remained unlabeled. After 24-h incubation, label appeared in gentamicins C_1, C_{1a}, and C_2 as well as gentamicins A and X_2 and antibiotic G-418. These results support the proposal that gentamicins A and X_2 are precursors of gentamicins C_1, C_{1a}, and C_2 and that antibiotic G-418 is a precursor of gentamicins C_1 and C_2. Further evidence that gentamicin C_2 is a precursor of gentamicin C_1 was presented by DANIELS et al. (1977).

The unexpected observation (LEE et al., 1976a) that when [G-^{14}C]gentamicins C_1, C_{1a}, and C_2 biosynthesized from *L*-[*methyl*-^{14}C]methionine were incubated with *M. purpurea* they label gentamicin X_2 and antibiotic G-418 to a considerable degree emphasizes the need for a more detailed examination of the relationship between these antibiotics. Gentamicin X_2 and antibiotic G-418 could be produced from gentamicins C_1, C_{1a}, and C_2 either directly or via a hydrolysis mechanism.

The mechanism for biosynthesis of the complex amino sugar components which involves a preformed pseudotrisaccharide is intriguing. From the biosyntheses of other complex sugars it would be expected that nucleotide-diphosphate-linked intermediates would be involved in modification of the sugar moiety, and subsequent transfer to deoxystreptamine. Thus, the tentative conclusions drawn regarding both gentamicin and sisomicin biosynthesis below, are surprising and highlight an area where more investigation is required.

VII. Sisomicin

Sisomicin (Fig. 5), produced by *Micromonospora inyoensis*, is 4′,5′-dehydrogentamicin and it is assumed that its biosynthesis parallels closely that of the gentamicins. Using techniques similar to those used in their experiments on gentamicin biosynthesis, TESTA and TILLEY (1975) have also examined sisomicin biosynthesis. In this study a deoxystreptamine-idiotroph of *M. inyoensis* was shown to synthesize sisomicin when incubated with a number of deoxystreptamine derivatives. The pathway for sisomicin biosynthesis in Figure 16 is based on these results. Gentamicin A was shown to be converted to sisomicin, which was rigorously identified; in all other cases sisomicin identification was based on chromatographic evidence. Also, it was not shown whether the added sisomicin precursors were incorporated directly into sisomicin. Thus, a mechanism which involves the hydrolysis of the precursors followed by incorporation of the liberated deoxystreptamine into sisomicin cannot be excluded.

Two methylation steps were involved in the conversion of gentamicin A_2 to sisomicin. LEE et al. (1976b) have demonstrated that label from *L*-[*methyl*-^{14}C]-methionine was incorporated into sisomicin by *M. inyoensis* and suggest that the amino acid provides the methyl groups of this antibiotic. Shortly after the addition of *L*-[*methyl*-^{14}C]methionine to *M. inyoensis* cultures, label appeared in gentamicin A and antibiotic 66-40 B and, following further incubation, ^{14}C label appeared in sisomicin also. From these results it was proposed that gentamicin A and antibiotic 66-40 B are precursors for sisomicin biosynthesis.

VIII. Streptomycin

The biosynthesis of streptomycin (Fig. 7) has been the subject of a number of recent reviews (WALKER, 1971; HORNER, 1967; DEMAIN and INAMINE, 1970; GRISEBACH, 1978) and for this reason is discussed only briefly here. Early investigations using the streptomycin-producing organism *Streptomyces griseus* (KAROW et al., 1952) demonstrated that glucose is the precursor for the carbon skeleton of streptomycin; HUNTER and HOCKENHULL (1955) showed later that *D*-glucose is incorporated into all three subunits approximately equally. Specifically labeled glucose has also been utilized in the study of all of the subunits of streptomycin. Thus, results obtained by SILVERMAN and RIEDER (1960) and by BRUTON et al. (1967) suggest that the conversion of *D*-glucose into *N*-methyl-*L*-glucosamine occurs via multiple epimerizations similar to those proposed by VOLK (1959) for the formation of *D*-arabinose from *L*-arabinose. The two groups provided evidence that glucose is converted to *N*-methyl-*L*-glucosamine as a unit, with the glucose carbons becoming the corresponding amino-sugar carbons, although some scrambling of the label from C-1 to C-6 has been reported (AKAMATSU and ARAI, 1967). *L*-Glucose was not incorporated into *N*-methyl-*L*-glucosamine (BRUTON et al., 1967), whereas [^{15}N]glucosamine was (TOVAROVA et al., 1966), thus suggesting glucosamine as an intermediate in the conversion of glucose into *N*-methyl-*L*-glucosamine. The *N*-methyl group was shown to arise from the methyl group of *L*-methionine (CANDY et al., 1964). HEDING and BAJPAI (1973) have suggested that this methylation does not occur until after the synthesis of *N*-demethylstreptomycin or *N*-demethyldihydrostreptomycin. These workers demonstrated that, when [*methyl*-^{14}C]methionine and either *N*-demethyldihydrostreptomycin or *N*-demethyldihydrostreptomycin and *N*-demethylstreptomycin together were incubated with *S. griseus*, labeled dihydrostreptomycin or dihydrostreptomycin together with streptomycin, respectively, was produced. However, the position of the ^{14}C-label was not determined and scrambling of label among the other precursors by catabolism and anabolism cannot be excluded. In addition, a high level of *N*-demethyldihydrostreptomycin or *N*-demethylstreptomycin (five times the normal level for that strain of *S. griseus*) was used and this may also influence the observation.

The streptose unit is also biosynthesized from glucose, with carbons 1, 2, 3, and 6 of glucose providing carbons 1, 2, 3′, and 5 of streptose, respectively (CANDY et al., 1964; CANDY and BADDILEY, 1965; BRUTON and HORNER, 1969; BRUTON and HORNER, 1966). The involvement of such potential formyl precursors as *L*-[*methyl*-^{14}C]methionine and sodium [^{14}C]formate in the biosynthesis of the formyl (C-3′) group of streptose was excluded by earlier studies (CANDY et al., 1964; HORNER, 1966). The conversion of glucose into streptose occurs via an intramolecular carbon-carbon rearrangement involving deoxythymidine 5′-diphosphoglucose (dTDP-glucose), which is converted into 4-keto-4,6-dideoxy-*D*-glucose and then into dihydrostreptose and *L*-rhamnose (Fig. 17). Evidence for this pathway was provided by the demonstration that a cell-free extract of *S. griseus* could convert dTDP-*D*-[U-^{14}C]glucose, in the presence of NADPH, into dTDP-dihydrostreptose, dTDP-4-keto-4,6-dideoxy-*D*-glucose and dTDP-*L*-rhamnose (ORTMANN et al., 1974). In the absence of NADPH, the cell-free extract synthesized only dTDP-4-keto-4,6-dideoxyglucose. Furthermore, the extract which converts dTDP-4-keto-4,6-dideoxyglucose into dTDP-*L*-dihydrostreptose was separated into two fractions. These were a 3,5-epimerase and 'dTDP-*L*-dihydrostreptose synthase' (WAHL et al., 1975). The exact mechanism of the molecular rearrangement is unknown, as is the stage at which dihydrostreptose is oxidized to streptose, although work by KNIEP and GRISEBACH (1976) and MAIER et al. (1975) suggests that this occurs following incorporation of the sugar into either a partially assembled streptomycin precursor or, more likely, dihydrostreptomycin.

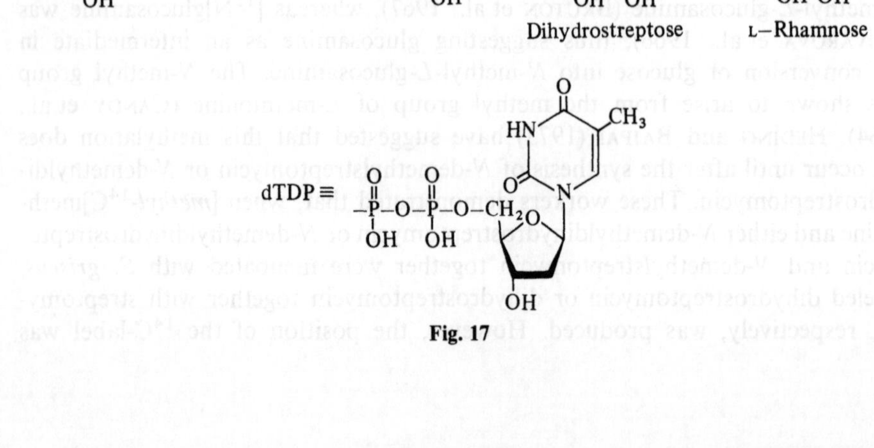

Fig. 17

Early work on streptidine biosynthesis by BRUCE et al. (1968) and by HORNER and RUSS (1971) showed that glucose is incorporated into streptidine, with C-1 of glucose providing C-5 of streptidine. The guanidino groups of streptidine were shown to be donated by arginine (SEVERINA et al., 1960; EGOROV, 1960; GALANINA and AGATOV, 1960; MAJUMDAR and KUTZNER, 1962a).

Using *D*-[6-^{13}C]glucose as a biosynthetic precursor, MUNRO et al. (1975) demonstrated labeling of C-6 of *N*-methyl-*L*-glucosamine, C-5 of streptose, and C-6 of streptidine. These results confirm the previously reported observations using radioactive precursors.

There are marked differences between the biosynthesis of streptidine and that of 2-deoxystreptamine. Thus, although *myo*-inositol does not seem to be involved in the production of the latter compound (FALKNER, 1969), it has been shown to be a precursor for streptidine (MAJUMDAR and KUTZNER, 1962b; HORNER, 1964).

The steps currently thought to be involved in the conversion of *myo*-inositol to streptidine are outlined in Figure 18. Interestingly, streptidine appears to be produced by two consecutive series of five similar enzymatic steps from *myo*-inositol – oxidation, amination, phosphorylation, carbamidinylation, dephosphorylation. The initial step in streptidine biosynthesis probably involves the cyclization of D-glucose, via 6-phosphate, to inositol-1-phosphate, which is dephosphorylated to produce *myo*-inositol. *Myo*-inositol is then oxidized to *myo*-inosose-2 and aminated to produce *scyllo*-inosamine (WALKER and WALKER, 1968, 1969). *Scyllo*-inosamine is then phosphorylated (WALKER and WALKER, 1967a) and the amino group *para* to the phosphate is carbamidinated, with arginine providing the carbamidinyl group. The phosphate is then removed.

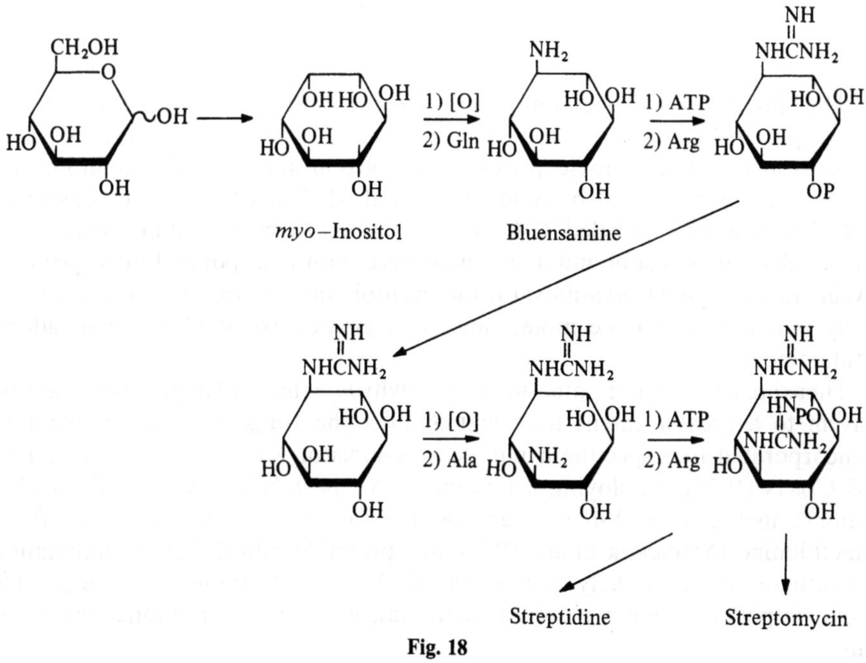

Fig. 18

The second guanidinyl group is introduced in a similar manner. Thus, the 3-hydroxyl group is oxidized to a keto function, which is then aminated by a different enzyme from the one responsible for aminating the 1-position (WALKER and WALKER, 1969). Phosphorylation of the amino product is catalyzed by the same enzyme that is responsible for phosphorylating *scyllo*-inosamine (WALKER and WALKER, 1967a; 1967c) and again is *'para'* to the amino group. The final carbamidinylation also uses arginine as the carbamidinyl group donor (WALKER and WALKER, 1965), the reaction being catalyzed by an enzyme which differs from the one involved in the first transfer (PLA, 1971).

Dephosphorylation of streptidine phosphate probably does not occur until after it is incorporated into streptomycin phosphate. Evidence suggesting this has been reported by a number of workers (BARABAS et al., 1974; WALKER and WALKER, 1966, 1967b; NOMI et al., 1966, 1967, 1968). Further evidence that streptidine phosphate and not free streptidine is an intermediate in streptomycin biosynthesis was provided by KNIEP and GRISEBACH (1976), who showed dihydrostreptose could be transferred from dTDP-*L*-dihydrostreptose to streptidine phosphate but not to streptidine. This work also suggests that the first step in the assembly of the three subunits is the formation of 4-*O*-(α-*L*-dihydrostreptosyl)-streptidine phosphate.

It has been shown that streptidine is incorporated into streptomycin (NAGAOKA and DEMAIN, 1975) by a mutant of *S. griseus*; this probably occurs via the phosphorylated derivative.

IX. Spectinomycin

The biosynthesis of spectinomycin (Fig. 6), an antibiotic produced by *Streptomyces spectabilis,* has been studied by MITSCHER et al. (1971). These workers demonstrated that *D*-glucose provides the carbon skeleton of spectinomycin, an observation confirmed by STROSHANE et al. (1976), who also demonstrated that C-6 of glucose labeled C-6 of actinamine. MITSCHER et al. (1971) also showed that *myo*-inositol and actinamine were both incorporated into spectinomycin. In the case of *myo*-inositol, the cyclitol was shown to be incorporated solely into the actinamine moiety and to a greater extent (47%) than added actinamine (6.6%).

There are a number of potential reasons why *myo*-inositol might label spectinomycin to a greater extent than actinamine. The suggestion that actinamine is incorporated into spectinomycin via *myo*-inositol was excluded by SLECHTA and COATS (1974), employing a mutant of *S. spectabilis*. These workers also demonstrated that the *N*-methyl groups, previously shown to be derived from *L*-methionine (MITSCHER et al., 1971), are probably added last in actinamine biosynthesis. It seems likely that *myo*-inositol labels spectinomycin to a greater extent simply because it is more efficiently taken up by the antibiotic-producing cells.

X. Validamycin

Glucose has been shown to provide the carbon source for the monoaminocyclitol-containing antibiotic validamycin A (Fig. 9) (KAMEDA et al., 1975). Also, it was demonstrated that [^{14}C]validoxylamine A was incorporated into validamycin A with little detectable label in the *D*-glucose moiety. On this basis it was suggested that glucose is added last in the biosynthetic assembly, although the possibility that validoxylamine A was degraded and then resynthesized was not excluded.

XI. Plasmids

The involvement of plasmids in the biosynthesis of antibiotics has been suggested by various authors (OKANISHI et al., 1970; KIRBY et al., 1975; AKAGAWA et al., 1975; WRIGHT and HOPWOOD, 1976). Recent reports have indicated that the presence of plasmids may, in particular, be essential for the biosynthesis of some aminocyclitol antibiotics. Thus, SHAW and PIWOWARKSI (1977) have demonstrated that acridine or ethidium bromide treatment of *S. bikiniensis* resulted in the loss of ability to produce streptomycin in some of the survivors. Interestingly, the non-producing isolates were also sensitive to low concentrations of streptomycin.

Using similar procedures, HOTTA et al. (1977) showed plasmids may be involved in kanamycin biosynthesis by *S. kanamyceticus*. The non-producers were found to be able to synthesize kanamycin when cultured in the presence of deoxystreptamine, suggesting that acriflavin was eliminating the ability to produce this subunit.

More direct evidence for the involvement of plasmids in neomycin biosynthesis was obtained by YAGISAWA et al. (1978). These workers showed that acridine treatment of *S. fradiae* led to the loss of the ability to produce neomycin, an observation made independently by BYRNE and RINEHART (unpublished results). In addition, the former workers showed that two isolates which were sensitive to neomycin had no detectable phosphotransferase [APH(3′)]. Neither of these organisms contained either of the two plasmids isolated from the original strain. A third non-producing strain, which was originally able to produce phosphotransferase, and could produce neomycin when incubated with deoxystreptamine, on continuous subculture became sensitive to neomycin and lost both the ability to produce phosphotransferase and the ability to convert deoxystreptamine to neomycin, suggesting a further link between phosphotransferase activity and neomycin biosynthesis.

It seems premature to conclude that plasmids are involved in aminocyclitol antibiotic biosynthesis. However, these reports indicate that this hypothesis is attractive and deserves further investigation.

XII. Conclusion

The great improvement in our knowledge of the biosynthesis of aminocyclitol antibiotics over the past few years can be attributed to a large extent to experiments involving the use of deoxystreptamine idiotrophs. Furnishing biosynthetic information, these organisms have been used to produce novel semi-synthetic antibiotics, some of which have properties greatly superior to the parent compound. For example, hydroxygentamicin produced by the D^- mutant of *M. purpurea* has essentially the same activity as gentamicin but much reduced toxicity (ROSI et al. 1977).

Evidence produced by the use of these mutant organisms, together with labeling studies, has led to the proposal of novel, unpredicted pathways for some of the aminocyclitol antibiotics (e.g., sisomicins and gentamicin) and has provided invaluable clues to the biosynthesis of deoxystreptamine. However, there is still much experimental work to be carried out both in exploring as yet ignored areas and in testing many of the theories currently proposed.

References

Akagawa H, Okanishi M, Umezawa H (1975) A plasmid involved in chloramphenicol production in *Streptomyces venezuelae*: evidence from genetic mapping. J Gen Microbiol 90:336–346

Akamatsu N, Arai T (1967) On the origin of *N*-methyl-*L*-glucosamine in the molecule of streptomycin. Biochim Biophys Acta 141:650–652

Bandyophadhyay SK, Majumdar SK (1974) Regulation of the formation of alkaline phosphatase during neomycin biosynthesis. Antimicrob Agents Chemother 5:431–434

Barabas G, Szeszak F, Szabo G (1974) Transamidinase activity of hyphal fractions of a streptomycin-producing *Streptomyces griseus* strain and enhancement of enzyme activity in a non-producing mutant. Antimicrob Agents Chemother 6:11–15

Baud HA, Betencourt A, Peyre H, Penasse L (1977) Ribostamycin, as an intermediate in the biosynthesis of neomycin. J Antibiot 30:720–723

Bruce RM, Ragheb HS, Weiner H (1968) Biosynthesis of streptomycin: origin of streptidine from D-glucose. Biochim Biophys Acta 158:499–500

Bruton J, Horner WH (1966) Biosynthesis of streptomycin. III. Origin of the carbon atoms of streptose. J Biol Chem 241:3142–3146

Bruton J, Horner WH (1969) Biosynthesis of streptomycin. V. Origin of the formyl carbon atom of streptose. Biochim Biophys Acta 184:641–642

Bruton J, Horner WH, Russ GA (1967) Biosynthesis of streptomycin. IV. Further studies on the biosynthesis of streptidine and *N*-methyl-*L*-glucosamine. J Biol Chem 242:813–818

Byrne KM, Rinehart KL Jr (1978) Utilization of deoxythymidine-diphospho-*D*-glucose by *Streptomyces fradiae*. 78th Annu Meet Am Soc Microbiol. Las Vegas, Nevada, Abstracts 46, K37

Candy DJ, Baddiley J (1965) The biosynthesis of streptomycin. The origin of the C-formyl group of streptose. Biochem J 96:526–529

Candy DJ, Blumson NL, Baddiley J (1964) The biosynthesis of streptomycin. Incorporation of ^{14}C-labeled compounds into streptose and *N*-methyl-*L*-glucosamine. Biochem J 91:31–35

Chen Y-M, Walker JB (1977) Transaminations involving keto- and amino-inositols and glutamine in actinomycetes which produce gentamicin and neomycin. Biochem Biophys Res Commun 77:688–692

Claridge CA, Bush JA, Defuria MD, Price KE (1974) Fermentation and mutation studies with a butirosin-producing strain of *Bacillus circulans*. Dev Ind Microbiol 15:101–113

Comb DG, Roseman S (1956) Glucosamine 6-phosphate deaminase. Biochim Biophys Acta 21:193–194

Daniels PJL, Yehaskel A, Morton JB (1976) The biosynthetic origin of the methyl groups of the gentamicin antibiotics. 16th Intersci Conf Antimicrob Agents Chemother. Chicago, Abstract 45

Daniels PJL, Weinstein J, Condon RG, Lee BD (1977) The biosynthetic relationship between gentamicins C_2 and C_1. 17th Intersci Conf Antimicrob Agents Chemother. New York, Abstract 156

Daum SJ, Rosi D, Goss WA (1977) Mutational biosynthesis by idiotrophs of *Micromonospora purpurea*. II. Conversion of non-amino containing cyclitols to aminoglycoside antibiotics. J Antibiot 30:98–105

Demain AL, Inamine E (1970) Biochemistry and regulation of streptomycin and mannosidostreptomycinase (α-*D*-mannosidase) formation. Bacteriol Rev 34:1–19

Egorov NS (1960) The effects of compounds containing a guanidine group and of inosite on the biosynthesis of streptomycin. Antibiotiki H, 265 (1959); Chem Abstr 54:2488e

Eisenberg F Jr, Bolden AH, Loewus FA (1964) Inositol formation by cyclisation of glucose chain in rat testis. Biochim Biophys Res Commun 14:419–424

Falkner FC (1969) Studies on the biosynthesis of neomycin. PhD Thesis, University of Illinois, Urbana

Feingold DS, Nevfeld EF, Hassid WA (1960) The 4-epimerization and decarboxylation of uridine diphosphate *D*-glucuronic acid by extracts from *Phaseolus aureus* seedlings. J Biol Chem 235:910–913

Foght JL (1963) Biosynthetic studies on the neomycins. PhD Thesis, University of Illinois, Urbana

Galanina LA, Agatov PA (1960) Effect of some chemical compounds on function of streptomycin by LS-1 strain of *Actinomyces streptomycini*. Dokl Akad Nauk SSSR 127:450 (1959); Chem Abstr 54:2406h

Grisebach H (1978) Biosynthesis of sugar components of antibiotic substances. In: Tipson RS, Horton D (eds) Advances in carbohydrate chemistry and biochemistry, pp 81–126. Academic Press, London New York

Heding H, Bajpai K (1973) The last step in the biosynthesis of streptomycin: *N*-methylation of *N*-demethylstreptomycin. J Antibiot 26:725–727

Hessler EJ, Jahnke HK, Robertson JH, Tsuji K, Rinehart KL Jr, Shier WT (1970) Neomycins D, E and F. Identity with paromamine, paromomycin I and paromomycin II. J Antibiot 23:464–466

Horner WH (1964) Biosynthesis of streptomycin. II. *Myo*-inositol, a precursor of the streptidine moiety. J Biol Chem 239:2256–2258

Horner WH (1966) The role of methionine in streptomycin biosynthesis. In: Herold M, Gabriel Z (eds) Antibiotics – advances in research, production and clinical use, p 612. Butterworths & Co, London

Horner WH (1967) Streptomycin. In: Gottlieb D, Shaw PD (eds) Antibiotics. II. Biosynthesis, pp 373–399, 447–448. Springer, Berlin Heidelberg New York

Horner WH, Russ GA (1971) Biosynthesis of streptomycin. VII. Stereospecificity of the enzymatic dehydrogenation of 1-guanidine-1-deoxy-*scyllo*-inositol. Biochim Biophys Acta 237:123–127

Hotta K, Okami Y, Umezawa H (1977) Elimination of the ability of a kanamycin-producing strain to biosynthesize deoxystreptamine moiety by acriflavin. J Antibiot 30:1146–1149

Hunter GD, Hockenhull DJD (1955) Actinomycete metabolism. Incorporation of ^{14}C-labeled compounds into streptomycin. Biochem J 59:268–272

Kameda Y, Horii S, Yamano T (1975) Microbial transformation of validamycins. J Antibiot 28:298–306

Karow EO, Peck RL, Rosenblum C, Woodbury DT (1952) Microbiological synthesis of ^{14}C-labeled streptomycin. J Am Chem Soc 73:3056–3059

Kirby R, Wright LF, Hopwood DA (1975) Plasmid-determined antibiotic synthesis and resistance in *Streptomyces coelicolor*. Nature (London) 254:265–267

Kniep B, Grisebach H (1976) Enzymic synthesis of streptomycin. Transfer of *L*-dihydrostreptose from dTDP-*L*-dihydrostreptose to streptidine-6-phosphate. FEBS Lett 65:44–46

Kojima M, Satoh A (1973) Microbial semi-synthesis of aminoglycoside antibiotics by mutants of *S. ribosidificus* and *S. kanamyceticus*. J Antibiot 26:784–786

Kojima M, Yamada Y, Umezawa H (1968) Studies on the biosynthesis of kanamycins. I. Incorporation of ^{14}C-glucose or ^{14}C-glucosamine into kanamycins and kanamycin-related compounds. Agric Biol Chem 32:467–473

Kojima M, Yamada Y, Umezawa H (1969) Studies on the biosynthesis of kanamycins. II. Incorporation of the radioactive degradation products of kanamycin A or related metabolites into kanamycin A. Agric Biol Chem 33:1181–1185

Lee BK, Testa RT, Wagman GH, Liu CM, McDaniel L, Schaffner C (1973) Incorporation of *L*-methionine-methyl-^{14}C into gentamicins. J Antibiot 26:728–731

Lee BK, Condon RG, Wagman GH, Byrne K, Schaffner C (1974) Incorporation of *L*-methionine-methyl-^{14}C into gentamicins. II. Large-scale preparation of methyl-^{14}C-gentamicins. J Antibiot 27:822–825

Lee BK, Condon RG, Wagman GH, Katz E (1976a) *Micromonospora*-produced gentamicin components. Antimicrob Agents Chemother 9:151–159

Lee BK, Condon RG, Wagman GH, Weinstein MJ, Katz E (1976b) *Micromonospora*-produced sisomicin components. J Antibiot 29:677–684

Magasanik B (1962) Biosynthesis of purine and pyrimidine nucleotides. In: Gunsalus IC, Stanier RY (eds) The bacteria. III. Biosynthesis, pp 295–334. Academic Press, London New York

Maier S, Matern U, Grisebach H (1975) On the role of dihydrostreptomycin in streptomycin biosynthesis. FEBS Lett 49:317–319

Majumdar SK, Kutzner HJ (1962a) Studies on the biosynthesis of streptomycin. Appl Microbiol 10:157–168

Majumdar SK, Kutzner HJ (1962b) *Myo*-inositol in the biosynthesis of streptomycin by *Streptomyces griseus*. Science 135:734

Majumdar MK, Majumdar SK (1969) Amino sugar antibiotic as phosphoamide from *Streptomyces fradiae*. J Antibiot 22:174–175

Majumdar MK, Majumdar SK (1970) Isolation and characterization of three phosphoamido-neomycins and their conversion into neomycin by *Streptomyces fradiae*. Biochem J 120:271–278

Majumdar MK, Majumdar SK (1971) Relationship between alkaline phosphatase and neomycin formation in *Streptomyces fradiae*. Biochem J 122:397–404

Mitscher LA, Martin LL, Feller DR (1971) The biosynthesis of spectinomycin. Chem Commun 1541–1542

Munro MHG, Taniguchi M, Rinehart KL Jr, Gottlieb D, Stoudt TH, Rogers TO (1975) Carbon-13 evidence for the inositol pathway in streptomycin biosynthesis. J Am Chem Soc 97:4782–4783

Nagaoka K, Demain AL (1975) Mutational biosynthesis of a new antibiotic, streptomutin A, by an idiotroph of *Streptomyces griseus*. J Antibiot 28:627–635

Nomi R, Nimi O, Miyazaki T, Matsuo A, Kiyohara H (1966) Biosynthesis of streptomycin. II. Isolation of a natural precursor and an enzymatic substance transforming the precursor to streptomycin. Agric Biol Chem 30:1269–1276

Nomi R, Nimi O, Miyazaki T, Matsuo A, Kiyohara H (1967) Biosynthesis of streptomycin. III. Liberation of inorganic phosphate from a natural precursor in transformation of the precursor to streptomycin. Agric Biol Chem 32:973–978

Nomi R, Nimi O, Kado T (1968) Biosynthesis of streptomycin. IV. Accumulation of a streptomycin precursor in the culture broth and partial purification of the precursor. Agric Biol Chem 32:1256–1260

Okanishi M, Ohta T, Umezawa H (1970) Possible control of formation of aerial mycelium and antibiotic production in *Streptomyces* by episomal factors. J Antibiot 23:45–47

Ortmann R, Matern U, Grisebach H, Stadler P, Sinnwell V, Paulsen H (1974) NADPH-dependent formation of thymidine diphosphodihydrostreptose from thymidine diphospho-*D*-glucose in a cell-free system from *Streptomyces griseus* and its correlation with streptomycin biosynthesis. Eur J Biochem 43:265–271

Pearce CJ (1977) Studies on the biosynthesis of neomycins. PhD Thesis, University of Southampton

Pearce CJ, Akhtar M, Anthony C, Barnett JEG, Gero SD (1976) The role of the pseudodisaccharide neamine as an intermediate in the biosynthesis of neomycin. Biochem J 159:601–606

Pearce CJ, Akhtar M, Barnett JEG, Mercier D, Sepulchre A-M, Gero SD (1978) Sub-unit assembly in the biosynthesis of neomycin. The synthesis of 5-*O*-*β*-*D*-ribofuranosyl and 4-*O*-*β*-*D*-ribofuranosyl-2,6-dideoxystreptamines. J Antibiot 31:74–81

Perlman D, O'Brien E (1953) Studies on utilization of lipids and polysaccharides by *Streptomyces fradiae*. Bacteriol Proc A25

Pla LC (1971) Streptomycin biosynthesis. I. Existence of two amidino-transferase activities in *Streptomyces griseus*. Biochim Biophys Acta 242:541–548

Reuter G, Koster H, Liebermann B (1977) Physiologie und Biochemie der Streptomyceten. XIII. Biosynthese von Paromomycin unter Einsatz von ^{14}C-Glucose, -Glucosamin, -2-Deoxystreptamine und Ribose durch *Streptomyces albus* var. *metamycinus nov.* var. Z Allg Mikrobiol 17:543–547

Rinehart KL Jr (1977) Mutasynthesis of new antibiotics. Pure Appl Chem 49:1361–1384

Rinehart KL Jr, Malik JM, Nystrom RS, Stroshane RM, Truitt ST, Taniguchi M, Rolls JP, Haak WJ, Ruff BA (1974a) Biosynthetic incorporation of [1-^{13}C]glucosamine and [6-^{13}C]glucose into neomycin. J Am Chem Soc 96:2263–2265

Rinehart KL Jr, Stroshane RM, Shier WT, Truitt ST, Taniguchi M, Malik JM, Schaefer PC, Rolls JP, Haak WJ (1974b) Biosynthesis of aminocyclitol antibiotics and application to synthesis of new antibiotics. 168th Nat Meet Am Chem Soc. Atlantic City, NJ, Abstract MICR 19

Rinehart KL Jr, Stroshane RM (1976) Biosynthesis of aminocyclitol antibiotics. J Antibiot 29:319–353

Rolls JP, Ruff BD, Haak WJ, Rinehart KL Jr, Stroshane RM (1975) Use of precursors labeled with stable isotopes to study the biosynthesis of neomycin. 75th Annu Meet Am Soc Microbiol. New York, Abstract 95-0.12

Rosi D, Goss WA, Daum SJ (1977) Mutational biosynthesis by idiotrophs of *Micromonospora purpurea*. I. Conversion of aminocyclitols to new aminoglycoside antibiotics. J Antibiot 30:88–97

Satoh A, Ogawa H, Satomura Y (1975a) Role and regulation mechanism of kanamycin acetyltransferase in kanamycin biosynthesis. Agric Biol Chem 39:2311–2336

Satoh A, Ogawa H, Satomura Y (1975b) Effect of sclerin on production of the aminoglycoside antibiotics accompanied by salvage function in *Streptomyces*. Agric Biol Chem 39:1593–1598

Satoh A, Ogawa H, Satomura Y (1976) Regulation of *N*-acetylkanamycin amidohydrolase in the idiophase in kanamycin fermentation. Agric Biol Chem 40:191–196

Schatz A, Bugie E, Waksman S (1946) Streptomycin, a substance exhibiting antibiotic activity against gram-positive and gram-negative bacteria. Proc Soc Exp Biol Med 55:66–69

Schimbor FR (1966) The microbiological incorporation of labeled intermediates into the neomycin antibiotics. PhD Thesis, University of Illinois, Urbana

Severina VO, Gorskaya SV, Gracheva SV (1960) Amino acids in streptomycin biosynthesis. Vopr Med Khim 5:448 (1959); Chem Abstr 54:10047e

Shaw PD, Piwowarski J (1977) Effects of ethidium bromide and acriflavin on Streptomycin production by *Streptomyces bikiniensis*. J Antibiot 30:404–408

Shier WT (1970) The hybrimycins. PhD Thesis, University of Illinois, Urbana

Shier WT, Rinehart KL Jr, Gottlieb D (1969) Preparation of four new antibiotics from a mutant of *Streptomyces fradiae*. Proc Natl Acad Sci USA 63:198–204

Shier WT, Rinehart KL Jr, Gottlieb D (1972) Method of making antibiotics containing the aminocyclitol subunit. US Patent 3,669,838, Chem Abstr 77:150584x

Shier WT, Schaefer PC, Gottlieb D, Rinehart KL Jr (1974) Use of mutants in the study of aminocyclitol antibiotic biosynthesis and the preparation of the hybrimycin C complex. Biochemistry 13:5073–5078

Silverman M, Rieder SV (1960) The formation of *N*-methyl-*L*-glucosamine from *D*-glucose by *Streptomyces griseus*. J Biol Chem 235:1251–1254

Slechta L, Coats JH (1974) Studies of the biosynthesis of spectinomycin. 14th Intersci Conf Antimicrob Agents Chemother, San Francisco, Abstract 294

Stroshane RM, Taniguchi M, Rinehart KL Jr, Rolls JP, Haak WJ, Ruff BA (1976) Spectinomycin biosynthesis studied by carbon magnetic resonance spectroscopy. J Am Chem Soc 98:3025–3027

Takeda K, Aihara K, Furumai T, Ito Y (1978a) An approach to the biosynthetic pathway of butirosins and the related antibiotics. J Antibiot 31:250–253

Takeda K, Kinumaki A, Furumai T, Yamaguchi T, Ohshima S, Ito Y (1978b) Mutational biosynthesis of butirosin analogues. J Antibiot 31:247–249

Taylor HD, Schmitz H (1976) Antibiotics derived from a mutant of *Bacillus circulans*. J Antibiot 29:532–535

Testa RT, Tilley BC (1975) Biotransformation, a new approach to aminoglycoside biosynthesis. I. Sisomicin. J Antibiot 28:573–579

Testa RT, Tilley BC (1976) Biotransformation, a new approach to aminoglycoside biosynthesis. II. Gentamicin. J Antibiot 29:140–146

Tovarova II, Kornitskaja EJ, Pliner SA, Puchkov VA, Wulfson NS, Khokhlov AS (1966) Studies on the biosynthesis of streptomycin. 4th Int Symp Chem Nat Prod IUPAC, Stockholm, Abstract 3-3

Volk WA (1959) The enzymatic formation of *D*-arabinose 5-phosphate from *L*-arabinose and adenosine triphosphate by *Propionibacterium pentosaceum*. J Biol Chem 234:1931–1936

Wahl HP, Matern U, Grisebach H (1975) Two enzymes in *Streptomyces griseus* for the synthesis of dTDP-*L*-dihydrostreptose from dTDP-6-deoxy-*D*-*xylo*-4-hexosulose. Biochem Biophys Res Commun 64:1041–1045

Walker JB (1971) Enzymatic reactions involved in streptomycin biosynthesis and metabolism. Lloydia 34:363–371

Walker JB, Walker MS (1967a) Enzymatic synthesis of streptidine from *scyllo*-inosamine. Biochemistry 6:3821–3829

Walker JB, Walker MS (1967b) Streptomycin biosynthesis. Enzymatic synthesis of O-phosphorylstreptidine from streptidine and adenosine-triphosphate. Biochim Biophys Acta 148:335–341

Walker JB, Walker MS (1968) Streptomycin biosynthesis. Enzymatic synthesis of *scyllo*-inosose and *L*-glutamine. Biochim Biophys Acta 170:219–220

Walker JB, Walker MS (1969) Streptomycin biosynthesis. Transamination reactions involving inosamines and inosadiamines. Biochemistry 8:763–770

Walker MS, Walker JB (1965) Evidence for participation of a phosphorylated derivative of streptidine in streptomycin biosynthesis. Biochim Biophys Acta 97:397–398

Walker MS, Walker JB (1966) Enzymic studies on the biosynthesis of streptomycin. Transamidination of inosamine and streptamine derivatives. J Biol Chem 241:1262–1269

Walker MS, Walker JB (1967c) Streptomycin biosynthesis. Conversion of *myo*-inositol to *O*-phosphorylstreptidine. Biochim Biophys Acta 136:272–279

Wolfe JB, Britton BB, Nakada HI (1957) Glucosamine degradation by *Escherichia coli*. III. Isolation and studies of "phosphoglucosaminisomerase". Arch Biochem Biophys 66:333–339

Wright LF, Hopwood DA (1976) Identification of the antibiotic determined by the SCP1 plasmid of *Streptomyces coelicolor* A3(2). J Gen Microbiol 95:96–106

Yagisawa M, Huang T-S R, Davies JE (1978) Possible involvement of plasmids in biosynthesis of neomycin. J Antibiot 31:809–813

Biosynthesis of β-Lactam Antibiotics

J. O'SULLIVAN and E.P. ABRAHAM

I. Introduction

A. Penicillins and Cephalosporins Produced by Microorganisms

Penicillins are N-acyl derivatives of 6-aminopenicillanic acid (6-APA) (I), which has a fused β-lactam-thiazolidine ring system (see Fig. 1). *Penicillium chrysogenum* produces 6-APA, isopenicillin N (Fig. 2) (which has a δ-linked L-α-aminoadipyl side chain [(II), $RCO = {}^{-}O_2CCH(\overset{+}{N}H_3)(CH_2)_3CO$] and a number of penicillins with non-polar side chains [RCO in (II)] derived from mono substituted acetic acids whose nature depends on the precursors present in the fermentation medium. For example, when phenoxyacetic acid is added, phenoxymethylpenicillin (penicillin V) is produced [(II), $RCO = C_6H_5OCH_2CO$]. At least eight other fungal genera are known to produce penicillins in this manner (KITANO et al., 1975).

The cephalosporins from *Cephalosporium* sp. are N-acyl derivatives of 7-aminocephalosporanic acid (7-ACA) which contains a fused β-lactam-dihydro-thiazine ring system. They have structure III (Fig. 3), where RCO is predominantly δ-linked D-α-aminoadipyl [$^{-}O_2CCH(\overset{+}{N}H_3)(CH_2)_3CO$] and R′ is H in deacetoxycephalosporin C, OH in deacetylcephalosporin C, and $OCOCH_3$ in cephalosporin C. The fungus *C. acremonium* has a fermentation pattern different

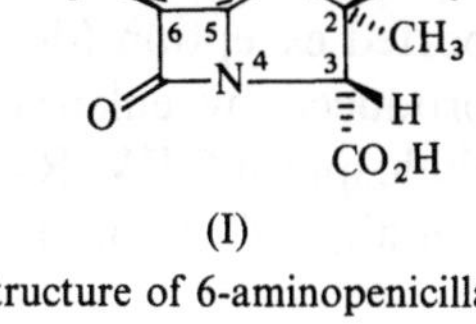

(I)

Fig. 1. Structure of 6-aminopenicillanic acid

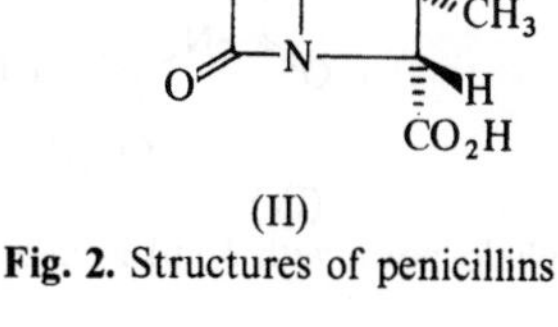

(II)

Fig. 2. Structures of penicillins

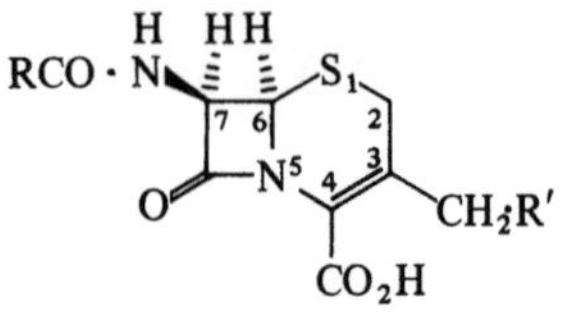

(III)

Fig. 3. Structures of cephalosporins

from that of *Penicillium,* in that the side chain of the antibiotic produced is not changed by the addition of different side chain precursors and that isopenicillin N does not accumulate. The fermentation typically yields penicillin N, which has a δ-linked D-α-aminoadipyl side chain [II, RCO = $^{-}O_2CCH(\overset{+}{N}H_3)(CH_2)_3CO$], and cephalosporin C. However, the α-aminoadipyl side chain is replaced by N-acetyl-D-α-aminoadipyl [III, RCO = $CH_3CONHCH(COOH)(CH_2)_3CO-$; R′ = H] in the deacetoxycephalosporin produced by a mutant of *C. acremonium* (TRAXLER et al., 1975) and by glutaryl in the cephalosporins [III, RCO = $^{-}O_2C(CH_2)_3CO$; R′ = H, OH or $OCOCH_3$] produced by certain strains of *C. chrysogenum* (KITANO et al., 1976a), while certain *Paecilomyces* species have been found to produce a penicillin with a 6-(5-hydroxy-n-valeramido) side chain [II, RCO = $HOCH_2(CH_2)_3CO-$] in addition to penicillin N and cephalosporins (KITANO et al., 1976b). More recently, a mutant of *C. acremonium* which requires lysine for growth and synthesizes no α-aminoadipic acid has been shown to produce a penicillin with a D-S-carboxymethylcysteine side chain [II, RCO = $^{-}O_2C.CH(\overset{+}{N}H_3)CH_2.S.CH_2CO-$] when the corresponding L-amino acid, which is isosteric with α-aminoadipic acid, is added to the medium (TROONEN et al., 1976).

Other mutants of *C. acremonium* produce cephalosporins with δ-linked D-α-aminoadipic acid side chains [RCO in III, Fig. 3] but with novel substituents at R′ in (III), that is, R′ = SCH_3, (KANZAKI et al., 1974a), S_2O_3H, (FUJISAWA et al., 1975) and $SC.(CH_3)_2.CH(NH_2)COOH$ (KANZAKI et al., 1976) which may be formed from methane thiol, thiosulphate (derived from methionine), and penicillamine (D-β-thiolvaline), respectively.

Streptomycetes can produce penicillin N (HIGGENS and KASTNER, 1971) and a range of cephalosporins (NAGARAJAN et al., 1971). All the cephalosporins obtained so far from *Streptomyces* have a δ-linked D-α-aminoadipyl side chain (Fig. 4, IV) and, with one reported exception (deacetoxycephalosporin C), they differ from cephalosporins produced by eukaryotes in having a 7α-methoxy group, as in the 7-methoxycephalosporin C [IV, R = OCH_3] produced by *Streptomyces lipmanii* (NAGARAJAN et al., 1971), or a carbamoyl function in place

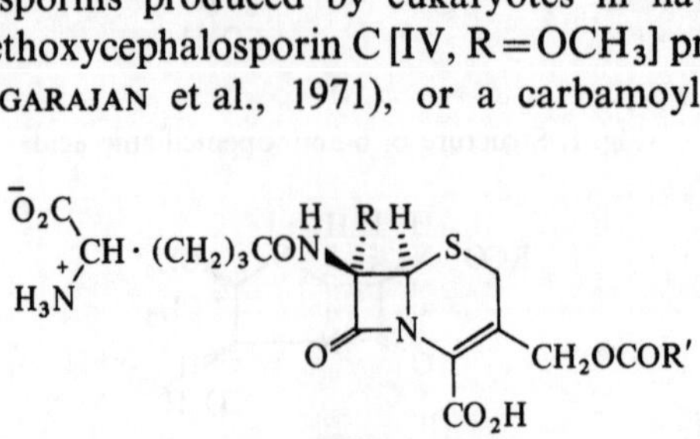

(IV)

Fig. 4. Structure of a cephalosporin with δ-linked D-α-aminoadipyl side chain

of an 0-acetyl group as in (IV) [R=H; R′=NH_2] from *S. clavuligerus*. The latter organism also produces a cephalosporin with both a 7-methoxy group and a carbamoyl function [IV, R=OCH_3; R′=NH_2] named cephamycin C. Cephamycin A [IV, R=OCH_3; R′=−C(OCH_3=CH.C_6H_4OH] and cephamycin B [IV, R=OCH_3; R′=C(OCH_3)=CH.C_6H_4.OSO_3H], which are 7α-methoxycephalosporins with cinnamoyl groups, are produced by eight species of *Streptomyces* (STAPLEY et al., 1972). Two further species have also been found to produce a substance that only differs from cephamycin B in having a second hydroxyl group on the cinnamoyl ring (FUKASE et al., 1976) [IV, R=−OCH_3; R′=−C(OCH_3)=CH.$C_6H_3(OH)_2$].

B. Other Naturally Occurring β-Lactam Compounds

In addition to the substances based on the penam or cephem nucleus, a series of new β-lactam antibiotics have now been discovered. Clavulanic acid, containing a fused β-lactam-oxazolidine ring system (Fig. 5, V), is produced by *S. clavuligerus*. It has low antibacterial activity but is a deactivator of certain β-lactamases (BROWN et al., 1976). Thienamycin (Fig. 6, VI) is a broad spectrum and highly potent antibiotic produced by *S. cattleya* (KAHAN et al., 1976) which

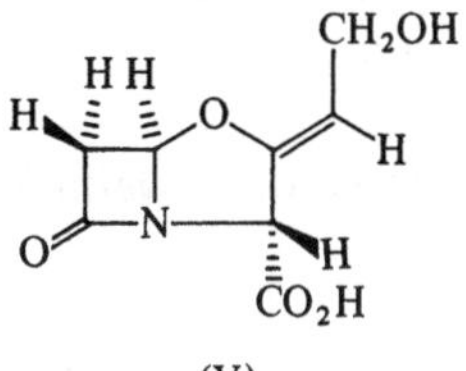

(V)

Fig. 5. Structure of clavulanic acid

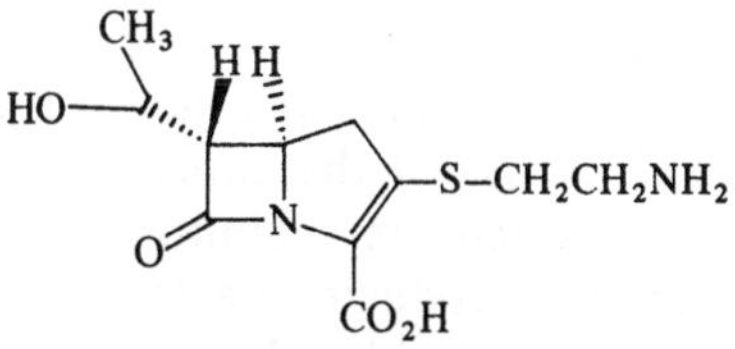

(VI)

Fig. 6. Structure of thienamycin

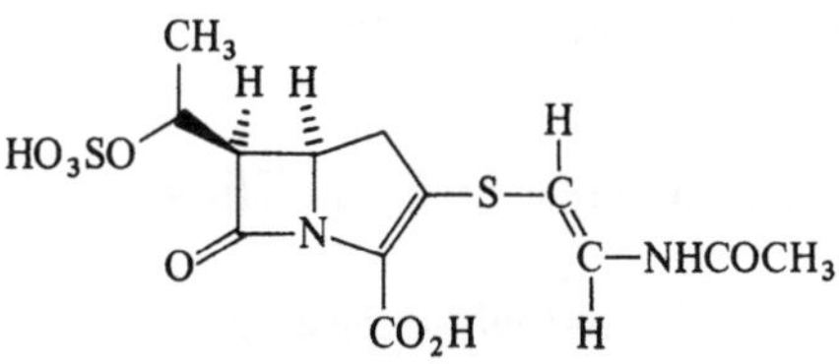

(VII)

Fig. 7. Structure of olivanic acid

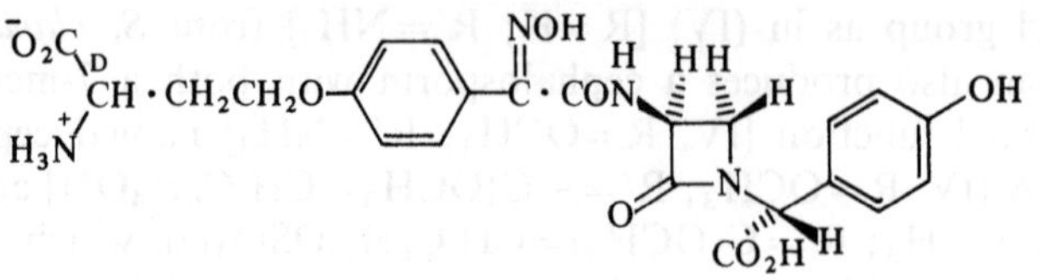

(VIII)

Fig. 8. Structure of nocardicin A

contains sulphur outside, but not in, the ring system and an unsaturated five-membered ring fused to the β-lactam ring. Two thienamycin-like compounds (VII, Fig. 7 and its sulphoxide) have been found in cultures of *S. olivaceus* and named olivanic acids (BROWN et al., 1977); they are both deactivators of β-lactamases. A compound similar to VII, but with CH_3CH_2 attached to the β-lactam ring, has also been found to be a metabolite of a *Streptomyces* sp. (OKAMURA et al., 1978). Unlike the penicillins and cephalosporins, compounds V, VI, and VII do not contain an N-acyl side chain.

Nocardicin A (Fig. 8, VIII) is the major component of a family of at least seven nocardicins produced by *Nocardia uniformis* and is a monocyclic β-lactam compound (AOKI et al., 1976). Other monocyclic β-lactam compounds have been reported to occur in nature, including the alkaloids pachystermine A and B (KIKUCHI and UYEO, 1967), tabtoxin, the agent of wildfire disease in tobacco plants (STEWART, 1971) and (S)-alanyl-3-[-α-(S)-chloro-3-(S)-hydroxy-2-oxo-3-azetidinyl-methyl]-(S)-alanine, which closely resembles tabtoxin and is produced by a streptomycete (SCANNELL et al., 1975).

C. Screening Methods

The recent dramatic increase in both the range of known β-lactam antibiotics and in the number of known producing organisms is partly due to the development of new and more sensitive screening techniques. Supersensitive mutants of *Pseudomonas aeruginosa* (KITANO et al., 1974) and *Escherichia coli* (AOKI et al., 1976) are now available which allow the assay of cephalosporins and penicillins with α-aminoadipyl side chains at concentrations below 1 μg/ml. The nocardicins were discovered by use of the supersensitive *E. coli* (AOKI et al., 1976). β-Lactam compounds which are inhibitors of β-lactamases have been found by the use of β-lactamase-producing bacteria in solid media containing subinhibitory concentrations of penicillin. In the presence of an inhibitor of the β-lactamase, the penicillin is no longer subinhibitory and a zone of inhibition results; clavulanic acid (Fig. 5, V) and the olivanic acid (Fig. 7, VII) were discovered in this way (BROWN et al., 1976, 1977).

II. Amino Acid Precursors of Penicillins and Cephalosporins

A. α-Aminoadipic Acid

The involvement of α-aminoadipic acid in penicillin N and cephalosporin production was clear from the structure of these antibiotics, but its role in the biosynthesis of penicillins with non-polar side chains was less obvious. However, free DL-α-aminoadipic acid was found to stimulate the production of benzyl penicillin by *P. chrysogenum* (SOMERSON et al., 1961). L-α-aminoadipic acid is an intermediate in the pathway to lysine in fungi and lysine inhibited penicillin biosynthesis by feedback inhibition of homocitrate synthase, an enzyme involved in the formation of α-aminoadipic acid (DEMAIN and MASUREKAR, 1974). Lysine auxotrophs of *P. chrysogenum* blocked before α-aminoadipate failed to make benzylpenicillin when grown in the presence of lysine unless α-aminoadipic acid was added (GOULDEN and CHATTAWAY, 1968). These facts suggested that an intermediate containing an α-aminoadipic acid residue was involved in the biosynthesis of penicillins with non-polar side chains.

Whether α-aminoadipic acid has a role in the biosynthesis of all the penicillins and cephalosporins that can be produced by the *Cephalosporium* type of fermentation must be questioned since the findings that cephalosporins having glutaryl side chains, in addition to others with an α-aminoadipyl side chain, are produced by *C. chrysogenum* and that a penicillin with a 6-(5-hydroxy-n-valeryl) side chain is produced by a *Paecilomyces* sp. together with penicillin N and cephalosporin C (KITANO et al., 1976a, b). It has not been established whether these new compounds are derived from a normal cephalosporin and from penicillin N respectively, or from precursors of these antibiotics, or whether they are produced without the involvement of α-aminoadipic acid.

The production of a penicillin with a D-S-carboxy-methyl-cysteine side chain by a mutant of *C. acremonium* auxotrophic for lysine and fed with L-S-carboxymethylcysteine (TROONEN et al., 1976) shows that the specificity of the enzymes involved in the incorporation of an α-aminoadipyl side chain is not absolute. Nevertheless, in the mutant concerned, normal cephalosporins were produced on addition of α-aminoadipic acid to the growth medium, although they were not detected when L-S-carboxymethylcysteine was added alone.

B. Valine

L-Valine is the precursor of the D-penicillamine fragment of penicillins (STEVENS et al., 1956; ARNSTEIN and CLUBB, 1957; WARREN et al., 1967) and is incorporated into the αβ-dehydrovaline fragment of cephalosporin C (TROWN et al., 1963). D-Valine was found to be a poorer precursor than L-valine in low-yielding strains of *P. chrysogenum* (ARNSTEIN and MARGREITER, 1958) and *C. acremonium* (TROWN et al., 1963). With a high-producing strain of *P. chrysogenum* both isomers were incorporated into benzylpenicillin to a similar extent (BYCROFT et al., 1975b).

Studies of the incorporation of chirally labelled [^{13}C]valines (IX) into penicillin N and cephalosporin C by *C. acremonium* and into phenoxymethylpenicillin by *P. chrysogenum* have established that the ^{13}C of (2S, 3S)-[4-^{13}C]valine was incorporated into the 2α-methyl group of penicillin N in *C. acremonium* (KLUENDER et al., 1973) (Fig. 9), and the ^{13}C of (2RS, 3R)-[4-^{13}C]valine was incorporated into the 2β-methyl group of phenoxymethyl penicillin in *P. chrysogenum* (NEUSS et al., 1973). Further, by use of chirally labelled CD_3 valines and mass spectrometric analysis it was shown that all three deuterium atoms of each methyl group of valine were incorporated into penicillin N (KLUENDER et al., 1974). Hence, incorporation of the chiral isopropyl group of valine into penicillins is stereospecific and occurs with retention of configuration. Similarly, the ^{13}C of (2S, 3S)-[4-^{13}C]valine was incorporated exclusively into the exocyclic methylene of cephalosporin C at C-17 and that of (2RS, 3R)-[4-^{13}C]valine into the C-2 of cephalosporins (KLUENDER et al., 1973). Two deuterium atoms from (3S)-[4,4,4-$^{2}H_3$]valine and from 3R-[4,4,4-$^{2}H_3$]valine were incorporated into the exocyclic methylene and into the C-2 position of cephalosporin C, respectively (KLUENDER et al., 1974).

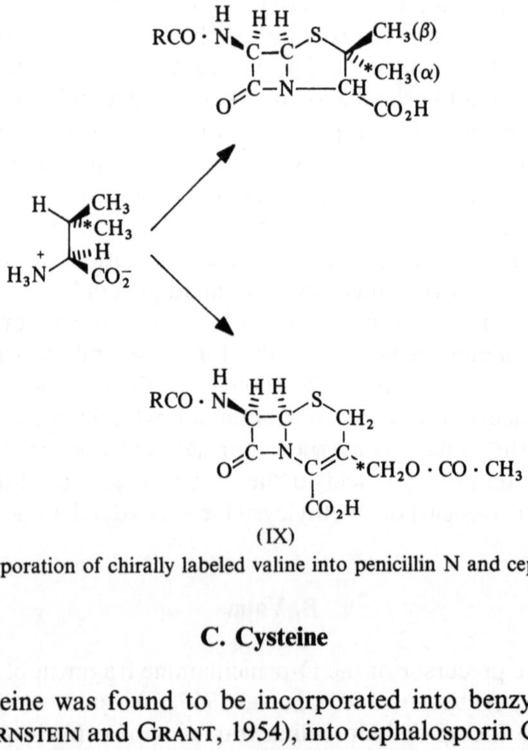

(IX)

Fig. 9. Incorporation of chirally labeled valine into penicillin N and cephalosporin C

C. Cysteine

Labeled cysteine was found to be incorporated into benzylpenicillin in *P. chrysogenum* (ARNSTEIN and GRANT, 1954), into cephalosporin C in *C. acremonium* (TROWN et al., 1963), and into cephamycin C in *S. clavuligerus* (WHITNEY et al., 1972). ARNSTEIN and CRAWHALL (1957) found that the ^{3}H from DL-[2,2'-^{3}H]cysteine and half of the ^{3}H from DL-[3,3'-$^{3}H_2$]cysteine was incorporated into the C-6 and C-5, respectively, of benzylpenicillin and concluded that β-lactam ring formation did not involve an $\alpha\beta$-dehydrocysteine-containing intermediate. This conclusion has been confirmed by recent work (BYCROFT et al., 1975a; MORECOMBE and YOUNG, 1975). The stereochemistry of L-cysteine incorporation into benzylpenicillin in *P. chrysogenum* has been determined by experiments with (2RS, 2'RS, 3R, 3'R)-3, 3'-$^{3}H_2$]cystine and (2RS, 2'RS, 3S, 3'S)-[3,3'-$^{3}H_2$]cystine in one case (ABERHART et al., 1975) and (2R, 3S)-[U-^{14}C, 3-$^{3}H_1$]cysteine and (2R, 3R)-[U-^{14}C, 2,3-$^{3}H_2$]cysteine in another (YOUNG et al., 1977). These experiments have shown that there is loss of the 3-*pro*-S and

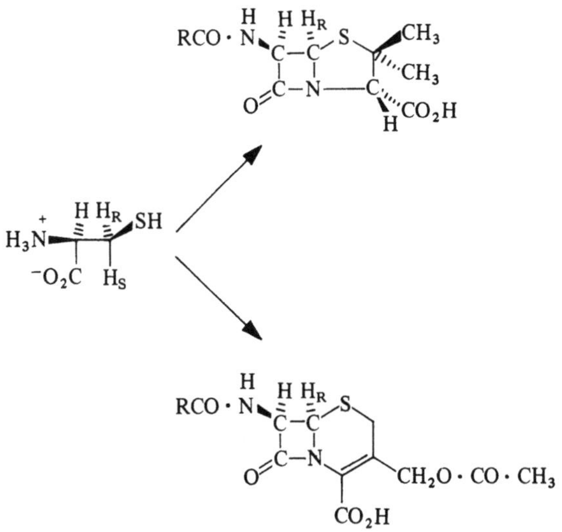

(X)

Fig. 10. Incorporation of chirally labeled cysteine into benzylpenicillin and cephalosporin C

retention of the 3-*pro*-R hydrogen of cysteine and, therefore retention of configuration at C-5 during β-lactam ring formation (Fig. 10).

Experiments with (2R, 3S)-[U-^{14}C, 3-^{3}H]cysteine HCl and (2R, 3R)-[U-^{14}C, 2,3-$^{3}H_2$]cysteine HCl (X) in suspensions of *C. acremonium* and degradation of the labeled cephalosporin C to δ-(D-α-aminoadipyl-[1-^{14}C]glycine (JEFFERY et al., 1960) have indicated that the 3-*pro*-R hydrogen is also predominantly incorporated at C-6 of the cephalosporin ring system (HUDDLESTON et al., 1978) (Fig. 10).

III. Methionine and the Sulphur Supply

Methionine was found to act as a stimulant of penicillin N and cephalosporin C production in *C. acremonium* by MILLER et al. (1956), the D-isomer being more effective than the L-isomer, but the precise nature of its action has not yet been established. In contrast, methionine did not stimulate the production of benzylpenicillin by *P. chrysogenum*. In a study of the effect of methionine on some 42 cephalosporin-producing fungi, KITANO (1977) found that cephalosporin production was markedly stimulated by methionine in some strains of *Cephalosporium* and *Emericellopsis*, but that no stimulation was observed in other strains of these two genera, or in certain strains of *Paecilomyces, Arachnomyces, Anixiopsis*, and *Spiroidium*. Moreover, methionine inhibited the production of cephalosporins by certain strains of all these genera with the exception of *Anixiopsis*. D'AMATO and PISANO (1976) also found that cephalosporin production by *Paecilomyces persicinus* was inihibited by methionine.

KITANO (1977) tested the effect of cysteine, S-methylcysteine, and sodium sulfate, in addition to methionine, on cephalosporin production. Cysteine stimulated production by some strains, inhibited it by others, and in yet others had no effect. There was no correspondence between the strains in which production was affected by cysteine and methionine respectively, but in the strains affected by S-methyl-cysteine production was affected similarly by methionine.

Sodium sulfate inhibited cephalosporin production by some strains, but was not found to stimulate it significantly in any of the strains tested. It seems clear, therefore, that the role of methionine and other sulfur-containing compounds in cephalosporin production is complicated and may vary from strain to strain. In the species most studied, *C. acremonium,* methionine can act as the supplier of sulfur (CALTRIDER and NISS, 1966), but its stimulatory effect on cephalosporin C production can be mimicked in defined media by the non-sulfur-containing, norleucine, with which it is isosteric (DEMAIN et al., 1963). This suggested that methionine exerted a regulatory function by affecting an enzyme involved in cephalosporin biosynthesis (DREW and DEMAIN, 1973; DEMAIN, 1974).

IV. α-Aminoadipylcysteinyl Peptides

Following the isolation of penicillin N (ABRAHAM et al., 1954), the finding that δ-(α-aminodipyl) cysteinylvaline (ACV) was present in minute quantities in *P. chrysogenum* (ARNSTEIN and MORRIS, 1960), was a significant development in our understanding of penicillin and cephalosporin biosynthesis. LODER and ABRAHAM (1971) subsequently isolated a tripeptide from the mycelium of *C. acremonium* and showed that it was δ-(L-α-aminoadipyl)-L-cysteinyl-D-valine; and more recently, the configuration of the tripeptide from *P. chrysogenum* has also been found to be LLD (ADRIAENS et al., 1975; FAWCETT et al., 1976; CHAN et al., 1976). The dimer of the LLD tripeptide and the disulfide of this tripeptide and methanethiol have been found in the culture filtrates (KANZAKI et al., 1974b) of antibiotic-negative mutants of *C. acremonium.*

It has been established that an αβ-dehydrovalinyl intermediate is not involved in LLD-tripeptide formation from L-valine in *C. acremonium* (HUANG et al., 1975) and experiments with a cell-free system have indicated that the peptide is synthesized from δ-(L-α-aminoadipyl)-L-cysteine and valine (LODER and ABRAHAM, 1971).

In addition to this tripeptide, two related peptides were identified in *C. acremonium* (LODER and ABRAHAM, 1971). Both were tetrapeptides and contained glycine. One also contained α-aminoadipic acid, cysteine and valine, but in the other, the valine was replaced by β-hydroxyvaline.

An analysis of the peptides present in the mycelium of the prokaryotic *S. lipmanii* and *S. clavuligerus* has revealed a pattern different from that of the eukaryotes (FAWCETT et al., 1979). After oxidation of the cysteine-containing peptides with performic acid and electrophoresis on paper at pH 1.8 the following sulfonic acids were identified: δ-(α-aminoadipyl)cysteicylvaline, δ-(α-aminoadipyl) cysteic acid, γ-glutamylcysteic acid, cysteic acid, and penicillaminic acid. Glutathione and the tetrapeptides found in *C. acremonium* (LODER and ABRAHAM, 1971) were not present in amounts detectable by ninhydrin in either species.

V. Tripeptide Incorporation into Penicillin

The ACV tripeptide, with its structural relationship to isopenicillin N and penicillin N, seemed to be a likely intermediate in penicillin and cephalosporin biosynthesis. On feeding [^{14}C]valine to *C. acremonium*, the tripeptide was rapidly labeled at a time when antibiotic production was about to begin (WARREN et al., 1967). LEMKE and NASH (1972), using a mutant of *C. acremonium* auxotrophic for lysine, found that neither the tripeptide nor the antibiotics, penicillin N and cephalosporin C, were synthesized when this mutant was grown in the presence of lysine, but that both the tripeptide and antibiotics were produced on addition of α-aminoadipic acid. These findings were consistent with a role for the tripeptide in β-lactam antibiotic biosynthesis.

Earlier attempts to determine whether the tripeptide was a precursor of penicillin N were frustrated because the peptide was not taken up by mycelial cells of *C. acremonium* and by the difficulty of obtaining cell-free extracts in which any synthesis of antibiotic could be detected. However, in a system prepared by the lysis of protoplasts of *C. acremonium* (FAWCETT et al., 1973) ^{3}H was found to be incorporated into a compound which behaved like penicillin N or isopenicillin N from the LLD tripeptide labeled in either the methyl groups or in the α position of its valine residue. This incorporation was specific for the LLD isomer, since ^{3}H was not incorporated from the LLL and DLD tripeptides, at least to a comparable extent (FAWCETT et al., 1976). More recently, by use of LLD tripeptide labeled in both its α-aminoadipic acid and valine residues, it has been shown that ring closure takes place without hydrolysis of the tripeptide and that the immediate product of the reaction is isopenicillin N (O'SULLIVAN et al., 1979b) Using a microbiological assay KONOMI et al. (1979) also concluded that isopenicillin N was the first product of cyclization of the LLD-tripeptide.

In *S. clavuligerus* the intact tripeptide was not taken up by the mycelium, nor was it hydrolysed at the cell surface (O'SULLIVAN and ABRAHAM, 1979). However, the organism was highly susceptible to disruption by ultrasonic treatment and brief sonication yielded an extract in which ^{3}H from the LLD tripeptide labeled in the methyl groups of its valine residue was incorporated into a substance which yielded penicillaminic acid upon performic acid oxidation. Thus, in this extract, as in that from protoplasts of *C. acremonium*, the LLD tripeptide appeared to function as a precursor of the penicillin ring system.

VI. Isopenicillin N and 6-APA

Enzymes which are acylases, or transacylases, or both, can be considered in relation to the terminal stages of penicillin biosynthesis in the *Penicillium* type of fermentation. Members of a family of penicillin acylases catalyse a reversible removal of N-acyl groups from biosynthetic penicillins with non-polar side chains to yield 6-APA. Enzymes of this type, which are found in a variety of bacteria and fungi, have been reported not to hydrolyze penicillin N or isopenicillin N. Benzylpenicillin is a better substrate than phenoxymethylpenicillin for the bacterial acylases but the reverse is true for the enzymes from fungi (HAMILTON-MILLER, 1966).

Acyl transferases which transfer an acyl group from one penicillin with a non-polar side chain to another, or from an acyl coenzyme A to 6-APA, have been found in *Penicillia* (PRUESS and JOHNSON, 1967; GATENBECK and BRUNSBERG, 1968; BRUNNER et al., 1968; FAWCETT et al., 1975) and the levels of these enzymes are said to be increased in high-yielding mutants (VANDAMME, 1977).

SPENCER and MAUNG (1970) obtained an enzyme preparation from *P. chrysogenum* which showed the following activities: penicillin acyltransferase, 6-APA acyltransferase, penicillin acylase, and phenylacetyl-Co A hydrolase. This preparation gave a single band after disc gel electrophoresis. All four activities were reported to show similar stability to pH and temperature, to be inhibited by N-ethylmaleimide and to be produced at the same stage of the fermentation. On the other hand, an acyl transferase from *P. chrysogenum* described by GATENBECK and BRUNSBERG (1968) was said to have no penicillin acylase activity.

Whilst these studies indicated that 6-APA might have a role in the biosynthesis of benzylpenicillin by *P. chrysogenum,* they did not reveal a function for isopenicillin N. However, in a subsequent experiment with a crude extract of *P. chrysogenum,* ^{14}C from phenylacetyl-Co A was reported to be incorporated into benzylpenicillin in the presence of isopenicillin N (LODER, 1972). That isopenicillin N, as well as 6-APA, was a substrate for an acyl transferase was later confirmed by labeling these compounds with ^{3}H in the 2β-methyl group of the ring system. In both cases, ^{3}H was incorporated by the extract into benzylpenicillin (FAWCETT et al., 1975). Later, it was found that 6-APA and isopenicillin N acyltransferase activities in *P. chrysogenum* did not separate during a purification process involving ammonium sulfate fractionation, gel filtration, and chromatography on DEAE cellulose (FISHER and ABRAHAM, 1979).

These results are consistent with a model for penicillin biosynthesis in which isopenicillin N is a precursor of penicillins with non-polar side chains, but it is not yet clear whether free 6-APA is an intermediate in the reaction concerned.

VII. Final Stages of Cephalosporin Biosynthesis

Cephalosporins are known to be derived from L-α-aminoadipic acid, L-cysteine, and L-valine in both eukaryotes and prokaryotes. As with penicillin biosynthesis, the tripeptide, δ-(L-α-aminoadipyl)-L-cysteinyl-D-valine, appears to be involved. HUANG et al. (1975) fed (2S, 3S)-valine-^{15}N, 3-methyl-d_3 to washed cells of *C. acremonium* and found that the skeleton of the molecule was incorporated intact into penicillin N and cephalosporin C. The isotopic ratios of the valinyl moieties in the two antibiotics were very similar, despite considerable deamination of the valine. This finding is consistent with the view that both penicillin N and cephalosporin C are derived from a common tripeptide.

There are two hypothetical pathways from the tripeptide to cephalosporins: the first is branched, the cephalosporin branch involving more oxidative steps than the penicillin branch, while in the second penicillin N is a precursor of cephalosporin C. A branched pathway appeared to be consistent with the finding that D-valine inhibited penicillin N production but not cephalosporin production (WARREN et al., 1967). However, the apparent failure to find mutants that were blocked in penicillin N production but could synthesize cephalosporins, although mutants blocked only in cephalosporin production could be isolated, was readily explicable if penicillin N were a precursor of the cephalosporins (LEMKE and NASH, 1972).

KOHSAKA and DEMAIN (1976) reported that a substance with cephalosporin-like properties was formed in a protoplast lysate system from *C. acremonium* containing penicillin N. This substance was not formed in the presence of a penicillinase type of β-lactamase and it could be destroyed by a cephalosporinase type of β-lactamase. These findings suggested that penicillin N was indeed converted to a cephalosporin.

Certain mutants of *C. acremonium* which failed to produce cephalosporin C were found to accumulate deacetylcephalosporin C in the culture filtrate (FUJISAWA et al., 1975b). Since there was no difference in the cephalosporin C acetyl hydrolase activity between the parents and the mutant, it was unlikely that deacetylcephalosporin C was a product of hydrolysis of cephalosporin C and, indeed, cephalosporin C was not detected at any stage of the fermentation (FUJISAWA et al., 1973). In addition, the failure to detect an acetyl Co A deacetylcephalosporin C acetyl transferase in cephalosporin C negative mutants, although it was present in the parent, indicated that deacetylcephalosporin C was a precursor of cephalosporin C.

An extract obtained from *Streptomyces clavuligerus* by ultrasonic treatment has been found to transfer a carbamoyl group from carbamoyl phosphate to the 3-hydroxymethyl group of deacetyl-7α-methoxycephalosporin C (BREWER et al., 1977). The product of this reaction is cephamycin C (IV, $R = OCH_3$; $R' = NH_2$).

Deacetoxycephalosporin C is present in the fermentations of a wide range of fungi and in *S. lipmanii* and *S. clavuligerus* (HIGGENS et al., 1974; KITANO et al., 1974). That it was a precursor of cephalosporin C seemed likely when it was found to be produced by mutants of *C. acremonium* which lacked the ability to synthesize deacetylcephalosporin C and cephalosporin C (FUJISAWA et al., 1975a; QUEENER et al., 1974; LIERSCH et al., 1976). The utilization of molecular oxygen in cephalosporin C biosynthesis was established by the production of the antibiotic in the presence of ^{18}O. Analysis of the dimethyl ester of N-acetylcephalosporin C by mass spectrometry showed that one atom of ^{18}O had been incorporated at the exocyclic methylene (STEVENS et al., 1975). Other evidence for the involvement of molecular oxygen was presented by LIERSCH et al. (1976) who reported that extracts of *C. acremonium* contained a hydroxylase and acetyl transferase that converted deacetoxycephalosporin C to cephalosporin C. A further analysis of the hydroxylation, which was followed by measurement of the incorporation of ^3H from [3-methyl-^3H]deacetoxycephalosporin C into deacetylcephalosporin C, has shown that the enzyme concerned, in both *C. acremonium* and *S. clavuligerus,* is a dioxygenase and requires 2-oxoglutarate, ascorbate, and Fe^{2+} for activity (TURNER et al., 1978).

It is clear, therefore, that the final steps in cephalosporin C biosynthesis proceed from deacetoxycephalosporin C through deacetylcephalosporin C to cephalosporin C.

VIII. Biosynthesis of 7α-Methoxycephalosporins

The 7α-methoxycephalosporins, which are produced by some species of *Streptomyces,* are derived from α-aminoadipic acid, cysteine, and valine, and the methyl group of methionine provides the methyl of their methoxyl group (WHITNEY et al., 1972).

The oxygen in the 7α-methoxyl group of cephamycin C was shown to be derived from molecular oxygen (O'SULLIVAN et al., 1979a) Cephamycin C produced by aqueous suspensions of *S. clavuligerus* in the presence of $^{18}O_2$ was converted to its N-acetyl dimethyl ester. Chemical ionization mass spectrometry of the ester showed that one atom of $^{18}O_2$ was incorporated into the methoxyl group as well as one into the group attached to the exocyclic methylene at C-3.

The incorporation of a 7α-methoxyl group into cephalosporin C, or the carbamoyl derivative of deacetylcephalosporin C, has been shown to occur in cell-free extracts of *S. clavuligerus* when S-adenosylmethionine is used as a methyl donor and when the cofactors α-oxogluterate, ferrous ion, and reducing agents are present (O'SULLIVAN and ABRAHAM, 1980). The reaction presumably occurs in two steps, an initial hydroxylation followed by methyl transfer.

IX. Mechanisms of Ring Closure

The mechanisms by which the bicyclic ring systems of penicillins and cephalosporins are formed have still to be determined. No intermediate between the LLD tripeptide and isopenicillin N has yet been found and it is not known whether the β-lactam is the first ring to be formed. Nevertheless, the information that is now available about the incorporation of valine and cysteine into the penicillin and cephalosporin ring systems makes some hypotheses untenable and raises problems with respect to others.

The formation of the penicillin thiazolidine ring was long thought to involve the formation of a dehydrovaline residue and the addition of the thiol of the cysteine residue to the double bond (ARNSTEIN and CRAWHALL, 1957; BIRCH and SMITH, 1958). But the finding that tritium in the α-position of the valine residue in the LLD tripeptide was retained when the tripeptide was incorporated into a penicillin was not consistent with this hypothesis (FAWCETT et al., 1976). Moreover, no double bond was formed between the carbon atoms of the valine isopropyl group since this group was incorporated into penicillin N intact.

The isolation from *C. acremonium* of minute amounts of a tetrapeptide related to the LLD tripeptide, but containing a β-hydroxyvaline residue in place of a valine residue, raised the question whether the mechanism of ring closure involved oxygenation of a valine residue at C-3 and subsequent displacement of oxygen by sulfur (LODER and ABRAHAM, 1971). However, for this mechanism to be clearly consistent with the fact that the valine isopropyl group is incorporated into penicillin with retention of configuration it would be necessary to postulate two successive inversions at C-3. BALDWIN and WAN (1979) have pointed out that hydroxylation catalysed by certain enzymes may involve a carbon radical intermediate (GROVES et al., 1978). They have suggested that the generation of a carbon radical at C-3 of the tripeptide valine residue is followed by its intramolecular trapping by a peptide disulfide linkage. If the trapping were faster than rotation of the carbon radical the configuration of the isopropyl would be retained during formation of the thiazolidine ring.

It is now certain that the formation of the penicillin β-lactam ring does not involve an αβ-dehydrocysteine intermediate. The mechanisms postulated by ARNSTEIN and CRAWHALL (1957) for the formation of this ring involved the oxidation of a cysteine thiol group to a thioaldehyde and subsequent attack of an amide nitrogen on the resulting electrophilic centre at the cysteine C-3. Since the 3-*pro*-S hydrogen is lost during the incorporation of cysteine into penicillin (YOUNG et al., 1977; ABERHART et al., 1975; HUDDLESTON et al., 1978) the stereochemistry would differ from that in the enzymic oxidation of alcohols to aldehydes, in which the hydrogen lost is *pro*-R. Moreover, an attempt to demonstrate the reaction with a chemical model was unsuccessful (CHENEY et al., 1974). An inversion at C-3 would be expected to occur (BRUCE and KIRBY, 1968; HANSON et al., 1968), although in fact the configuration at this center is retained. An alternative suggestion (BIRCH and SMITH, 1958) is that oxidation at the amide nitrogen renders the latter susceptible to attack by a negatively charged C-3 of a cysteine residue. Ring closure has been shown to occur in a model hydroxamate sulphone upon treatment with potassium t-butoxide (SCOTT et al., 1976).

In the formation of the dihydrothiazine ring of the cephalosporins only one hydrogen atom is lost from the methyl group of 2-S, 3-*pro*-R valine during the establishment of the carbon-sulfur bond. It follows that oxidation of a valine methyl group to the level of an aldehyde does not occur during ring closure and that a Δ-2 cephalosporin is unlikely to be an intermediate in the reaction (KLUENDER et al., 1974). Whether hydroxylation of the methyl group of a valine residue occurs during the formation of deacetoxycephalosporin C remains to be investigated.

X. Genetic Aspects of Biosynthesis

It has already been mentioned that the use of blocked mutants of *P. chrysogenum* and *C. acremonium* has helped to throw light on the role of α-aminoadipic acid in the biosynthesis of benzylpenicillin and on the late steps in the biosynthesis of cephalosporin C (GOULDEN and CHATTAWAY, 1968; FUJISAWA et al., 1975a, b; QUEENER et al., 1974; LIERSCH et al., 1976). But it has been pointed out that the potential for acquiring genetic knowledge relating to antibiotic production is far greater than that so far obtained and applied (HOPWOOD and MERRICK, 1977).

The discovery of the parasexual cycle in *P. chrysogenum* (PONTECORVO and SERMONTI, 1953) raised the hope that its use would lead to rational breeding programs, resulting in higher yields of penicillin, as well as to a clearer understanding of the genetics of penicillin production. Nevertheless, industrial strains of *P. chrysogenum* and *C. acremonium* have been largely derived by mutation and selection and the contribution of formal genetics has not so far been extensive. The behavior of heterokaryons has indicated that penicillin production in *P. chrysogenum* is largely under the control of the nucleus (SERMONTI, 1959a; MACDONALD et al., 1963a). The genetic analysis of high-titer industrial strains is impeded by an inadequate recovery of recombinants among segregants from diploids (MACDONALD et al., 1965), and by somatic instability (ELANDER, 1967), although these difficulties can be diminished by the selection of suitable parental strains (BALL, 1971).

Aspergillus nidulans has a sexual as well as a parasexual cycle and its formal genetics are well established (PONTECORVO et al., 1953), but it produces only low levels of penicillin. Unlike *P. chrysogenum,* where mutations that increase penicillin titer are normally recessive (SERMONTI, 1959b; MACDONALD et al., 1963b), *A. nidulans* may yield mutants that are recessive, dominant, or semidominant (DITCHBURN et al., 1976). In a study of wild type isolates of *A. nidulans,* it was found that an additive increase in penicillin titer could be achieved by hybridization and selection (MERRICK, 1975).

C. acremonium has been examined genetically by parasexual techniques (NÜESCH et al., 1973), but difficulty was found in forming and handling heterokaryons and diploids. *Emericillopsis* has a sexual cycle and has been used to study the genetics of penicillin N production (FANTINI, 1962); heterokaryosis was infrequent and meiotic recombination rare. One approach to the problem of low heterokaryon formation involves the use of cell protoplasts. Intraspecific fusion of protoplasts of *A. nidulans* auxotrophs (FERENCZY et al., 1975) and of *Penicillium* sp and *C. acremonium* (ANNÉ and PEBERDY, 1976) led to high heterokaryon formation, and interspecific hybrid formation between *P. chrysogenum* and *P. roquefortii* was shown to occur (ANNÉ et al., 1976). HAMLYN and BALL (1979) hybridized closely related and divergent strains of *C. acremonium* by protoplast fusion. They isolated a recombinant which showed improved cephalosporin C production, growth rate, and sporulation when compared with its highest titer parent.

The discovery of viruses containing double-stranded RNA in *P. chrysogenum* (BANKS et al., 1969) and in *C. acremonium* (DAY and ELLIS, 1971) was followed by a report of direct correlation between viral titer and penicillin yield in *P. chrysogenum* (BOBKOVA et al., 1975). The results of other investigations, however, suggest that viruses have no direct role in the synthesis of β-lactam antibiotics (LEMKE et al., 1973).

Methods for the genetic analysis of *Streptomyces* sp are well established (HOPWOOD et al., 1973) and preliminary work with cephamycin producers suggest that *S. clavuligerus* is a suitable organism for genetic mapping and possibly for strain improvement through genetic recombination (AHARONOWITZ and DEMAIN, 1977; KIRBY, 1978).

XI. Conclusion

Despite certain remaining gaps in our knowledge, our view of the biosynthetic pathway to penicillin and cephalosporins is now substantially clearer than it was in 1967 when the previous volume on the biosynthesis of antibiotics appeared. Figure 11 gives a summary of the pathway as we now see it. Greater understanding will be possible when more active cell-free systems have been obtained, when some of the key enzymes have been purified, and when further compounds have been tested on these systems as intermediates. Further progress could be made by the production of permeabilized cells which would allow the entry of intermediates that are not transported into normal cells (MIOZZARI et al., 1978), or by the fusion of cell protoplasts with liposomes in which intermediates

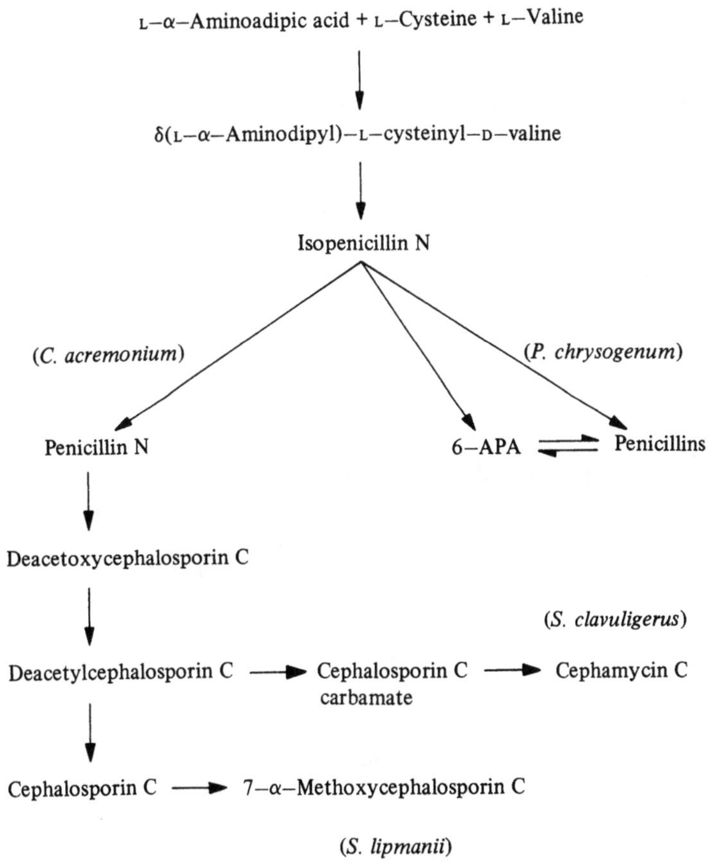

Fig. 11. Possible pathways to penicillins and cephalosporins

have been enclosed (BANGHAM, 1978). More knowledge of the individual steps in the biosynthetic pathways could facilitate the elucidation of the unknown biochemical and genetic factors on which the regulation of biosynthesis depends.

XII. Biosynthesis of Thienamycin, Clavulanic Acid, and Nocardicin

Very little has been revealed about the biosynthesis of thienamycin (Fig. 6, VI) and the olivanic acids (Fig. 7, VII), although it has been reported that thienamycin is derived from acetate and L-glutamate (ALBERS-SCHÖNBERG et al., 1976) and the exocyclic sulfur is presumably supplied by cysteine, or cysteamine.

ELSON and OLIVER (1978) recently described the use of ^{13}C-labeled compounds to study the origins of the carbon skeleton of clavulanic acid (V). 1,3-$^{13}C_2$-glycerol was added to *Streptomyces clavuligerus* fermentations and the clavulanic acid produced was isolated as the benzyl ester and analysed by ^{13}C NMR spectroscopy. It was found that the carbon of the glycerol was incorporated intact into the three carbons of the β-lactam ring. Similarly, by feeding [1-^{13}C]acetate, [2-^{13}C]acetate, and [1,2-^{13}C]acetate it was concluded that the remaining five carbons of clavulanic acid were probably derived from α-oxoglutarate. It thus seems unlikely that a tripeptide such as α-aminoadipylserinylnorvaline is involved in the biosynthesis of clavulanic acid, although the test organism also produces penicillin N and cephalosporins.

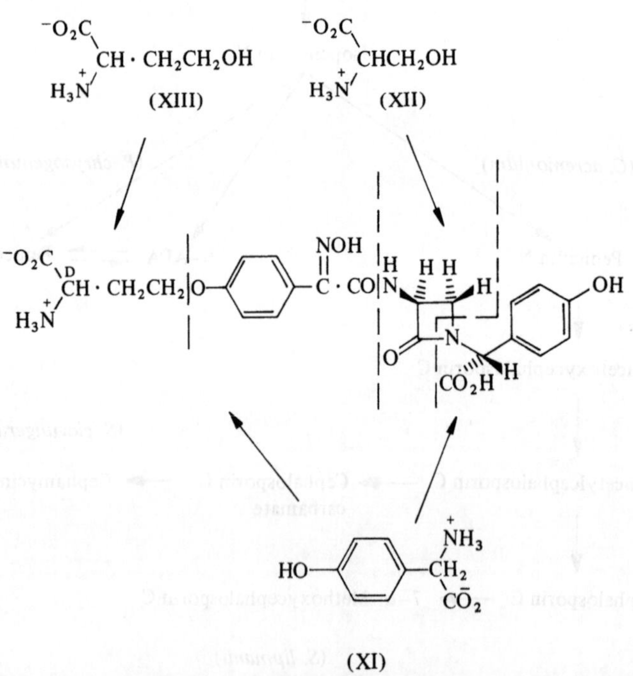

Fig. 12. Biosynthetic origin of nocardicin A

HOSODA et al. (1977) studied the incorporation of L-tyrosine, L-serine-[U-^{14}C], and L-[U-^{14}C]-homoserine into nocardicin A (VIII) by cultures of *N. uniformis* in complex media. The distribution of radioactivity in the product was determined after enzymic hydrolysis, alkali hydrolysis, and reductive degradation. From an analysis of the degradation products it was concluded that radioactivity in the two benzene rings was derived from tyrosine, that radioactivity from serine enters the β-lactam ring only, and that the 3-amino-3-carboxypropoxy moiety is derived from homoserine. A large number of amino acids were tested for their effect on antibiotic production during the fermentation, and tyrosine, shikimic acid, the p-hydroxyphenyl derivatives of pyruvic acid, glyoxylic acid and glycine, and DL-p-hydroxymandelic acid were all found to stimulate. Both the D- and L-forms of tyrosine were effective, but only the L-form of p-hydroxyphenylglycine. The results suggested that nocardicin A was derived from 2 moles of L-p-hydroxyphenylglycine (XI) and one mole each of L-serine (XII) and L-homoserine (XIII) (Fig. 12). There was no indication of peptide intermediates in this study of nocardicin A biosynthesis and it thus remains unclear to what extent the pathway is analogous to the biosynthesis of penicillins and cephalosporins.

References

Aberhart DJ, Lin LJ, Chu JY-R (1975) Studies on the biosynthesis of β-lactam antibiotics. II. Synthesis and incorporation into penicillin G, of (2RS, 2′RS, 3R, 3′R)−[3,3′-$^3H_2$]−cystine and (2RS, 2′RS, 3S, 3′S)−[3,3′-$^3H_2$]cystine. J Chem Soc Perkin I:2517–2523

Abraham EP, Newton GGF, Hale CW (1954) Purification and some properties of cephalosporin N, a new penicillin. Biochem J 58:94–102

Adriaens P, Meesschaert B, Wuyts W, Vanderhaeghe H, Eyssen H (1975) Presence of δ-(L-α-aminoadipyl)-L-cysteinyl-D-valine in fermentations of *Penicillium chrysogenum*. Antimicrob Agents Chemother 8:638–642

Aharonowitz Y, Demain AL (1977) Genetic recombination in the cephamycin producer *Streptomyces clavuligerus*. Eur J Appl Microbiol 4:125–130

Albers-Schönberg G, Arison BH, Kaczka E, Kahan FM, Kahan JS, Lago B, Maiese WM, Rhodes RE, Smith JL (1976) Thienamycin. A new β-lactam antibiotic. III. Structure, determination and biosynthetic data. Abstr 229, 16th Intersci Conf Antimicrob Agents Chemother, Chicago Ill

Anné J, Peberdy JF (1976) Induced fusion of fungal protoplasts following treatment with polyethylene glycol. J Gen Microbiol 92:413–417

Anné J, Eyssen H, DeSomer P (1976) Somatic hybridisation of *Penicillium roquefortii* with *P. chrysogenum* after protoplast fusion. Nature (London) 262:719–721

Aoki H, Sakai H, Kohsaka M, Konomi T, Hosoda J, Kubochi Y, Iguchi E, Imanaka H (1976) Nocardicin A, a new monocyclic β-lactam antibiotic. I. Discovery, isolation and characterization. J Antibiot 29:492–500

Arnstein HRV, Clubb ME (1957) The biosynthesis of penicillin. 5. Comparison of valine and hydroxyvaline as penicillin precursors. Biochem J 65:618–627

Arnstein HRV, Crawhall JC (1957) The biosynthesis of penicillin. 6. A study of the mechanism of the formation of the thiazolidine-β-lactam rings, using tritium-labelled cystine. Biochem J 67:180–187

Arnstein HRV, Grant PT (1954) The biosynthesis of penicillin. I. The incorporation of some amino acids into penicillin. Biochem J 57:353–359

Arnstein HRV, Margreiter H (1958) The biosynthesis of penicillin. 7. Further experiments on the utilization of L- and D-valine and the effect of cysteine and valine analogues on penicillin biosynthesis. Biochem J 68:339–348

Arnstein HRV, Morris D (1960) The structure of a peptide, containing α-aminoadipic acid, cystine and valine, present in the mycelium of *Penicillium chrysogenum*. Biochem J 76:357–361

Baldwin JE, Wan TS (1979) Penicillin biosynthesis. A model for carbon-sulphur bond formation. J Chem Soc Chem Commun 79:249–250

Ball C (1971) Haploidization analysis in *Penicillium chrysogenum*. J Gen Microbiol 66:63–69

Bangham AD (1978) Properties and uses of lipid vesicles: an overview. Ann NY Acad Sci 308:2–7

Banks GT, Buck KW, Chain EB, Darbyshire JE, Himmelweit F (1969) Virus-like particles in penicillin producing strains of *Penicillium chrysogenum*. Nature (London) 223:89–90

Birch AJ, Smith H (1958) Oxidative formation of biologically active compounds from peptides. In: Wolstenholme GEW, O'Conner CM (eds) Amino acids and peptides with antimetabolic activity, pp 247–257. Churchill, London

Bobkova AF, Velikodvorskaya GA, Tikhonenko GI, Lebed ES, Egorov AA, Bartoshevich YE (1975) Viruses infective for bacteria in strains of *Penicillium chrysogenum* with various antibiotic activity. Antibiotiki 7:600–606

Brewer SJ, Boyle TT, Turner MK (1977) The carbamoylation of the 3-hydroxymethyl group of 7α-methoxy-7β-(5-D-aminoadipamido)-3-hydroxymethyl-ceph-3-em-4-carboxylic acid (des-acetyl-7α-methoxy-cephalosporin C) by homogenates of *Streptomyces clavuligerus*. Biochem Soc Trans 5:1026–1029

Brown AG, Butterworth D, Cole M, Hanscomb G, Hood JD, Reading C, Rolinson GN (1976) Naturally-occurring β-lactamase inhibitors with antibacterial activity. J Antibiot 29:668–669

Brown AG, Corbett DF, Eglington AJ, Howarth TT (1977) Structures of olivanic acid derivatives MM 4550 and MM 13902; two new, fused β-lactam isolated from *Streptomyces olivaceus*. J Chem Soc Chem Commun 523–525

Bruce IT, Kirby GW (1968) Stereochemistry of protonation and hydroxylation in the biosynthesis of norpluvine and lycorine. J Chem Soc Chem Commun 207–208

Brunner R, Röhr M, Zinner M (1968) Zur Biosynthese des Penicillins. Untersuchungen zur enzymatischer Aktivierung von Phenylessigsäure und Phenoxyessigsäure sowie zur Bildung von Penicillin aus 6-Amino-penicillansaure und aktivierter Seitenkettensäure durch Mycelhomogenate und zellfreie Extrakte von *Penicillium chrysogenum*. Hoppe-Seylers Z Physiol Chem 349:95–103

Bycroft BW, Wels CM, Corbett K, Lowe DA (1975a) Incorporation of [α-^{2}H]- and [α-^{3}H]-L-Cystine into Penicillin G and the location of the label using isotope exchange and ^{2}H nuclear magnetic resonance. J Chem Soc Chem Comm 123–125

Bycroft BW, Wels CM, Corbett K, Maloney AP, Lowe DA (1975b) Biosynthesis of Penicillin G from D- and L-[^{14}C]- and [α-^{3}H]-valine. J Chem Soc Chem Comm 923–924

Caltrider PG, Niss HF (1966) Role of methionine in cephalosporin synthesis. Appl Microbiol 14:746–753

Chan JA, Huang F-C, Sih CJ (1976) The absolute configuration of the amino acids in δ-(α-aminoadipyl) cysteinylvaline from *Penicillium chrysogenum*. Biochemistry 15:177–180

Cheney J, Moores CJ, Raleigh JA, Scott AI, Young DW (1974) Synthesis and reactions of α-thioformyl dipeptides, possible biogenetic precursors of penicillin. J Chem Soc Perkin I:986–998

D'Amato RF, Pisano MA (1976) A chemically defined medium for cephalosporin C production by *Paecilomyces persicinus*. Antonie van Leeuwenhoek 42:299–308

Day LE, Ellis LF (1971) Virus-like particles in *Cephalosporium acremonium*. Appl Microbiol 22:919–920

Demain AL (1974) Biochemistry of penicillin and cephalosporin fermentations. Lloydia 37:147–167

Demain AL, Masurekar PS (1974) Lysine inhibition of in vivo homocitrate synthesis in *Penicillium chrysogenum*. J Gen Microbiol 82:143–151

Demain AL, Newkirk JF, Hendlin D (1963) Effect of methionine, norleucine, and lysine derivatives on cephalosporin C formation in chemically defined media. J Bacteriol 85:339–344

Ditchburn P, Holt G, Macdonald KD (1976) The genetic location of mutations increasing penicillin yield in *Aspergillus nidulans*. Macdonald KD (ed) 2nd Int Symp Genet Ind Microorg, pp 213–227. Academic Press, London New York

Drew SW, Demain AL (1973) Methionine control of cephalosporin C formation. Biotechnol Bioeng 15:743–754

Elander RP (1967) Enhanced penicillin biosynthesis in mutant and recombinant strains of *Penicillium chrysogenum*. Abh d Dtsch Akad Wiss Berlin. Kl Med 2:403–423

Elson SW, Oliver RS (1978) Studies on the biosynthesis of clavulanic acid. I. Incorporation of ^{13}C-labelled precursors. J Antibiot 31:586–592

Fantini AA (1962) Genetics and antibiotic production of *Emericellopsis* species. Genetics 47: 161–177

Fawcett PA, Loder PB, Duncan MJ, Beesley TJ, Abraham EP (1973) Formation and properties of protoplasts from antibiotic-producing strains of *Penicillium chrysogenum* and *Cephalosporium acremonium*. J Gen Microbiol 79:293–309

Fawcett PA, Usher JJ, Abraham EP (1975) Behaviour of tritium-labelled isopenicillin N and 6-aminopenicillanic acid as potential penicillin precursors in an extract of *Penicillium chrysogenum*. Biochem J 151:741–746

Fawcett PA, Usher JJ, Huddleston JA, Bleaney RC, Nisbet JJ, Abraham EP (1976) Synthesis of δ-(α-aminoadipyl)cysteinylvaline and its role in penicillin biosynthesis. Biochem J 157:651–660

Fawcett PA, Kilbride L, O'Sullivan J, Abraham EP (1979) Unpublished experiments

Ferenczy L, Kevei F, Szegedi M (1975) High-frequency fusion of fungal protoplasts. Experientia 31:1028–1030

Fisher A, Abraham EP (1979) Unpublished experiments

Fujisawa Y, Shirafuji H, Kida M, Nara K, Yoneda M, Kanzaki T (1973) New findings on cephalosporin C biosynthesis. Nature (London) 246:154–155

Fujisawa Y, Kitano K, Kanzaki T (1975a) Accumulation of deacetoxycephalosporin C by a mutant of *Cephalosporium acremonium*. Agric Biol Chem 39:2049–2055

Fujisawa Y, Shirafuji H, Kida M, Nara K, Yoneda M, Kanzaki T (1975b) Accumulation of deacetylcephalosporin C by cephalosporin C negative mutants of *Cephalosporium acremonium*. Agric Biol Chem 39:1295–1301

Fujisawa Y, Kitano K, Katamoto K, Nara K, Kanzaki T (1976) Unpublished data (1975) cited by Kanzaki T, Fujisawa Y. Adv Appl Microbiol 20:159–201

Fukase H, Hasegawa T, Hatano K, Iwasaka H, Yoneda M (1976) C-2801X, a new cephamycin-type antibiotic. II. Isolation and characterization. J Antibiot 29:113–120

Gatenbeck S, Brunsberg U (1968) Biosynthesis of penicillins. Isolation of a 6-aminopenicillanic acid acyltransferase from *Penicillium chrysogenum*. Acta Chem Scand 22:1059–1061

Goulden SA, Chattaway FW (1968) Lysine control of α-aminoadipate and penicillin synthesis in *Penicillium chrysogenum*. Biochem J 110:55

Groves JT, McClusky GA, White RE, Coon MJ (1978) Aliphatic hydroxylation by highly purified liver microsomal cytochrome P-450. Evidence for a carbon radical intermediate. Biochem Biophys Res Commun 81:154–160

Hamilton-Miller JMT (1966) Penicillinacylase. Bacteriol Rev 30:761–771

Hamlyn PF, Ball C (1979) Recombination studies with *Cephalosporium acremonium*. In 3rd Int Symp Genet Ind Microorg. Sebek OK, Laskin AI (eds). (1979) American Soc Microbiol, Washington, pp 185–191

Hanson JR, Hough A, White AF (1968) The mevalonoid origin of some hydrogen atoms in the tetracyclic diterpenes. J Chem Soc Chem Commun 467–468

Higgens CE, Kastner RE (1971) *Streptomyces clavuligerus* sp. nov., a β-lactam antibiotic producer. Int J Syst Bacteriol 21:326–331

Higgens CE, Hamill RL, Sands TH, Hoehn MM, Davis NE, Nagarajan R, Boeck LD (1974) The occurrence of deacetoxycephalosporin C in fungi and streptomycetes. J Antibiot 27:298–300

Hopwood DA, Merrick MJ (1977) Genetics of antibiotic production. Bacteriol Rev 41:595–635

Hopwood DA, Chater KF, Dowding JE, Vivian A (1973) Advances in *Streptomyces coelicolor* genetics. Bacteriol Rev 37:371–405

Hosoda J, Tani N, Konomi T, Ohsawa S, Aoki H, Imanaka H (1977) Incorporation of ^{14}C-amino acids into Nocardicin A by growing cells. Agric Biol Chem 41:2007–2012

Huang F-C, Chan JA, Sih CJ, Fawcett P, Abraham EP (1975) The non-participation of α, β-dehydrovalinyl intermediates in the formation of δ-(L-α-aminoadipyl)-L-cysteinyl-D-valine. J Am Chem Soc 97:3858–3859

Huddleston JA, Abraham EP, Young DW, Morecombe DJ, Sen PK (1978) The stereochemistry of β-lactam formation in cephalosporin biosynthesis. Biochem J 169:705–707

Jeffery JDA, Abraham EP, Newton GGF (1960) Further degradation products of cephalosporin C. Isolation and synthesis of 2-(4-amino-4-carboxybutyl)thiazole-4-carboxylic acid. Biochem J 75:216–223

Kahan JS, Kahan FM, Goegelman R, Currie SA, Jackson M, Stapley EO, Miller JW, Miller AK, Hendlin D, Mochales, S, Hernandez S, Woodruff HB (1976) Thienamycin, a new β-lactam antibiotic. I. Discovery and isolation. 16th Intersci Conf Antimicrob Agents Chemother

Kanzaki T, Fukita T, Shirafugi H, Fujisawa Y, Kitano K (1974a) Occurrence of a 3-methylthiomethylcephem derivative in a culture broth of *Cephalosporium* mutant. J Antibiot 27:361–362

Kanzaki T, Shirafuji H, Fujisawa Y, Fukita T, Nara K, Kitano K, Kida M (1974b) New aspects of cephalosporin C biosynthesis. Abstr 2nd Int Symp Genet Ind Microorg, p 32

Kanzaki T, Fukita T, Kitano K, Katamoto K, Nara K, Nakao Y (1976) Occurrence of a novel cephalosporin compound in the culture broth of a *Cephalosporin acremonium* mutant. J Ferment Technol 54:720–725

Kikuchi T, Uyeo S (1967) Pachysandra alkeloids. VIII. Structures of pachystermine-A and -B, novel type alkaloids having a β-lactam ring. Chem Pharm Bull 15:549–570

Kirby R (1978) Genetic mapping of *Streptomyces clavuligerus*. FEMS Microbiol Letts 3:177–180

Kitano K (1977) Studies on the production of β-lactam antibiotics. J Takeda Res Lab 36:105–192

Kitano K, Kintaka K, Suzuki S, Katamoto K, Nara K, Nakao Y (1974) Production of cephalosporin antibiotics by strains belonging to the genera *Arachnomyces, Anixiopsis* and *Spiroidium*. Agric Biol Chem 38:1761–1762

Kitano K, Kintaka K, Suzuki S, Katamoto K, Naro K, Nakao Y (1975) Screening of microorganisms capable of producing β-lactam antibiotics. J Ferment Technol 53:327–338

Kitano K, Fujisawa Y, Katamoto K, Nara K, Nakao Y (1976a) Occurrence of 7β-(4-carboxybutanamido)-cephalosporin compounds in the culture broth of some strains of the genus *Cephalosporium*. J Ferment Technol 54:712–719

Kitano K, Kintaka K, Suzuki S, Katamoto K, Nara K, Nakao Y (1976b) A novel penicillin produced by strains of the genus *Paecilomyces*. J Ferment Technol 54:705–711

Kluender H, Bradley CH, Sih CJ, Fawcett P, Abraham EP (1973) Synthesis and incorporation of (2S, 3S)-[4-^{13}C]valine into β-lactam antibiotics. J Am Chem Soc 95:6149–6150

Kluender H, Huang F-C, Fritzberg A, Schnoes H, Sih CJ, Fawcett P, Abraham EP (1974) Studies on the incorporation of (2S, 3R)-[4,4,4-$^{2}H_3$]valine and (2S, 3S) – [4,4,4-$^{2}H_3$]valine into β-lactam antibiotics. J Am Chem Soc 96:4054–4055

Kohsaka M, Demain AL (1976) Conversion of penicillin N to cephalosporin(s) by cell-free extracts of *Cephalosporium acremonium*. Biochem Biophys Res Commun 70:465–473

Konomi T, Herchen S, Baldwin JE, Yoshida M, Hunt N, Demain AL (1979) Cell-free conversion of δ-(L-α-aminoadipyl)-L-cysteinyl-D-valine into an antibiotic with the properties of isopenicillin N in *Cephalosporium acremonium*. Biochem J 184:427–430

Lemke PA, Nash CH (1972) Mutations that effect antibiotic synthesis by *Cephalosporium acremonium*. Can J Microbiol 18:255–259

Lemke PA, Nash CH, Pieper SW (1973) Lytic plaque-formation and variation in virus titre among strains of *Penicillium chrysogenum*. J Gen Microbiol 76:265–275

Liersch M, Nüesch J, Treichler HJ (1976) Final steps in the biosynthesis of cephalosporin C. Macdonald KD (ed) 2nd Int Symp Genet Ind Microorg, pp 179–195. Academic Press, London New York

Loder PB (1972) Selected aspects of the biosynthesis of penicillins and cephalosporins. Postepy Hig Med Dosw 26:493–500

Loder PB, Abraham EP (1971) Isolation and nature of intracellular peptides from a cephalosporin C-producing *Cephalosporium* sp. Biochem J 123:471–476

Macdonald KD, Hutchinson JM, Gillett WA (1963a) Heterokaryon studies and the genetic control of penicillin and chrysogenin production in *Penicillium chrysogenum*. J Gen Microbiol 33:375–383

Macdonald KD, Hutchinson JM, Gillett WA (1963b) Formation and segregation of heterozygous diploids between a wild-type strain and derivatives of high penicillin yield in *Penicillium chrysogenum*. J Gen Microbiol 33:385–394

Macdonald KD, Hutchinson JM, Gillett WA (1965) Heterozygous diploids of *Penicillium chrysogenum* and their segregation patterns. Genetica 36:378–397

Merrick MJ (1975) Hybridization and selection for increased penicillin titre in wild-type isolates of *Aspergillus nidulans*. J Gen Microbiol 91:278–286

Miller GA, Kelly BK, Newton GGF (1956) Cephalosporin production. Br Patent No 759.624

Miozzari GF, Niederberger P, Hütter R (1978) Permeabilization of microorganisms by Triton X-100. Anal Biochem 90:220–233

Morecombe DJ, Young DW (1975) Synthesis of chirally labelled cysteines and the steric origin of C(5) in penicillin biosynthesis. J Chem Soc Chem Commun 198–199

Nagarajan R, Boeck LD, Gorman M, Hamill RL, Higgens CE, Hoehn M, Stark WM, Whitney JG (1971) β-lactam antibiotics from *Streptomyces*. J Am Chem Soc 93:2308–2310

Neuss N, Nash CH, Baldwin JE, Lemke PA, Grutzner JB (1973) Incorporation of (2RS, 3S)-[4-^{13}C]valine into cephalosporin C. J Am Chem Soc 95:3797–3798, 6511

Nüesch J, Treichler HJ, Liersch M (1973) The biosynthesis of cephalosporin C. Vaněk Z, Hošťálek Z, Cudlin J (eds) 1st Int Symp Genet Ind Microorg, pp 309–334. Elsevier, Amsterdam London New York

Okamura K, Hirata S, Okumura Y, Fukagawa Y, Shimauchi Y, Kuono K, Ishikura T (1978) PS-5, a new β-lactam antibiotic from *Streptomyces*. J Antibiot 31:480–482

O'Sullivan J, Abraham EP (1979) Unpublished experiments

O'Sullivan J, Abraham EP (1980) The conversion of cephalosporins to 7α-Methoxy-cephalosporins by cell-free extracts of Streptomyces clavuligerus. Biochem J 186:613–616

O'Sullivan J, Aplin RT, Stevens CM, Abraham EP (1979a) Biosynthesis of a 7α-methoxycephalosporin. Incorporation of molecular oxygen. Biochem J 1979:47–52

O'Sullivan J, Bleaney RC, Huddleston JA, Abraham EP (1979b) Incorporation of ^{3}H from D-(L-α-amino[4,5-^{3}H]adipyl)-L-cysteinyl-D-[4,4-^{3}H]valine into isopenicillin N. Biochem J 184:421–426

Pontecorvo G, Sermonti G (1953) Recombination without sexual reproduction in *Penicillium chrysogenum*. Nature (London) 172:126

Pontecorvo G, Roper JA, Hemmons LM, Macdonald KD, Bufton AL (1953) The genetics of *Aspergillus nidulans*. Adv Genet 5:141–253

Pruess DL, Johnson MJ (1967) Penicillin acyltransferase in *Penicillium chrysogenum*. J Bacteriol 94:1502–1508

Queener SW, Capone JJ, Radue AB, Nagarajan R (1974) Synthesis of deacetoxycephalosporin C by a mutant of *Cephalosporium acremonium*. Antimicrob Agents Chemother 6:334–337

Scannell JP, Pruess DL, Blount JF, Ax HA, Kellett M, Weiss F, Demny TC, Williams JH, Stempel A (1975) Antimetabolites produced by microorganisms. XII. (S)-Alanyl-3-[α-(S)-Chloro-3-(S)-hydroxy-2-oxo-3-azetidinylmethyl]-(S)-alanine, a new β-lactam containing natural product. J Antibiot 28:1–6

Scott AI, Yoo SE, Chung SK, Lacadie JA (1976) Reactivity of peptide hydroxamates: a model for the biosynthesis of β-lactam antibiotics. Tetrahedron Lett 1137–1140

Sermonti G (1959a) Genetics of *Penicillium chrysogenum*. III. Cytoplasmic inheritance in Penicillium. Sel Sci Pap 1st Super Sanita 2:407–415

Sermonti G (1959b) Genetics of penicillin production. Ann NY Acad Sci 81:950–966

Somerson NL, Demain AL, Nunheimer TD (1961) Reversal of lysine inhibition of penicillin production by α-aminoadipic or adipic acid. Arch Biochem Biophys 93:238–241

Spencer B, Maung C (1970) Multiple activities of penicillin acyltransferase of *Penicillium chrysogenum*. Biochem J 118:29

Stapley EO, Jackson M, Hernandez S, Zimmerman SB, Currie SA, Mochales S, Mata JM, Woodruff HB, Hendlin D (1972) Cephamycins, a new family of β-lactam antibiotics. I. Production by actinomycetes, including *Streptomyces lactamdurans* sp. n. Antimicrob Agents Chemother 2:122–131

Stevens CM, Inamine E, DeLong CW (1956) The rates of incorporation of L-cystine and D- and L-valine in penicillin biosynthesis. J Biol Chem 219:405–409

Stevens CM, Abraham EP, Huang F-C, Sih CJ (1975) Incorporation of molecular oxygen at C-17 of cephalosporin C during its biosynthesis. Fed Proc 34:625

Stewart WW (1971) Isolation and proof of structure of wildfire toxin. Nature (London) 229:174–178

Traxler P, Treichler HJ, Nüesch J (1975) Synthesis of N-acetyldeacetoxycephalosporin C by a mutant of *Cephalosporium acremonium*. J Antibiot 28:605–606

Troonen H, Roelants P, Boon B (1976) RIT 2214, a new biosynthetic penicillin produced by a mutant of *Cephalosporium acremonium*. J Antibiot 29:1258–1267

Trown PW, Smith B, Abraham EP (1963) Biosynthesis of cephalosporin C from amino acids. Biochem J 86:284–291

Turner MK, Farthing JE, Brewer SJ (1978) The oxygenation of [3-methyl-^{3}H]desacetoxycephalosporin C [7β-(5-D-aminoadipamido)-3-methylceph-3-em-4-carboxylic acid) to [3-hydroxymethyl-^{3}H]desacetylcephalosporin C by 2-oxoglutarate-linked dioxygenases from *Acremonium chrysogenum* and *Streptomyces clavuligerus*. Biochem J 173:839–850

Vandamme EJ (1977) Enzymes involved in β-lactam antibiotic synthesis. Perlman D (ed) Adv Appl Microbiol, vol 21, pp 89–123. Academic Press, London New York

Warren SC, Newton GGF, Abraham EP (1967) The role of valine in the biosynthesis of penicillin N and cephalosporin C by a *Cephalosporium* sp. Biochem J 103:902–912

Whitney JG, Brannon DR, Mabe JA, Wicker KJ (1972) Incorporation of labelled precursors into A16886B, a novel β-lactam antibiotic produced by *Streptomyces clavuligerus*. Antimicrob Agents Chemother 1:247–251

Young DW, Morecombe DJ, Sen PK (1977) The stereochemistry of β-lactam formation in penicillin biosynthesis. Eur J Biochem 75:133–147

Biosynthesis of Methylenomycin A: A Plasmid-Determined Antibiotic

ULFERT HORNEMANN and DAVID A. HOPWOOD

Although knowledge of the genetic control of actinomycete antibiotic production is still scanty, three patterns are apparent. In the first, exemplified by actinorhodin in *Streptomyces coelicolor* A3(2), all mutations specifically interrupting the biosynthesis are chromosomal and serve to identify a group of closely linked structural genes, perhaps an operon (WRIGHT and HOPWOOD, 1976a; RUDD and HOPWOOD, 1979); plasmids are apparently not involved. In the second type of control, represented by several antibiotics, including oxytetracycline in *S. rimosus*, chloramphenicol in *S. venezuelae*, holomycin in *S. clavuligerus*, and turimycin in *S. hygroscopicus* (reviewed by HOPWOOD, 1978), some or all of the structural genes are chromosomal, while putative plasmids influence their expression in an as yet undefined way. Methylenomycin A in *Streptomyces coelicolor* A3(2) represents the first example of a third situation in which all the information specifically required for synthesis of the antibiotic is carried by a plasmid, SCP1.

SCP1 was first defined genetically by VIVIAN (1971) as a self-transmissible plasmid able to promote chromosomal recombination. Having characterized strains by their recombination properties as SCP1$^+$ (then called IF) or SCP1$^-$ (UF), he noted that SCP1$^+$ cultures inhibited the development of SCP1$^-$ cultures by producing a diffusible inhibitor. Evidently the presence of SCP1 in a strain caused it to produce, and to be resistant to, this material. The agent was first thought to inhibit only the development of aerial mycelium and spores on the sensitive SCP1$^-$ culture, but this later turned out to be incorrect: even very young growth of SCP1$^-$ strains was found to be sensitive. The inhibitor was later shown to be an antibiotic of comparatively low molecular weight and with a wide spectrum of activity against gram-positive bacteria and some gram-negative strains, notably *Proteus* (KIRBY et al., 1975), and was identified, mainly on mass spectral and chromatographic evidence (WRIGHT and HOPWOOD,

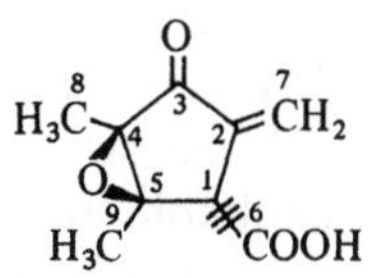

(I)

Fig. 1. Methylenomycin A

1976a), as methylenomycin A (I) (HANEISHI et al., 1974a, b). The structure of methylenomycin A has been determined by chemical and spectroscopic studies and was supported by X-ray analysis. The absolute configuration has not been established. Syntheses of (±)-methylenomycin A (SCARBOROUGH and SMITH, 1977) and of the (+) isomer (J. JERNOW et al., personal communication) have been achieved. A number of methylenomycin A analogs, some of which possessed improved potency over the parent compound, have been reported (HANEISHI et al., 1974c).

In view of its importance as a genetic determinant of antibiotic production, it is relevant to review the evidence for the existence of the SCP1 plasmid. The genetic evidence is substantial. Fertility states can be recognized amongst derivatives of *S. coelicolor* A3(2) with the properties expected if a sex factor is absent ($SCP1^-$), autonomous ($SCP1^+$ or SCP1′), or chromosomally integrated (NF and other high frequency donors of chromosomal genes). The SCP1′ strains (HOPWOOD and WRIGHT, 1976b), analogous with F′ strains of *Escherichia coli*, provide particularly strong evidence for SCP1 as a genetic element capable of autonomous existence. SCP1′ can be transferred by mating into appropriate auxotrophic mutants of two other species, *S. lividans* and *S. parvulus*, with which *S. coelicolor* has little chromosomal homology. Heterozygous prototrophic strains result in which segments of the *S. coelicolor* chromosome can be inherited and expressed indefinitely without, presumably, being integrated into the chromosome of the recipient species but the recessive chromosomal marker continues to segregate when the plasmid is lost (HOPWOOD and WRIGHT, 1976a). Further, circumstantial, evidence for the plasmid nature of SCP1 is provided by a phenomenon likened to lethal zygosis promoted by the F plasmid of *E. coli*. This phenotype is expressed, in almost identical form, by both SCP1 and the second sex factor of *S. coelicolor* A3(2), SCP2, which has been well characterized physically (BIBB et al., 1977).

Physical data on the nature of SCP1 have been hard to obtain; evidently, in common with several other streptomycete plasmids, it cannot be isolated by methods which readily recover most eubacterial and some other streptomycete plasmids. However, physical evidence for its existence as DNA has recently come from hybridization experiments between $SCP1^+$ and $SCP1^-$ strains of *S. coelicolor* A3(2) (a negative selection for sequences present only in the $SCP1^+$ strain) or between $SCP1^+$ *S. coelicolor* and $SCP1^+$ *S. parvulus* (a positive selection for those sequences common to both strains); these studies gave a molecular weight for SCP1 in the region of 100 million assuming a single copy per chromosome (WESTPHELING and BYERS, 1978).

Evidence that structural, rather than regulatory, genes for the production of methylenomycin A are carried on SCP1 is of two kinds. One type of evidence comes from the ability to transfer SCP1 to other species. It is particularly relevant that *S. parvulus* ATCC 12434, which normally produces actinomycin D as the only identified antibiotic (WILLIAMS and KATZ, 1977), makes an antibiotic chromatographically indistinguishable from methylenomycin A when SCP1 is mated into it (KIRBY and HOPWOOD, 1977). The second, and more direct, evidence comes from the isolation of mutations (*mmy*) derived from *S. coelicolor* A3(2) strains carrying SCP1 in the integrated or autonomous ($SCP1^+$ or SCP1′)

state which have lost the ability to make methylenomycin. Had there been chromosomal genes specifically required for its synthesis, these should have been revealed, but all 28 *mmy* mutations so far isolated (KIRBY and HOPWOOD, 1977; U. HORNEMANN and D.A. HOPWOOD, unpublished observations) are linked to SCP1 rather than to the chromosome.

The *mmy* mutants have so far yielded relatively little information on the biosynthetic pathway of the antibiotic, partly because cosynthetic reactions between pairs of mutants are few. Only one mutant (R39) acts as a converter, and it does so with the great majority of the other mutants, which function as secretor. Cosynthesis therefore defines only three classes of *mmy* mutations. The class not involved in any cosynthetic reactions could include regulatory mutations and deletions as well as point mutations in single structural genes, some of which might be polar.

The large secretor class of *mmy* mutants was subdivided into three groups (KIRBY and HOPWOOD, 1977) on the basis of differences in pigmentation. One mutant (SCP1-*orange*) in the original series of 16 mutations, and another (U15) isolated subsequently, produced an orange diffusible pigment, presumed to be related to the methylenomycin pathway rather than to those of the pigmented antibiotics of *S. coelicolor* A3(2), especially because the orange pigment was made by *S. parvulus* carrying SCP1-*orange*. The remaining members of the secretor class were classified into two groups on the basis of their synthesis of red mycelial pigments. These are now known to include two unrelated compounds: actinorhodin in its acidic, poorly soluble form (proto-actinorhodin), and a second poorly soluble red pigment (RUDD, 1978). Under conditions when methylenomycin A is made, for example, on the 'complete medium' used for *S. coelicolor* propagation, SCP1$^-$ strains produce the red pigments earlier and more copiously than SCP1$^+$ strains, and it is therefore likely that methylenomycin tends to inhibit their synthesis (SCP1-*orange* strains also lack red pigments on media supporting methylenomycin production). Many of the *mmy* secretor mutants resembled SCP1$^-$ strains in their pigmentation, but some had the pale color characteristic of SCP1$^+$ cultures, suggesting that they might be accumulating a precursor of methylenomycin which, like the antibiotic itself, interfered with red pigment synthesis. However, it remains to be seen whether the two classes of secretor mutants are really genetically distinct or whether, for example, the non-pigmented mutants might simply be slightly leaky members of other mutant classes.

The immediate precursor of methylenomycin A appears to be an antibiotically inactive compound recently characterized as desepoxy-4,5-didehydro-methylenomycin A (II) (HORNEMANN and HOPWOOD, 1978) and produced by *mmy*$^+$ strains in comparable quantities to methylenomycin A itself: it is the 'Spot C' of WRIGHT and HOPWOOD (1976a). When fed to an SCP1$^+$ strain or to the R39 converter *mmy* mutant, but not to an SCP1$^-$ culture, or to the secretor mutants R40 and U17, it is converted (Fig. 3) to methylenomycin A (HORNEMANN and HOPWOOD, 1978). II is not the compound responsible for cosynthesis by any members of the secretor class of *mmy* mutants since they show no chromatographic evidence for the accumulation of this material (KIRBY and HOPWOOD, 1977). On the other hand, it could explain the conversion to antibiotic

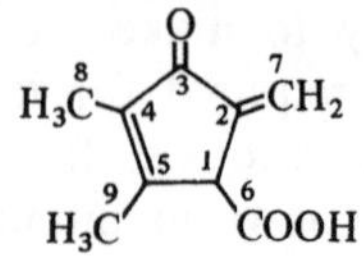

(II)

Fig. 2. Desepoxy-4,5-didehydro methylenomycin A

by R39 seen in Petri dish tests of material secreted by an SCP1$^+$ strain (KIRBY and HOPWOOD, 1977).

In an effort to complement the genetic studies on methylenomycin A biosynthesis with chemical and biochemical information, tracer feeding experiments were undertaken using *S. coelicolor* A3(2) strains 104 (VIVIAN and HOPWOOD, 1970) and U9, derived from B229 (RUDD, 1978), which carry the wild type SCP1 plasmid. Strain 104 occasionally produced fairly large amounts of actinorhodin besides methylenomycin A which interfered with the analyses of precursor incorporation into the latter; therefore several of the biosynthetic studies were carried out with Strain U9 which does not produce the pigment while producing high titers of methylenomycin A. Precursors were added to 3-day-old cultures started from a spore suspension and incubated at 30° on a rotary shaker in a complete medium (CM). The cultures were harvested one day later by filtration, acidification of the broth to pH 2, and extraction of I and its co-metabolite II with ethyl acetate. I and II were then purified either by thin layer chromatography or by column chromatography (HORNEMANN and HOPWOOD, 1978). Incorporation of the radioactive precursors listed in Table 1 was determined either using autoradiography or radiochromatogram scanning. Since II has been recognized as a precursor of I, the incorporation rates listed in the table apply to both compounds.

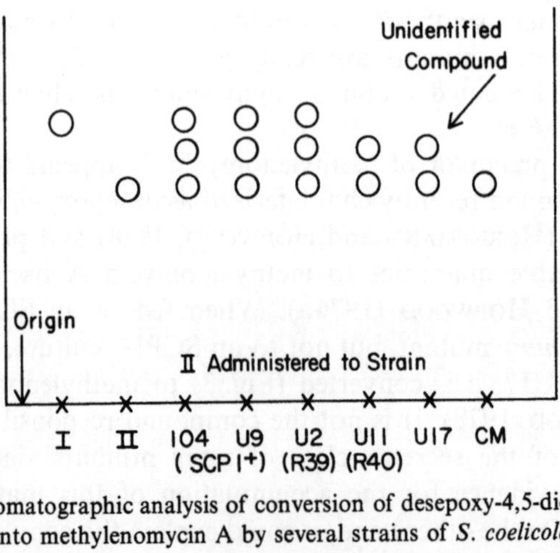

Fig. 3. Thin-layer chromatographic analysis of conversion of desepoxy-4,5-didehydro methylenomycin A into methylenomycin A by several strains of *S. coelicolor* A3(2)

Table 1. Feeding experiments with labeled precursors

Precursor	Incorporation into I plus II (%)
Sodium [1-^{14}C]acetate	9.3
Sodium [2-^{14}C]acetate	8.4
[2-^{14}C]Glycine	5.8
Sodium [3-^{14}C]pyruvate	3.9
Sodium [2,3-^{14}C]succinate	2.0
L-[U-^{14}C]Aspartic acid	2.5
L-[$^{14}CH_3$]Methionine	<0.1
D,L-[2-^{14}C]Mevalonic acid DBED salt	<0.1
Sodium [2-^{14}C]propionate	<0.1
L-[U-^{14}C]Tyrosine	<0.1

Approximately 5 µmol of labeled compound containing $1.1 \cdot 10^7$ dpm ^{14}C were administered to 3-day-old shake cultures of strains 104 or U9 one day before harvest

Table 2. Competition feeding experiments

Precursor	Incorporation into I plus II (%)
[2-^{14}C]Glycine	8.4
[2-^{14}C]Glycine and 500 µmoles unlabeled sodium acetate	2.1
Sodium [3-^{14}C]pyruvate	3.9
Sodium [3-^{14}C]pyruvate and 500 µmoles unlabeled sodium acetate	0.3
Sodium [2,3-^{14}C]succinate	2.0
Sodium [2,3-^{14}C]succinate and 500 µmoles unlabeled sodium acetate	0.4
Sodium [1-^{14}C]acetate	5.3
Sodium [1-^{14}C]acetate and 500 µmoles unlabeled sodium succinate	5.2
Sodium [1-^{14}C]acetate and 500 µmoles unlabeled glycine	3.1

Approximately 5 µmol of labeled compound containing $1.1 \cdot 10^7$ dpm ^{14}C were administered, together with nonlabeled compound where indicated, to 3-day-old shake cultures of strains 104 or U9 one day before harvest

It is apparent from the data presented in Table 1 that acetate, glycine, pyruvate, succinate, and aspartate are efficient precursors, while L-[$^{14}CH_3$]methionine D,L-[2-^{14}C]mevalonic acid DBED salt, [3-^{14}C]propionic acid and L-[U-^{14}C]tyrosine fail to label I and II. Thus it is quite clear that the methyl groups of methylenomycin and its co-metabolite do not arise from methionine through C-methylation or from mevalonic acid via an isoprene unit; furthermore, pathways involving propionic acid or tyrosine can be excluded. Since all the actual precursors listed in Table 1 can be metabolically converted into acetate it was of interest to examine the effect of excess acetate on the incorporation of these compounds. The results of parallel competition feeding experiments are shown in Table 2. While acetate at the level added does not by itself reduce the amount of I and II produced, it clearly lowers the amount of radioactivity incorporated from added glycine, pyruvate, and succinate, presumably by preventing the

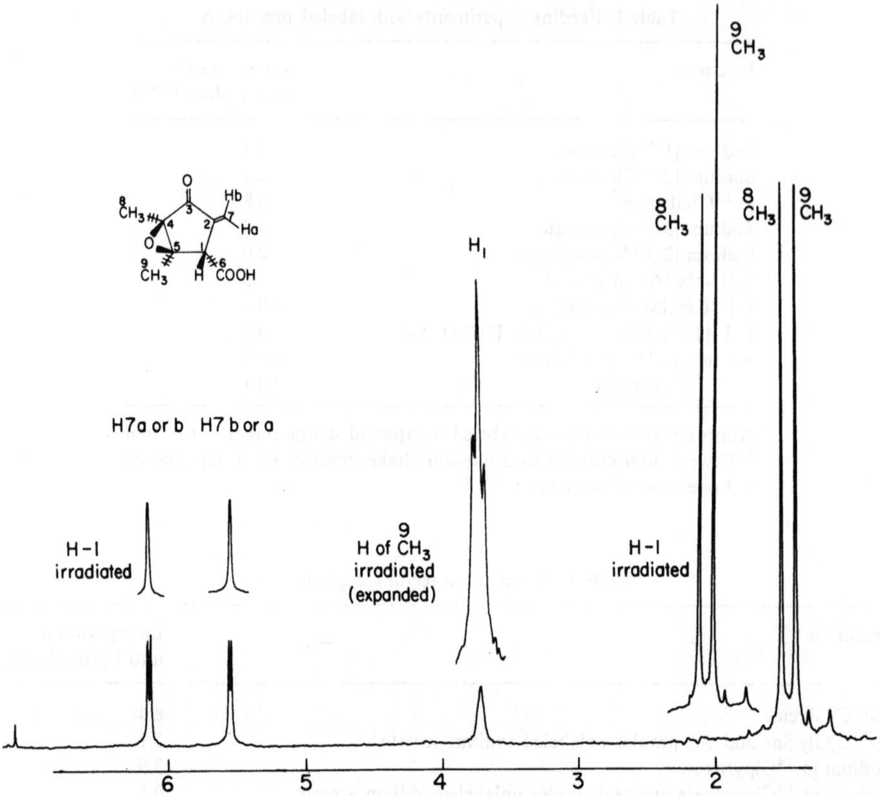

Fig. 4. 100 MHz proton NMR spectrum of methylenomycin A: assignment of methyl protons on basis of long-range coupling with H_1

incorporation of these precursors into 'acetate positions' of I and II. Conversely succinate and glycine do not appear significantly to alter acetate incorporation. Additional experiments will need to be carried out to evaluate the significance of the residual incorporation of glycine, pyruvate, and succinate which presumably occurs into positions different from 'acetate positions' and to locate the atoms of I and II labeled by these compounds.

Since the feeding experiments with radioactive precursors clearly indicated an important role of acetate in methylenomycin A biosynthesis, ^{13}C labeled acetates were administered and the atoms introduced from this precursor were identified by ^{13}C NMR analysis. The assignment of the nine carbon atoms of methylenomycin A was achieved on the basis of known functional group chemical shift data, long-range coupling data from the proton NMR spectrum of the antibiotic, and a feeding experiment with [1,2-$^{13}C_2$]acetate. The high-field methyl group in the ^1H NMR spectrum (HANEISHI et al., 1974b, Fig. 4) shows long-range coupling with H-1, which also shows long-range coupling with H-7a and H-7b causing the signal for H-1 to appear as a broad envelope. Irradiation of H-1 causes the small coupling between H-1 and H-7a and H-1 and H-7b to collapse while the height, but not the integral of the high-field methyl group increases. As expected, irradiation of the high-field methyl group simplifies

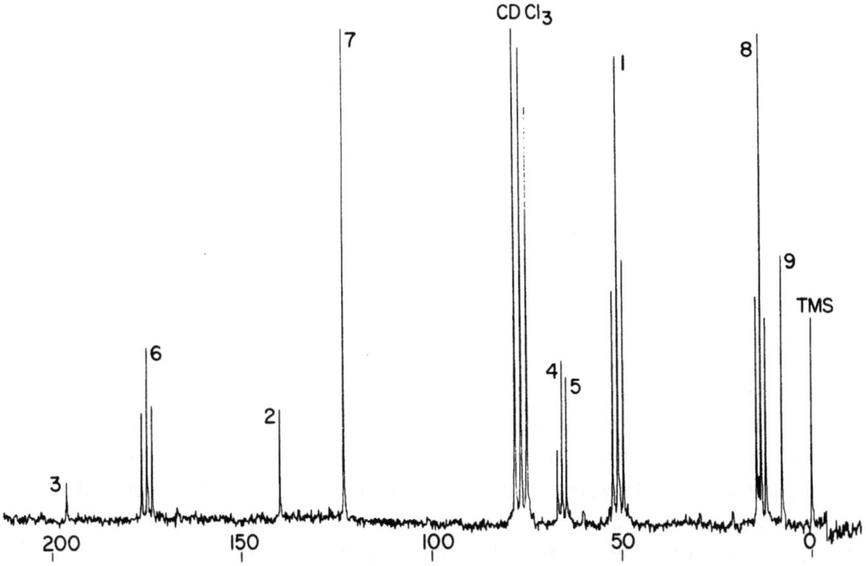

Fig. 5. Proton noise decoupled pulse Fourier transform 25.2 MHz ^{13}C NMR spectrum showing incorporation of sodium [1,2-$^{13}C_2$]acetate (100 mg, 90 atom % ^{13}C enrichment, administered to 3-day-old 500-ml culture of *S. coelicolor* A3(2) strain B 229-SCP1$^+$ for 1 day at 28° C) into methylenomycin A. Enrichment factors (%): C-1, 1.3; C-4, 1.1; C-6, 1.6; C-8, 1.1, determined by the procedure of McInnes et al. (1974)

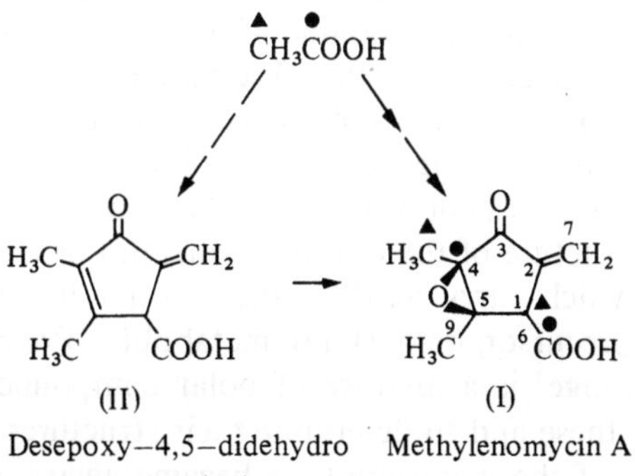

Fig. 6. Precursors of methylenomycin A

the signal of the H-1 proton to a distorted triplet (doublet of doublets), therefore the high-field methyl group is assigned as C-9. Selective heteronuclear decoupling experiments in the methyl region show that the high-field methyl in the proton spectrum is also the high-field methyl in the carbon spectrum. C-4 was identified as the carrier of the low-field methyl group (C-8) on the basis of the observation that both these carbons were labeled from [1,2-$^{13}C_2$]-acetate and showed characteristic carbon-carbon coupling.

The feeding experiment with sodium [1,2-$^{13}C_2$]acetate revealed enrichment of and coupling between C-1 and C-6 besides enrichment of and coupling between C-4 and C-8 (Fig. 5), thus indicating that two intact acetate units are incorporated into methylenomycin as shown in Figure 6 which summarizes the presently available information on methylenomycin A biosynthesis. It was somewhat unexpected to find that C-4 and C-8 in I rather than C-5 and C-9 are labeled by sodium [1,2-$^{13}C_2$]acetate. This observation at first sight is not in harmony with the previously considered possibility that acetoacetyl CoA may function as a precursor in methylenomycin A biosynthesis by providing C-9, C-5, C-1, and C-6 (HORNEMANN et al., 1978). An involvement of acetoacetyl CoA was suggested based on the labeling of II from [1-^{13}C]acetate at C-5 and C-6 when the precursor was added to 2-day-old cultures for 2 days (U. HORNEMANN, unpublished observations) and based on the knowledge that II is a precursor of I. However, the possibility exists that acetate provides label predominantly to C-9 and C-5 besides C-1 and C-6 at relatively early stages in the fermentation when II may be produced as the major product, and that acetate may label I predominantly at later stages of the fermentation and then predominantly at C-8 and C-4 besides C-1 and C-6. Thus acetoacetyl CoA or a related metabolite would be a viable precursor without precluding the possibility that acetate also functions as the progenitor of C-8 and C-4.

The biosynthetic results obtained so far in addition to demonstrating a precursor role of II for I, clearly indicate the biosynthetic origin of C-1 and C-6 and C-8 and C-4 from acetate and suggest a role of acetate as a precursor for C-9 and C-5, but the origin of the remaining three carbons is presently unknown. It will be of interest to examine whether or not pyruvate can provide C-2, C-3, and C-7 as suggested by the observation that incorporation of this acid remains significant even in the presence of a large excess of nonlabeled acetate added in the same feeding experiment (Table 2).

Future studies on methylenomycin biosynthesis would presumably be aided considerably if the structure of the orange pigment(s) produced by strains 2235 and U15, both of which carry SCP1-orange, could be elucidated, since the pigment may be a precursor or a shunt metabolite. Preliminary experiments have shown that 'orange' is a mixture of polar compounds and attempts are under way to purify these and to determine their structures.

After submission of the manuscript we became aware of a paper by SAKAI et al. (1979) reporting the absolute stereochemistry of methylenomycin A as 1(R), 4(S), 5(S) methylenomycin A. Thus methylenomycin A is the mirror image of the structures shown in this chapter and in the previously published literature.

Acknowledgments. The scientific contributions of D.P. HONOR and J.F. KOZLOWSKI and help with the assignment and measurement of the CMR spectra by Drs. C.J. CHANG, this Department, J.B. GRUTZNER, Department of Chemistry, and R.K. HARRIS, University of East Anglia, Norwich, United Kingdom, as well as financial support (to U.H.) through the 1976 Pfeiffer Award by the American Foundation for Pharmaceutical Education, Eli Lilly and Company, and the National Cancer Institute, DHEW, through research grant CA 14378, are gratefully acknowledged.

References

Bibb MJ, Freeman RF, Hopwood DA (1977) Physical and genetical characterisation of a second sex factor, SCP2, for *Streptomyces coelicolor*. Mol Gen Genet 154:155–166

Haneishi T, Kitahara N, Takiguchi Y, Arai M, Sugawara S (1974a) New antibiotics, methylenomycins A and B. I. Producing organism, fermentation and isolation, biological activities and physical and chemical properties. J Antibiot 27:386–392

Haneishi T, Terahara A, Arai M, Hata T, Tamura C (1974b) New antibiotics, methylenomycins A and B. II. Structures of methylenomycins A and B. J Antibiot 27:393–399

Haneishi T, Terahara A, Hamano K, Arai M (1974c) New antibiotics, methylenomycins A and B. III. Chemical modifications of methylenomycin A and structure-activity correlations in methylenomycins. J Antibiot 27:400–407

Hopwood DA (1978) Extrachromosomally determined antibiotic production. Annu Rev Microbiol 32:373–392

Hopwood DA, Wright HM (1976a) Interactions of the SCP1 plasmid with the chromosome of *Streptomyces coelicolor* A3(2). In: Macdonald KD (ed) 2nd Int Symp Genet Indust Microorg, pp 607–619. Academic Press, London New York

Hopwood DA, Wright HM (1976b) Genetic studies on SCP1-prime strains of *Streptomyces coelicolor* A3(2). J Gen Microbiol 95:107–120

Hornemann U, Hopwood DA (1978) Isolation and characterization of desepoxy-4,5-didehydro-methylenomycin A, a precursor of methylenomycin A in $SCP1^+$ strains of *Streptomyces coelicolor* A3(2). Tetrahedron Lett 2977–2978

Hornemann U, Honor DP, Hopwood DA (1978) Studies on the biosynthesis of methylenomycin by *Streptomyces coelicolor* A3(2). Abstr No 77 3rd Int Symp Genet Ind Microorg, Madison, Wisconsin, American Society for Microbiology, Washington DC

Kirby R, Hopwood DA (1977) Genetic determination of methylenomycin synthesis by the SCP1 plasmid of *Streptomyces coelicolor* A3(2). J Gen Microbiol 98:239–252

Kirby R, Wright LF, Hopwood DA (1975) Plasmid-determined antibiotic synthesis and resistance in *Streptomyces coelicolor*. Nature (London) 254:265–267

McInnes AG, Smith DG, Walter JA, Vining LC, Wright LC (1974) New techniques in biosynthetic studies using ^{13}C nuclear magnetic resonance spectroscopy. The biosynthesis of tenellin enriched from singly and doubly labeled precursors. JCS Chem Commun 282–284 (1974)

Rudd BAM (1978) Genetics of pigmented secondary metabolites in *Streptomyces coelicolor* A3(2). PhD Thesis, University of East Anglia, Norwich

Rudd BAM, Hopwood DA (1979) Genetics of actinorhodin biosynthesis by *Streptomyces coelicolor* A3(2). J Gen Microbiol 114:35–43

Sakai K, Amemiya S, Inoue K, Kojima K (1979) The conversion of methylenomycin A to natural botryodiplodin and their absolute configurations. Tetrahedron Lett 2365–2368

Scarborough RM Jr, Smith III AB (1977) A stereospecific total synthesis of (±)-methylenomycin A. A novel antibiotic possessing a α-methylene ketone functionality. J Am Chem Soc 99:7085–7087

Vivian A (1971) Genetic control of fertility in *Streptomyces coelicolor* A3(2): plasmid involvement in the interconversion of UF and IF strains. J Gen Microbiol 69:353–364

Vivian A, Hopwood DA (1970) Genetic control of fertility in *Streptomyces coelicolor* A3(2): The IF fertility type. J Gen Microbiol 64:101–117

Westpheling J, Byers M (1978) Detection of SCP1 by nucleic acid hybridization. John Innes Annu Rep p 67

Williams WF, Katz E (1977) Development of a chemically defined medium for the synthesis of actinomycin D by *Streptomyces parvulus*. Antimicrob Agents Chemother 11:281–290

Wright LF, Hopwood DA (1976a) Identification of the antibiotic determined by the SCP1 plasmid of *Streptomyces coelicolor* A3(2). J Gen Microbiol 95:96–106

Wright LF, Hopwood DA (1976b) Actinorhodin is a chromosomally determined antibiotic in *Streptomyces coelicolor* A3(2). J Gen Microbiol 96:289–297

Biochemical Mechanisms in the Biosynthesis of the Erythromycins

JOHN W. CORCORAN

I. Introduction

A number of reviews on macrolide antibiotics have appeared since they were first reviewed in this series (VANĚK and MAJER, 1967): the subject was recently included in a more detailed account of macrolides (MASAMUNE et al., 1977) as well as in an annual report on the subject of antibiotics (CORCORAN, 1977). A detailed discussion of the 16-membered group of macrolides appears in Chapter 8 of this volume. Of all the other possible models, the family of the erythromycins has been the subject of the most biochemical and enzymatic study, and far more knowledge is available about the detailed mechanisms involved in their biosynthesis than about any other macrolide type of antibiotic. Many natural products, including antibiotics, are made from the same (or similar) common intermediates of metabolism as are employed in the formation of the erythromycins, and the nature of the enzymatic reactions occurring in the formation of these precursors and in the synthesis of the complex natural product have implications for our understanding of biosynthesis beyond that of the model system (e.g., erythromycins) used for their elucidation. Therefore,

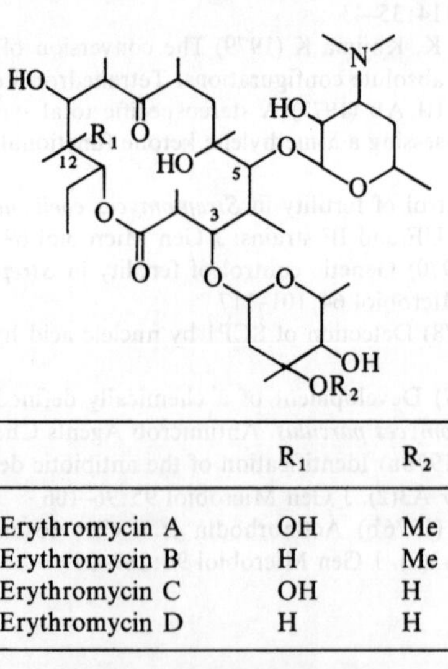

	R_1	R_2
(Ia) Erythromycin A	OH	Me
(Ib) Erythromycin B	H	Me
(Ic) Erythromycin C	OH	H
(Id) Erythromycin D	H	H

Fig. 1. The erythromycins

this chapter analyzes in detail the present state of knowledge concerning the biosynthesis of the erythromycins (Fig. 1) and presents and discusses some general aspects of biosynthesis with this model system as an example.

II. Historical Aspects

Work starting in the late 1950s (cf. CORCORAN and CHICK, 1966; VANĚK and MAJER, 1967) showed that the erythromycins known at that time (A, B and C; Ia, Ib and Ic of Fig. 1) were formed by the combination of two biosynthetic pathways. One of these utilizing intermediates of the oxidative metabolism of glucose and of amino acid metabolism led to the formation of a 21-carbon macrolide lactone which appeared to be a result of the polymerization of seven *propionate** subunits (Fig. 2). The best evidence from experiments using the intact mycelium of *Streptomyces erythreus,* the principle producer of the erythromycins, is that the enzyme system (synthase) operating is similar in structure and function to fatty acid synthases; it utilizes one molecule of propionyl Co A (*propionate*) as a 'starter' or 'primer' for the biosynthesis and employs six units of 2-methylmalonyl Co A (*2-methylmalonate*) for chain growth leading to the pentahydroxy-oxo-hexamethylpentadecanoic acid whose lactone (13 → 1) is found in erythromycins D and B (cf. CORCORAN, 1965, 1977).

The *propionate* used for the biosynthesis of the erythromycins could arise from the oxidative metabolism of *pyruvate* (*via succinate*), from the breakdown of odd carbon fatty acids, from branch-chain amino acids (valine, isoleucine), or from amino acids such as threonine and methionine. In reality the physiological source probably varies with the experimental conditions. However, in one situation where the 'average' source could be estimated during a long-term fermentation with glucose as the sole source of carbon, the majority of the

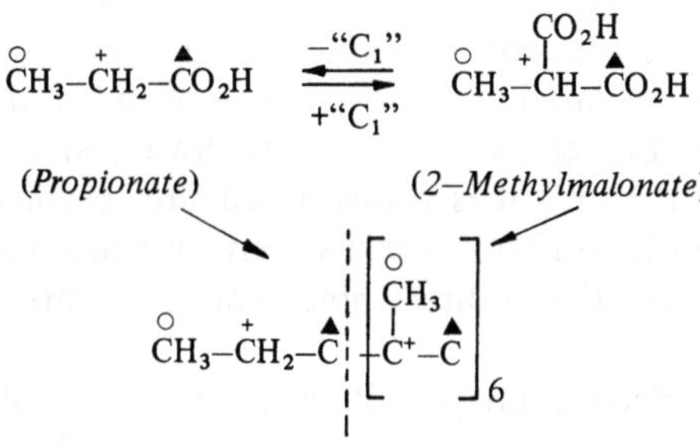

Fig. 2. Biosynthetic pathway leading to erythronolide

---

* In this chapter the use of italicized names of simple organic molecules (like *propionate, acetate* etc.) implies that the actual reactant in the enzymatic step is 'formally' related to the simple molecule, but may be and probably is some activated molecule derived from it. For instance, the term *acetate* would be used in describing enzymatic reactions that may employ either acetyl coenzyme A (Co A) as the reactive species or the carboxylated form of this substrate, malonyl Co A.

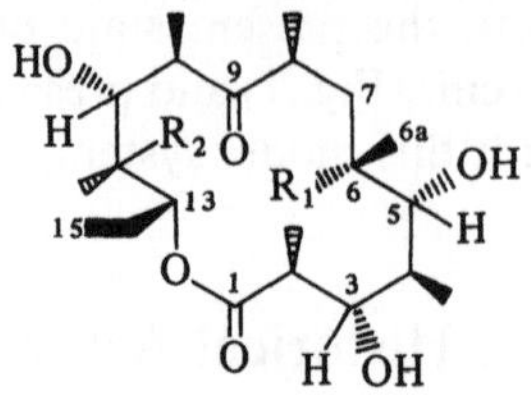

	R_1	R_2
(IIa)	–OH	–OH
(IIb)	–OH	–H
(IIc)	–H	–H

propionate used for the formation of erythromycin A appeared to be derived from the breakdown of the branch-chain amino acids (BUTTE and CORCORAN, 1963).

The second biosynthetic pathway operating to support the biosynthesis of the erythromycins generates the deoxy sugars present in the antibiotic glycosides (Fig. 1). The amino sugar of the erythromycins, D-desosamine, and the two branch-chain neutral sugars, L-mycarose and L-cladinose (cf. Section VI, below), are formed from D-glucose without obligatory breakage of its carbon chain (BUTTE and CORCORAN, 1962), and the branch-methyl group in the neutral sugars as well as the N- and O-methyl groups in them comes from the amino acid L-methionine (cf. Fig. 1).

The sequence of steps leading to the bis-glycosides in the family of the erythromycins could not be deduced from early work. The first evidence came from the study of blocked mutants of *S. erythreus* by MARTIN (cf. CORCORAN, 1977), and it was proposed that the first enzyme-free macrolide lactone is 6-deoxyerythronolide B (IIc). This lactone after hydroxylation at position six becomes erythronolide B (IIb) which is then transformed into the monoglycoside 3-O-mycarosyl erythronolide B (IV). With the isolation of erythromycin D by MAJER et al. (1977) it was possible to define this biologically-active bis-glycoside as the next stable intermediate in the biosynthesis of the erythromycins. Erythromycin D stands at a branch point in the pathway, since by O-methylation of its neutral sugar (at C-3″) it is transformed into erythromycin B (Ib) and by hydroxylation at position 12 it is, alternatively, transformed into erythromycin C (Ic). The erythromycin C is a direct precursor of erythromycin A (Ia) (CORCORAN, 1975).

The results summarized so far permitted the definition of a general pathway for the biosynthesis of the erythromycins (Fig. 3). Subsequent work, which will be discussed in some detail below, has studied the enzymes involved in each step of the pathway. The results on the lactone synthase have been disappointing. However, the biochemical mechanisms for the hydroxylation and transmethylation steps have been defined either in a preliminary or relatively detailed fashion. Some limited work has been done on the biosynthesis of the sugars of the erythromycins, and some insight into the regulation of the overall pathway has been gained.

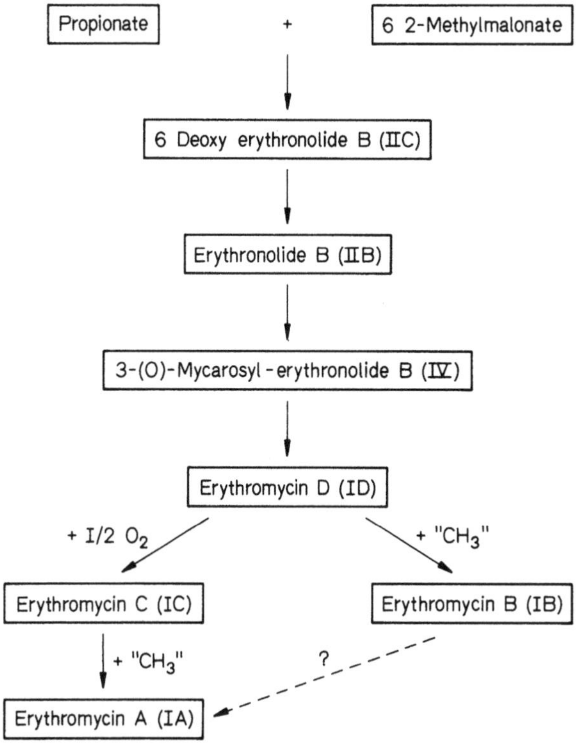

Fig. 3. Biosynthetic pathway leading to the erythromycins

III. Structures, Stereochemistry and Nomenclature of Intermediates in the Biosynthetic Pathway Leading to the Erythromycins

(with Dr. DAVID R. MITCHELL)

The trivial name erythromycin A (Ia) was assigned to the first antibiotic glycoside isolated from cultures of *S. erythreus* (cf. review by MASAMUNE et al., 1977). At least four other erythromycins are now known which seem to possess the same 13-hexamethylpentadecanolide backbone as does (Ia). The lactones present in the erythromycins generally have been called erythronolides. Two forms of erythronolide are found in the biologically active bis-glycosides; the A form in erythromycins A and C (Ia and Ic) and the B form found in erythromycins B and D (Ib and Id). Erythronolides A and B are similar, differing only in the substituent at C-12 which is hydrogen in the B form (IIb) and hydroxyl in the A species (IIa). Numerous other forms of erythronolide are known from studies of blocked mutants of *S. erythreus* as well as from chemical work. One, 6-deoxyerythronolide B (IIc) is an obligate intermediate in the biosynthesis of the erythromycins (Sections II and V) and others are shunt metabolites (MARTIN and ROSENBROOK, 1967; MARTIN and PERUN, 1968; MARTIN and EGAN, 1970; MARTIN et al., 1972).

The use of trivial names like erythromycins and erythronolides is useful and satisfactory for naming some of these compounds, but serious problems with nomenclature arise in naming many of their derivatives and some of the abnormal metabolites. The use of a 'semisystematic' nomenclature is recommended for such cases (IUPAC-IUB: Commission on Biochemical Nomenclature, 1967) and this author proposes that one be adopted for the lipid aglycon of the erythromycins. His suggestion is specific for this example, but in light of the marked structural and configurational similarity among the macrolides (CELMER, 1971) a related and compatible 'semisystematic' nomenclature could probably be developed readily for other antibiotics of the 14-member macrolide class, and possibly also for the 16-member groups (oleandomycin, pikromycin, narbomycin, tylosins, carbomycins, leucomycins, etc.).

The aglycons of the erythromycins are lipids and their biological formation appears to resemble that of long-chain fatty acids. As recommended for other lipids, the 'semisystematic' nomenclature proposed is based on the structure of the most highly reduced lactone present in these antibiotics. The name *erythranolide* is suggested for this hypothetical macrolide (III). The structure of

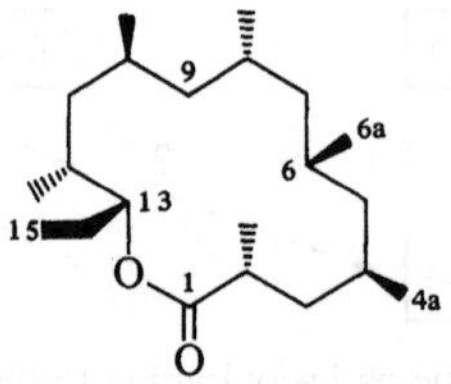

(III)

erythromycin A (Ia) has been defined unambiguously by a combination of chemical (MASAMUNE et al., 1977) and X-ray (HARRIS et al., 1965) analysis. The 13-hexamethylpentadecanolide backbone of erythromycin B (Ia) has been related (HUNG et al., 1965) to the same portion of erythronolide B (IIa), 3-(O)-α-*L*-mycarosylerythronolide B (IV) (MARTIN et al., 1966), 5-(O)-β-*D*-desosaminylerythronolide B (V), 6-deoxyerythronolide B (IIc) (MARTIN and ROSENBROOK, 1967), and other metabolites of *S. erythreus* (Table 1: VI, VII, and VIII) (MARTIN and PERUN, 1968; MARTIN and EGAN, 1970; MARTIN et al., 1972) by a combination of chemical, spectral and biological criteria (MASAMUNE et al., 1977; PERUN, 1971). All the evidence available suggests that this partial structure is identical to the 'erythr*a*nolide' moiety in erythromycins A and C where it has been defined unambiguously because of their proven structures. Thus, *erythranolide* (III) is the name chosen as the basis for the 'semisystematic' nomenclature for the erythr*o*nolides. Erythr*a*nolide may also be called a 'stereoparent' for this family of compounds (Chemical Abstracts, 1972). Erythranolide (III) is the 14-member macrolide that would be formed by the removal of all non-lactone oxygen atoms from the aglycon present in erythromycins A and C (Ia and Ic). To construct the name of any given derivative of (III) a substitutive system of indicating functional groups is used, and the rules proposed by the IUPAC Commission on the naming of organic compounds is followed (IUPAC Nomenclature of Organic Chemistry Sections A, B, and C, 1969). The glycosidic deriva-

Table 1. Trivial and semisystematic names of compounds related to the biosynthetic pathways leading to the erythromycins

Compound	Trivial name	Semisystematic name
IIa	Erythronolide A	3(*L*), 5(*L*), 6(*D*), 11(*L*), 12(*D*)-pentahydroxyerythranolide-9-one
IIb	Erythronolide B	3(*L*), 5(*L*), 6(*D*), 11(*L*)-tetrahydroxyerythranolide-9-one
IIc	6-deoxyerythronolide B	3(*L*), 5(*L*), 11(*L*)-trihydroxyerythranolide-9-one
VI	5-deoxy-5-oxo-erythronolide B	3(*L*), 6(*D*), 11(*L*)-trihydroxyerythranolide-5,9-dione
VII	5,6-dideoxy-5-oxoerythronolide B	3(*L*), 11(*L*)-dihydroxyerythranolide-5,9-dione
VIII	(8S)-8-hydroxy-5,6-dideoxy-5--oxo-erythronolide B	3(*L*), 8(*D*), 11(*L*)-trihydroxyerythranolide-5,9-dione
IV	3-α-L-mycarosylerythronolide B	3(*L*)-α-L-mycarosyloxy, 5(*L*), 6(*D*), 11(*L*)-trihydroxyerythranolide-9-one
V	5-β-D-desosaminylerythronolide B	5(*L*)-β-D-desosaminyloxy, 3(*L*), 6(*D*), 11(*L*)-trihydroxyerythranolide-9-one
Ia	Erythromycin A	3(*L*)-α-L-cladinosyloxy, 5(*L*)-β-D-desosaminyloxy, 6(*D*), 11(*L*), 12(*D*)-trihydroxyerythranolide-9-one
Ic	Erythromycin C	3(*L*)-α-L-mycarosyloxy, 5(*L*)-β-D-desosaminyloxy, 6(*D*), 11(*L*), 12(*D*)-trihydroxyerythranolide-9-one
Id	Erythromycin D	3(*L*)-α-L-mycarosyloxy, 5(*L*)-β-D-desosaminyloxy, 6(*D*), 11(*L*)-dihydroxyerythranolide-9-one
Ib	Erythromycin B	3(*L*)-α-L-cladinosyloxy, 5(*L*)-β-D-desosaminyloxy, 6(*D*), 11(*L*)-dihydroxyerythranolide-9-one
IX	Megalomicin A	3(*L*)-α-L-mycarosyloxy, 5(*L*)-β-D-desosaminyloxy, 6(*D*)-α-L-megalosaminyloxy, 11(*L*), 12(*D*)-dihydroxy-erythranolide-9-one

tives of an erythranolide structure are named using the proper glycosyloxy radical term as appropriate (cf., Table 1).

The ring numbering system previously used for the naturally-occurring erythronolides is retained with (III) since it emphasizes the biological origin of the carbon chain by giving the highest number to the methyl position in the acyl Coenzyme A monomer that presumably initiates the biosynthesis (propionyl Co A in the case of erythr*a*nolides). The branch-methyl groups in erythranolide are numbered as being subsidiary to the ring carbon to which they are attached (e.g., C-2a, -4a, -6a, etc.).

Definition of the stereochemistry at asymmetric centers in derivatives of *erythranolide* is by the method of KLYNE (based on the Fischer convention) (KLYNE, 1951; CELMER, 1971), in which each substituent at an asymmetric center is defined as *D* or *L* depending on whether it projects to the right or left of the ring when viewed from the front (lactone oxygen atom to the rear) with carbon position one at the top (Fig. 4). This method for definition of

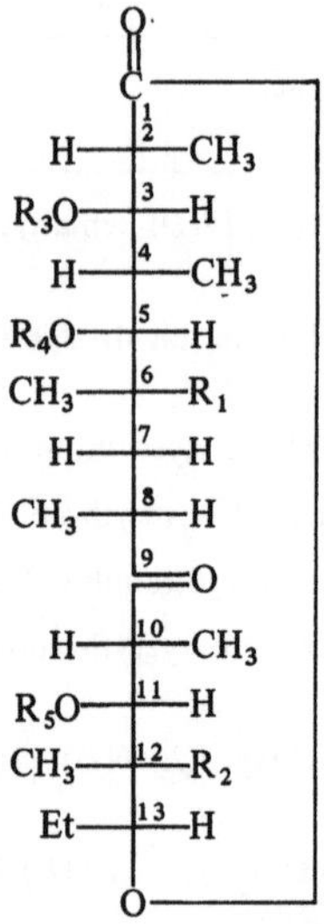

(R/S System)	(Klyne/Celmer)
–	–
R	L
S	L
S	L
R	L
R	D
–	–
R	D
–	–
R	L
R	L
S	D
R	D

(Ia): $R_1 = R_2 = OH$, R_3 = L-cladinose, R_4 = D-desosamine, $R_5 = H$
(Ib): $R_1 = OH$, $R_2 = R_5 = H$, R_3 = L-cladinose, R_4 = D-desosamine
(Ic): $R_1 = R_2 = OH$, R_3 = L-mycarose, R_4 = D-desosamine, $R_5 = H$
(Id): $R_1 = OH$, $R_2 = R_5 = H$, R_3 = L-mycarose, R_4 = D-desosamine
(IX): $R_1 = R_2 = OH$, R_3 = L-mycarose, R_4 = D-desosamine, R_5 = L-megalosamine.
(IV): $R_1 = OH$, $R_2 = R_4 = R_5 = H$, R_3 = L-mycarose
(V): $R_1 = OH$, $R_2 = R_3 = R_5 = H$, R_4 = D-desosamine
(IIa): $R_1 = OH$, $R_2 = R_3 = R_4 = R_5 = H$
(IIb): $R_1 = R_2 = OH$, $R_3 = R_4 = R_5 = H$
(IIc): $R_1 = R_2 = R_3 = R_4 = R_5 = H$

(The assignment shown is that for erythronolide A (IIa). Some assignments change with other structures. The indication of (*D*) or (*L*) is based on the substituent introduced into erythranolide (III) with the group -OR taking priority over -H or -alkyl)

Fig. 4. Substituted erythranolides according to the convention of CAHN/INGOLD/PRELOG and KLYNE/CELMER

stereochemistry is not affected by the projection formulae used or uncertainties about crystal or solution conformation of the derivatives. By way of comparison, the configurational assignments (R or S) arrived at for erythronolide A (IIa) by use of the alternate Cahn, Ingold, and Prelog system of stereochemical nomenclature (CAHN et al., 1966) are listed in Figure 4. This method is not recommended for the substituted erythr*a*nolides since the notation at a given center may change because of a configurational change at an adjacent position (e.g., C-5 changes from S to R when a hydroxyl group is substituted at C-6). This could cause considerable confusion in making biochemical comparisons, and the R/S system of notation should be used only when a 'fully systematic' name is being constructed. The other alternative method of identifying the stereochemistry at an asymmetric center as *alpha* or *beta* is not useful with the erythr*a*nolides since the assignments at some carbon positions depend on how the projection formula is constructed (this contrasts with small ring or fused ring systems like those of terpenes, sterols etc.).

Table 1 lists most compounds of the erythronolide family which have commonly-accepted trivial names together with the new 'semisystematic' names being proposed. In spite of the slightly longer new name, the similarities and differences among these structures are clearly indicated. This is true not only for the sugar-free compounds, but also for the glycosides. For instance, it is easy to see the type of oxygen substitution and the number of hydroxyl and/or oxo functions from the 'semisystematic' name, whereas this is not so when the trivial or common names are compared. For glycosides, the potential advantages of the proposed nomenclature may be even greater since, for example, names like erythromycins A, B, C, and D do not describe any differences. In another example, the close relationship of megalomicin A (IX) to the erythromycins (THANG et al., 1978) is completely obscured by the use of a trivial nomenclature.

It is hoped that the proposed nomenclature for the derivatives of erythr*a*nolide will facilitate communication of information about this potentially extremely large group of natural and semisynthetic substances. It is convenient, however, to continue to use the trivial names for the naturally occurring and well-known examples like 6-deoxyerythronolide B (IIc), erythronolide B (IIb), and erythronolide A (IIa).

IV. Biosynthesis of the Lactones in the Erythromycins

A. General Aspects

From early work employing radioactive substrates and the whole mycelium of *S. erythreus* it was concluded that the macrolide lactone of erythromycin A (Ia) was formed from one 'primer' unit of *propionate* and six chain-extending molecules of *2-methylmalonate* (Fig. 3, MASAMUNE et al., 1977). It was assumed at an early date that the enzymatic mechanism for the biosynthesis of the erythronolide moiety in the erythromycins was similar to that established for the biosynthesis of saturated fatty acids from *acetate* and *malonate*. For this reason, considerable attention has been given to a study of the enzymes that form and metabolize the presumed substrates for both enzyme systems. These enzymes activate acetate and propionate and interconvert the products with the carboxylated forms, malonyl- and 2-methylmalonyl Co A respectively.

B. Variation of the Biosynthetic Enzymes with the Age of the *S. erythreus*

From the outset of cell-free studies on the biosynthesis of the erythromycins conducted in the author's laboratory, it was apparent that the activity of each enzyme depends largely on the age of the mycelium from which it is isolated. Most likely, the strain of *S. erythreus* used and the culture conditions employed will also have great quantitative effects on this variation (time in hours, relative specific activities of enzymes, etc.), but these parameters have not been studied in any detail as yet. Unless specified otherwise, the observations reported here

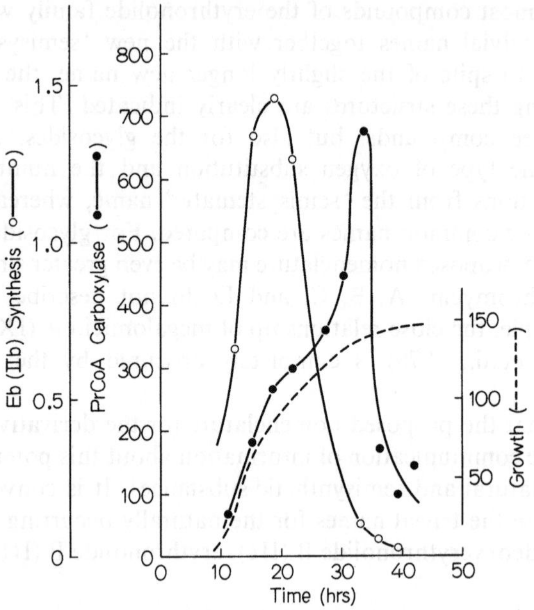

Fig. 5. Time dependency of relative biosynthesis of erythronolide B (IIb) and activity of propionyl coenzyme A carboxylase in *S. erythreus:* CA340

Apparent biosynthesis of erythronolide B is measured as CPM of ^{14}C-propionate incorporated into a trapping pool of (IIb) by washed mycelium and is expressed as CPM/mg dry weight; Pr–Co A carboxylase activity is expressed as CPM $^{14}C-HCO_3^-$ fixed into non-volatile acids/mg crude enzyme protein/30 min; growth is expressed as mg mycelium/5 ml fermentation broth

pertain to *S. erythreus* (CA340: Abbott), a former (primative) production strain cultured as described by CORCORAN (1975). Using these conditions, it was found that fatty acid synthase activity measured with acetyl- and malonyl Co A was almost absent when cultures were collected after 20-h of growth. A time-course study showed that there is a biphasic high peak of 'apparent' specific activity (measured for each enzyme tested as the specific incorporation of an obligate precursor, acetate in this case, by washed aliquots of *S. erythreus* under standard conditions as described by KANEDA et al. (1962) with the main peak occurring between 10 and 12 h of growth. The shoulder peak is probably an artefact reflecting increased metabolic activity of the innoculum of *S. erythreus* just prior to the start of exponential cell growth. When the time dependency of the erythronolide synthase was measured similarly, using radiolabeled propionate, the same variation in 'apparent' specific activity was noted (Fig. 5). The variation in the formation of the erythromycins with time (assayed as the incorporation of ^{14}C-methyl-L-methionine into trapping pools of the erythromycins A, B, and C) was similar, but delayed by about 2 h.

Work on the erythronolide synthase has used measurement of the incorporation of radioactive propionate into a product of the synthase, originally thought to be erythronolide B (IIb) (SPÍŽEK et al., 1966). Erythronolide B is an obligate intermediate in the biosynthesis of the erythromycins and a small 'trapping pool' of (IIb) was added to the assay system to minimize losses of the lactone product by further metabolism to the glycosides (Ia, b, c, and d, IV). With the recent development of HPLC* analysis in which we have been able to separate (IIb) from its precursor 6-deoxyerythronolide B (IIc) we have discovered that when radioactive propionate is incubated with *S. erythreus* and a small amount of non-radioactive erythronolide B (IIb), the bulk of the radioactive product is 6-deoxyerythronolide B (IIc) rather than (IIb). The lack of significant conversion of (IIc) into (IIb) in these experiments is probably explained by the fact (cf. Sect V. C.3.a. and VIII. B., below) that (IIb) is a potent inhibitor of the C-6 hydroxylase of *S. erythreus*. Fortunately, earlier results using the assay when recovered (IIb) was diluted further with carrier material and crystallized to constant specific activity (CORCORAN et al., 1967; SPÍŽEK et al., 1966) seem to have reflected the correct biosynthetic pattern, presumably because the 6-deoxyerythronolide B product (IIc) co-crystallized with the large amount of (IIb) present. Until now (IIc) has only been reported (MARTIN and ROSENBROOK, 1967) as a product of a mutant strain of *S. erythreus* (Abbott 9EI262) or found in normal cultures (CA340) when grown in the presence of an inhibitor of an NADPH-specific reductase of the cholesterol synthase system (CORCORAN and VYGANTAS, unpublished results).

C. Source and Nature of the Substrates Used for the Biosynthesis of the Erythronolides

1. The Propionyl Coenzyme A Carboxylase in Stationary Phase Cultures of *S. erythreus*

In a strict sense the activation of propionate, and especially the formation of 2-methylmalonyl Co A from the propionyl Co A produced, represents the first steps in the biosynthesis of an erythronolide from its ultimate precursors. The propionyl- and 2-methylmalonyl Co A molecules which presumably donate their activated acyl moieties to the erythronolide synthase may well be formed as such by the intermediary metabolism of the mycelium. Alternatively, propionyl Co A (and also acetyl Co A) can be formed by the direct activation of the free acid, either via a phosphate intermediate or via direct exchange between the acid and another thioester like succinyl Co A. In addition, 2-methylmalonyl Co A and (subsequently) propionyl Co A can be formed directly from succinyl Co A by a cobalamin-dependent mutase [it is assumed in this chapter that all the enzymes of this pathway exist in *S. erythreus* CA340 and also that the two forms of 2-methylmalonyl Co A (R and S) are interconvertible]. Other

* The usual abbreviations for analytical and chromatographic techniques (UV, IR, Mass, TLC, GLC, HPLC, etc.) will be used in this chapter, and the similar abbreviations for coenzymes etc. (NADH, NADPH, etc.) and substrates common to papers published in The Journal of Biological Chemistry and Biochemistry will be employed.

possible sources of propionyl- and 2-methylmalonyl Co A are the amino acid biosynthetic and catabolic pathway: L-valine (or the alpha-oxo-isovalerate formed from two molecules of pyruvate) yields 2-methylmalonyl Co A; L-isoleucine, L-threonine, and L-methionine can presumably give propionyl Co A. Propionyl Co A is also the product of the metabolism of fatty acids with odd numbers of carbons. The two acyl Co A precursors of erythronolide thus may be formed independently from carbohydrate, protein, and/or lipid precursors.

It is also well known that propionyl- and 2-methylmalonyl Co A may be formed from each other (Fig. 2). The interconversion can occur by either of two well-studied routes: the action of propionyl Co A carboxylase or by 2-methylmalonyl Co A, pyruvate transcarboxylase. Much has been made of a possible correlation between the activity of enzymes which form propionyl Co A or convert it into 2-methylmalonyl Co A and the ability of *S. erythreus* to form erythronolides. As RACZYŃSKA-BOJANOWSKA et al. (1970b) reported the activation of propionate has been correlated with increased production of erythromycin by normal strains of *S. erythreus* and by mutants whose already high production of erythromycin is stimulated by propanol and by citrate. The activation described is a two-step process involving ATP and the initial formation of propionyl phosphate (RUCZAJ et al., 1969). The kinase for propionate is not able to activate acetate, and in *S. erythreus* it is very much more active than the acetate kinase (13:1), whereas in other microorganisms the relative activities are either nearly the same (e.g. *S. noursei*, which forms polyene macrolides made from *acetate, malonate, 2-methylmalonate,* etc.) or disproportionate in the opposite sense (1:10 in *E. coli*). The propionate kinase also increases in specific activity in late stages of mycelial growth when erythromycin accumulation is also increasing, while the acetate kinase diminishes in activity after cell growth ceases. RACZYŃSKA-BOJANOWSKA et al. (1970b, 1976) have also studied the carboxylation of propionyl Co A, and seem to have ruled out transcarboxylase as an important enzyme in this process. They report that the propionyl Co A carboxylase activity in their strain of *S. erythreus* is time-dependent and peaks when erythromycin accumulation is high. Erythromycin does not inhibit the carboxylase. Taken alone this work is hard to evaluate in terms of the authors' thesis that propionyl Co A carboxylase is an important enzyme in the pathway for the biosynthesis of the erythromycins, but when considered with other results (cf. Section IV. D.) the suggestion is interesting.

A related study was reported by WAWSZKIEWICZ and LYNEN (1964) who found, in addition to a weak protein-dependent exchange between 2-methylmalonyl Co A and ^{14}C-bicarbonate (assumed to reflect reversibility of the first condensation step in the biosynthesis of erythronolide), an ATP-dependent, avidin-sensitive, propionyl Co A carboxylase activity in cell-free extracts of a strain of *S. erythreus* that was a poor producer of erythromycins. No evidence was found of a significant transcarboxylase activity. These results also did not clarify the role (if any) of propionyl Co A carboxylation in the biosynthesis of erythronolide.

A study initiated in the author's laboratory attempted to elucidate the importance of propionyl Co A carboxylase in the biosynthesis of 6-deoxyerythronolide B (IIc). First, the time course of the carboxylase activity in relationship to the 'apparent' specific activity of the erythronolide synthase was determined (Fig. 5). Initially a crude cell-free enzyme (48,000 *g* supernatent fraction) prepared from the sonicated mycelium of the *S. erythreus* was used, and the activity of the propionyl Co A carboxylase (Reaction 1) showed a

$$\text{propionyl CoA} + {}^{14}\text{C-HCO}_3^- + \text{ATP} \rightleftharpoons {}^{14}\text{C-(COOH)-2-methylmalonyl-CoA} + \text{P}_i + \text{ADP}$$

(Reaction 1)

maximum (at about 32 h) following completion of the exponential phase of growth and long after the 'apparent' specific activity of the erythronolide synthase had reached its maximum and then declined. A minor peak of activity in the carboxylase assay was noted at about the time of maximal 'apparent' activity of the lactone synthase, and it is not obvious whether this is an artefact reflecting physiological change in the innoculum prior to exponential growth or if it reflects instead an activity of the same or a different acyl Co A carboxylase (cf. discussion in Section IV, D). The propionyl Co A carboxylase was then purified about twentyfold by ammonium sulfate precipitation (bulk of the activity precipitates between 30 and 50% of saturation) followed by gel filtration chromatography, using first Sepharose 4B and then Biogel A-5 m columns. The partially purified carboxylase activity (about a 30% yield) was used to study the reaction. The peak of carboxylase activity from the 30-to-40-h mycelium eluted from the gel columns at the same time as did the lesser carboxylase activity found in the 12-to-18-h growths, and it also coincided with vigorous 2-methylmalonyl Co A: propionyl Co A exchange and 2-methylmalonyl Co A decarboxylase activities (cf. Section IV. C. 2) which showed maximal specific enzymatic activities in the younger mycelium. It is not yet known whether all these activities reflect different enzymes or the same enzyme following a complex 'apparent' activity pattern (caused by varying ratios of synthesis to degradation, the variable presence of activators and inhibitors, or some other factor).

When the purified propionyl Co A carboxylase from a 40-h culture of *S. erythreus* was assayed for activity, using either the ATP-dependent fixation of radioactive bicarbonate into acid stable counts (2-methylmalonate) or an HPLC ion exchange column (Whatman Partisil-10/25-SAX; 0.1 M phosphate; pH 4.5) for direct measurement of reactant and product amounts, it was found to behave like similar carboxylases from other sources (CORCORAN, J.W., MITCHELL, D.R., and NISHIKIORI, T., unpublished results). The K_m value of 2.95×10^{-4} M is close to those (1.5–2.6×10^{-4} M) reported for propionyl Co A carboxylases from liver mitochondria, pig heart, and goose uropygial gland and somewhat higher than that of *Mycobacterium smegmatus* (5.2×10^{-5} M). The activity is rather low and the rate of the forward reaction is only about ten times that of the backwards reaction, in contrast to a difference of nearly 70-fold reported by KAZIRO et al. (1961) for the same enzyme from pig heart. The propionyl Co A carboxylase of *S. erythreus* is specific for propionyl Co A, requires ATP and magnesium ions, and is inhibited strongly by avidin, iodoacetamide, and p-chloromercuribenzoate. No activation is noted when citrate is added to the assay system.

2. Propionyl Co A Carboxylase Activity in Exponentially-Dividing Cultures of *S. erythreus*

A small peak of propionyl Co A carboxylase activity is noted when *S. erythreus* taken from exponentially-growing cultures is assayed. The activity co-purifies with the carboxylase described in Section IV.D.1, which it resembles in its dependency on ATP and magnesium ions and its inhibition by avidin. The same preparation also has some acetyl Co A carboxylase activity and without further purification it was not possible to decide whether this 'second' propionyl Co A carboxylase activity is that of a truly independent enzyme, different from the one appearing in the older cultures, or whether it is caused by the acetyl Co A carboxylase lacking substrate specificity.

3. 2-Methylmalonyl Co A Exchange with Propionyl Co A and Decarboxylase Activities in Exponentially Dividing Cultures of *S. erythreus*

Some exchange is detectable between propionyl- and 2-methylmalonyl Co A when the purified propionyl Co A carboxylase obtained from stationary phase cultures of *S. erythreus* is assayed (Table 2). However, the exchange is much more vigorous when the enzyme is obtained from exponentially dividing *S. erythreus* (assayed with mixtures of propionyl- and 2-methylmalonyl Co A via the ion-exchange HPLC method described above). The same enzyme fraction also possesses a very active 2-methylmalonyl Co A decarboxylase activity (ATP-independent) which depends on propionyl Co A. The exchange reaction and the decarboxylase activity may be due to the same enzyme, a propionyl Co A carboxylase, and if so would reflect the second of the two partial reactions (Reactions 2 and 3) summarized by the overall stoichiometry for the carboxylase shown as Reaction 1 (cf. KAZIRO and OCHOA, 1961).

Table 2. Rates of reactions catalyzed by propionyl-coenzyme A carboxylase of *S. erythreus* CA340

Reaction measured	Rate (µmole/min/unit)
(a) Pr-Co A carboxylation	1.53
(b) 2-MeMal–Co A decarboxylation	0.18
(c) Pr-Co A-1-^{14}C:2-MeMal-Co A exchange	2.14

The reaction mixtures were: (**a**) Pr-Co A carboxylation; 0.1 ml with (µmoles) Tris-HCl buffer (10, pH 9.0), $MgCl_2$ (1.5), $NaHCO_3$ (6), ATP (0.5), 1-^{14}C-propionyl Co A (291,000 d.p.m./µmole, 0.2), enzyme (1 unit), (**b**) 2-MeMal-Co A decarboxylation; Tris-HCl (10), $MgCl_2$ (1.4), P_i (1.4), ADP (0.5), 2-methylmalonyl-Co A (148,000 d.p.m./µmole, 0.2), enzyme (1 unit), (**c**) Exchange; Tris-HCl (10), 1-^{14}C-propionyl Co A (0.2), 2-methylmalonyl Co A (0.2), and enzyme (1 unit). Incubations were for 10 min at 35° C. The radioactivity in substrate and product was directly measured by HPLC as described in the text

$$\text{ATP} + \text{HCO}_3^- + \text{enzyme} \xrightleftharpoons{\text{Mg}^{2+}} \text{enzyme-(HCO}_3) + \text{ADP} + \text{P}_i$$

(Reaction 2)

$$\text{propionyl CoA} + \text{enzyme-(HCO}_3) \rightleftharpoons \text{2-methylmalonyl CoA} + \text{enzyme}$$

(Reaction 3)

However, an alternative explanation for our results is suggested by the work of RACZYŃSKA-BOJANOWSKA et al. (1973) who have shown (indirectly) that acetyl Co A carboxylase activity is high in exponentially dividing cultures of *S. erythreus*, whereas propionyl Co A carboxylase is most active in a stationary phase culture. If generally true for *S. erythreus*, this could support our suggestion that at least two enzyme activities are present in our young (12-to-17-h) cultures. One would be an acetyl Co A carboxylase enzyme. If this enzyme is also active with propionyl Co A (or if there is a weak propionyl Co A carboxylase present as a separate entity) our observed propionyl Co A carboxylase as well as the 2-methylmalonyl Co A exchange and decarboxylase activities could be rationalized. However, since there is extremely vigorous, bulk decarboxylation of the 2-methylmalonyl Co A and the exchange is also quite rapid, it seems easier to explain all the phenomena by a second enzyme. The work of BUCKNER and KOLATTUKUDY (1975a) has shown that a substrate-specific malonyl Co A decarboxylase is present in the uropygial gland of the goose, and it co-purifies with an enzyme that carboxylates both acetyl- and propionyl Co A. A regulatory role in determining the ratio of n- and branch-chain fatty acids in the gland of the goose was demonstrated for the malonyl Co A decarboxylase. If a similar regulatory mechanism exists in *S. erythreus* it might require the presence of a potent 2-methylmalonyl Co A decarboxylase (cf. discussion in Section IV.D.3).

D. The Erythronolide Synthase

1. Studies with Whole Mycelium of *S. erythreus*

A number of questions about the biosynthesis of erythronolides could be answered by the continued use of systems of whole *S. erythreus* (e.g., the stereochemistry of the polymerization steps could possibly be determined with the aid of stereospecifically labeled enantiomers of 2-methylmalonyl Co A). However, the best chance for a detailed understanding of the properties of the synthase rests with the development of a purified, cell-free, enzyme system that makes an erythronolide. Probably for this reason little work has been done (or at least reported) with intact cultures of the producing organism. Studies of mutants by MARTIN and his colleagues showed that 6-deoxyerythronolide B (IIc) is a stable intermediate and that erythronolide B (IIb) is a metabolite of (IIc). The studies with mutants failed to reveal any other obligatory intermediates, and the possible conclusion that (IIc) may be the first synthase-free product in the biosynthesis of the erythronolides rests solely on negative evidence. This argument is not persuasive, and a definitive answer must await studies with other mutants or, better, cell-free purified enzyme systems.

In one useful study with the intact mycelium of *S. erythreus* (MCALPINE, J.B., NOURSE, J.G., ROBERTS, J.D. and CORCORAN, J.W., unpublished results) ^{13}C NMR analysis provided further information on the possible mechanism of erythronolide formation. A mutant of *S. erythreus* that accumulates erythronolide B (IIb) was grown in the presence of propionate-1-^{13}C, and the recovered (IIb) converted to the 3,5,11-tri-acetyl derivative. This substance when analyzed by NMR (cf. NOURSE and ROBERTS, 1975; TERUI et al., 1975; ŌMURA et al., 1976) showed a significant enrichment of ^{13}C in the single carbon position (C-13) which is derived from the carboxyl group of *propionate* if the biosynthesis of (IIb) is as depicted in Figure 2 (Section II). In one short-term experiment the enrichment of ^{13}C in position 13 was about 25% compared with those positions (C-1, -3, ··· -11) derived from the activated carboxyl group of 2-methylmalonate. The nearly uniform enrichment of the six units of (IIb) believed to be derived from the 2-methylmalonate is compatible with the hypothesis that the whole lactone (IIb) is formed by the rapid concerted polymerization of a single *propionate* and six *2-methylmalonate* building blocks. This result is to be expected if a fatty acid-like synthase is responsible for the biosynthesis of (IIb), and it tends to rule out the formation of erythronolides from two or more preformed units (e.g., C_9+C_{12}) or by other less likely mechanisms.

Another limited study done with an intact culture of a streptomycete showed that companion metabolites produced together with pikromycin and narbomycin by *S. venezuelae* had structures indicating that enzymes typical of fatty acid synthases had played a role in their biosynthesis (MAJER and CORCORAN, 1973; MAJER et al., 1976). These macrolides are very similar to the erythromycins and thus the results also support the idea that the erythronolides are the result of fatty acid synthase-like enzymatic activity.

2. Cell-Free Studies

The possibility that an intermediate in the biosynthesis of an erythronolide is formed in a cell-free system from *S. erythreus* was first reported by CORCORAN et al. (1967). Attempts to study and purify the synthase (CORCORAN, J.W., VYGANTAS, A.M., MITCHELL, D.R., unpublished results) have been disappointing and recent work has emphasized the study of the enzymes responsible for supplying substrates to the putative synthase (Section IV.D, above) and of the fatty acid synthase(s) of *S. erythreus*. The partial definition of a fatty acid synthase which is a multienzyme complex (ROSSI and CORCORAN, 1973) and the possibility that the lactone synthase is of similar molecular size has kept attention focused on experimental approaches that might decide whether these two synthases are identical or very similar.

Some time ago, it was suggested (CORCORAN, 1965) that the erythronolide synthase might be identical with the fatty acid synthase of *S. erythreus*: according to the chain-extending monomer utilized by the synthase, which could be a random matter determined by the relative concentrations of acetyl- and propionyl Co A and malonyl- or 2-methylmalonyl Co A present and the respective K_m values for each, the synthase could become 'committed' to the formation either of n-saturated fatty acids or of the branch-chain polymer resulting from use of 2-methylmalonyl Co A units. [The speculative approach could not explain why 'mixed' cases are known in which both malonyl Co A and 2-methylmalonyl Co A units participate in the biosynthetic reactions, and clearly such can occur because the structures of some closely-related macrolides (pikronolide, narbonolide, methynolide, etc.) have one or more of the propionate-derived units substituted by acetate-derived ones.] The *S. erythreus* situation is not yet understood, and of the two other examples one tends to support the speculative hypothesis while the other does not.

An interesting series of reports by BUCKNER and KOLATTUKUDY (1975a, b, 1976) on the fatty acid synthase isolated from the uropygial gland of the goose have appeared. This enzyme, which represents an astounding one-third to one-sixth of the total protein of the uropygial gland, is readily purified by gel filtration chromatography (Sepharose 4B) to an extremely high degree of homogeneity. The enzyme consists of two polypeptide chains with multienzymatic activities. The synthase has a molecular weight of 547,000 Daltons, and is dissociable into two partially active polypeptides of equal molecular weight (269,000 Daltons). The subunits each possess a 4′-phosphopantetheine residue. This synthase forms either n-saturated fatty acids (n-C_{16} and n-C_{18} in 4:1 ratio) from acetyl- and malonyl Co A substrates, or a mixture of 2,4,6,8-tetramethyl-decanoic and -undecanoic acids from propionyl- and 2-methylmalonyl Co A. Apparently, the initial choice (random) of the first chain-extending unit determines the type of product formed, since no 'mixed' products (ones reflecting use of both malonyl- and 2-methylmalonyl Co A as chain-extending substrates) were reported. The synthase actually prefers acetyl Co A as a 'primer' since when supplied with an equimolar mixture of acetyl- and propionyl Co A plus 2-methylmalonyl Co A the major branch-fatty acid product is that derived from acetyl- and 2-methylmalonyl Co A. The enzyme system utilizes malonyl Co A more readily than 2-methylmalonyl Co A (eight-fold lower K_m value) but the formation of product is driven towards the branch-chain side by the action of a powerful malonyl Co A decarboxylase which keeps the concentration of this intermediate low while at the same time maintaining the acetyl Co A pool. The decarboxylase which is not sensitive to avidin is without significant effect on 2-methylmalonyl Co A. A similar mechanism may be involved in regulating the biosynthesis of erythronolides and fatty acids by *S. erythreus* (cf. IV.D.3, below).

The highly interesting work on the synthase of the goose may have implications for the synthesis of branch-chain fatty acids like the erythronolides, but since the products of the goose gland lack oxygen functionality (except for the carboxyl position) they may be more analogous to the branch-chain fatty acids of the tubercle bacillus and to the singly branched shorter fatty acids produced by the parasite *Ascaris lumbricoides* etc., than to the erythronolides. Nonetheless, as the first report of a purified fatty acid synthase making lipid products from *2-methylmalonate* this work must be taken seriously.

Results which perhaps would argue against the participation of the same fatty acid-like synthase in the formation of both n-saturated fatty acids and the erythronolides has been reported by DIMROTH et al. (1970) and SCOTT et al.

(1974). In these studies concerning the biosynthesis of 6-methylsalicylate by *Penicillium patulum* they found that two separable multi-enzyme complexes are responsible for the different biosyntheses. Even though this result may suggest a basic difference between the fatty acid synthase of *S. erythreus* and its lactone synthase, it is still possible that both synthases in the penicillium have a great deal of evolutionary homology and that the two biosynthetic functions became separated after relatively recent genetic change.

3. Regulation of Erythronolide and Fatty Acid Synthesis in *S. erythreus*

We can only speculate on the biochemical mechanisms that operate to affect the time course of accumulation of the erythronolides (e.g., 6-deoxyerythronolide B, IIc) and the relationship of this process to the biosynthesis of n-saturated fatty acids like palmitic. An unequivocal answer must await detailed study of all the enzymes involved in both pathways, as well as possibly other work on side branches and alternate routes. However, the evidence now available from study of *S. erythreus* and some other possibly similar biological systems permits a highly speculative discussion of possible regulatory mechanisms at the enzymatic level.

The 'apparent' peak of enzymatic activity for biosynthesis of both palmitic acid and erythronolide in *S. erythreus* occurs early in the growth of the mycelium at a time when the biomass is beginning to increase at an exponential rate (Fig. 5). This 'apparent' activity is measured in a non-physiological manner with resuspended aliquots of mycelium under conditions where the biomass remains almost unchanged (KANEDA et al., 1962). It is not known yet what effect this has on the amount and activity of enzymes involved with fatty acid or erythronolide biosynthesis, but it is quite likely that the results of the assays reflect substrate stability or availability as much (or more) than they do the absolute amount of enzyme protein present. When both the fatty acid and lactone synthase enzyme activities show a similar dependency on time, it is difficult to explain the rapid synthesis of n-fatty acids in the exponentially-growing mycelium and the accumulation of 6-deoxyerythronolide B (IIc), erythronolide B (IIb), and glycosides of (IIb) (Fig. 6) at the middle and especially the late stages of growth (CORCORAN, J.W., GOMM, J., and MITCHELL, D.R., unpublished results). One seemingly rational explanation is available, if the studies on the metabolism of substrates for the lactone synthase both in *S. erythreus* and in other systems (above) can be applied. The argument is developed here with the hope of stimulating further experimental work.

There is a strong requirement for the synthesis of n-fatty acids during the rapid growth of cells to ensure development of cell membranes and essential metabolites, and the observed correlation of acetate kinase and acetyl Co A carboxylase activities with this phase of growth fits with a need to supply the fatty acid synthase of *S. erythreus* with substrates. The declining need for the fatty acid product as growth slows down agrees with a very much lower synthase activity, which may be due to either a decrease in the amount of the synthase protein or to a reduced supply of acetyl- and malonyl Co A units.

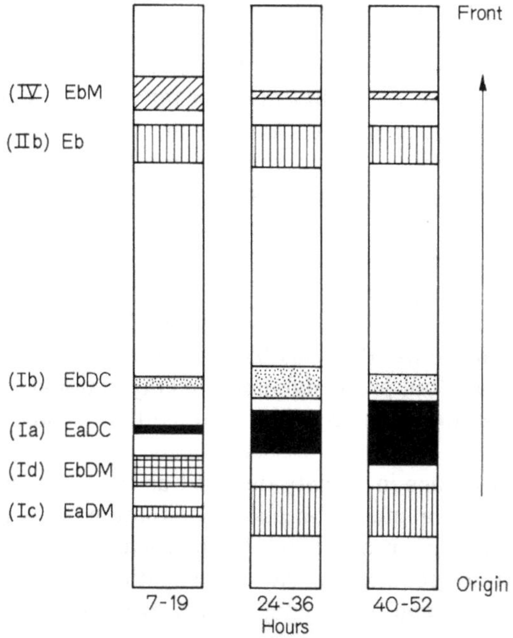

Fig. 6. Composite TLC chromatogram of metabolites present in fermentation beer of *S. erythreus* during three time periods

Aliquot of beer extracted with methylene chloride and chromatographed on silica gel using a methylene chloride/methanol/benzene/formamide (80:20:20:2.5 V/V) system. Substances identified by color reactions and comparison of mobilities with reference standards

Although this was not investigated with *S. erythreus*, it is possible that the amount of fatty acid synthase does not decrease as much as the 'apparent' activity (Fig. 5), and the decline in product formed is caused by both reduced acetyl Co A synthesis and the development of a strong malonyl Co A decarboxylase activity (cf. BUCKNER and KOLATTUKUDY, 1975a). The low rate of accumulation of erythronolide products during exponential growth, either from a unique synthase or from the fatty acid synthase itself, using the alternate substrates propionyl- and 2-methylmalonyl Co A could well be caused by a relative lack of these substrates because of low propionate kinase and propionyl Co A carboxylase activities (RACZYŃSKA-BOJANOWSKA et al., 1973; CORCORAN, J.W., MITCHELL, D.R. and NISHIKIORI, T., unpublished results), and also because of a potent 2-methylmalonyl Co A decarboxylase activity which shows its maximal activity in this time period (CORCORAN, J.W., MITCHELL, D.R. and WILSON, J.B., unpublished results). The increased accumulation of the erythronolide products seen in older (stationary phase) cultures of *S. erythreus* would then reflect increased availability of the three- and four-carbon substrates from amino acid breakdown, and the propionyl Co A carboxylase activity which appears in such cultures (CORCORAN, J.W., MITCHELL, D.R. and NISHIKIORI, T., unpublished results). This explanation leads to the conclusion that the amount of the lactone synthase protein may not be directly related to the 'apparent' time course of its activity

(Fig. 5) and that the relationship seen is caused mostly by substrate availability. This conclusion implies that the lactone synthase is present at times (early stages of growth) when its product is not formed rapidly. While this explanation is feasible, the alternative possibility that the fatty acid and lactone synthases are one and the same is attractive. As with the fatty acid synthase from the uropygial gland of the goose, all experimental results on n-fatty acid and erythronolide biosynthesis in *S. erythreus* could be nicely explained by a single protein complex with multiple activities whose products are regulated primarily by the availability of substrates. When acetyl- and malonyl Co A are the predominant species and 2-methylmalonyl Co A is at low concentration (because of a specific and active decarboxylase as well as weak propionate activation) the major product would be n-fatty acids like palmitic. When acetyl- and malonyl Co A are not abundant, but propionyl- and 2-methylmalonyl Co A, the alternate substrates, are, the major products of the same synthase would be the erythronolides.

Whether the variations in activity depicted as Figure 5 reflect the amounts of synthase protein or a more complicated situation in which the activities of other enzymes cause a strong time-dependent variation in the concentrations of alternate substrates requires further investigation of the synthase(s) (fatty acid and erythronolide) and of the enzymes involved in substrate metabolism.

V. The Transformation of 6-Deoxyerythronolide B into Erythronolide B by a Cytochrome P450-Dependent Mixed Function Oxidase

A. Studies With Mutants of *S. erythreus*

In 1964 Tardrew and Nyman reported the isolation of erythronolide B (IIb) from (presumably) normal cultures of *S. erythreus* that also produced the erythromycins. This intermediate has also been found as a product of blocked mutants of *S. erythreus,* and by using an HPLC assay system (Section IV,B) erythronolide B is detectable at all stages of growth in the culture filtrate of strain CA340 as used in the author's laboratory. Hung et al. (1965) as well as Spížek et al. (1966) proposed that erythronolide B was an obligatory intermediate in the biosynthesis of the erythromycins.

Soon after, Martin and Rosenbrook (1967) reported the isolation from a mutant strain of *S. erythreus* (Abbott 9EI262) of the presumed precursor of erythronolide B, a C-6 deoxy analog which they named 6-deoxyerythronolide B (IIc). The proof provided for the role of (IIc) in the biosynthesis of erythronolide B rested mainly on the apparent biotransformation of (IIc) into biologically active erythromycins. Chemical proof for the structure of (IIc) was not unequivocal and the production of the structurally and stereochemically defined erythronolide A nucleus (in erythromycin A as defined by Harris et al., 1965) was used as an argument for the structure and stereochemistry of 6-deoxyerythronolide B (IIc). The hydroxylation at C-6 of (IIc) was assumed to take place with retention of the configuration at C-6 (in agreement with most hydroxylations of natural products that had been reported). It was reasonable, using these assumptions, to describe the transformation of (IIc) into (IIb) by Reaction 4.

$$\text{6-deoxyerythronolide B (IIc)} + \tfrac{1}{2}O_2 \rightarrow \text{erythronolide B (IIb)}$$

(Reaction 4)

B. Characterization of the C-6 Erythranolide Hydroxylase System

1. Identification of 6-Deoxyerythronolide B (IIc) in Intact *S. erythreus*

6-Deoxyerythronolide B (IIc) was first found in normal cultures of *S. erythreus* grown in the presence of GEB [3-β-(2-dimethylaminoethoxy)-androst-5-ene-17-one], an inhibitor of an NADPH-specific Δ^{24}-reductase activity in the biosynthesis of the isooctyl side chain of cholesterol. Radioactive propionate was also added and significant amounts of highly radioactive (IIc) accumulated and were isolated by adsorption on XAD-2 resin (Rohm and Haas Corporation) and purified after elution with ethanol by TLC chromatography (VYGANTAS and CORCORAN, 1974). Proof of the structure of the (IIc) was based on comparison with a reference standard and by GLC-MASS analysis (CORCORAN, J.W., VYGANTAS, A.M. and TAKAHASHI, S., unpublished results). Following the initial detection of (IIc) in cultures of *S. erythreus* grown in the presence of GEB the same intermediate was routinely detected also in normal cultures.

2. Transformation of 6-Deoxyerythronolide B into Erythronolide B by Crude Cell-Free Preparation from *S. erythreus*

When radioactive 6-deoxyerythronolide B (IIc) was incubated with a crude cell-free preparation made from *S. erythreus* (VYGANTAS and CORCORAN, 1974) the accumulation of radioactive erythronolide B was noted. The enzymatic activity was found in the supernatant fraction of the mycelial extract (148,000 *g*) and the only product detected was (IIb). No hydroxylation of other positions on the erythranolide ring seemed to occur [no hydroxylation at C-12 to yield erythronolide A (IIa)]. The hydroxylase activity seemed to be correlated with the specific content of a cytochrome P450 moiety, and in addition it was inhibited by extreme anaerobiosis as well as by carbon monoxide. Some dependency on NADPH was also seen.

3. Studies on the Stereo- and Regiospecificity of the C-6 Erythranolide Hydroxylase and Development of an Alternate Substrate, 9-(*D*)-dihydro-6-deoxyerythronolide B (X)

a) Hydroxylation of Methynolide. When methynolide (XII), a 12-member macrolide lactone whose structure and stereochemistry in the region of C-3

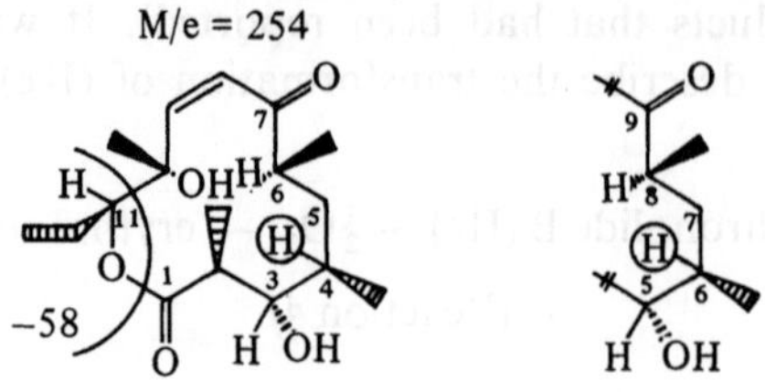

XII IIc

Fig. 7. Comparison of methynolide (XII) and 6-deoxyerythronolide B (IIc) as substrates for the erythranolide C-6 hydroxylase

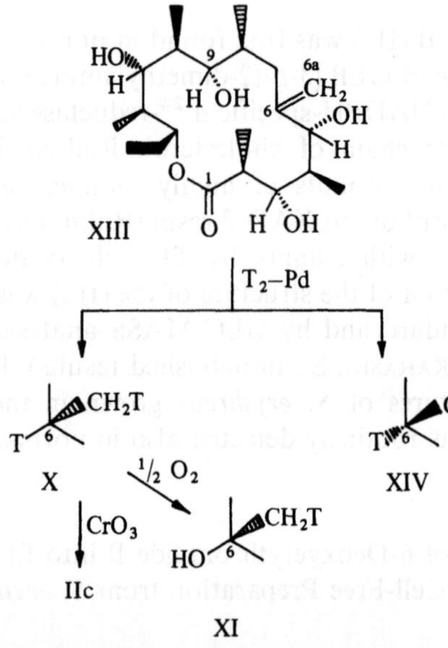

Fig. 8. Synthesis of tritiated substrates for study of the erythranolide C-6 hydroxylase: chemical partial synthesis of 6-deoxy erythronolide B (IIc) from derivatives of erythronolide B

through C-7 is identical to that of (IIc) in the C-5 to C-9 section, was added to the crude hydroxylase system a new product that absorbed UV light and had a M/e fragment at 270 mass units in its mass spectrum was formed (Fig. 7). This fragment is 16 mass units heavier than the fragment formed from methynolide itself (M/e = 254), and it is likely therefore that methynolide is hydroxylated (at the C-4 carbon?) by the erythranolide C-6 hydroxylase.

b) Activity of the Erythranolide C-6 Hydroxylase with 9-(D)-dihydro-6-deoxy-erythronolide B [3(L), 5(L), 9(D), 11(L)-tetrahydroxy-erythranolide (X)]. A chemical partial synthesis of 6-deoxyerythronolide B (IIc) from erythronolide B (IIb) was developed (CORCORAN, J.W., MITCHELL, D.R. and TAKAHASHI, S., unpublished results; CORCORAN and TAKAHASHI, 1975) and has proved to be extremely useful for the preparation of substrates used to study the C-6 hydroxylase reaction (Fig. 8). The key intermediate, [C-6, 6a-didehydro-3(*L*),

5(*L*), 9(*D*), 11(*L*)-tetrahydroxyerythranolide, (XIII)] could be reduced with tritium gas in the presence of a palladium catalyst to yield a mixture of (X) and (XIV), its epimer at C-6 (3:1 ratio). The desired C-6 normal product (X) was purified by LH-20 and HPLC chromatography. Chromic acid oxidation of (X) yields 6-deoxyerythronolide B (IIc) with two atoms of tritium, one at C-6 and the other on C-6a. The action of the hydroxylase enzyme system specifically removes the tritium atom at C-6, and the loss of radioactivity is a measure of the hydroxylase action (Reaction 5). The alternate substrate (X)

$$\text{C-6, 6a-ditritio-(IIc)} \xrightarrow{\frac{1}{2}O_2} \text{C-6a-tritio-(IIb)} + {}^3H_2O$$

$$\text{C-6, 6a-ditritio-(X)} \xrightarrow{\frac{1}{2}O_2} \text{C-6a-tritio-(XI)} + {}^3H_2O$$

(Reaction 5)

was used to study the specificity of the crude C-6 erythranolide hydroxylase with respect to C-9 and it was found that the intermediate with the reduced oxo function (X) was fully active. This is the 9-(S)-derivative using the Cahn-Ingold-Prelog nomenclature. Because of the improved stability to acid, both of the substrate and the hydroxylated product, and the very much higher radiochemical yield of (X) as compared with its chromic acid oxidation product (IIc), (X) was the substrate of choice for further studies of the mechanism of the C-6 hydroxylase.

Other work on the stereospecificity of the hydroxylase showed that (XIV) the C-6 epimer of (X) is not reactive (Corcoran, J.W. and Wiegand, R., unpublished results). It has not yet been determined whether the hydroxylase system has activity with the 9-(*L*)-dihydro derivative of 6-deoxyerythronolide B.

c) Biotransformation of [C-6, 6a-didehydro-3(L), 5(L), 9(D), 11(L)-tetrahydroxyerythranolide, (XIII)] by S. erythreus. A study of the biotransformation of (XIII) also sheds some light on the substrate specificity of the C-6 erythrano-

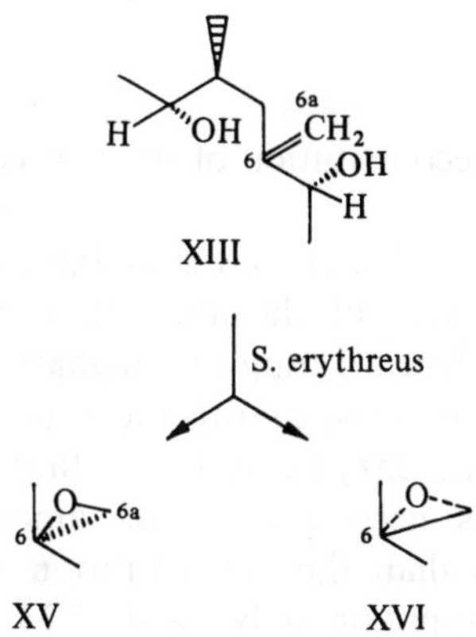

Fig. 9. Biotransformation of C-6, 6a-didehydro derivative of 6-deoxyerythronolide B (IIc) into epimeric C-6, 6a-oxido products

lide hydroxylase. When this C-6, 6a didehydro compound (XIII) was added to growing cultures of *S. erythreus* at least three new compounds were detected (CORCORAN, J.W., TAKAHASHI, S., MAJER, J. and ARORA, K.L., unpublished results) of which two are possible products of the hydroxylase. These structures were tentatively identified (Fig. 9) as the two different C-6, 6a-oxido compounds (XV and XVI) resulting when the epoxide ring is formed from one side of the C-6, 6a-ene (XIII) or the other. If the hydroxylase mediates the formation of these putative oxido compounds it is likely that the 'active' oxygen species involved may yield some intermediate at C-6 that can react in two alternative ways. Study of the oxido compounds may be useful later in working out the details of the enzymatic mechanism.

C. Mechanistic Studies of the C-6 Erythranolide Hydroxylase Using Purified Enzymes

1. Dependency of Erythranolide Hydroxylase and Cytochrome P450 Moiety of *S. erythreus* on the Age of the Mycelium

Prior to work on the fractionation of the C-6 hydroxylase activity, the dependency of the enzymatic activity on the age of the culture of *S. erythreus* from which it was obtained was studied. The activity was measured with a crude cell-free preparation with the alternate substrate (X) (Section V.B.3.b.). As the results show (Fig. 10), the hydroxylase activity depends sharply on the age of the mycelium, with the maximum between 12 and 20 h of growth. This time period is more or less the same as that of the peak for 'apparent' synthesis of the substrate, 6-deoxyerythronolide B (IIc) (Fig. 5). The specific content of a cytochrome P450 moiety in the mycelium (measured spectrally as the carbon monoxide adduct of the enzyme solution after treatment with dithionite) likewise depended on the age of the culture. For further work on the hydroxylase, the enzyme protein was derived from a mycelium harvested during the 'apparent' peak of activity (16–20 h).

2. Fractionation and Reconstitution of the C-6 Hydroxylase Activity

a) Assay of the Hydroxylase Activity. Assay of the C-6 erythranolide hydroxylase was based on measurement of the amount of radioactive hydroxylated product, generally (XI), produced during an incubation period that was determined empirically to be short enough for the rate of the hydroxylation to depend on the activity of the enzyme system rather than on the amount of substrate present. This was necessary as the amount of substrate added (3.6×10^{-8} M) is much less than the concentration required to saturate the hydroxylase activity (K_m is approximately 4×10^{-6} M measured with the crude enzyme). Although the details of the incubations vary somewhat with the experiments (cf. legends to Tables and Figures), in general the mixture consisted

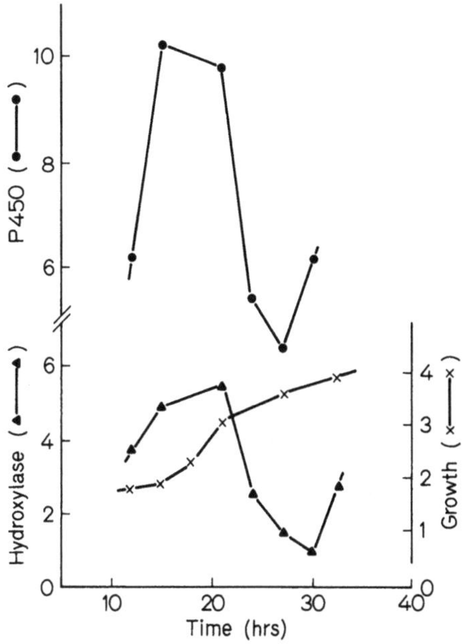

Fig. 10. Time dependency of erythranolide C-6 hydroxylase and cytochrome P450 content in *S. erythreus*

Hydroxylase activity in units $\times 10^2$/g cells; P450 in nmoles/g cells; growth in g wet weight/100 ml of medium

of radioactive substrate (X) (1.3×10^6 DPM; 7.2 nmoles) together with enzyme protein (4–5 mg), an NADPH-generating system (3.3 μmoles $NADP^+$, 26.6 nmoles glucose-6-phosphate, 4 units glucose-6-phosphate dehydrogenase), and buffer (phosphate; 0.05 M; pH 7.4) in a total volume of 2.0 ml. The reaction was started by adding the NADPH system to the other (preincubated) components and allowed to proceed without shaking at 35–37° C for the appropriate time (10–30 min). The reaction was terminated by the addition of non-radioactive product (XI) (0.02 mg) in acetonitrile (0.1 ml). The resultant mixture was passed through a column (1×5 cm) of Amberlite XAD-2 resin, and the column was washed with water (15 ml) to remove proteins and hydrophilic substances. Lipophilic substances adsorbed on the resin, including the product (XI) and unreacted substrate (X), were then eluted with acetone (12 ml) and concentrated by evaporation. The residue remaining was applied to a TLC plate (silica gel; 5×10 cm) which was then developed with an ethyl acetate and benzene solvent system (3:1; V/V). Reference lanes containing substrate and product were visualized by use of an anisaldehyde spray reagent. The silica gel from the experimental lanes was removed in horizontal sections (0.5 cm) and the radioactivity in each determined by liquid scintillation spectrometry. The calculation of enzyme activity was based on the assumption that radioactivity present in the substrate (X) is equally distributed between the C-6 and -6a positions, and that the product (XI) has half the specific radioactivity of the substrate. Equal recovery of product and unreacted substrate was assumed. Relative enzyme activity is calculated as:

$$(\text{ACTIVITY})_{\text{relative}} = 100\,\text{X}\,\frac{2\times[\text{Total CPM in (XI)}]}{[\text{Total CPM in (X)} + 2(\text{Total CPM in (XI)}]}$$

A unit of enzyme activity is defined as that amount which catalyzes the conversion of one picomole (pmole) of substrate (X) to product (XI) in 1 h at 35° C, and the specific activity is the number of units per milligram of enzyme protein.

b) Ammonium Sulfate Fractionation of the Hydroxylase. The crude enzyme used in defining the hydroxylase activity was prepared by rupture of the mycelium of *S. erythreus* in a French Pressure Cell and dialysis of the 48,000 *g* fraction of the centrifuged material against a dilute phosphate buffer (0.05 M; pH 7.4). Further purification was effected by treatment of this crude enzyme with solid ammonium sulfate. The fraction insoluble between 30 and 60% of saturation contained the bulk of the hydroxylase activity, and it was used for further column purification procedures (NISHIKIORI et al., 1978; CORCORAN, J.W.; NISHIKIORI, T.; unpublished results).

c) Fractionation of the Hydroxylase Activity by DEAE-Sepharose 6B-CL Column Chromatography. The crude enzyme from the precipitation step with ammonium sulfate was chromatographed using columns of DEAE-Sepharose 6B-CL ion exchange medium and elution (stepwise) with solutions of increasing molarity in potassium chloride. It was determined that three separate components, each being required for hydroxylase activity, were eluted from the column. The first component eluted together with a cytochrome P450 moiety in the 0.1 M KCl solution. The second component was found in the 0.2 M KCl eluate, and a third substance required for the activity emerged with the 0.6 M salt fraction. As shown in Table 3, all three components are required for hydroxylase activity. In addition, the full activity of the reconstituted system depends abso-

Table 3. Erythranolide C-6 hydroxylation by a reconstituted three component enzyme system derived from *S. erythreus*

System	Hydroxylase activity (pmoles/h)
Complete	130.5
Complete + Fe^{2+} (0.5 µmole)	136.0
Complete − $P450_{ery}$	6.9
Complete − 2nd Component	3.4
Complete − 3rd Component	8.1
Complete − FAD	29.3
Complete − NADPH regenerating system	3.3

Standard assay modified by substitution of P450 (1.26 mg protein), 2nd component (1.07 mg protein), and 3rd component (0.035 mg protein) for crude enzyme, and preincubation of 2nd component with FAD (50 nmoles) for 10 min

Table 4. Correlation of specific content of a cytochrome P450 moiety and the erythranolide C-6 hydroxylase activity during purification of the enzyme system

Preparation	Total protein (mg)	P450 (nmoles/mg)	Hydroxylase activity (pmoles/h/mg)	Fold purification	
				P450	Hydroxylase
Crude extract	13,790	0.025	8.8	1	1
Ammonium sulfate ppt. (30–60% sat'n)	11,900	0.036	7.4	1	1
DEAE-Sepharose					
(1st column)	462	0.35	174.0	14	20
(2nd column)	31	2.76	1,126.0	110	128
Bio Gel P-150	14	3.16	1,428.0	127	162

Standard assay with the reconstituted enzyme system (P450, ca. 0.18 nmoles; 2nd component, 3.83 mg protein; 3rd component, large excess

lutely on an NADPH-generating system (bulk NADPH is much less effective and NADH shows no activity). Also, maximal activity of the system is only seen if the second component is pre-incubated with FAD. This second component lacks significant flavin content as isolated.

d) Further Purification of the First Component, a Cytochrome P450 Heme Protein. Repeated ion exchange chromatography of the first component (0.1 M KCl) using DEAE-Sepharose 6B-Cl and subsequent gel filtration using Biogel P-150 gave a highly purified material (Table 4). This product was purified approximately 160-fold with respect to the hydroxylase activity and nearly the same (130-fold) in terms of its specific content of the heme protein. Disc gel electrophoretic analysis of this purified preparation showed the presence of one major and 4–5 minor bands of protein-containing material. Only the major band had the cytochrome P450 moiety ($P448_{ery}$) and it was also the only fraction showing hydroxylase activity after elution from the gel. This presumed cytochrome P450 heme protein is judged to be perhaps 80% pure on the basis of its apparent content of protein. The molecular weight of the $P448_{ery}$ heme protein was estimated by gel filtration behavior to be about 47,000 Daltons.

3. Mechanistic Studies of the C-6 Erythranolide Hydroxylase Using Purified Enzymes

a) Role of the Cytochrome P448-containing Component. The possibility that one component of the fractionated enzyme system was a P450 heme protein was first suggested circumstantially by experiments with a crude enzyme system (VYGANTAS and CORCORAN, 1974). It was supported by the physical evidence that the highly purified first component appears to be a heme protein which after reduction with dithionite forms an adduct with carbon monoxide that absorbs light at 448 nm. Evidence that the P448 moiety is essential for the

Table 5. Erythranolide C-6 hydroxylase activity in a reconstituted system depending on the cytochrome P450 moiety of *S. erythreus* and combinations of homologous and heterologous cytochrome reductases and non-heme iron proteins

Cytochrome reductase	Non-heme iron protein	Hydroxylase activity (pmoles/h)
S. erythreus (0.54 mg)	*S. erythreus* (35 μg)	73
S. erythreus (0.54 mg)	spinach ferredoxin (100 μg)	9
S. erythreus (0.54 mg)	Clostridium pasteurianum ferredoxin (100 μg)	14
spinach (0.24 units)	*S. erythreus* (35 μg)	132
spinach (0.24 units)	spinach ferredoxin (100 μg)	139
spinach (0.24 units)	*Cl. pasteurianum* ferredoxin (100 μg)	138

Standard assay using $P450_{ery}$ (1.26 mg protein, 0.82 nmole) and the combinations of cytochrome reductases and non-heme iron proteins indicated as replacements for the second and third components, respectively

function of the first component was provided by data showing that the activity of the hydroxylase was markedly inhibited by carbon monoxide in the range of 80–100%, and that inhibitors specific for cytochrome P450 moieties in other hydroxylase systems (SKF-525, metyrapone, cumene hydroperoxide) strongly inhibited the function of the product. Other inhibitors of cytochrome P450-dependent hydroxylases such as p-chloromercuribenzoate (which accelerates formation of an inactive P420 decomposition product) showed only modest inhibitory action when tested with the erythranolide hydroxylase.

Another potent inhibitor of the overall hydroxylase system proved to be the product, 9-(*D*)-dihydroerythronolide B (XI). Kinetic studies indicate that the inhibition is competitive in nature (K_i is approximately 2×10^{-5} M).

Additional evidence that the P448 heme protein plays an essential role in the C-6 erythranolide hydroxylase system is that it will couple with a heterologous cytochrome P450 reductase from spinach (Table 5).

In summary, the properties of the first component indicate it to be a heme protein of the P450 type. The P448 heme protein of *S. erythreus* is stable, present in the soluble fraction of the mycelium, and part of a constitutive system. Only two other cytochrome P450-linked hydroxylases which are soluble have been studied extensively. One is that found in *Pseudomonas putida* (TYSON et al., 1972) and the other is in a yeast, *Candida tropicalis* (DUPPEL et al., 1973).

b) The Second Component, a Flavin-Linked Pyridine Nucleotide Reductase. The second component isolated from the crude hydroxylase and found in the 0.2 M KCl eluate from the DEAE-Sepharose column is a protein, molecular weight estimated at about 61,000 Daltons that absorbs light weakly at 280 nM and 415 nM. The protein is not active as a cytochrome c reductase (NADPH-dependent) and it contains no apparent flavin moiety. The activity of this second component is greatly increased by pre-incubation with FAD (Table 3) and it is likely that as isolated this protein is the *apo* form of an FAD-specific, pyridine nucleotide-dependent, cytochrome P450 reductase. If the second component is not pretreated with FAD, ferrous ions will greatly increase the activity of the reconstituted system, but when treated with FAD the metal ions produce no additional stimulation (Table 3). A commercial cytochrome P450 reductase isolated from spinach will substitute for the second component in the hydroxylase reaction (Table 5).

c) The Third Component (a Ferredoxin Type of Non-heme Iron Protein?) The third component, recovered in the 0.6 M KCl eluate from the ion exchange column has not been purified extensively. It is unstable to heat, is not extracted into lipid solvents like chloroform, and has only a slight yellow color with no sharp absorption maximum. There is some evidence that it possesses acid-labile sulfur, and the properties of the active component are comparible with its being a non-heme iron protein of the ferredoxin type. The ability of ferredoxins obtained from spinach or from *Clostridium pasteurianum* to substitute for the third component in the hydroxylase reaction supports this conclusion (Table 5).

d) The Overall Reaction Mechanism. Although it is premature to propose a final reaction mechanism for the C-6 hydroxylase, the data available suggest at least one possibility. The high degree of specificity shown with respect to the pyridine nucleotide (NADPH) and flavin (FAD) moiety plus the rigid requirement for at least three catalytic components, each of which belongs to a type known to be involved in other better-studied hydroxylase systems, suggest strongly that the overall mechanism for the reaction may be compatible with that shown as Reaction 6.

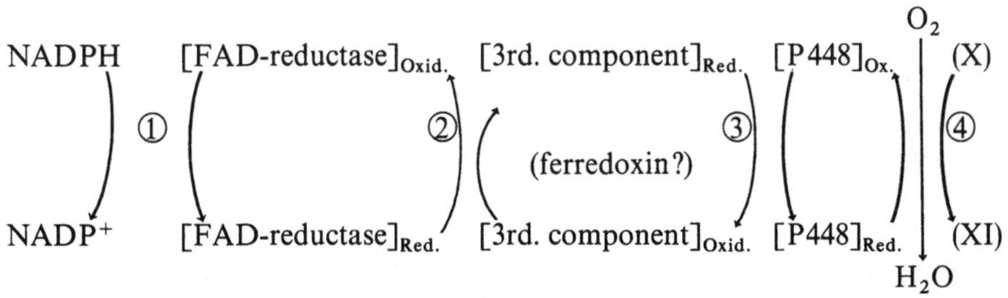

(Reaction 6)

The reaction sequence may not be as suggested here or, if similar, it could be more complex. For example, the third component (ferredoxin) might be both an essential link in the electron-transfer chain from NADPH to oxygen and an effector active in binding the reduced cytochrome P448 moiety to substrate (cf. TYSON et al., 1972).

The C-6 hydroxylase of *S. erythreus* is not inhibited by cyanide, but is inhibited strongly by cytochrome c and 2,6-dichloroindophenol. The behavior of the erythranolide hydroxylase towards inhibitors is typical of hepatic, fungal, and bacterial mono-oxygenases that depend on a cytochrome P450 heme protein. The system from *P. putida* is apparently similar to that of *S. erythreus,* although some heterologous ferredoxins will function in the system, whereas the one from the *Pseudomonas* is specific for putidaredoxin. Another solubilized bacterial hydroxylase (from *P. oleovorans*) does not utilize a cytochrome P450 moiety at all and functions instead with two non-heme iron proteins in the electron transport sequence (RUETTINGER et al., 1974).

The C-6 erythranolide hydroxylase of *S. erythreus* appears to be an important system for further investigation of the mechanistic aspects of the activation of molecular oxygen and the actual intermediates in the substrate-level insertion of activated oxygen. The complex structure and stereochemistry of the substrates (IIc or X) contrast sharply with those of substrates in other systems being studied, and the substitution at a tertiary center is also unique. The apparent activity of a C-6, 6a-didehydro derivative (XIII) of the substrate and the production of epimeric C-6, 6a-oxido products (XV and XVI) also suggests that the erythranolide C-6 hydroxylase system will be extremely useful in the study of the mechanism of action of cytochrome P450-linked heme proteins in biological hydroxylations, including some of those active in the biosynthesis of antibiotics.

The apparent constitutive nature of the C-6 erythranolide hydroxylase makes it an interesting exception to the general rule that such enzyme systems require induction by their substrate. This may be misleading, however, in the present example for it must be noted that the mycelium is also producing the substrate for the hydroxylase and induction could be of an autocatalytic nature.

VI. The Biosynthesis of Erythromycin D

A. Formation of Neutral Glycosides of Erythronolide B

1. Studies with Normal and Mutant Strains of *S. erythreus*

a) Historical Aspects. Studies employing strains of intact *S. erythreus* revealed that the sugars present in the biologically active bis-glycosides (I, a–d) are derived from intact D-glucose, activated S-methyl groups, and a source of nitrogen. Nothing could be deduced from this work about the identity of the sugars being transferred to a lactone acceptor, although it was (and still is) assumed that the donor is some form of nucleoside diphospho sugar. A detailed search for possible donors in *S. erythreus* was made by PAPE and GRISEBACH (1965), but no nucleoside derivatives of L-mycarose (XVII) or L-cladinose (XVIII)

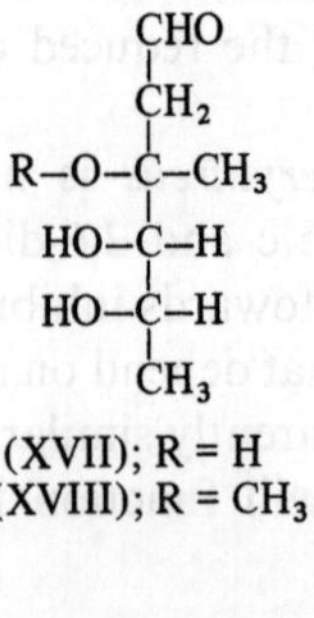

(XVII); R = H
(XVIII); R = CH_3

were detected. Similar studies in the author's laboratory were also negative. Using a sensitive radioisotopic dilution technique, it was not possible to detect any significant amounts of free or bound L-mycarose or L-cladinose in the mycelium of *S. erythreus* (Strain 233.1 Ky3, Eli Lilly), and it was concluded that these sugars appear in detectable amounts only as glycosides of erythronolides B and A (CORCORAN, J.W., VANĚK, Z., unpublished results).

SPÍŽEK et al. (1965) proposed that the biosynthetic pathway leading to the glycosides of erythronolide B and A might be complicated and that alternative routes for formation of an end product might exist. For instance, if the sequence of addition of the neutral and amino sugars is random and if the substrate specificity for hydroxylation of the lactone (at C-12) is independent of the presence of sugars, multiple alternate biosynthetic routes from erythronolide B to the erythromycins would be possible.

b) Identification of 3-(O)-α-(L)-mycarosylerythronolide B [3(L)-(α-L-mycarosyloxy), 5(L), 6(D), 11(L)-trihydroxyerythranolide-9-one] as an Intermediate in the Biosynthesis of the Erythromycins. Work by MARTIN et al. (1966) with a blocked mutant strain of *S. erythreus* (Abbott 8EI57) showed that an intermediate monoglycoside of erythronolide B and the neutral branch-chain sugar L-mycarose (XVII) accumulates in the growth medium and that this product, 3-(O)-α-*L*-mycarosylerythronolide B (IV) is an intermediate in the biosynthesis of the biologically active erythromycins. No other intermediate monoglycosides were found during Martin's extensive study of blocked mutants, and it is possible that the biosynthesis of (IV) occurs by the direct glycosylation of erythronolide B in a reaction in which some activated form of L-mycarose is the donor of the sugar (Reaction 7).

erythronolide B (IIb) + [X]-L-mycarose → 3-(O)-α-L-mycarosylerythronolide B (IV) + [X]

(Reaction 7)

The failure to find any significant amounts of a substance behaving like the postulated activated L-mycarose in the mycelium of *S. erythreus* (cf. Section VI.A.1.a) does not rule this mechanism out, since it is possible that synthesis of the activated sugar intermediate is rate-limiting and that no significant steady-state amount of 'free' [X]-(*L*)-mycarose ever accumulates. However, it is also quite likely that the synthesis of (IV) is more complicated than is suggested by Reaction 7, and perhaps the first product is some different monoglycoside in which the sugar is a precursor of L-mycarose, perhaps one lacking the branch methyl group. Such a possibility is supported by the work of COLLUM et al. (1976) which defined two 'aberrant' metabolites in the pathway for the biosynthesis of the erythromycins. These are monoglycosides of erythronolide B with (*L*)-2,6-dideoxyaldohexoses lacking a branch-methyl group. The two new metabolites (XIX), [3-(O)-(2′,6′-dideoxy-α-(*L*)-*Ribo*-hexopyranosyl)-erythronolide B], and (XX), [3-(O)-(2′,6′-dideoxy-α-(*L*)-*Arabino*-hexopyranosyl)-erythronolide B], could be derived from a common monoglycoside (e.g., XXI). Perhaps the precursor of (XIX) and (XX) has an oxo functional group at C-3 and normally a Reformatzky-type of C-methylation (at C-3) occurs in the biosynthesis of

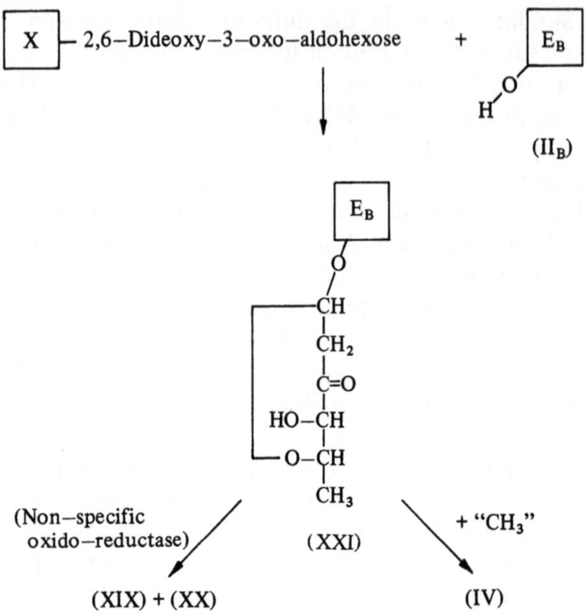

Fig. 11. Hypothetical scheme for the biosynthesis of glycosides of erythronolide B

(IV) from (XXI) (Figure 11). If true, perhaps a methyl cobalamin species is the donor of the required methyl group. This mechanism differs from that usually assumed to operate in the formation of (IV), in which a methyl group is supposedly inserted at a position with an activated hydrogen atom (e.g., a methylene carbon position adjacent to an oxo function at C-2 or C-4).

2. Mycelium-Free Studies of the Biosynthesis of 3-(O)-α-(*L*)-Mycarosyl-erythronolide B (IV)

Attempts to define a mycelium-free system for the biosynthesis of 3-(O)-α-(*L*)-mycarosylerythronolide B (IV) have been made in which the assay system employed erythronolide B (radioactive and non-radioactive) together with a crude mycelium-free extract of *S. erythreus*. Assuming the presence of a transferase activity in the crude extract, various cell fractions obtained by separate growth of the actinomycete with radioactive (methyl-labeled S-adenosyl-L-methionine) substrates were tested to see if they stimulated the synthesis of (IV). In particular the cell fractions tested were those containing nucleoside diphosphate sugars. No evidence was obtained of the accumulation of a new radioactive product similar to (IV) (CORCORAN, J.W., VANĚK, Z. and FUJII, A., unpublished results).

Attention was next focused on demonstrating the biosynthesis of some activated form of L-mycarose (or of a precursor) from D-glucose. PAPE and BRILLINGER (1973) have reported that cell-free extracts from *S. rimosus*, a producer of the 16-member macrolide antibiotic tylosin, specifically transform thymidine diphospho glucose (TDP-glucose) into L-mycarose bound to the same carrier

(TDP-mycarose). This transformation depends partly on S-adenosyl-L-methionine (SAM). These workers did not report any attempts to use their purified TDP-mycarose as a possible donor in a biosynthetic system with desmycosin, the presumed acceptor in the biosynthesis of tylosin (CORCORAN et al., 1977b), or with erythronolide B (IIb), the acceptor in the biosynthesis of (IV). This approach was therefore tried in the author's laboratory, and using an extract from *S. erythreus* and the methods described by PAPE and BRILLINGER (1973), the isolation of biologically-formed TDP-mycarose was attempted. It was planned to use the TDP-mycarose as a substrate with an extract of *S. erythreus* and the acceptor lactone (IIb). However, no TDP-mycarose seemed to be formed by *S. erythreus,* and although all the available nucleoside diphospho derivatives of D-glucose were metabolically active, there was no unique reactivity seen with the TDP-derivative and there was no evidence that any sort of activated L-mycarose was formed (CORCORAN, J.W. and FUJII, A., unpublished results). The proof of structure of the TDP-mycarose isolated by PAPE and BRILLINGER appears sound, and it thus is possible that *S. erythreus* and *S. rimosus* are metabolically different. The TDP-mycarose isolated from the latter organism indeed may not be a normal intermediate in the biosynthesis of tylosin, and it may instead be an abnormal metabolite that accumulates when the normal pathway is blocked. Perhaps the normal biosynthesis of L-mycarose is like that postulated above (Fig. 11) for the erythromycins, and the activated sugar accepted by desmycosin, the lactonic aglycon, is a TDP-derivative of an (*L*)-2,6-dideoxy-3-oxo-aldohexose which is normally not C-methylated until after it is attached in glycosidic linkage to the desmycosin (Fig. 12). If this attachment is blocked, as it might be in a cell-free system, and if the SAM present can react (directly or via a cobalamin carrier) with the TDP-oxo-sugar precursor, a TDP-mycarose molecule could be formed. Perhaps in *S. erythreus* a similar mechanism exists but with a different nucleotide carrier and the branch-reaction

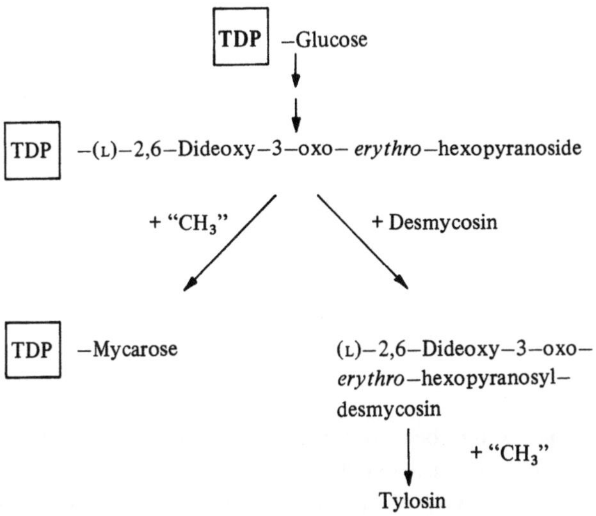

Fig. 12. Hypothetical scheme for the biosynthesis of TDP-mycarose and tylosin by *S. rimosus*

leading to the formation of the nucleoside diphospho L-mycarose derivative does not operate.

3. Specificity for the Substrate in the Glycosylation of Erythronolide B

A number of experiments have indicated that the enzyme system which attaches the neutral sugar to the C-3 position of erythronolide B has a very broad specificity with respect to the lactone acceptor. A large number of derivatives of erythronolide B have been prepared by chemical partial synthesis (Abbott Laboratories, unpublished results; CORCORAN, J.W., MCALPINE, J.B., TAKAHASHI, S., unpublished results). In addition, several other modified forms of erythronolide B have been isolated from blocked mutants and are apparently 'shunt' metabolites (MARTIN and PERUN, 1968; MARTIN and EGAN, 1970; MARTIN et al., 1972). Many of these modified erythronolides are transformed (cf. GOLDSTEIN et al., 1978) into neutral monoglycosides [usually the 3-(O)-α-*L*-mycarosyl-derivative] when added to growing cultures of *S. erythreus* (either normal strains or mutants blocked at an early step in the biosynthetic pathway). Work in the author's laboratory has shown that the C-6, 6a-didehydro-derivative (XIII) of 6-deoxyerythronolide B (IIc) is transformed into a neutral monoglycoside (CORCORAN, J.W., TAKAHASHI, S., MAJER, J. and ARORA, K.L., unpublished results).

A few mixed studies have been made employing either lactones produced by different species of *Streptomyces* together with *S. erythreus* (cf. GOLDSTEIN et al., 1978) or an erythronolide together with a strain of *Streptomyces* which normally produces a similar, but different macrolide (LEMAHIEU et al., 1976). In the former case lactones related to lankamycin were not glycosylated, although some biotransformation of the lactones themselves did occur. In the latter example, an erythronolide B derivative was added to a streptomycete that normally makes oleandomycin (a close relative of erythromycin) and the non-branched sugar L-oleandrose (XXII) was attached to the C-3 position of the lactone (oleandolide).

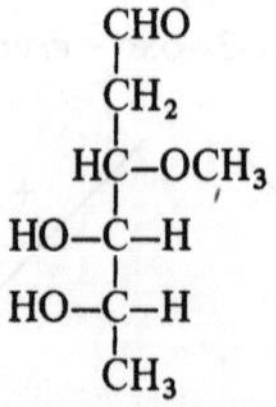

(XXII)

Although little work has been done, it seems that the presence of a sugar moiety at the C-5 position of the erythronolide ring system prevents attachment of a neutral sugar at C-3. For instance, 5-(O)-desosaminylerythronolide B (V) is not reactive.

B. Attachment of the Amino Sugar to 3-(O)-α-*L*-Mycarosylerythronolide B

1. General Description of the Reaction

Relatively little is known about the enzymatic nature of the next step in the biosynthesis of erythromycin D. From the structures involved, the reaction, namely, the addition of the basic dimethylamino sugar D-desosamine (XXIII)

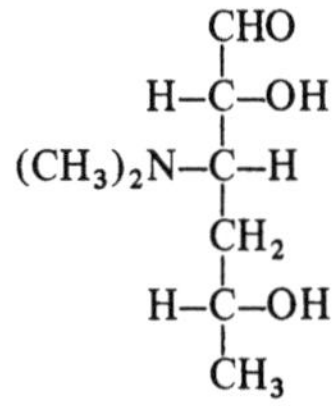

(XXIII)

to the C-5 position of (IV) as the *β*-(*D*)-*Xylo*-hexapyranoside, looks deceptively simple. Like the L-mycarose the ultimate origin of the D-desosamine moiety is D-glucose. The two N-methyl groups come efficiently from the methyl position of L-methionine and the nitrogen atom arises from an unknown source. Presumably, the D-desosamine is made from some nucleoside diphospho derivative of D-glucose, but no data are available either about the biosynthesis of the activated D-desosamine or its transfer to the formal acceptor, 3-(O)-α-L-mycarosylerythronolide B (IV).

The 5-(O)-*β*-(*D*)-desosaminylerythronolide B structure (V) is available from acid treatment of erythromycin B, and it is known that (V) cannot serve as a substrate in the biosynthesis of erythromycin B. This was used as an argument (Section VI.A.3.) for a rigid order for the enzymatic addition of sugars to erythronolide B. In the experiments with *S. erythreus* there is as yet no evidence to suggest formation of any abnormal monoglycosides between erythronolides and D-desosamine. This also tends to support the conclusion that the order of addition of the sugars is under strict control.

2. Substrate Specificity of the D-Desosamine: 3-(O)-α-*L*-Mycarosyl-erythronolide B Transferase

a) Specificity for the Lactone Moiety. Many neutral monoglycosides are known (Section VI.A.3.) in which the chemical nature of the lactone entity varies. Of these, the only one that seems transformable into an erythromycin is the 11-(O)-methyl-derivative of the normal intermediate (IV) (Martin, J.R., private communication). This suggests strongly that the transferase in *S. erythreus* which promotes the formation of erythromycin D (Id) from (IV) and activated D-desosamine (or its precursor) has a much stricter specificity for the structure of the lactone-containing substrate than does the transferase for the neutral sugar. However, a study in a related system suggests that some further flexibility with respect to the lactone structure may be expected. *Streptomyces narbonensis* is an actinomycete which produces narbomycin (XXIV), while *S. zaomyceticus* produces pikromycin (XXV) (C-12-hydroxy-narbomycin), and

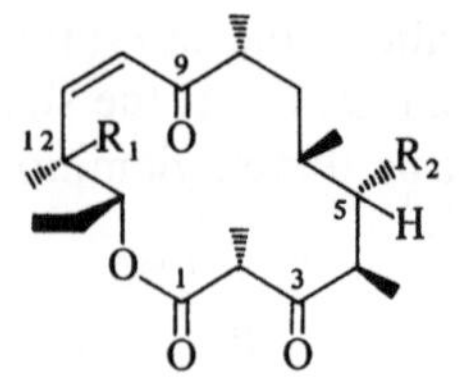

XXIV; R_1 = H, R_2 = Desosamine
XXV; R_1 = OH, R_2 = Desosamine

S. venezuelae can produce both antibiotics (MAEZAWA et al., 1973). Work with these strains has shown that D-desosamine (present in each antibiotic as a substituent at C-5) can be attached either to the normal or 9-dihydro form of narbonolide (XXIV, R_2=H) or of pikronolide (XXV, R_2=H). These lactones resemble the erythronolides and it seems that the specificity of the transferase in these organisms is not strict with respect to the oxygen substitution pattern at C-3, -6, -9, or -12, and the presence or absence of a bulky substituent group (neutral sugar) at C-3. The situation with *S. erythreus* may be different, for it is known (CORCORAN, J.W. and VYGANTAS, A.M., unpublished results) that no hydroxylation occurs at C-12 with the neutral monoglycoside (IV). Unequivocal proof awaits a study of the 5-(O)-desosaminyl derivative of erythronolide A as a possible substrate for the transferase system in *S. erythreus*.

b) Specificity for the Amino Sugar. In the case of *S. erythreus* there is no evidence yet of the attachment of a basic sugar other than D-desosamine to the acceptor neutral monoglycoside (IV). The possibility that the substrate specificity for the sugar donor may not be completely rigid comes again from the work of MAEZAWA et al. (1976) which showed that in a fermentation with *S. platensis* [producer of 16-member macrolides in which D-mycaminose (XXVI)

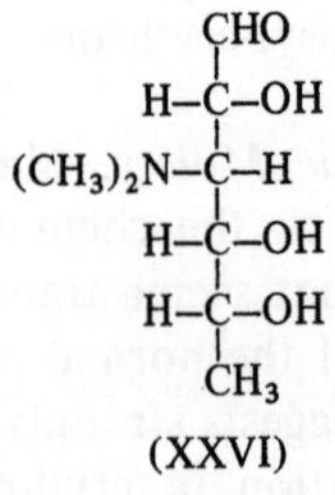

(XXVI)

replaces D-desosamine] the normal and 9-dihydro forms of narbonolide are transformed into 5-(O)-mycaminosyl derivatives.

VII. The Metabolism of the Erythromycins

A. Biosynthesis of Erythromycin C by Hydroxylation (at C-12) of Erythromycin D

1. Hydroxylation of 9-(*L*)-tritio-9-(*D*)-dihydroerythromycin D (XXVIII)

The transformation of erythromycin D to C merely requires a substitution of the hydrogen atom at C-12 by a hydroxyl group with retention of configuration. Superficially, this is the same reaction that is carried out by the C-6 erythranolide hydroxylase (Section E) and it was considered possible that the same enzyme system might be involved. However, no evidence was obtained of action of the C-6 hydroxylase or any other subcellular fraction on any center in the erythranolide molecule except C-6. Examination of the hydroxylation product of 6-deoxyerythronolide B (IIc) and its 9-(*D*)-dihydro derivative (X) was made using column, TLC, and GLC chromatography [Corcoran, J.W. and Vygantas, A.M., 1977; unpublished results]. Next, attention was turned to the possibility that the same or a different hydroxylase might act at the level of a mono- or bis-glycoside, and a study was made of these possibilities. Lacking adequate amounts of the radioactive forms of the 'natural' glycosidic intermediates (with the C-9 oxo function) a series of specifically tritiated possible substrates was made by reducing the 'natural' forms with borotritiide (Fig. 13). It was hoped that the substrate specificity of the C-12 hydroxylase would, as with the C-6 hydroxylase, be sufficiently broad to permit the use of a 9-(*D*)-dihydro derivative as a reactant in the hydroxylation. When the purified 9-(*D*)- and 9-(*L*)-tritio dihydroglycosides were examined for C-12 hydroxylase activity, using a crude cell-free preparation from *S. erythreus,* only one of the possible glycoside intermediates was metabolized. This proved to be 9-(*L*)-tritio-9-(*D*)-dihydroerythromycin D (XXVIII). The 9-(*D*)- and 9-(*L*)-tritio derivatives of 3-(O)-mycarosylerythronolide B (XXXIa, b) and the 9-(*L*)-tritio-9-(*D*)-dihydroerythromycin B failed to react. The products detected when the derivative of erythromycin D was the substrate were the 9-(*L*)-tritio-9-(*D*)-dihydro derivatives of erythromycin C (XXIX) and of erythromycin A (XXX). The formation of the latter is consistent with the presence of a SAM : erythromycin C(O)-methyltransferase activity in the crude extract (Corcoran, 1975).

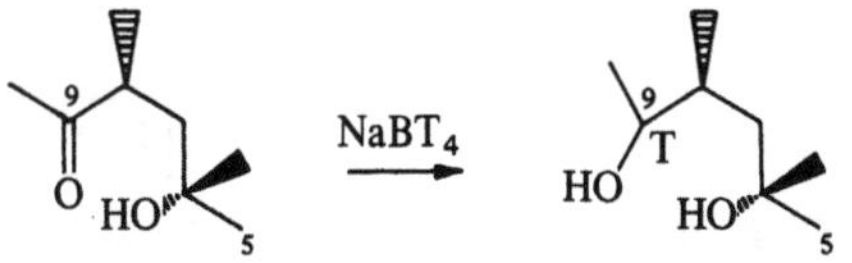

(Ib, Id, IIb, IV) (XXVII, XXVIII, XXIX, XXX, XXXIa, XXXIb)

Fig. 13. Preparation of tritiated substrates for the definition of the C-12 erythranolide hydroxylase

Although the unique reactivity of the 9-(*D*)-dihydro form of erythromycin D (XXVIII) among the similar derivatives of the other glycosides of erythronolide B suggests very strongly that erythromycin D is the 'natural' substrate for hydroxylation of the erythranolide ring system at C-12, this conclusion will not be proven formally until reactivity of the normal intermediate, erythromycin D itself, is demonstrated.

2. Properties of the C-12 Hydroxylase of *S. erythreus*

The nature of the C-12 erythranolide hydroxylase of *S. erythreus* has not been much investigated yet (CORCORAN and VYGANTAS, 1977). However, the enzymatic activity is apparently quite different from that of the C-6 hydroxylase. The C-12 hydroxylase does not seem to depend on a cytochrome P450 moiety; it is associated with the membranous fraction of the mycelium and is precipitated by much lower concentrations of ammonium sulfate (0–40%) than is the C-6 hydroxylase.

B. The Biosynthesis of Erythromycins B, A, and E

1. Properties of the S-Adenosyl-L-Methionine: Erythromycin C and D(O)-Methyl Transferase

The relationship between erythromycin A (Ia) and C (Ic) was studied (CORCORAN and MCALPINE, 1971) to settle a long-standing controversy about the role of the C form in the biosynthesis of erythromycin A. Although the structures of (Ia) and (Ic) suggested that the former would be made by O-methylation of (Ic) at C-3″, HUNG et al. (1965) had come to the opposite conclusion. The results of this investigation (cf. CORCORAN, 1975) showed conclusively that cell-free extracts of *S. erythreus* have a stable S-adenosyl-L-methionine (SAM): erythromycin C (O)-methyltransferase activity (Fig. 14) and that the product of the enzymatic reaction is erythromycin A (Ia). No reversibility of this trans-

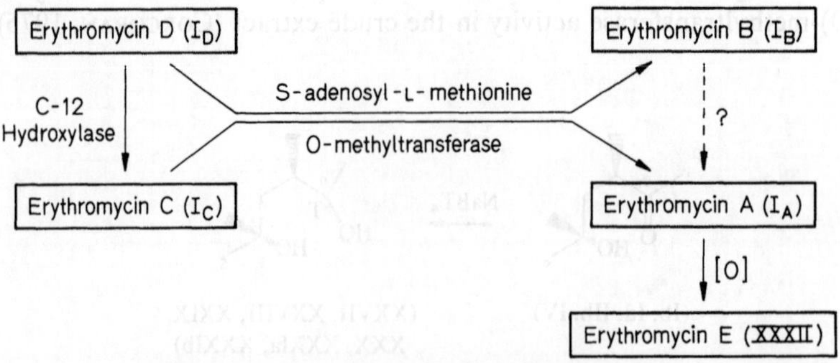

Fig. 14. Terminal metabolism of the erythromycins

methylase was observed. When erythromycin D (Id) was isolated and the key role it might play in the biosynthesis of both erythromycins B and C had been proposed (CORCORAN and MAJER, 1975; MAJER et al., 1974, 1977), the reactivity of erythromycin D in the transmethylase reaction was studied (CORCORAN, 1975; CORCORAN, J.W. and NAMKUNG, H.J., unpublished results). It was found that erythromycin D (Id) was a good substrate for transmethylase activity and the product proved to be erythromycin B (Ib). The K_m and V_{max} values for the two substrates (Ic and Id) are similar. The two erythromycin products as well as S-adenosyl-L-homocysteine are inhibitors of the enzymatic activity, and the erythromycins exhibit cross inhibitory actions. These findings, taken together with an observed parallel increase in the two transmethylase activities on limited purification, and a similar loss in the activities on partial heat inactivation of the enzyme, leads to the tentative conclusion that a single (O)-methyltransferase activity is responsible for the formation of both erythromycin A from C and erythromycin B from D (Fig. 14).

The SAM: erythromycin C, D (O)-methyltransferase of *S. erythreus* is associated with the particulate fraction, and it has not been much purified. The substrate specificity of the enzyme seems quite strict. If only one (O)-methyltransferase activity is present, its known substrates are erythromycin D and C and (probably) the 9-(*D*)-dihydro derivatives of both (cf. Section VII.A.1.). No other compound containing an L-mycarose entity has been reactive when tested with the crude enzyme system.

2. The Biosynthesis of Erythromycin E from A

Although early reports indicated that erythromycin A was a stable end product of the fermentation of *S. erythreus,* erythromycins A and B added to washed mycelial suspensions rapidly disappeared (CORCORAN, J.W., unpublished results). MARTIN and GOLDSTEIN (1970) reported that at least two biologically active metabolites of erythromycin A are formed by mutant strains of *S. erythreus,* and of these one, the so-called erythromycin E (XXXII), has

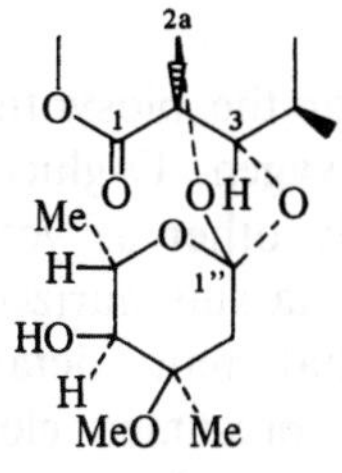

XXXII

been defined structurally (MARTIN et al., 1975). The formation of erythromycin E clearly follows oxidative attack (a still different hydroxylase perhaps) on the C-2a branch-methyl group as well as at the C-1'' position of the cladinosyl moiety present in erythromycin A (Ia). Although interesting the mechanism of this and other further metabolic changes to the erythromycins are not part of the formal biosynthetic pathway leading to the 'classical' antibiotics of this family.

3. Concerning the Direct Formation of Erythromycin A from B

A puzzling discrepancy exists between the results of cell-free studies on the biosynthesis of erythromycins A and B and observations made by MARTIN and GOLDSTEIN (1970) on intact mutant and production strains of *S. erythreus* during long-term fermentations. In the former (CORCORAN, 1975; CORCORAN, J.W., unpublished results) there is no positive evidence for a direct transformation of erythromycin B into the A form. Similar results were obtained by the same workers when washed mycelial suspensions were utilized. However, the studies of MARTIN's group indicated a transformation of erythromycin B into A. If the proof of formation of the erythromycin A is sound, and if the transformation is direct rather than indirect (it is always possible that the cladinosyl and/or deosaminyl moieties of the erythromycin B are removed by a hydrolytic mechanism and erythromycin D is formed *de novo* from the erythronolide B nucleus thus generated) these results suggest that some other mechanism may exist for hydroxylation of erythromycin B at the C-12 position. Substrate specificity studies done on the cell-free C-12 hydroxylase (Section VII.A.) have indicated that erythromycin B is not a substrate for this hydroxylase. However, it is possible with a different strain of *S. erythreus* or when conditions for the growth are other than the extremely limited ones described (CORCORAN, 1975) that a different C-12 hydroxylase is induced and becomes active. Until some of these questions are answered the conditions under which direct transformation of erythromycin B into A occurs must remain obscure.

VIII. Summary of the Biosynthesis of the Erythromycins

A. Review of the Entire Pathway

In summary, the pathway for the biosynthesis of the erythromycins from *propionate, 2-methylmalonate,* oxygen, D-glucose, S-adenosyl-L-methionine, a source of nitrogen, and possibly other as yet unidentified precursors is that in Figure 3. The experimental data summarized in Sections I–VII support this pathway, although it is clear that many details are still lacking. The nature of the lactone synthase and its presumed close relationship to a fatty acid synthase, although supported by much circumstantial data, is basically still a mystery. Likewise, the mechanisms by which D-glucose is transformed into the first neutral sugar, L-mycarose, and the basic sugar, D-desosamine, are obscure, and the postulated dependency on some nucleoside carrier is based mostly on analogy with other well-studied systems for the biosynthesis of deoxy sugars. It is unfortunate, since we would wish to know as much as possible about the unique facets of macrolide antibiotic biosynthesis, that the most detailed biochemical understanding we have at present concerns minor changes or modifications made to the macrolide lactones or the sugar entities attached to them. Quite a number of these so-called minor metabolic alterations may still be unknown, for instance, those between the first synthase-free lactone (or its open-chain precursor) and 6-deoxyerythronolide B (IIc). In spite of a wealth of information, and it is likely that the knowledge we have far exceeds that available for any other antibiotic of its class, it is obvious that these are only the first steps towards a full understanding in biochemical detail of biosynthesis of the erythromycins.

B. Regulation of the Biosynthesis of the Erythromycins

Several steps in the biosynthetic pathway leading to the erythromycins are inhibited by their products. For instance, erythronolide B (IIb) seems to inhibit its own formation in intact cultures (SPÍŽEK et al., 1966) and (IIb) is a potent inhibitor of the C-6 erythranolide hydroxylase that is responsible for its formation from 6-deoxyerythronolide B (IIc) (Section V). Whether (IIb) is also an inhibitor of the overall lactone synthase as well as of the C-6 hydroxylase is not yet known, although preliminary results with the putative lactone synthase have suggested that it is.

Two other steps in the biosynthetic pathway are also subject to product inhibition. The (O)-methyltransferase which promotes the transformation of erythromycin D into B and C into A is strongly inhibited by these two antibiotic products as well as by S-adenosyl-L-homocysteine, the other product of the reaction (Fig. 14). Since erythromycins A and B accumulate in the culture broth of *S. erythreus* (reaching final concentrations in excess of several mg/ml) the actinomycete must have some mechanism to permit continued operation of the transmethylase in the presence of these potent inhibitors. One possibility is a physical separation of the product erythromycins from the (O)-methyltransferase, and another is a rapid recycling of the S-adenosyl-L-homocysteine back to the active methioninyl form. Indeed, isotopic tracer studies indicate that both L-methionine and the S-adenosyl form of this amino acid may be present in very low concentrations and that the turnover of SAM is rapid.

The biosynthetic pathway is also regulated by a variable dependency of selective parts of the enzymatic apparatus on time. Section IV.B. speculated on the possibility that this sort of mechanism regulates the availability of *propionate* and *2-methylmalonate* for the lactone synthase. The apparent maximal activity of those enzymes varies with time and could cause accumulation of erythronolide-containing products at a late stage in the growth of *S. erythreus* even though the enzymes themselves are present and capable of activity at early stages of growth. Experimental evidence (CORCORAN, J.W., GOMM, J. and MITCHELL, D.R., unpublished results) shows that the overall erythromycin pathway is also regulated by two other enzyme activities: the erythromycin B, C: SAM (O)-methyltransferase, and; the C-12 erythranolide hydroxylase. In early stages of the growth cycle products accumulate (Fig. 6) which are made from the action of the lactone synthase and the attachment of L-mycarose and D-desosamine. These are mostly (IV) and (Id), the mono- and bis-glycoside of erythronolide B. Later in the fermentation, a rapid change in the distribution of products is seen, with accumulation of erythromycins B and A at the expense of the D form and (IV). One explanation for this could be that activity of the (O)-methyltransferase and the C-12 hydroxylase is low in the early time periods and then the two enzymes develop as the culture approaches the stationary phase of growth. Clearly, the two enzymes which act on the same substrate, erythromycin D, also compete and it is not obvious what determines the ratio of the products.

Information about the regulation of the pathway for the biosynthesis of the erythromycins is useful both for theoretical and practical reasons. Very often when a biosynthetic pathway leads to a family of closely related products one member is the desired product and the ability to manipulate the pathway to favor its production is an exceedingly important commercial goal. Although this degree of understanding of the pathway leading to the erythromycins has not quite been reached, it is now within reach.

References

Buckner JS, Kolattukudy PE (1975a) Lipid Biosynthesis in sebaceous glands; Regulation of the synthesis of n- and branched fatty acids by malonyl-coenzyme A decarboxylase. Biochemistry 14:1768–1773

Buckner JS, Kolattukudy PE (1975b) Lipid biosynthesis in the sebaceous glands: synthesis of multibranched fatty acids from methylmalonyl-coenzyme A in cell-free preparations from the uropygial gland of goose. Biochemistry 14:1774–1782

Buckner JS, Kolattukudy PE (1976) One-step purification and properties of a two-peptide fatty acid synthetase from the uropygial gland of the goose. Biochemistry 15:1948–1957

Butte JC, Corcoran JW (1962) The biogenesis of desosamine, an amino-trideoxy-sugar in erythromycin. Fed Proc 21:89

Butte JC, Corcoran JW (1963) The origin of propionate, used by *Streptomyces erythreus* for erythronolide-A synthesis. Fed Proc 22:355

Cahn RS, Ingold C, Prelog V (1966) Specification of molecular chirality. Angew Chem Int Ed Engl 5385–5415

Celmer WD (1971) Stereochemical problems in macrolide antibiotics. Pure Appl Chem 28:413–453

Celmer WD (1972) Chem Abstr 76: Index Guide Sect IV, 841–1011

Collum P, Egan RS, Goldstein AW, Martin JR (1976) 3-O-(2″,6″-dideoxy-α-L-*Ribo*-hexopyranosyl) erythronolide B and 3-O-(2″,6″-dideoxy-α-L-*Arabino*-hexopyranosyl)erythronolide B, aberrant erythromycin biogenetic metabolites with defective sugar moieties. Tetrahedron 32:2375–2378

Corcoran JW (1965) Speculation on the origin of macrolide antibiotics. In: Biogenesis of antibiotic substances, pp 131–142. Czech Academy of Sciences, Prague

Corcoran JW (1975) S-Adenosylmethionine: Erythromycin C O-methyltransferase. In: Hash JH (ed) Methods in enzymology, vol XLIII, pp 487–497. Antibiotics. Academic Press, London New York

Corcoran JW (1977) Biosynthesis of antibiotics. In: Clarke FH (ed) Annu Rep Med Chem, vol XII, pp 130–139, Academic Press, London New York

Corcoran JW, Chick M (1966) Biochemistry of the macrolide antibiotics. In: Snell JF (ed) Biosynthesis of antibiotics, pp 149–201. New York: Academic Press, London New York

Corcoran JW, Majer J (1975) Erythromycin D, A key intermediate in the biogenesis of the erythromycins. Federation Proc 34:589

Corcoran JW, McAlpine TS (1971) Enzymatic O-methylation of erythromycin C as the final step in the biogenesis of erythromycin A. Fed Proc 30:1168

Corcoran JW, Takahashi S (1975) Acid catalyzed reactions of 9-(S)-dihydro-erythronolides A and B: structures of Wiley's dehydration products A and B and analogous products derived from erythromycin B. 15th Intersci Conf Antimicrob Agents Chemother Abstr 425

Corcoran JW, Vygantas AM (1977) Hydroxylation steps in erythromycin biogenesis. Fed Proc 36:663
Corcoran JW, Chick M, Darby FJ (1967) The biogenesis of fatty acids and erythronolide-like substances in mycelium-free extracts of *Streptomyces erythreus*. In: Proc. 5th Int Congr Chemother, p 35. Abstracts of Communications, Wien
Corcoran JW, Huber MLB, Huber FM (1977) Relationship of Ribosomal Binding and Antibacterial Properties of Tylosin-Type Antibiotics. J. Antibiotics, 30:1012–1014
Dimroth P, Walter H, Lynen F (1970) Biosynthese von 6-Methylsalicylsaure. Eur J Biochem 13:98–110
Duppel W, Lebeault J-M, Coon MJ (1973) Properties of a yeast cytochrome P-450-containing enzyme system which catalyzes the hydroxylation of fatty acids, alkanes, and drugs. Eur J Biochem 36:583–592
Goldstein AW, Egan RS, Mueller SL, Martin JR (1978) Biotransformation of lankamycin, darcanolide, and 11-acetyllankolide by a blocked mutant of the erythromycin producing organism *Streptomyces Erythreus*. J Antibiot 31:63–69
Harris DR, McGeachin SG, Mills HH (1965) The structure and stereochemistry of erythromycin A. Tetrahedron Lett 679–685
Hung PP, Marks CL, Tardrew PL (1965) The biosynthesis and metabolism of erythromycins by *Streptomyces Erythreus*. J Biol Chem 240:1322–1326
IUPAC Nomenclature of Organic Chemistry (1969) Sect A, B, C, pp 85–115. Butterworths, London
IUPAC-IUB (1967) Commission on Biochemical Nomenclature. The nomenclature of lipids. J Biol Chem 242:4845–4849
Kaneda T, Butte JC, Taubman SB, Corcoran JW (1962) Actinomycete antibiotics III. The biogenesis of erythronolide. The C_{21} branched chain lactone in erythromycin. J Biol Chem 237:322–328
Kaziro Y, Ochoa S (1961) Mechanism of the propionyl carboxylase reaction. I. Carboxylation and decarboxylation of the enzyme. J Biol Chem 236:3131–3136
Kaziro Y, Ochoa S, Warner RL, Chen J-Y (1961) Metabolism of propionic acid in animal tissues. VIII. Crystalline propionyl carboxylase. J Biol Chem 236:1917–1923
Klyne W (1951) Nomenclature of some stereoisomeric compounds, specification of configurations. Chem Ind 1022–1025
Lemahieu RA, Ax HA, Blount JF, Carson M, Despreaux CW, Pruess DL, Scannell JP, Weiss F, Kierstead RW (1976) A new semisynthetic macrolide antibiotic, 3-O-oleandrosyl-5-O-desosaminyl-erythronolide A oxime. J Antibiot 29:728–734
Maezawa I, Hori T, Kinumaki A, Suzuki M (1973) Biological conversion of narbonolide to picromycin. J Antibiot 26:771–775
Maezawa I, Kinumaki A, Suzuki M (1976) Biological glycosidation of macrolide antibiotics I. Isolation and characterization of 5-O-mycaminosyl narbonolide and 9-Dihydro-5-O-mycaminosyl narbonolide. J Antibiotics 29:1203–1208
Majer J, Corcoran JW (1973) Macrolide biosynthesis in *Streptomyces Venezuelae*. Fed Proc 32:468
Majer J, Martin JR, Corcoran JW (1974) Erythromycin D, properties and structure. 14th Interscience Conference on Antimicrobial Agents and Chemotherapy, San Francisco, Calif. Abstract # 200
Majer J, McAlpine JB, Egan RS, Corcoran JW (1976) Antibiotic glycosides. VII 10,11-dihydropicromycin: Another metabolite of *Streptomyces Venezuelae*. J Antibiot 29:769–770
Majer J, Martin JR, Egan RS, Corcoran JW (1977) Antibiotic glycosides VIII. Erythromycin D, a new macrolide antibiotic. J Am Chem Soc 99:1620–1622
Martin JR, Egan RS (1970) 5,6-Dideoxy-5-oxoerythronolide B, a shunt metabolite of erythromycin biosynthesis. Biochemistry 9:3439–3445
Martin JR, Goldstein AW (1970) Final steps in erythromycin biosynthesis. In: Progress in antimicrobial and antitumor chemotherapy, Univ. Tokyo Press, pp 1112–1116. Tokyo
Martin JR, Perun TJ (1968) Studies on the biosynthesis of the erythromycins. III. Isolation and structure of 5-Deoxy-5-Oxoerythronolide B, a shunt metabolite of erythromycin biosynthesis. Biochemistry 7:1728–1733
Martin JR, Rosenbrook W (1967) Studies on the biosynthesis of the erythromycins. II. Isolation and structure of a biosynthetic intermediate, 6-Deoxyerythronolide B. Biochemistry 6:435–440
Martin JR, Perun TJ, Girolami RL (1966) Studies on the biosynthesis of the erythromycins. I. Isolation and structure of an intermediate glycoside, 3-α-L-mycarosylerythronolide B. Biochemistry 5:2852–2856

Martin JR, Perun TJ, Egan RS (1972) (8S)-8-Hydroxy-5,6-Dideoxy-5-oxoerythronolide B, a shunt metabolite of erythromycin biosynthesis. Tetrahedron 28:2937–2948

Martin JR, Egan RS, Goldstein AW, Collum P (1975) Extension of the erythromycin biosynthetic pathway: Isolation and structure of erythromycin E, Tetrahedron 31:1985–1989

Masamune S, Bates GS, Corcoran JW (1977) Macrolides. Recent progress in chemistry and biochemistry. Angew Chem (Int Ed Engl) 16:585–607

Nishikiori T, Wiegand RJ, Martens MG, Corcoran JW (1978) Further characterization of the erythranolide C-6 hydroxylase of *Streptomyces erythreus*. Fed Proc 37:1721

Nourse JG, Roberts JD (1975) Nuclear magnetic resonance spectroscopy. Carbon-13 spectra of some macrolide antibiotics and derivatives, substituent and conformational effects. J Am Chem Soc 97:4584–4594

Ōmura S, Takeshima H, Nakagawa A, Miyazawa T (1976) The biosynthesis of picromycin using ^{13}C-enriched precursors. J Antibiot 29:316–317

Pape H, Brillinger GU (1973) Stoffwechselprodukt von Microorganismus. 113. Mitteilung. Biosynthese von Thymidin diphospho-mycarose durch ein Zellfreie System aus *Streptomyces rimosus*. Arch Microbiol 88:25

Pape H, Grisebach H (1965) Untersuchungen über Nucleotidzucker und freie Nucleotide in *S. erythreus*. Biochem Z 343:154–175

Perun TJ (1971) The chemistry and conformation of erythromycin. In: Mitsuhashi S (ed) Drug action and drug resistance in bacteria. 1. Macrolide antibiotics and lincomycin, pp 123–152. Univ Tokyo Press, Tokyo

Raczyńska-Bojanowska K, Ruczaj Z, Ostrowska-Krysiak B, Roszkowski J, Gaworowska-Michalik J, Sawnor-Korszyńska D (1970) Precursors and control in erythromycin biosynthesis. Acta Microbiol Pol Ser B 2(19):103–110

Raczyńska-Bojanowska K, Rafalski A, Ostrowska-Krysiak B (1976) Carboxylation of propionyl-Co A in erythromycin biosynthesis. Acta Biochem Pol 17:331–338

Raczyńska-Bojanowska K, Ruczaj Z, Sawnor-Korszyńska D, Rafalski A (1973) Limiting reactions in activation of acyl units in biosynthesis of macrolide antibiotics. Antimicrob Agents Chemother 3:162–167

Rossi A, Corcoran JW (1973) Identification of a multienzyme complex synthesizing fatty acids in the actinomycete *Streptomyces erythreus*. Biochem Biophys Res Commun 50:597–602

Ruczaj Z, Sawnor-Korszyńska D, Raczyńska-Bojanowska K (1969) Propionate and acetate kinase in *Streptomyces*. Bull Acad Pol Sci 17:531–533

Ruettinger RT, Olson ST, Boyer RF Jr, Coon MJ (1974) Identification of the ω-hydroxylase of *Pseudomonas Oleovorans* as a nonheme iron protein requiring phospholipid for catalytic activity. Biochem Biophys Res Commun 57:1011–1017

Scott AI, Beadling LC, Georgopapadakou NH, Subbarayan CR (1974) Biosynthesis of polyketides. Purification and inhibition studies of 6-Methylsalicylic acid synthase. Bioorg Chem 3:238–248

Spížek J, Chick M, Corcoran JW (1966) The biogenetic relationship of the erythromycins and the lactone of erythromycin B. Antimicrob Agents Chemother 1965:138–143

Tardrew PL, Nyman MA (1964) Hypocholesterolemic agent M-850 and method of preparation, US Patent 3, 127, 315

Terui Y, Tori K, Nagashima K, Tsuji N (1975) C-13 nuclear magnetic resonance spectra of erythromycins. Tetrahedron Lett 2583–2586

Thang TT, Lukacs G, Ōmura S, Bartner P, Boxler DL, Brambilla R, Mallams AK, Morton JB, Reichert P, Sancilio FD, Surprenant H, Tomalesky G (1978) Megalomicins. 6. Tertiary glycosidic macrolide antibiotics. A structural revision by carbon-13 nuclear magnetic resonance and X-ray crystallography. J Am Chem Soc 100:663–666

Tyson CA, Lipscomb JD, Gunsalus IC (1972) The roles of putidaredoxin and $P450_{Cam}$ in methylene hydroxylation. J Biol Chem 247:5777–5784

Vaněk Z, Majer J (1967) Macrolide antibiotics. In: Gottlieb D, Shaw PD (eds) Antibiotics II. Biosynthesis, pp 154–188. Springer, Berlin Heidelberg New York

Vygantas AM, Corcoran JW (1974) Hydroxylation of 6-Deoxyerythronolide B by a soluble enzyme system from *Streptomyces Erythreus*. Fed Proc 33:1233

Wawszkiewicz EJ, Lynen F (1964) Propionyl-Co A dependent $H^{14}CO_3^-$ exchange into methylmalonyl-Co A in extracts of *Streptomyces erythraeus*. Biochem Z 340:213–227

Biosynthesis of 16-Membered Macrolide Antibiotics

SATOSHI ŌMURA and AKIRA NAKAGAWA

I. Classification of 16-Membered Macrolide Antibiotics Based on the Skeleton of Lactone Ring

To date 57 components of the structurally known 16-membered macrolide antibiotics have been identified (ŌMURA and NAKAGAWA, 1975; MORIN and GORMAN, 1967; CELMER, 1971; MALLAMS, 1978). Some of the macrolide antibiotics, including leucomycin, spiramycin, and acetylspiramycin have clinical applications and/or are used as supplements in animal feeds. The currently known macrolides can be classified biosynthetically into four groups, on the basis of the pattern of glycosidation of each sugar to the aglycone moiety, the varieties of constituent sugar, and the carbon skeleton of the aglycones (ŌMURA and TAKESHIMA, 1977) (Fig. 1). The first group is represented by the clinically important antibiotics magnamycin and leucomycin. The characteristic features of the antibiotics belonging to this group are the acyl group at the 3-position on the lactone ring, the acyl group at the 4″-position of the mycarose moiety, the structure of the 9–13 positions in the lactone ring, and their combinations. The total number of such macrolides has reached 36.

The second group of antibiotics is represented by tylosin. Among those in this group, only tylosin is used for the preservation of food and as a supplement in animal feed. The macrolides of this group possess a variety of sugars such as mycinose, angolasamine, desosamine (which also is a constituent sugar of the 14-membered macrolides), cinerulose, chalcose, aldgarose, mycaminose and mycarose. The antibiotics such as rosamicin, cirramycin, and angolamycin that belong to the tylosin group have a methyl group in the 4- and 12-positions, mycinose linked via the hydroxymethyl group at the 14-position and an ethyl group in the 15-position of the lactone ring.

Juvenimicin A_2, a component of the juvenimicin complex belongs to the third group of 16-membered macrolides. Although the aglycone moiety of these antibiotics resembles that of the tylosin group, to which they could therefore be assigned, they differ from the tylosin group in having a methyl group in place of the ethylformyl group at the 6-position on the lactone ring.

The last group of antibiotics, the chalcomycin group, includes neutramycin and aldgamycin and is characterized by a neutral sugar, chalcose or aldgarose, respectively, in place of mycaminose. Neutramycin is especially interesting because it has no methyl group at the 6-position. Structural differentiation between

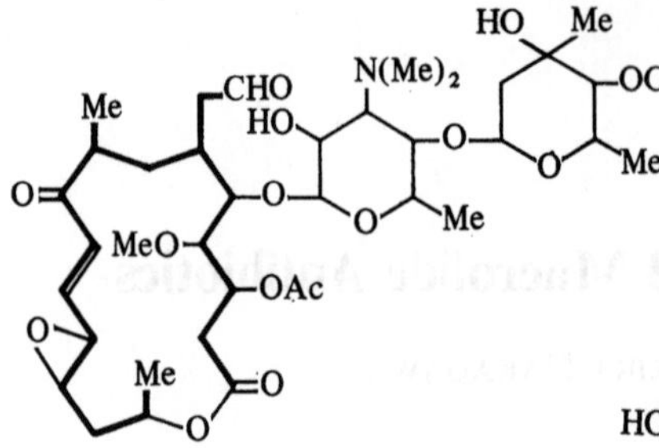

Magnamycin A

Magnamycins (Carbomycins)	TANNER et al., 1952; WOODWARD et al., 1965
Leucomycins	HATA et al., 1953; ŌMURA et al., 1967
Spiramycins	PINNERT-SINDICO et al., 1954/55; KEUHNE et al., 1965; ŌMURA et al., 1969
Niddamycins	HUBER et al., 1962
Maridomycins	MUROI et al., 1972a, b
Espinomycins	MACHIDA et al., 1972
Midecamycins	INOUYE et al., 1971
Platenomycins	SUZUKI et al., 1971a, b
Deltamycins	SHIMAUCHI et al., 1978

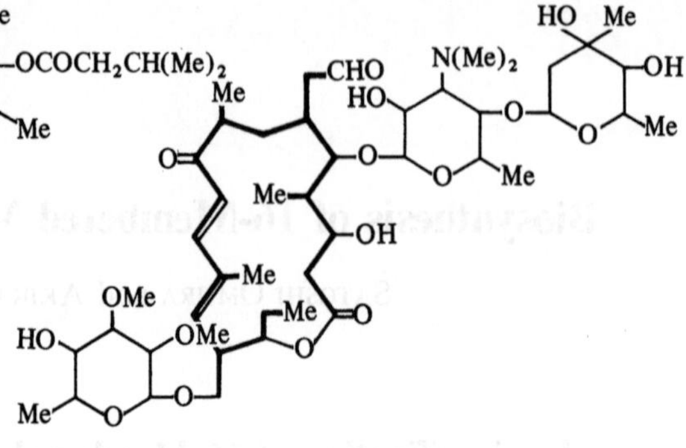

Tylosin McGUIRE et al., 1961; MORIN et al., 1970; ŌMURA et al., 1975c

Cirramycins	KOSHIYAMA et al., 1963; TSUKIURA et al., 1969
Rosamicin	WAGMAN et al., 1972; REIMAN and JARET, 1972
Angolamycin (Shincomycin)	KINUMAKI and SUZUKI, 1972
Relomycin	WHALEY et al., 1964
Macrocin	HAMILL and STARK, 1964
B-58941	SUZUKI, 1963
M-4365	FURUMAI et al., 1977; KINUMAKI et al., 1977
Juvenimicins	HATANO et al., 1976; KISHI et al., 1976

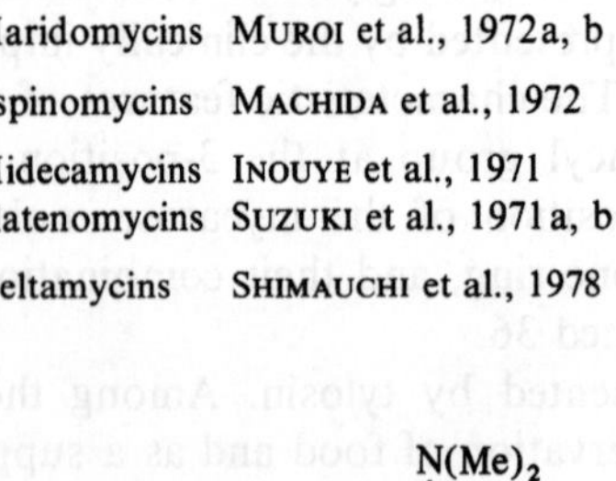

Juvenimicin A_2 HATANO et al., 1976

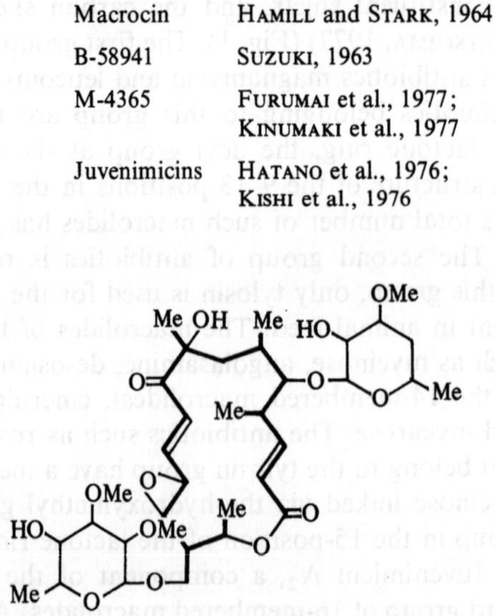

Chalcomycin	Woo et al., 1964
Neutramycin	LEFEMINE et al., 1964; MITSCHER et al., 1969
Aldgamycin	KUNSTMAN and KUNSTMAN, 1964; ACHENBACH and KARL, 1975

Fig. 1. Classification of 16-membered macrolide antibiotics based on the skeleton of lactone ring

the lactone rings of juvenimicin A_2 and of the chalcomycin group can be made by the presence of an ethyl or a methyl group at the 15-position, respectively.

There is a high probability that new related 16-membered macrolides may be discovered in the future, especially since new combinations are possible of the substituents on the lactone ring, the acyl groups, and sugar moieties.

II. Biosynthesis of the Aglycone Moiety

The biosynthetic origin of the carbon skeleton of the lactone ring in the 16-membered macrolides has been studied intensely using magnamycin A as a representative example and ^{14}C-precursors. WOODWARD (1957) first proposed an 18-membered lactone ring for the structure of magnamycin and suggested that its lactone ring moiety originates from nine acetate and one methionine unit. Subsequently the structure of magnamycin A was revised by KUEHNE et al. (1965) and WOODWARD et al. (1965). GRISEBACH and ACHENBACH (1962) and ACHENBACH and GRISEBACH (1964) and CORCORAN and CHICK (1966) had originally suggested that the lactone ring arises from four acetates and one propionate with the C-1 ~ 6 carbon positions and the ethylformyl group on the lactone ring being derived from some precursor other than acetate possibly one formed through the metabolism of glucose or succinate (Fig. 2a). On the other hand, SRINIVASAN and SRINIVASAN (1967) had reported that nine acetate units and one propionate residue were used for the lactone ring (Fig. 2b). The possibility that the formyl group originated from succinate was eliminated later by GRISEBACH and WEBER-SCHILLING (1968)

Recently, ONO et al. (1974) and GERSCH et al. (1977) have reported the incorporation of several ^{14}C-labeled compounds into maridomycin and turimycin, respectively, both of which belong to the magnamycin-leucomycin group. They

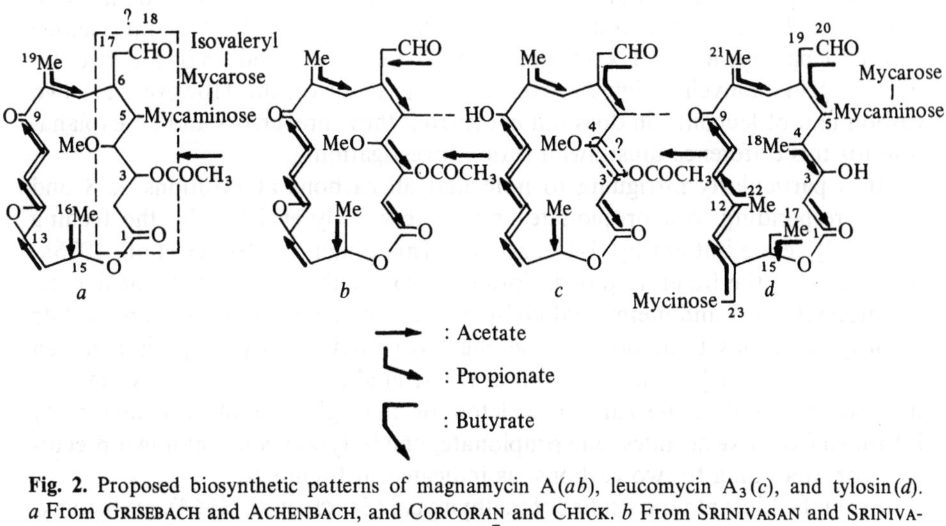

Fig. 2. Proposed biosynthetic patterns of magnamycin A(*ab*), leucomycin A_3(*c*), and tylosin(*d*). *a* From GRISEBACH and ACHENBACH, and CORCORAN and CHICK. *b* From SRINIVASAN and SRINIVASAN. *c*, *d* From ŌMURA et al.

suggested the efficient incorporation of butyrate into both aglycone moieties, although this did not confirm an explicit labeling site in the lactone ring.

In view of an unsatisfactory degradation scheme involving the use of ^{14}C-labeled compound, ^{13}C-magnetic resonance (CMR) spectroscopy and ^{13}C-labeled precursors have been introduced as an effective tool for studying the biosynthesis of the aglycone moiety of macrolide antibiotics such as leucomycin and tylosin. The carbon signal assignments of each 16-membered macrolide and the incorporation of ^{13}C-labeled precursors into leucomycin have been actively investigated by ŌMURA et al. (1975a, b, c, 1977a). The CMR spectra of leucomycin A_3 labeled with the [^{13}C]-acetate indicated that carbons 1, 2, 9–16, 20, and 21 are directly derived from the intact form of acetate. Furthermore the spectral observation of the weak enrichment of carbons 6, 7, 8, 18, and 19 by [^{13}C]acetate suggested that these five carbons are indirectly derived from acetate.

This result could be interpreted as a consequence of indirect incorporation of the precursor through propionate (C-7, 8, 19) and butyrate (C-6, 18 and C-5, 17). As expected, the addition of butyrate indicated strong enrichment only at C-5 and the weak incorporation was interpreted as the degradation of butyrate into acetate by β-oxidation, as seen in the biosynthetic studies of antibiotic X-537 A (WESTLEY et al., 1970, 1972, 1974; DAY et al., 1973). Further, the feeding of [4-^{13}C]2-ethylmalonate which arises from carboxylation of butyrate also produced a strong enrichment in C-17. The evidence that butyrate is a direct precursor for four carbons and that the formyl group which is characteristic of the basic 16-membered macrolides thus arises from C-4 of butyrate is consistent with the observation (FURUMAI et al., 1975) that an aglycone containing a methyl group in place of the formyl group was isolated from a mutant of the platenomycin-producing strain (described below). No enrichment in carbons 3 and 4 was observed after the addition of ^{13}C-labeled compounds, such as [1-^{13}C]glycine, diethyl [1-^{13}C]oxalate, [2-^{13}C]malonic acid, and diethyl[1,4-^{13}C]succinate. Two C_2 units in the molecule of geldanamycin (SASAKI, 1970), are structurally similar to the C_2 unit at C-3,4 of the lactone ring of leucomycin A_3. HABER et al. (1977) recently found that the two C_2 units in geldanamycin originate from glycolate or glycerate. However, the two carbon unit of leucomycin does not come from these precursors and an explanation for this difference must await future investigations.

It is particularly intriguing to note that all carbons at positions 7, 8 and 19, corresponding to a propionate unit, were weakly enriched by the feeding of [2-^{13}C]acetate but not by [1-^{13}C]acetate. This evidence (ŌMURA et al., 1976a) indicates that the building unit is formed through the tricarboxylic acid cycle via succinyl-Co A and methylmalonyl-Co A. A similar metabolism from acetate to propionate has been observed in the biosynthetic study of pyrindicin, an alkaloid produced by *Sm. griseoflavus* (IWAI et al., 1978). From these results, it is concluded that the carbon skeleton of the aglycone of leucomycin A_3 is formed from five acetates, one propionate, one butyrate, and unknown precursors corresponding to two carbons, as indicated in Figure 2c.

From the biosynthetic studies of methymycin (BIRCH et al., 1964), erythromycin (KANEDA et al., 1962; FRIEDMAN et al., 1964), and leucomycin (ŌMURA et al.,

Table 1. Incorporation of ^{13}C-labeled precursors into tylosin

Carbon atoms	Chemical shift δ (ppm) from $(CH_3)_4Si$	Enrichment factor[a]			Relative intensity[b] (%)
		[1-^{13}C] Acetate	[1-^{13}C] Propionate	[1-^{13}C] Butyrate	[4-^{13}C]2-ethylmalonate
C-1	173.9	2.8	0.8	1.7	
2	39.4	1.5	1.8	2.0	
3	68.2	0.1	3.8	9.8	
4	45.1	1.7	1.3	1.1	156
5	81.6	2.2	1.3	22.7	
6	32.2	0.1	1.9	2.5	
7	32.9	2.5	6.1	17.3	
8	40.3	1.3	1.3	0.8	133
9	202.8	3.9	1.6	3.2	
10	118.8	1.0	0.9	0.8	
11	148.0	2.0	6.0	17.0	
12	134.9	1.0	1.0	1.0	100
13	142.2	2.0	5.7	15.6	
14	44.7	1.4	1.5	0.7	233
15	75.3	1.2	4.0	9.7	
16	25.5	1.1	1.1	0.9	200
17	9.0	0.7	1.0	0.8	
18	9.6	1.1	1.0	0.6	
19	43.9	2.8	1.3	1.8	367
20	203.0	1.9	0.5	1.3	
21	17.4	1.1	1.3	1.3	
22	13.0	1.1	1.2	0.8	
23	69.5	0.8	0.7	2.3	

[a] Peak height $\frac{\text{enriched sample}}{\text{natural abundance}}$ from spectra run under essentially identical instrumental conditions

[b] The peak of C-12, as a reference, is taken for 100% and the height of the other peaks is compared with it. Under the experimental conditions of recording this spectrum the natural abundance peaks were not observed

1975b), it is expected that the lactone ring of tylosin, belonging to the second group in the classification of 16-membered macrolides, may be derived from two acetate units, five propionate units, and one butyrate unit. These precursors were, in fact, confirmed to be the building units for the lactone moiety of tylosin shown in (Fig. 2d). The signal assignments of the lactone ring and incorporation of ^{13}C-labeled precursors into tylosin are reported in Table 1 (Ōmura et al., 1975c).

Although the origin of carbons 3 and 4 of leucomycin still remains unknown, the corresponding carbons of tylosin originate from propionate. It should be noted that, in the feeding of [1-^{13}C]butyrate, a high degree of incorporation was observed not only in carbon 5 but also in carbons 3, 7, 11, 13, and 15, which should be derived from C-1 of propionate. Similarly, the addition of [1′-^{13}C]ethylmalonate enriched carbons 4, 8, 12, 14, and 16, which should arise from C-2 of propionate, as well as carbon 19. These results indicate that the latter two compounds are metabolized into propionyl-Co A or methylmalonyl-

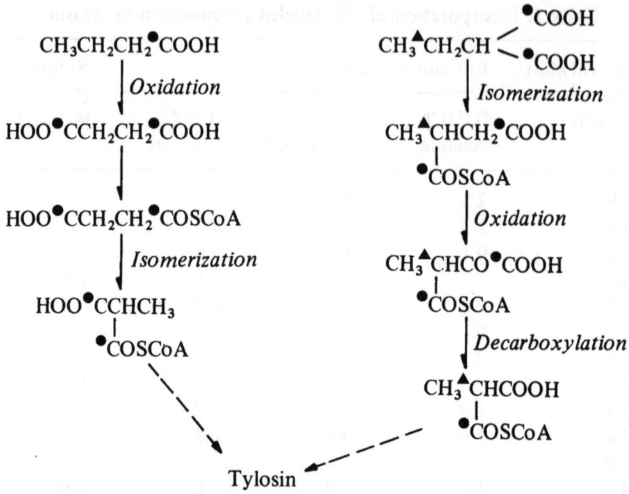

Fig. 3. Proposed pathways of butyric and 2-ethylmalonic acid into methylmalonyl-Co A. Symbols (● and ▲) indicate ^{13}C-enriched carbons

Co A, followed by incorporation into the lactone ring. A plausible metabolic pathway is summarized in Figure 3. To prove the metabolic pathway from [1-^{13}C]butyric acid to a propionate unit, [1,4-^{13}C]succinate was added to a tylosin fermentation. The results revealed enrichment of carbons 11, 13, and 15, which should be essentially derived from the carboxyl carbon of propionate (ŌMURA et al., 1976a). Further, [1,3,1′-^{13}C]2-ethylmalonic acid was added to the fermentation medium together with the [4-^{13}C]substrate to study the metabolism of 2-ethylmalonate by the double-labeling technique. The CMR spectrum of the tylosin revealed enrichment in carbons 5 and 19 as expected. In addition to these two carbons, enriched signals of carbon 11, 12, 13, 14, 15, and 16 were observed and each of these signals was accompanied by a doublet arising from vicinal ^{13}C-^{13}C coupling. These results suggested that [1,3,1′-^{13}C]2-ethylmalonate is also metabolized via a pathway involving methylmalonyl-Co A mutase, as illustrated in Figure 3 (ŌMURA et al., 1975).

A.K. GANGULY et al. (1976) and B.K. LEE et al. (1976) have reported on the biosynthesis of rosamicin (classified with the tylosin group) and using ^{13}C-NMR spectrometry obtained the same information as with tylosin. Thus, the application of ^{13}C-NMR spectrometry to biosynthesis is of interest because one can study the direct incorporation of precursor into secondary metabolites without degradation techniques and elucidate directly some metabolic pathways for simple organic compounds which are the building units of the metabolites.

With reference to the biosynthesis of juvenimicin A_2 and chalcomycin, having an ethyl instead of an ethylformyl group on the lactone ring, it is anticipated that these are built from two acetate and six propionate units, and four acetate and four propionate units, respectively, taking into consideration the structures of their lactone rings.

III. Biosynthesis of Macrolide Sugars

It is well known that the deoxysugar and aminosugar found in macrolide antibiotics are biosynthesized from D-glucose. With regard to the binding positions of the sugars to the aglycone moieties, an α-L-sugar must be linked to C-3 on the lactone ring, and a β-D-sugar at C-5. CELMER (1971) has proposed the presence of a 4,5-dehydrosugar in some common intermediate for macrolide sugars and suggests that the branch group of the L-sugars is derived from methionine (CORCORAN, 1961; CANTONI, 1963). Recently, PAPE and BRILLINGER (1973) have studied the biosynthesis of mycarose in a cell-free system from a tylosin-producing strain of *Sm. rimosus* and proposed that the biosynthetic sequence proceeds via TDP-4-keto-6-deoxy-D-glucose.

IV. Biosynthesis After the Formation of Aglycone Moiety

In the biosynthetic process for macrolide antibiotics, the lactone ring is formed by condensation of acetate, malonate, and their analogs followed by oxidation and reduction of the intermediates involved. It has been found that the sugar is subsequently bound to an intermediate which is again subjected to oxidation, reduction and acylation. Consequently, the possibility of so many of these reactions after the formation of the aglycone moiety suggests many possibilities for new macrolide antibiotics.

A. Biosynthetic Studies Using a Blocked Mutant Method

FURUMAI et al. (1973, 1975) have applied 'cosynthesis' devised by DELIC et al. (1969) and McCORMICK (1960) to the biosynthetic studies of the 16-membered macrolide, platenomycin. They obtained many non-platenomycin-producing blocked mutants by NTG treatment and/or UV irradiation of platenomycin-producing *Sm. platensis* subsp. *malvinus* and tested them for their capability for cosynthesis. Antibiotic cosynthesis with a pair of mutants ('secretor' and 'convertor') made it possible to detect the producer of a biosynthetic intermediate. Several platenomycin intermediates were isolated from the fermentation broth of the mutants and their structures were determined chiefly by means of mass spectrometry. To clarify the biosynthetic pathway of platenomycin, a biosynthetic correlation of the intermediates was made using growing cultures or the washed mycelium of a blocked mutant of *Sm. platensis*. It was revealed by these experiments that platenomycin was biosynthesized from its aglycone, platenolide I, via demycarosyl platenomycin and 4″-deacyl platenomycin by the pathways summarized in Figure 4.

In analogy with the biosynthesis of the erythromycins (14-membered macrolides) (TARDREW and NYMAN, 1964; HUNG et al., 1965; MARTIN et al., 1966, 1972; MARTIN and PERUN (1968); MARTIN and EGAN (1970); MAJER et al., 1977), it was confirmed that both sugars, mycaminose and mycarose in 16-

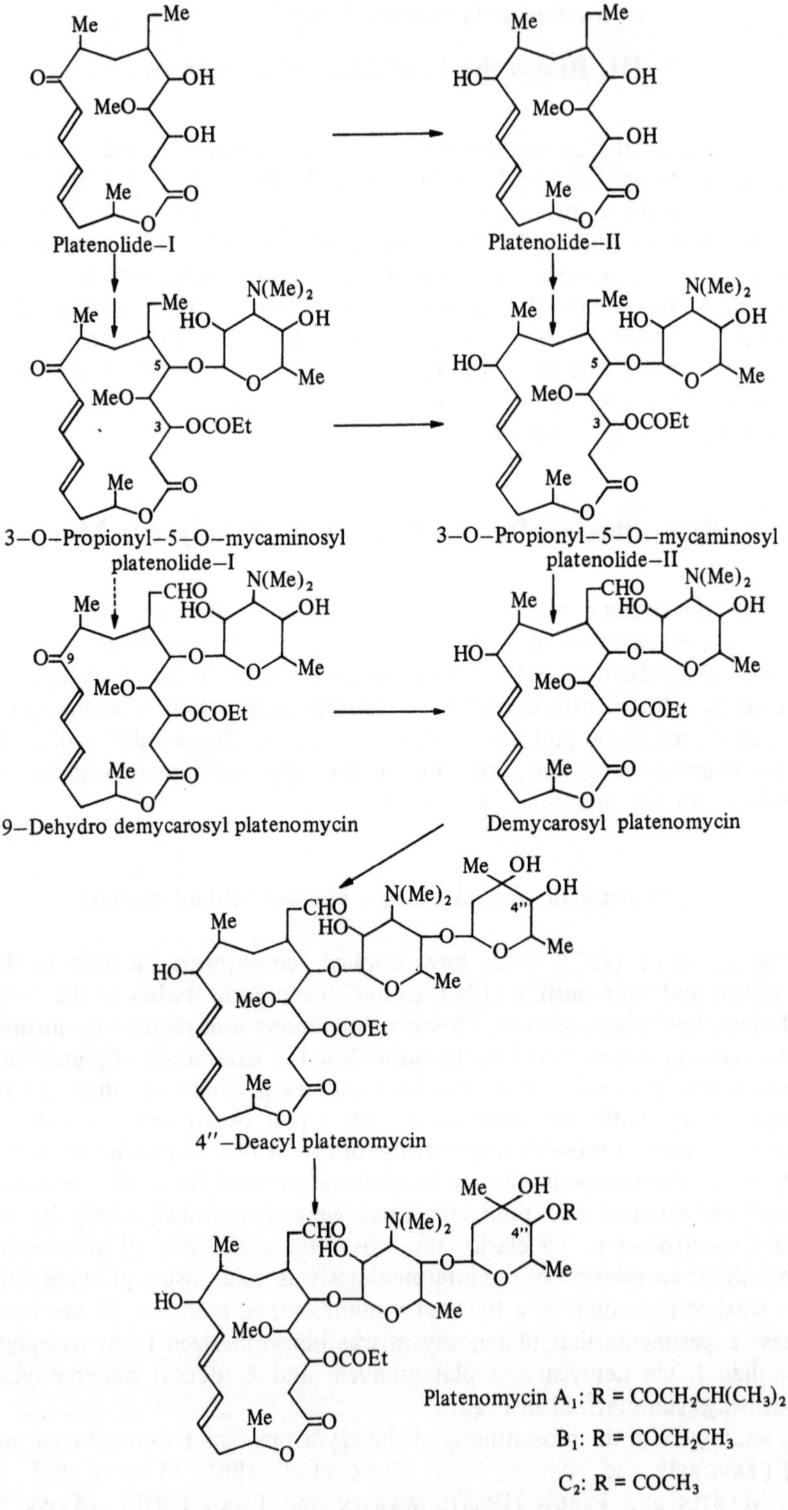

Fig. 4. Biosynthetic pathway of platenomycins

membered macrolides are linked to the aglycone after the formation of the lactone ring. Further, it should be noted that the aldehyde group in platenomycin was formed by the oxidation of a methyl group. These data are consistent with the results of the direct incorporation of butyrate into the lactone ring as shown by ^{13}C-NMR spectrometry (ŌMURA et al., 1975b, c).

With regard to the origin of the 4″-acyl group of the mycarose moiety, GRISEBACH and ACHENBACH (1963), FURUMAI et al. (1975) and ONO et al. (1974) suggested that the 4″-isovaleryl and 4″-propionyl units on the mycarose were derived from L-leucine and L-isoleucine, respectively. L-Valine is reported by REUTER and HÜTTER (1976) as a precursor of the isovaleryl group.

B. Bioconversion and Biosynthesis of the Antibiotics in the Terminal Stage

In place of the biosynthetic studies using a blocked mutant, ŌMURA et al. (1978, 1979) have reported the application of the fatty acid synthetase inhibitor, cerulenin, to the study of the biosynthesis of 16-membered macrolides. The antibiotic cerulenin is a specific inhibitor of what is called the 'condensing enzyme' which is involved in the condensing step between acyl-ACP and malonyl-ACP in the biosynthesis of fatty acids (NOMURA et al., 1972; VANCE et al., 1972; GREENSPAN et al., 1977; ŌMURA et al., 1976b). Cerulenin also inhibits the biosynthesis of metabolites such as leucomycin, tetracycline, and 6-methylsalicylic acid which are presumably synthesized via polyketide intermediates (ŌMURA and TAKESHIMA, 1974; OHNO et al., 1975; TAKESHIMA et al., 1977).

Under the conditions when cerulenin inhibits the formation of the aglycone moiety of macrolides, the bioconversion of the preformed lactone ring to the final product, tylosin, was examined by adding intermediates obtained chemically from tylosin to the culture medium of a tylosin-producing strain of *Sm. fradiae*. Tylosin and other substances were added to the culture broth at 48 h or 168 h of cultivation. The incubation was continued for an additional 24 h. The correlation between the sequence of aldehyde formation on the lactone ring and the order of glycosidic attachment of the neutral sugars, mycarose and mycinose during the course of tylosin biosynthesis is listed in Figure 6 (a). The structures of relomycin and its relatives are depicted in Figure 5. The production of tylosin in cultures of *Sm. fradiae* is always associated with the later appearance of relomycin which has a hydroxylmethyl group in place of a formyl group. Tylosin and relomycin were efficiently formed from mycaminosyl tylonolide and mycaminosyl relonolide, respectively. The conversion of alcohol to aldehyde is predominant in the early stage of incubation. However, in the later stage the reverse process is predominant.

On the other hand, SENO et al. (1977) have examined the terminal stages of tylosin biosynthesis, together with the relationship among the tylosin-like compounds, macrocin (HAMILL and STARK, 1964), desmycosin (=mycaminosyl tylonolide), lactenocin, and relomycin which are produced simultaneously with tylosin in fermentation broth of *Sm. fradiae*. The relationship in their biosynthetic pathway is presented in Figure 6 (b). The results obtained by the addition of the purified ^{14}C-labeled antibiotics to cultures of *Sm. fradiae* revealed that

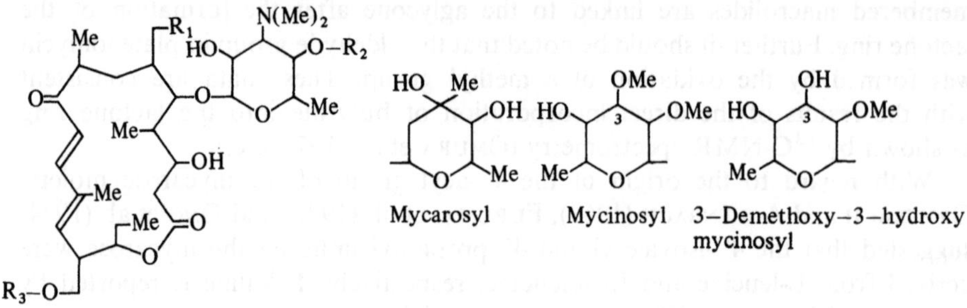

	R_1	R_2	R_3
Tylosin	CHO	Mycarosyl	Mycinosyl
Demycarosyl tylosin	CHO	H	Mycinosyl
Mycaminosyl tylonolide	CHO	H	H
Relomycin	CH_2OH	Mycarosyl	Mycinosyl
Demycarosyl relomycin	CH_2OH	H	Mycinosyl
Mycaminosyl relonolide	CH_2OH	H	H
Macrocin	CHO	Mycarosyl	3-Demethoxy-3-hydroxy mycinosyl
Lactenocin	CHO	H	3-Demethoxy-3-hydroxy mycinosyl

Fig. 5. Structures of tylosin and its related compounds

macrocin and desmycosin were direct precursors of tylosin, whereas lactenocin was an immediate precursor of both macrocin and desmycosin. Incubation of these cultures with [^{14}C]tylosin resulted in an equal distribution of radioactive label between relomycin and an unidentified component. This transformation of tylosin to relomycin agrees with the results of the experiment using the enzymatic inhibitor cerulenin described above. It is also compatible with the report by JENSEN et al. (1964) who reported that tylosin appeared before relomycin in cultures of *Sm. hygroscopicus* and that the addition of tylosin to these

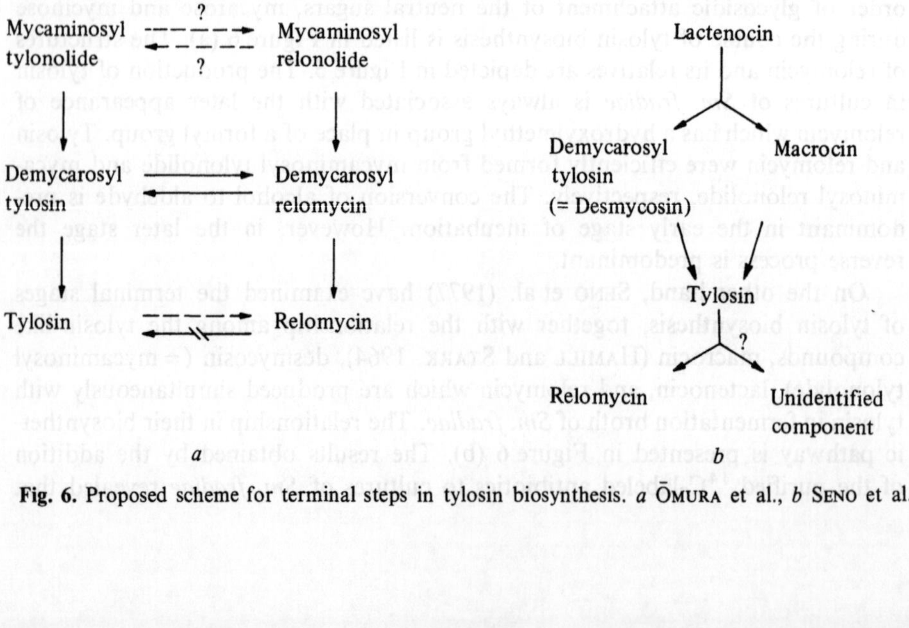

Fig. 6. Proposed scheme for terminal steps in tylosin biosynthesis. *a* ŌMURA et al., *b* SENO et al.

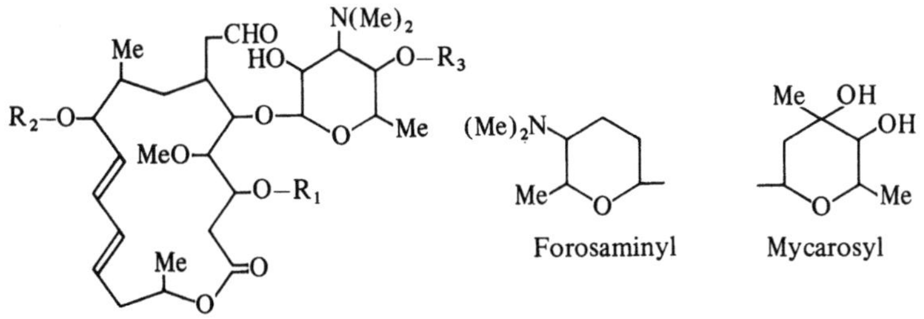

	R_1	R_2	R_3
Forocidin I	H	H	H
Forocidin III	COC_2H_5	H	H
Neospiramycin I	H	Forosaminyl	H
Neospiramycin III	COC_2H_5	Forosaminyl	H
Spiramycin I	H	Forosaminyl	Mycarosyl
Spiramycin III	COC_2H_5	Forosaminyl	Mycarosyl
Leucomycin V	H	H	Mycarosyl

Fig. 7. Structures of spiramycin-related compounds

cultures resulted in an increase of relomycin production. The similar bioconversion of tylosin to relomycin has been demonstrated in several species of *Streptomyces* and one *Nocardia* species by FELDMAN et al. (1964). Further, SENO et al. (1977) has studied the methylation of macrocin to tylosin by cell-free extracts of *Sm. fradiae* and demonstrated the requirement of S-adenosylmethionine or L-methionine and adenosin 5′-triphosphate as the methyl donor (CORCORAN, 1961; GRISEBACH et al., 1961) for the conversion of macrocin to tylosin. This relationship between macrocin and tylosin is analogous to that of erythromycin C and erythromycin A, the former being a demethylated form of the latter (CORCORAN, 1975; MARTIN and GOLDSTEIN, 1970).

On the other hand, ŌMURA et al. (1978) have reported the biosynthetic pathway of forocidin I, which was obtained by acidic hydrolysis of spiramycin I, into spiramycin III (Figs. 7 and 8). Forocidin I was converted into forocidin III, neospiramycin I, neospiramycin III, and spiramycin III. The remarkable result that forocidin I was not transformed into leucomycin V indicated that the linking of forosamine to C-9 of the aglycone predominates over that of

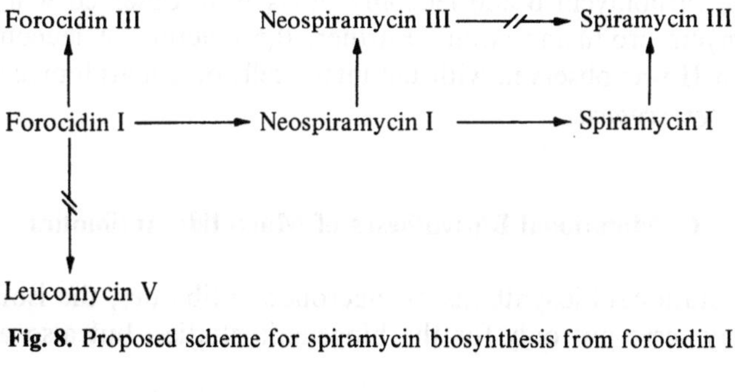

Fig. 8. Proposed scheme for spiramycin biosynthesis from forocidin I

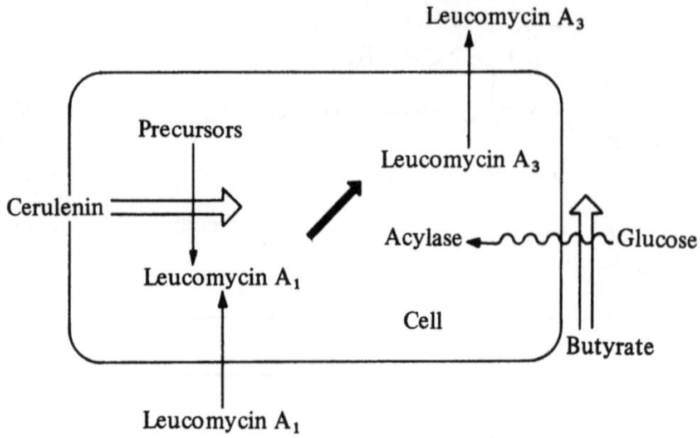

Fig. 9. Proposed action mechanism of butyrate on the bioconversion from leucomycin A_1 to leucomycin A_3 in the presence of cerulenin

mycarose to C-4′ of mycaminose. Spiramycin III was rapidly produced from spiramycin I, but not from neospiramycin III. These results suggested that the binding of forosamine to the lactone ring at C-3 occurs in the final step of spiramycin biosynthesis.

In the course of the biosynthetic studies on the leucomycins, it was noted that the transformation of leucomycin A_1 to A_3 was suppressed when butyrate was added to the fermentation broth of a leucomycin-producing strain of *Sm. kitasatoensis* (ŌMURA et al., 1976c, 1977b). Consequently, it was found that the production of the acylating enzyme catalyzing the acetylation at C-3 on the lactone ring of leucomycin A_1 is induced by glucose and is specifically inhibited by butyrate. The mechanism of action of butyrate on the bioconversion of leucomycin A_1 to leucomycin A_3 in the presence of cerulenin is illustrated in Figure 9. On the other hand, in the case of streptomycin it is known that α-D-mannosidase is repressed by glucose and induced by mannan (DEMAIN and INAMINE, 1970). Also, acetylhydrolase which converts cephalosporin C to desacetylcephalosporin C is repressed by glucose (HINNEN and NÜESCH, 1976). This is the first information about glucose induction of any enzyme related to secondary metabolite biosynthesis.

SUZUKI et al. (1977) have investigated the interconversions among leucomycin A_3, carbomycin A, carbomycin B, and maridomycin II caused by intact cells. The bioconversion of carbomycin A to maridomycin II and the reversible conversion between carbomycin B and leucomycin A_3 were observed with intact cells of a carbomycin-producing strain. Further, the reaction of leucomycin A_3 to maridomycin II was observed with the intact cells of a maridomycin-producing strain *Sm. hygroscopicus*.

C. Mutational Biosyntheses of Macrolide Antibiotics

In the mutational biosynthesis of macrolide antibiotics, the isolation of the aglycone may serve not only for the biogenetic studies, but also as a starting

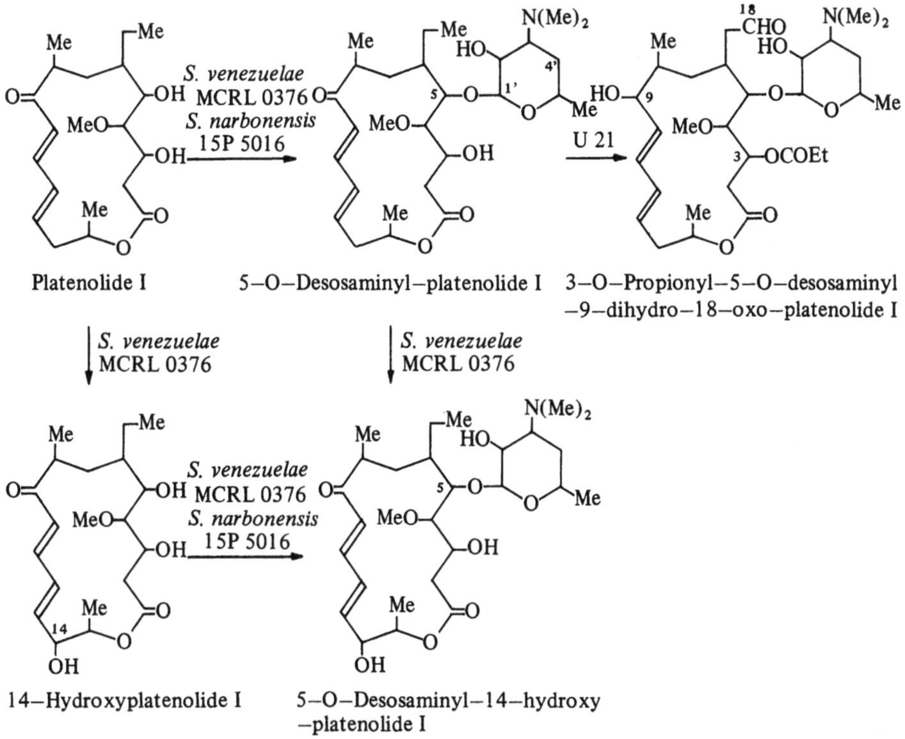

Fig. 10. Biological glycosidation of platenolide I

material for the construction of new macrolide antibiotics. LeMahieu et al. (1976) have reported the production of 3-O-oleandrosyl-5-O-desosaminyl-erythronolide A oxime by an oleandomycin-producing strain.

Maezawa et al. (1978) has attempted the biological glycosidation of platenolide I, a biosynthetic intermediate leading to the aglycone of platenomycin with a foreign amino sugar. The feeding of platenolide I to the fermentation broth of *Sm. narbonensis* producing narbomycin, a 14-membered macrolide antibiotic, gave a new product designated as 5-O-desosaminyl-platenolide I. Further, *Streptomyces venezuelae* (Maezawa et al., 1973) producing narbomycin and picromycin gave 5-O-desosaminyl platenolide I together with a second product, 5-O-desosaminyl 14-hydroxyplatenolide I as shown in Figure 10. These experiments led to an attractive result when the bioconversion of the non-antibiotic substance 5-O-desosaminyl platenolide I by a blocked mutant of *Sm. platensis* subsp. *malvinus*, a producer of platenomycin, gave an antibiotically active compound, 3-O-propionyl 5-O-desosaminyl-9-dihydro-18-oxo-platenolide I, as the main product.

On the other hand, the glycosidation of narbonolide, a 14-membered macrolide aglycone (Maezawa et al., 1976), with mycaminose (generally found only in 16-membered macrolides) was attempted by adding narbonolide during the fermentation of a platenomycin-producing strain of *Sm. platensis* and its blocked mutant. Two new products, 5-O-mycaminosyl narbonolide and 9-dihydro-5-O-mycaminosyl narbonolide, were isolated, but no compound possessing the disaccharide mycarosyl mycaminose was found.

References

Achenbach H, Grisebach H (1964) Zur Biogenese der Makrolide, XI. Weitere Untersuchungen zur Biogenese des Magnamycins. Z Naturforsch 19b (7):561

Achenbach H, Karl W (1975) Untersuchungen an Stoffwechselprodukten von Mikroorganisme, VIII. Aldgamycin F, ein neues Antibiotikum aus *Streptomyces lavendulae*. Chem Ber 108:772

Birch AJ, Djerassi C, Dutcher JD, Majer J, Perlan D, Pride E, Rickards RW, Thomson PJ (1964) Studies in relation to biosynthesis part XXXV. Macrolide antibiotics part XII. Methymycin. J Chem Soc 5274

Cantoni GL (1963) S-Adenosylmethionine, a new intermediate formed enzymatically from L-methionine and adenosine triphosphate. J Biol Chem 204:403

Celmer WD (1971) Stereochemical problems in macrolide antibiotics. Pure Appl Chem 28:413

Corcoran JW (1961) Actonomycete antibiotics, II. Participation of the methionine methyl group in the biogenesis of L-cladinose, a branched chain monosaccharide. J Biol Chem 236:27

Corcoran JW (1975) S-Adenosylmethionine: Erythromycin C O-methyltransferase. In: Hash JH (ed) Methods in enzymology, vol XLIII, Antibiotics, pp 487–497. Academic Press, London New York

Corcoran JW, Chick M (1966) Biochemistry of the macrolide antibiotics. In: Snell JF (ed) Biosynthesis of antibiotics, pp 149–201. Academic Press, London New York

Day LE, Chamberlin JW, Gordee EZ, Chen S, Gorman M, Hamill RL, Ness T, Weeks RW, Stroshan R (1973) Biosynthesis of monensin. Antimicrob Agents Chemother 4:410

Delić V, Pigac J (1969) Detection and study of co-synthesis tetracycline antibiotics by an agar method. J Gen Microbiol 55:103

Demain AL, Inamine E (1970) Biochemistry and regulation of streptomycin and mannosidostreptomycinase (α-D-mannosidase) formation. Bacteriol Rev 34:1

Feldman LI, Dill IK, Holmlund CE, Whaley HA, Patterson EL, Bohonos N (1964) Microbiological transformations of macrolide antibiotics. Antimicrob Agents Chemother 1963:54

Friedman SM, Kaneda T, Corcoran W (1964) Antibiotic glycosides. V. A comparison of 2-methylmalonate and propionate as precursor of the C_{21} branched chain lactone in erythromycin. J Biol Chem 239:2386

Furumai T, Suzuki M (1975a) Studies on the biosynthesis of basic 16-membered macrolide antibiotic, platenomycins. I. Selection of and cosynthesis by nonplatenomycin-producing mutants. J Antibiot 28:770

Furumai T, Suzuki M (1975b) Studies on the biosynthesis of basic 16-membered macrolide antibiotics platenomycins. II. Production, isolation and structure of 3-O-propionyl-5-O-mycaminosyl platenolides I and II, 9-dehydro demycarosyl platenomycin. J Antibiot 28:775

Furumai T, Suzuki M (1975c) Studies on the biosynthesis of basic 16-membered macrolide antibiotics, platenomycins. III. Production, isolation and structures of platenolides I and II. J Antibiot 28:783

Furumai T, Seki Y, Takeda K, Kinumaki A, Suzuki M (1973) An approach to the biosynthesis of macrolide antibiotic platenomycin. J Antibiot 26:708

Furumai T, Takeda K, Suzuki M (1975) Studies on the biosynthesis of basic 16-membered macrolide antibiotics, platenomycins. IV. Biosynthesis of platenomycins. J Antibiot 28:789

Furumai T, Maezawa I, Matsuzawa N, Yano S, Yamaguchi T, Takeda K, Okuda T (1977) Macrolide antibiotics M-4365 produced by micromonospora. I. Taxonomy, production, isolation, characterization and properties. J Antibiot 30:443

Ganguly AK, Lee BK, Brambilla R, Condon R, Sarre O (1976) Biosynthesis of rosamicin. J Antibiot 29:976

Gersch D, Bocker H, Thrum H (1977) Biosynthetic studies on the macrolide antibiotic turimycin using ^{14}C-labeled precursors. J Antibiot 30:448

Greenspan MD, Macknow RC, Ōmura S (1977) The effect of cerulenin on sterol biosynthesis in *Saccharomyces cerevisiae*. Lipid 12:729

Grisebach H, Achenbach H (1962a) Biogenesis of macrolide origin of the aldehyde group of magnamycin. Tetrahedron Lett 569

Grisebach H, Achenbach H (1962b) Zur Biogenese der Makrolide. III. Über den Einbau von Propionsäure-(1-^{14}C-3-T) und (2-^{14}C-3-T) in Magnamycin. Z Naturforsch 17b:6

Grisebach H, Achenbach H (1963) Über die Herkunft der Isovaleriansäure in Magnamycin. Experientia 19:6

Grisebach H, Weber-Schilling CA (1968) Zur Biosyntheses der Makrolide. XVI. Über den Einbau von Bernsteinsäure in Magnamycin. Z Naturforsch 23b:655

Grisebach H, Achenbach H, Hofheinz W (1961) Biogenesis of macrolides. Origin of the branched methyl groups in cladinose and mycarose. Tetrahedron Lett 234

Haber H, Johnson RD, Rinehart KL Jr (1977) Biosynthetic origin of the C_2 units of geldanamycin and distribution of label from D-[6-^{13}C]glucose. J Am Chem Soc 99:3541

Hamill RL, Stark WM (1964) Macrocin, a new antibiotic and lactenocin, an active degradation product. J Antibiot 17:133

Hata T, Sano Y, Ohki N, Yokoyama Y, Matsumae A, Ito S (1953) Leucomycin, a new antibiotic. J Antibiot 6:87

Hatano KE, Higashide, Shibata M (1976) Studies on juvenimicin, a new antibiotic I. Taxonomy, fermentation and antimicrobia properties. J Antibiot 29:1163

Hinnen A, Nüesch J (1976) Enzymatic hydrolysis of cephalosporin C by an extracellular acetylhydrolase of *Cephalosporium acremonium*. Antimicrob Agents Chemother 9:824

Huber G, Wallaheusser KH, Fries L, Steigler A, Weidenmueller UH (1962) Niddamycin, ein neues Makrolid-Antibioticum. Arzneim Forsch 12:1191

Hung PP, Marks CL, Tardrew PL (1965) The biosynthesis and metabolism of erythromycins by *Streptomyces erythreus*. J Biol Chem 240:1322

Inouye S, Tsuruoka T, Shomura T, Omoto S, Niida T (1971) Studies on antibiotic, SF-837, a new antibiotic. II. Chemical structure of antibiotic, SF-837. J Antibiot 24:460

Iwai Y, Kumano K, Ōmura S (1978) Biosynthetic studies of microbial alkaloid pyrindicin using C-13 labeled precursors. Chem Pharm Bull 26:736

Jensen AL, Darken MA, Schultz JS, Shay AJ (1964) Relomycin, flask and tank fermentation studies. Antimicrob Agents Chemother 1963:49

Kaneda T, Butte C, Taubman SB, Corcoran JW (1962) Actinomycete antibiotics. III. The biogenesis of erythronolide, the C_{21} branched chain lactone in erythromycin. J Biol Chem 237:322

Kinumaki A, Suzuki M (1972) Proposed structure of angolamycin (shinocomycin A) by mass spectrometry. J Antibiot 25:480

Kinumaki A, Harada K, Suzuki T, Suzuki M, Okuda T (1977) Macrolide antibiotics M-4365 produced by micromonospora. II. Chemical structures. J Antibiot 30:450

Kishi T, Harada S, Yamana H, Miyake A (1976) Studies on juvenimicin, a new antibiotic. II. Isolation, chemical characterization and structures. J Antibiot 29:1171

Koshiyama H, Okanishi M, Ohmori T, Miyaki T, Tsukiura H, Matsuzaki M, Kawaguchi H (1963) Cirramycin, a new antibiotic. J Antibiot 16:59

Kuehne ME, Benson BW (1965) The structures of the spiramycins and magnamycin. J Am Chem Soc 87:4660

Kunstman MP, Mitscher LA, Patterson EL (1964) Aldgamycin E, a new neutral macrolide antibiotic. Antimicrob Agents Chemother 1963:87

Lee BK, Condon RG, Patel M, Marquec JA, Wagman GH (1976) A method for the biosynthetic preparation of [methyl-1-^{14}C]rosamicin. J Appl Bacteriol 40:217

Lefemine DV, Barbatschi E, Dann M, Thomas SO, Kunstman MP, Mitscher LA, Bohonos N (1964) Neutramycin, a new neutral macrolide antibiotic. Antimicrob Agents Chemother 1963:41

LeMahieu RA, Ax HA, Blount JF, Carson M, Despreaux CW, Pruess DL, Scannell JP, Weiss F, Kierstead RW (1976) A new semisynthetic macrolide antibiotic 3-O-oleandrosyl-5-O-desosaminyl erythronolide A oxime. J Antibiot 29:728

Machida I, Shiozu S, Yokota K, Makino S, Kawaguchi T, Honda K (1972) Process for a new antibiotic. Japan Kokai Patent 47-25384

Maezawa I, Hori T, Kinumaki A, Suzuki M (1973) Biological conversion of narbonolide to picromycin. J Antibiot 26:708

Maezawa I, Kinumaki A, Suzuki M (1976) Biological glycosidation of macrolide aglycones. I. Isolation and characterization of 5-O-mycaminosyl narbonolide and 9-dihydro-5-O-mycaminosyl narbonolide. J Antibiot 29:1203

Maezawa I, Kinumaki A, Suzuki M (1978) Biological glycosidation of macrolide aglycones. II. Isolation and characterization of desosaminyl-platenolide I. J Antibiot 31:303

Majer J, Püza M, Doleziloa L, Vanek Z (1961) Methylation stages in the biosynthesis of erythromycin sugars. Chem Ind 669

Majer J, Martin JR, Egan RS, Corcoran JW (1977) Antibiotic glycosides VIII. Erythromycin D. A new macrolide antibiotic. J Am Chem Soc 99:1620–1622

Mallams AK (1978) In Kirk-Othmer Encyclopedia of Chemical Technology, John Wiley and Sons: New York 2nd ed. 2:937

Martin JR, Egan RS (1970) 5,6-Dioxy-5-oxoerythronolide B, a shunt metabolite of erythromycin biosynthesis. Biochemistry 9:3439

Martin JR, Goldstein AW (1970) Final steps in erythromycin biosynthesis. Proc 6th Int Congr Chemother, vol II, p 112. University of Tokyo Press, Tokyo

Martin JR, Perun TJ (1968) Studies on the biosynthesis of the erythromycins. III. Isolation and structure of 5-deoxy-5-oxo-erythronolide B, a shunt metabolite of erythromycin biosynthesis. Biochemistry 7:1728

Martin JR, Perun TJ, Grirolami RL (1966) Studies on the biosynthesis of the erythromycins. I. Isolation and structure of intermediate glycoside, 3-α-L-mycarosyl erythronolide B. Biochemistry 5:2852

Martin JR, Perun TJ, Egan RS (1972) (8S)-8-hydroxy-5,6-dideoxy-5-oxo-erythronolide B, a shunt metabolite of erythromycin biosynthesis-V. Studies on the biosynthesis of the erythromycins-V. Conformation of macrolide antibiotics-V. Tetrahedron 28:2937

McCormick JRD (1960) Cosynthesis of tetracyclines by pairs of *Streptomyces aureofaciens* mutants. J Am Chem Soc 82:5006

McGuire JM, Boniece WS, Higgens CE, Hoehn MM, Stark WM, Westhead J, Wolfe RN (1961) Tylosin, a new antibiotic. I. Microbiological studies. Antibiot Chemother 11:320

Mitscher LA, Kunstman MP (1969) The structure of neutramycin. Experientia 15:12

Morin R, Gorman M (1968) In Kirk-Othmer Encyclopedia of Chemical Technology, John Wiley and Sons: New York 2nd ed. 12:632

Morin RB, Gorman M, Hamill RL, DeMarco PV (1970) The structure of tylosin. Tetrahedron Lett 1970:4737

Muroi M, Izawa M, Ono H, Higashide E, Kishi T (1972a) Isolation of maridomycins and structure of maridomycin II. Experientia 28:878

Muroi M, Izawa M, Kishi T (1972b) Structure of maridomycins. I, III, IV, V and VI, macrolide antibiotics. Experientia 28:129

Niida T, Tsuruoka T, Ezaki N, Shomura T, Akita E, Inouye S (1973) A new antibiotics, SF-837. J Antibiot 24:319

Nomura S, Horiuchi T, Hata T, Ōmura S (1972) Inhibition of sterol and fatty acid biosynthesis by cerulenin in cell-free systems of yeast. J Antibiot 25:365

Ohno H, Harada S, Kishi T (1974) Maridomycin, a new macrolide antibiotic. VII. Incorporation of labeled precursors into maridomycin and preparation of ^{14}C-labeled 9-propionyl maridomycin. J Antibiot 27:442

Ohno H, Ohno T, Awaya J, Ōmura S (1975) Inhibition of 6-methylsalicylic acid synthesis by the antibiotics cerulenin. J Biochem 78:1149

Ōmura S (1976) The antibiotic cerulenin, a novel tool for biochemistry as an inhibitor of fatty acid synthesis. Bacteriol Rev 40:681

Ōmura S, Nakagawa A (1975) Chemical and biological studies on 16-membered macrolide antibiotics. J Antibiotics (Tokyo) 28:401

Ōmura S, Takeshima H (1974) Inhibition of the biosynthesis of leucomycin, a macrolide antibiotic, by cerulenin. J Biochem 75:193

Ōmura S, Takeshima H (1977) Kagaku to Seibutsu (Tokyo) 15:309

Ōmura S, Katagiri M, Hata T (1967) The structure of leucomycin A_4, A_5, A_6, A_7, A_8 and A_9. J Antibiotics (Tokyo) 20:234

Ōmura S, Nakagawa A, Otani M, Hata T, Ogura H, Furuhata K (1969) The structure of the spiramycins (foromacidines) and their relationship with the leucomycins and carbomycins (Magnamycins). J Am Chem Soc 91:3401

Ōmura S, Nakagawa A, Neszmelyi A, Gero SD, Sepulchre AM, Piriou F, Lukacs G (1975a) Carbon-13 nuclear magnetic resonance spectral analysis of 16-membered macrolide antibiotics. J Am Chem Soc 97:4001

Ōmura S, Nakagawa A, Takeshima H, Atsumi K, Miyazawa J, Piriou F, Lukacs G (1975b) Biosynthetic studies using ^{13}C enriched precursors on the 16-membered macrolide antibiotic leucomycin A_3. J Am Chem Soc 97:6600

Ōmura S, Nakagawa A, Takeshima H, Miyazawa J, Kitao C (1975c) A ^{13}C-nuclear magnetic study of the biosynthesis of the 16-membered macrolide antibiotic tylosin. Tetrahedron Lett 50:4503

Ōmura S, Takeshima H, Nakagawa A, Kanemoto N, Lukacs G (1976a) Studies on carboxylic acid metabolism in a macrolide producing microorganism using carbon-13 magnetic resonance. Bioorg Chem 5:451

Ōmura S, Miyazawa J, Takeshima H, Kitao C, Atsumi K, Aizawa M (1976b) Bioconversion of leucomycins and its regulation by butyrate in a producing strain. J Antibiot 29:1131

Ōmura S, Takeshima H, Nakagawa A, Miyazawa J, Piriou T, Lukacs G (1977a) Studies on the biosynthesis of 16-membered macrolide antibiotics using carbon-13 nuclear magnetic resonance spectroscopy. Biochemistry 16:2860

Ōmura S, Miyazawa J, Takeshima H, Kitao C (1977b) Induction of the bioconversion of leucomycins by glucose in a producing strain. J Antibiot 30:192

Ōmura S, Kitao C, Miyazawa J, Imai H, Takeshima H (1978b) Bioconversion and biosynthesis of 16-membered macrolide antibiotic, tylosin using enzyme inhibitor, cerulenin. J Antibiot 31:254

Ōmura S, Kitao C, Hamada H, Ikeda H (1978c) Bioconversion and biosynthesis of 16-membered macrolide antibiotics. X. Final steps in the biosynthesis of spiramycin using enzyme inhibitor, cerulenin. Chem Pharm Bull in press

Pape H, Brillinger GU (1973) Stoffwechselprodukt von Microorganismen. 113. Mitteilung. Biosynthese von Thymidin diphospho-mycarose durch ein zellfreies System aus *Streptomyces rimosus*. Arch Microbiol 88:25

Pinnert-Sindico S, Ninet L, Preud'Homme J, Cosar C (1954) A new antibiotic, spiramycin. Antibiot Ann 55:724

Reiman H, Jaret RS (1972) Structure of rosamicin, a new macrolide from *Micromonospora rosaria*. Chem Commun 1972:1270

Reuter G, Hütter R (1976) Valin und Leucin als mögliche Vorstufen von Isobuttersäure rest. Isovaleriansäure in Turimycin. Biochem Physiol Pflanz 169:1

Sasaki K, Rinehart KL Jr, Slomp G, Grostic MF, Olson EC (1970) Geldanamycin. I. Structure assignment. J Am Chem Soc 92:7591

Seno ET, Pieper RL, Huber FM (1977) Terminal stages in the biosynthesis of tylosin. Antimicrob Agents Chemother 455

Shimauchi Y, Kubo K, Ōsumi K, Okamura K, Fukugawa Y, Ishikura T, Lein J (1978) Deltamycins, new macrolide antibiotics. II. Isolation and physicochemical properties. J Antibiot 31:270

Srinivasan D, Srinivasan PR (1967) Study on the biosynthesis of magnamycin. Biochemistry 6:3111

Suzuki T (1970) The structure of an antibiotic, B-58941. Bull Chem Soc Jpn 43:292

Suzuki M, Takamori I, Kinumaki A, Sugawara Y, Okuda T (1971a) The structures of antibiotic, YL-704 C_1, C_2 and W_1. J Antibiot 24:904

Suzuki M, Takamori I, Kinumaki A, Sugawara Y, Okuda T (1971b) The structures of antibiotics. YL-704 A and B. Tetrahedron Lett 435

Suzuki M, Takamaki T, Miyagawa K, Ono H, Higashide E, Uchida M (1977) Interconversion among leucomycin A_3, carbomycin A, carbomycin B and maridomycin II. Agric Biol Chem 41:419

Takeshima H, Kitao C, Ōmura S (1977) Inhibition of the biosynthesis of leucomycin, a macrolide antibiotics, by cerulenin. J Biochem 81:1127

Tanner FW, English AR, Lees TM, Routien JB (1952) Some properties of magnamycin, a new antibiotic. Antibiot Chemother 2:441

Tardrew PL, Nyman MA (1964) Hypocholesterolemic agent M-850. US Patent 3.127,315

Tsukiura H, Konishi M, Saka M, Naito T, Kawaguchi H (1969) Studies on cirramycin A_1. III. Structure of cirramycin A_1. J Antibiot 22:89

Tsuruoka T, Inouye S, Shomura T, Ezaki N, Niida T (1971) Studies on antibiotic, SF-837, a new antibiotic. IV. Structure of antibiotic SF-837 A_2, A_3 and A_4. J Antibiot 24:526

Vance D, Gordberg I, Mitsuhashi O, Bloch K, Ōmura S, Nomura S (1972) Inhibition of fatty acid synthetase by the antibiotic cerulenin. Biochem Biophys Res Commun 48:649

Wagman GH, Waitz JA, Marquez J, Murawski A, Oden EM, Testa RT, Weinstein MJ (1972) A new micromonospora-produced macrolide antibiotic, rosamicin. J Antibiot 25:641

Westley JW, Evans RH Jr, Pruess DL, Stempel A (1970) Biosynthesis of antibiotic X-537A. Chem Commun 1970:1467

Westley JW, Pruess DL, Pitcher RG (1972) Incorporation of [1-^{13}C]butyrate into antibiotic X-537A. Chem Commun 1972:161

Westley JW, Evans RH Jr, Harvey G, Pitcher RG, Pruess DL, Stempel A, Berger J (1974) Biosynthesis of lasalocid. I. Incorporation of ^{13}C and ^{14}C labeled substrates into sasalocid A. J Antibiot 27:288

Whaley HA, Patterson EL, Dornbush AC, Backus EJ, Bohonos N (1964) Isolation and characterization of relomycin, a new antibiotic. Antimicrob Agents Chemother 1963:45

Woo PWK, Dion HW, Bartz QR (1964) The structure of Chalcomycin. Chem Commun 86:2726

Woodward RB (1957) Struktur und Biogenese der Makrolide. Eine neue Klasse von Naturstoffen. Angew Chem 69:50

Woodward RB, Wiler LS, Dutta PC (1965) The structure of magnamycin. J Am Chem Soc 87:4662

Biosynthesis of Some Unusual Macrolide Antibiotics

Heinz G. Floss and Ching-jer Chang

There is an abundance of antibiotics containing a macrocyclic lactone ring structure. The majority of these fall into one of a few major classes, e.g., the 12-, 14-, or 16-member macrolides, the ansamycins or the polyene antibiotics. The biosynthesis of these classes of compounds is discussed in several other chapters. There are also a few rather unusual macrolides which do not fit into any of these major categories. The biosynthesis of three of these, chlorothricin and the boron-containing macrodiolides aplasmomycin and boromycin, is the subject of this chapter.

I. Chlorothricin

A. Background

Chlorothricin (*1*) was isolated from *Streptomyces antibioticus* strain Tü 99 (Keller-Schierlein et al., 1969a). It co-occurs in a ratio of about 4:1 with the corresponding deschloro derivative (*2*), from which it could so far not be completely separated (Keller-Schierlein et al., 1969a). In a medium supplemented with 5 g/l KBr the same strain produces a bromo analog, bromothricin (*3*) (Keller-Schierlein et al., 1969b):

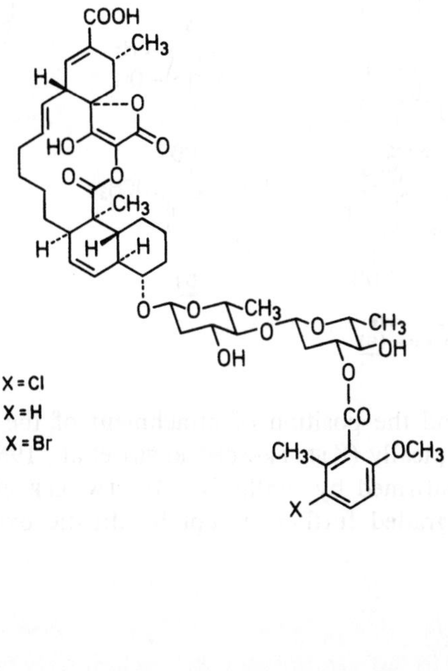

1: X = Cl
2: X = H
3: X = Br

Chlorothricin inhibits growth of gram-positive organisms, like *Bacillus subtilis,* on synthetic media, but not on complex rich media (KELLER-SCHIERLEIN et al., 1969a), indicating some form of an antimetabolite effect. The inhibitory effect can be overcome by lipoproteins and, in part, by acetate (SCHINDLER and ZÄHNER, 1972). Studies on the mode of interaction of chlorothricin with membrane phospholipids (PACHE and CHAPMAN, 1972) suggest that the antagonistic effect of lipoproteins may be a non-specific one due to lowering of the effective concentration of chlorothricin by hydrophobic interaction with the lipid moieties. In tracing the antagonistic effect of acetate, it was found (SCHINDLER and ZÄHNER, 1972) that the inhibition of *B. subtilis* by *1* on a defined glucose medium is due to an inhibition of the anaplerotic CO_2 fixation catalyzed by pyruvate carboxylase. In its binding to pyruvate carboxylase from *B. stearothermophilus,* chlorothricin antagonizes the activating effect of acetyl-coenzyme A on this enzyme (SCHINDLER and ZÄHNER, 1973). Different inhibition characteristics were observed for pyruvate carboxylases from different organisms (SCHINDLER and SCRUTTON, 1975), and, in an observed inhibition of porcine heart malate dehydrogenase, the antibiotic discriminated between the mitochondrial and the cytoplasmic isoenzyme (SCHINDLER, 1975). The mode of action of *1* is clearly quite different from that of other macrolide antibiotics.

The structure of chlorothin was determined by a combination of chemical and spectroscopic techniques, including a single-crystal X-ray analysis of a degradation product. Methanolysis of the antibiotic gave three major products (and the chlorine-free analog of one of them, resulting from the contaminating *2*): α-methyl-2-deoxy-D-rhamnoside (*4*), an acyl-α-methyl-2-deoxy-D-rhamnoside (*5*), and chlorothricolide methyl ester (*6*) (KELLER-SCHIERLEIN et al., 1969a):

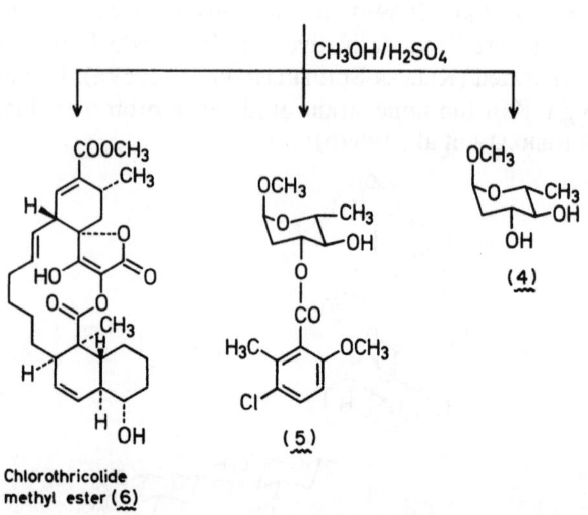

The structure and the position of attachment of the acyl moiety of *5* was deduced spectroscopically (KELLER-SCHIERLEIN et al., 1969a) and the structure of the acid was confirmed by synthesis (MUNTWYLER et al., 1970). Fragment *6* could not be degraded further, except by drastic oxidations to give some naphthalene and benzene derivatives. The structure and absolute configuration were eventually determined by an X-ray analysis of the cesium salt (BRUFANI et al., 1972). The result of the latter is supported by considerable spectroscopic and chemical work, which also defined the mode in which the fragments are joined together in the intact antibiotic (MUNTWYLER and KELLER-SCHIERLEIN, 1972). In a more recent paper from KELLER-SCHIERLEIN'S group (GERHARD et al., 1975), an interesting rearrangement reaction in the aglycone moiety of chlorothricin is described, which leads to a dihydronaphthalene derivative:

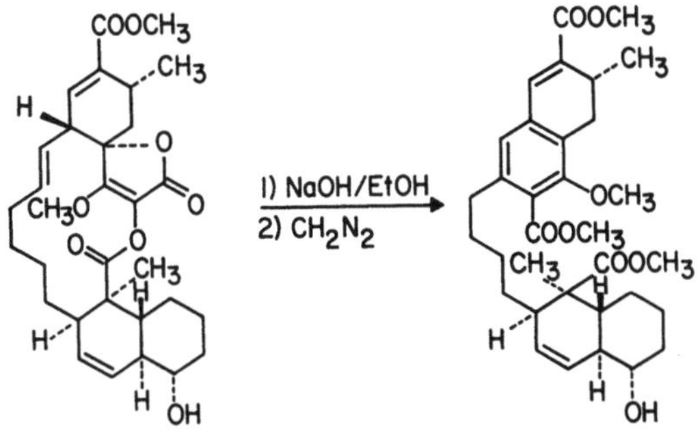

B. Assignment of the ^{13}C-NMR Spectrum of Chlorothricin

Studies on the biosynthesis of molecules of the complexity of chlorothricin are most efficiently carried out by the use of stable isotopes, like ^{13}C, followed by NMR spectroscopic analysis of the labeling pattern in the compound. However, an essential prerequisite, and often one of the most time-consuming tasks in the entire project, is the complete assignment of the ^{13}C-NMR spectrum of the compound to be investigated.

The ^{13}C-NMR spectrum of chlorothricin (Fig. 1) is rather complex, in part because of the presence of about 20% of *2* in even the purest samples. However, the task of assigning all the signals in this spectrum (MASCARETTI et al., 1979) is simplified by the possibility of breaking the molecule down to fragments *4*, *5*, and *6* by methanolysis. The spectra of these fragments were recorded and analyzed separately, and allowed assignment of the corresponding signals in the parent compound. Spectral analysis of *4* and *5* was straightforward, based on multiplicity, chemical shift theory, and long-range coupling patterns. In the aglycone portion, the downfield carbon signals could be assigned based on comparison of *6* with *1* and with various tetronic acids. For the assignment of the carbons of the decaline moiety, *6* was oxidized at C-7 to the ketone, which was rearranged to the corresponding α,β-unsaturated ketone, and the chemical shift changes accompanying these transformations were analyzed. The α,β-unsaturated ketone was exchanged with D_2O at C-6 and C-10, leading to characteristic decreases in intensity of the signals of the deuterated and adjacent carbons. Further assignments were made by measuring the ^{13}C–^{13}C one bond coupling constants of pairs of carbons in *1* and *6* derived biosyntheti-

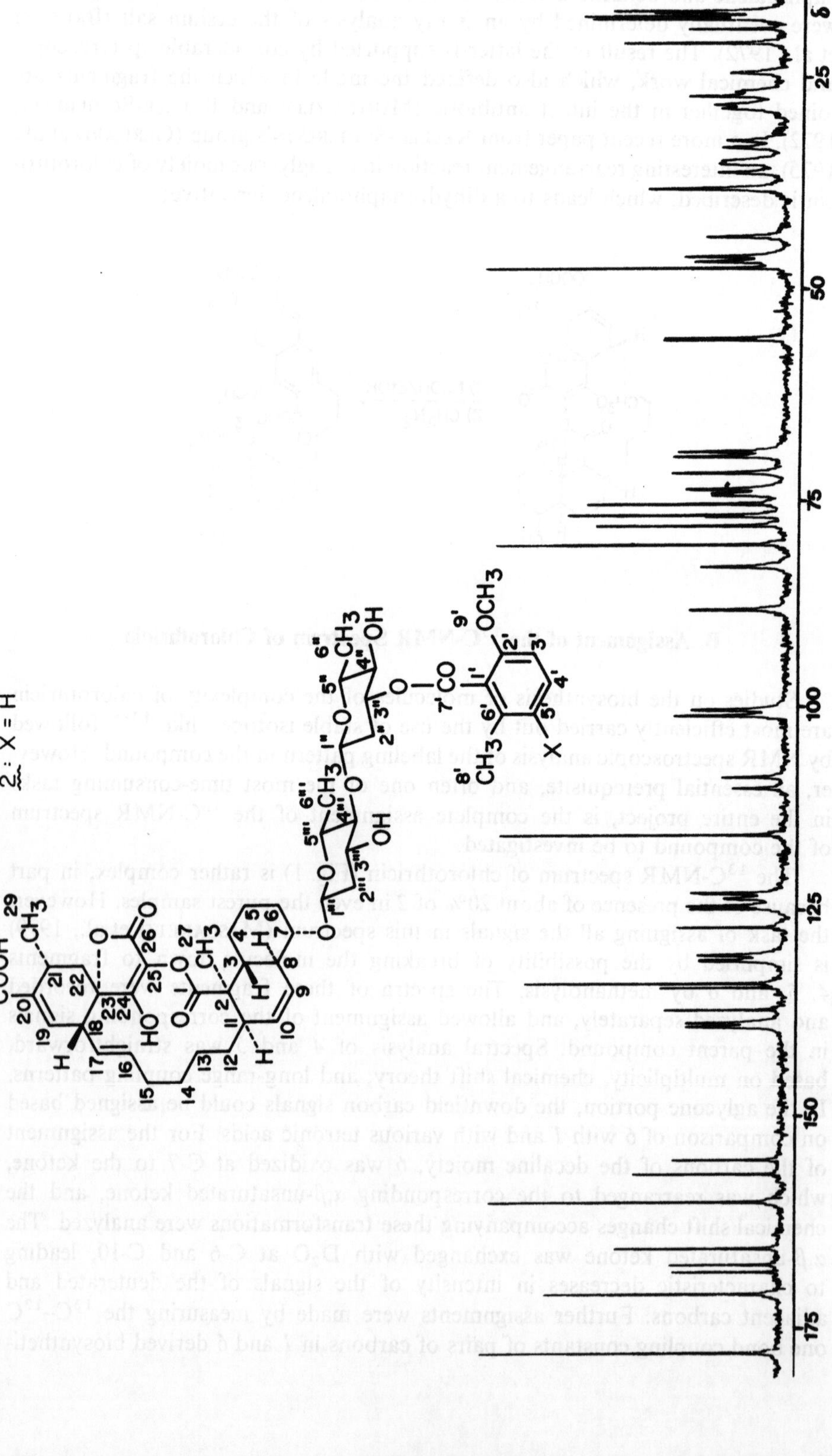

Fig. 1. Proton-decoupled carbon-13 NMR spectrum of *1* and *2* (4:1) in $CDCl_3$ solution

cally from $^{13}CH_3$–$^{13}COONa$. In this way a nearly complete assignment of all the carbon signals in the spectra of *1* and *6* could be made without using any biosynthetic assumptions as the basis for spectral interpretation (MASCARETTI et al., 1979). The chemical shift assignments are referred to in the following discussion of the biosynthetic results.

C. Biosynthesis of the Aglycone

A series of feeding experiments with radioactive precursors using strain Tü 99 of *S. antibioticus* were carried out in our laboratory and in that of Prof. H. PAPE, then at the University of Tübingen, to determine which compounds are utilized in the biosynthesis of *1* (HOLZBACH et al., 1978). The results are summarized in Table 1. Inspection of the structure of *6* together with our knowledge of the biosynthesis of other macrolides suggests that acetate, propionate, methionine, or even mevalonate are all potential precursors of the aglycone moiety of chlorothricin. All of these, with the exception of mevalonate, are efficiently incorporated (Table 1); all carbon atoms of acetate as well as propionate seem to be utilized. Degradation of *1* from these latter two precursors by methanolysis indicated that a major portion of the label was present in the aglycone moiety. In contrast, methanolysis of *1* from [methyl-^{14}C]methionine, gave *6* containing very little radioactivity and a Zeisel degradation of the same material gave methyl iodide, from the methoxy group of the acyl moiety, which had 101% of the specific radioactivity of the parent antibiotic. Thus, methionine does not seem to contribute to the formation of the aglycone, i.e., the C-methyl groups of the latter do not arise by C-methylation. This was confirmed by a Kuhn-Roth oxidation of *1* derived from [methyl-^{14}C]methionine, which gave non-radioactive acetic acid (HOLZBACH et al., 1978).

Further delineation of the mode of incorporation of acetate and propionate into the aglycone of *1* involved feeding [1-^{13}C]- and [2-^{13}C]acetate and [1-^{13}C]- and [3-^{13}C]propionate (FLOSS et al., 1978). The purified chlorothricin was analyzed by ^{13}C-NMR spectroscopy and then degraded by methanolysis to give *6* which was again subjected to ^{13}C-NMR spectroscopy. The results, which are summarized in Table 2, clearly indicate the incorporation of two molecules of propionate into the aglycone moiety. In one of these the methyl group has been oxidized to a carboxyl (C-28).

The labeling pattern from acetate is more complex. However, it is clearly discernible that C-29 and C-21 come from the methyl group and the carboxyl group of acetate, respectively, and that carbons 3 through 18 are alternatingly labeled by the carboxyl carbon and the methyl carbon of acetate, respectively. These results are indicative of a polyketide mode of biosynthesis, with a contiguous polyketide chain starting with an acetate unit at C-29/C-21, extended by a propionate unit (C-28/C-20/C-19), eight acetate units (C-18 to C-3), and another propionate unit (C-27/C-2/C-1). An experiment with [1,2-$^{13}C_2$]acetate confirmed that carbons 29, 21, and 18 through 3 are all derived from intact acetate units, by showing that the ^{13}C-NMR spectrum of *6* from this precursor displayed

Table 1. Incorporation of radioactively labeled precursors into chlorothricin by *Streptomyces antibioticus* strain Tü 99

Expt. No.	Precursor fed: Name	Spec radioact. [mCi/mmol]	Amount added [mmol/L]	Total radioact. added [mCi/L]	Chlorothricin formed: Yield [mmol/L]	Spec radioact. of purified antibiotic [mCi/mmol $\times 10^{-3}$]	Total radioact. [mCi/L $\times 10^{-3}$]	Incorp rate [%]	Dilution factor
1	Sodium [1-^{14}C]Acetate	8.7	0.023	0.2	0.226	9.0	2.03	1.02	967
2	Sodium [1-^{14}C]Acetate	0.0029	1.19	0.0035	0.120	2.91	0.349	9.98	1.0
3	Sodium [2-^{14}C]Acetate	0.0096	1.13	0.011	0.219	1.76	0.385	3.5	5.5
4	Sodium [1-^{14}C]Propionate	5.9	0.034	0.2	0.120	8.0	0.96	0.48	738
5	Sodium [1-^{14}C]Propionate	0.0134	1.12	0.015	0.331	0.07	0.023	0.15	191
6	Sodium [2-^{14}C]Propionate	0.010	1.0	0.010	0.228	0.81	0.185	1.8	12.3
7	Sodium [3-^{14}C]Propionate	3.2	0.063	0.2	0.243	3.5	0.85	0.43	914
8	Sodium [3-^{14}C]Propionate	0.0075	1.14	0.0086	0.233	1.30	0.30	3.5	5.8
9	[U-^{14}C]-D-Glucose	3.0	0.125	0.375	0.314	11.9	3.73	0.99	252
10	[1-^{14}C]-D-Glucose	>1	<0.01	0.0088	0.137	0.46	0.063	0.72	–
11	[6-^{14}C]-D-Glucose	2.9	0.172	0.5	0.299	20	5.98	1.20	145
12	[methyl-^{14}C]-L-Methionine	5.4	0.037	0.2	0.210	116	24.36	12.2	46.6
13	[methyl-^{14}C]-L-Methionine	0.0112	1.09	0.0122	0.146	3.2	0.467	3.8	3.5
14	[2-^{14}C]Mevalonate	6.3	0.032	0.204	0.151	0	0	0	
15	[U-^{14}C]Shikimic acid	>5	>0.001	0.0054	0.156	0.0006	0.0001	0.002	–
16	[U-^{14}C]-L-Tyrosine	0.0128	0.866	0.0111	0.286	0.308	0.088	0.79	41.6
17	[3-^{14}C]-D,L-Tyrosine	0.0144	0.795	0.0114	0.073	0.395	0.029	0.25	36.5
18	[2-^{14}C]-D,L-Tyrosine	0.0075	0.831	0.0062	0.114	0.35	0.040	0.64	21.4
19	[1-^{14}C]-L-Tyrosine	0.0147	0.818	0.012	0.197	0.013	0.0026	0.02	1131
20	[U-^{14}C]-L-Phenylalanine	0.0094	1.01	0.0095	0.167	0.345	0.058	0.61	27.2
21	[U-^{14}C]-L-Leucine	0.009	0.98	0.0088	0.189	0.779	0.147	1.67	11.6
22	[1-^{14}C]-L-Leucine	0.006	1.02	0.0059	0.193	0.100	0.019	0.32	60

Table 2. ^{13}C Chemical shifts of the aglycone portion of *1* and *6*, and ^{13}C distribution in *6* obtained biosynthetically from various ^{13}C-labeled precursors

Carbon number	Chemical shift[a]		Relative ^{13}C abundance in 6 derived from			
	1	*6*	Acetate		Propionate	
			[1-^{13}C]	[2-^{13}C]	[1-^{13}C]	[3-^{13}C]
C-1	177.3	177.5	1.20	2.20	4.25	
C-2	47.5	47.4	1.63	1.83		
C-3	37.9	37.6	4.40	1.47		
C-4	26.5	26.6	1.20	2.20		
C-5	24.3	24.1	4.00	1.47		
C-6	36.1	36.2	1.41	2.63		
C-7	83.0	73.3	5.01	1.89		
C-8	43.7	45.4[c]	1.10	2.83		
C-9	123.2	123.2	5.54	1.28		
C-10	130.0	129.9	1.46	2.44		
C-11	46.6	46.8	4.71	1.90		
C-12	33.1	33.0	1.83	2.70		
C-13	28.0[b]	28.0[b]	4.52	1.70		
C-14	28.4[b]	28.4[b]	1.34	2.31		
C-15	32.2	32.3	4.64	1.44		
C-16	138.1[c]	138.0	2.82	3.04		
C-17	124.5	124.4	5.43	1.10		
C-18	46.0	45.9[c]	1.10	1.82		
C-19	138.4[c]	136.5	5.07	2.11	5.86	
C-20	133.6	134.0	1.10	2.08		
C-21	26.9	27.1	4.11	1.30		
C-22	34.9	35.0	1.98	1.70		
C-23	80.4	80.4	0.90	1.15		
C-24	159.4	159.4	1.10	1.10		
C-25	115.5	115.5	1.10	1.83		
C-26	165.0	164.9	2.75	2.30		
C-27	16.7	16.6	1.51	2.79		5.6
C-28	170.1	166.5	1.00	2.00		4.4
C-29	20.7	20.7	1.63	3.47		
C-30 (COO$\underline{CH_3}$)	–	51.6	Standard: 1.10	1.10	1.10	1.10

[a] In ppm downfield from TMS
[b,c,d] These values in any vertical column may be reversed. The assignments listed are the ones compatible with biosynthetic theory

one bond ^{13}C–^{13}C couplings for each of these carbon signals (Mascaretti et al., unpublished results).

The origin of the remaining five carbon atoms (C-22 to C-26) is not as apparent. As shown in Table 1, under comparable conditions [U-^{14}C]-, [3-^{14}C]- and [2-^{14}C]tyrosine was efficiently incorporated into *1*, but not [1-^{14}C]tyrosine. To explore the possibility that, by some ring-cleavage pathway, two of the side-chain and three of the ring carbons of tyrosine might provide the remaining five carbons of *6*, we fed [2-^{13}C]-D,L-tyrosine and analyzed the resulting *1* and *6* by ^{13}C-NMR. Despite a specific incorporation (enrichment) of 6% obtained with this precursor, no particular signal in the spectrum appeared to be specifically enhanced (E.F. KREUTZER, M.S. thesis. Purdue University, 1976). Thus, label from tyrosine is presumably only incorporated following breakdown of the compound, perhaps via the homogentisate pathway, to acetate. The data in Table 2 indicates that of the five carbons which are not accounted for, C-23 and C-24 are clearly not labeled from either carbon of acetate, C-25 is labeled by the methyl group of acetate and C-22 and C-26 are labeled by C-1 and to a lesser extent also by C-2, of acetate. Significantly, the spectrum of *6* derived from [1,2-$^{13}C_2$]acetate reveals the presence of doublets with $^1J_{C-C}$ 90.3 Hz for carbons 25 and 26, indicating that these two carbon atoms must originate from a single acetate unit. The biosynthetic origin of the aglycone moiety of *1*, to the extent that it is known, can thus be summarized as follows:

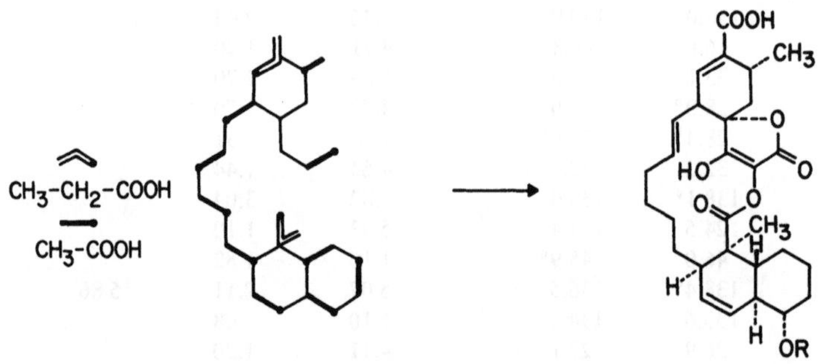

Many additional radioactively labeled compounds have been tested in order to identify a more specific precursor of the remaining three carbon atoms (22, 23, 24) of the aglycone moiety. In addition to the ones listed in Table 1, e.g., leucine, these included [1-^{14}C]ribose (0.42% incorp.), sodium [1-^{14}C]pyruvate (dilution 108), α-[U-^{14}C]ketoglutaric acid (0.09% incorp.), L-(U-^{14}C]lysine (0.15% incorp.), L-[1-^{14}C]ascorbic acid (0.03% incorp.), L-(U-^{14}C]malic acid (0.41% and 0.91% incorp.), [1-^{14}C]glyoxylic acid (0.05% incorp.), [2,3-^{14}C]succinic acid (1.42% incorp., dilution 4), and [1,4-^{14}C]succinic acid (0.28% incorp.). Evidently, of the compounds tested the C_4 dicarboxylic acids, malate and succinate, seem to be the most efficient precursors, and the center carbons of these are particularly well utilized. Whether this is due to a specific incorporation or represents breakdown of these compounds to acetate and/or propionate and incorporation of label via these established precursors remains to be determined.

From the above results and comparison with the structures and biosynthesis of other simpler tetronic acids, e.g., carolic and carlosic acids (LYBING and REIO, 1958; BENTLEY et al., 1962), one may speculate on the mode of formation of the tetronic acid moiety in chlorothricin. In analogy to carolic acid biosynthesis a precursor unit having all the necessary functionalities could be formed by condensation of oxalacetate and malonyl-Co A:

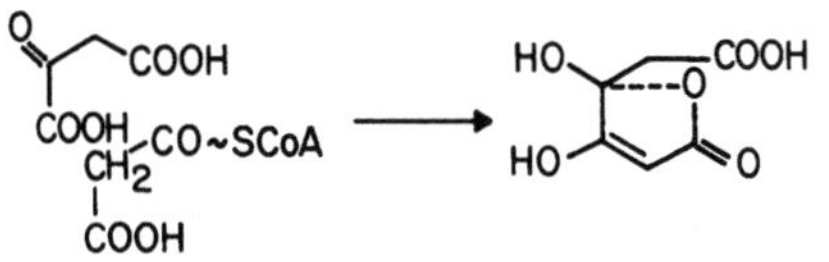

This compound would have to be functionalized at C-3 of the lactone ring or, in analogy to carlosic acid formation, may be acylated in that position by the carboxy terminus of the polyketide chain, followed by a Baeyer-Villiger oxidation. Even more attractive is the possibility that the main polyketide chain does not terminate with propionate, but rather with the acetate unit which gives rise to C-25/C-26:

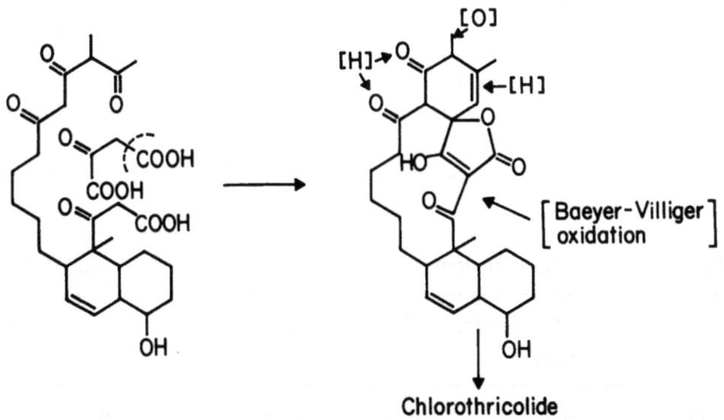

Obviously this is at the moment no more than a highly speculative working hypothesis to guide further experimentation.

It is also not known at which stage of the elaboration of the aglycone the sugar and the acyl moieties are attached. However, combination of the aglycone with these units does not seem to be the terminal step, because labeled chlorothricolide, the free acid corresponding to *6*, was not incorporated into *1* (MASCARETTI et al., unpublished results).

D. Biosynthesis of the Acyl and Sugar Moieties

The acyl moiety could either arise from shikimate or, in view of the substitution pattern more likely, from acetate via the polyketide pathway. The carbon of the methoxy group, as already indicated, is specifically derived from the methyl group of methionine. The non-incorporation of [U-^{14}C]shikimate favors a polyketide origin and this is confirmed by the ^{13}C distribution in the acyl moiety of *1* biosynthesized from [1-^{13}C]- and [2-^{13}C]acetate. The data, summarized in Table 3, were obtained by direct analysis of the ^{13}C spectra of *1*, and show the labeling of alternate carbons from C-1 and C-2 of acetate expected for a polyketide. In some of the experiments with ^{13}C propionate, a third

Table 3. ^{13}C Chemical shifts of the acyl portion of *1* and *5*, and ^{13}C distribution in the acyl portion of *1* obtained biosynthetically from ^{13}C acetate

Carbon number	Chemical shift[a]		Relative ^{13}C abundance in *1* derived from acetate	
	1	*5*	[1-^{13}C]	[2-^{13}C]
C-8′	16.8	16.9	1.2	2.1
C-6′	134.0	134.0	2.0	1.2
C-5′	126.8	126.8	1.3	2.4
C-4′	130.7	130.5	2.4	1.3
C-3′	109.9	109.8	1.4	3.1′
C-2′	154.4	154.4	1.8	1.2
C-1′	122.8	122.6	0.9	1.8
C-7′	166.7	167.2	2.6	1.0
C-9′	56.2	56.1	1.1	1.1

[a] In ppm downfield from TMS

Table 4. Incorporation of specifically labeled glucoses into chlorothricin and α-methyl-2-deoxy-D-rhamnoside

Position of label in glucose fed	T/^{14}C of glucose	Chlorothricin			α-methyl-2-deoxy-D-rhamnoside	
		^{14}C incorp. (%)	T/^{14}C	T-ret. (%)	T/^{14}C	T-ret. (%)
6-^{14}C, 1-T	1.45	0.7	0.21	14.4	0.98	67.5
6-^{14}C, 2-T	1.93	0.5	0.38	19.6	1.93	100.0
6-^{14}C, 3-T	1.81	1.2	0.13	7.1	0.19	10.4
6-^{14}C, 4-T	2.50	1.9	0.12	4.8	0.90	36.0
6-^{14}C, 5-T	3.97	2.3	0.04	1.0	0.13	3.2
6-^{14}C, 6-T	2.10	1.4	0.54	25.7	2.10	100.0

enriched peak was observed in the spectra of *1*, but not of *6*, which was absent in highly purified samples. It is speculated, although this has not been proven, that, in the presence of high levels of propionate, acetyl-Co A can to some extent be replaced by propionyl-Co A as starter unit for the formation of the acyl moiety, leading to contamination with small amounts of a highly enriched analog of *1* containing a C-ethyl instead of the C-methyl group in the acyl moiety.

The two 2-deoxy-D-rhamnose moieties presumably have an identical origin and are expected to arise from glucose. The specific incorporation of glucose samples labeled in various positions, as shown in Table 4, confirms this notion. The incorporation into the sugar moiety of, for example, [6-^{14}C, 2-T]glucose without change of the isotope ratio leaves little doubt that the biosynthesis of 2-deoxy-D-rhamnose involves intact conversion of the carbon skeleton of glucose. The biosynthetic origin of the acyl and the sugar moieties of *1* can thus be summarized as follows:

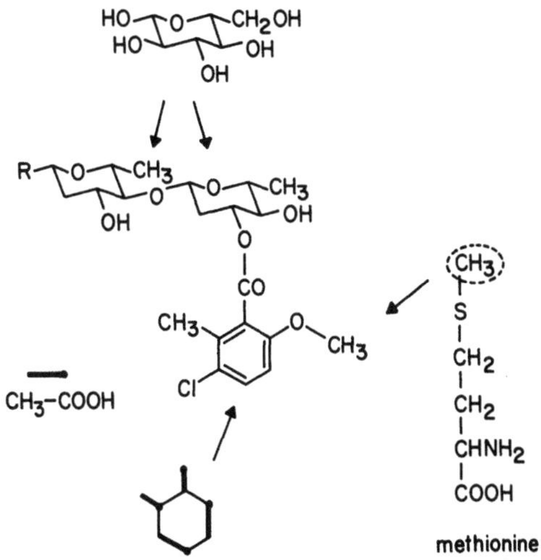

In the conversion of glucose to the 2-deoxy-D-rhamnose moieties of *1* the hydrogens at C-2 and C-6 are completely retained, those at C-1 and C-4 of glucose are partly retained whereas H-3 and H-5 are replaced by hydrogens from other sources. Furthermore, Kuhn-Roth oxidation of *1* derived from [6-^{14}C, 4-T]glucose gave acetic acid with 23% tritium retention relative to the starting glucose. This suggests strongly that in the transformation of glucose to 2-deoxy-D-rhamnose, tritium from C-4 of the sugar has migrated to C-6 of the deoxy sugar. This, as well as the loss of H-5, is typical of the dTDP-glucose oxidoreductase reaction (GABRIEL, 1973), implicating this enzyme in the first step of the formation of the 2-deoxy-D-rhamnose moiety. The results so far on the mode of formation of the sugar portions of *1* parallel entirely those obtained on the biosynthesis of the 2,6-dideoxyhexose moiety of the antibiotic granaticin (SNIPES et al., 1979) (see Chap. 8). Experiments are now underway to elucidate further the mode of transformation of glucose into 2-deoxy-D-rhamnose by determining the steric course of the reactions resulting in the replacement of the hydroxyl functions C-2 and C-6 by hydrogen.

II. Aplasmomycin

A. Background

Aplasmomycin (*7*) is a new antibiotic which was recently isolated from a strain of *Streptomyces griseus* obtained from shallow sea mud as part of a screening program for new metabolites from marine microorganisms (OKAMI et al., 1976). The compound inhibits the growth of gram-positive bacteria, including mycobacteria, in vitro and is active against *Plasmodium berghei* in vivo. The compound is produced in yields of 20–100 mg/l on media resembling sea

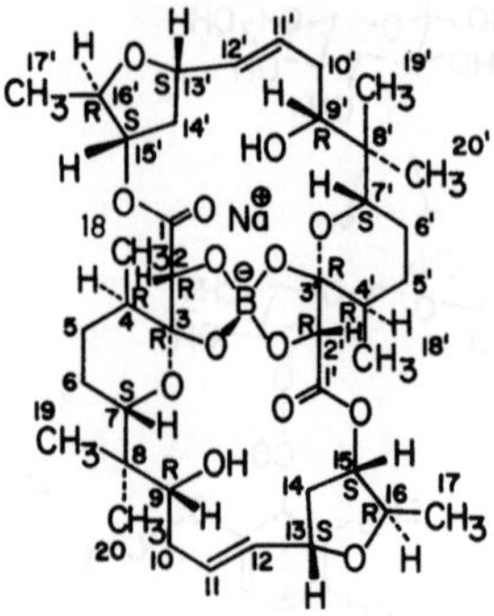

Aplasmomycin (7)

water, e.g., a medium consisting of 1% glucose, 1% Kobu-Cha (processed sea weed), and 3% NaCl (OKAMI et al., 1976). Aplasmomycin was originally thought to have the molecular formula $C_{41}H_{60}O_{14}Na$, but the subsequent structure determination by an X-ray analysis of the silver salt (NAKAMURA et al., 1977) showed that it contains only 40 carbon atoms and one boron. The compound, a macrodiolide, is a symmetrical dimer which closely resembles boromycin (*8*) (DUNITZ et al., 1971), the only other boron-containing natural product. Its 16 chiral centers have identical configurations in the two halves of the molecule and its stereochemistry corresponds to that of boromycin at all centers except C-9 in one half of the boromycin molecule. Recently, two minor components of the fermentation, aplasmomycins B and C, were isolated and identified as the mono-acetate (at C-9) and the diacetate (at C-9 and C-9′) of 7, respectively (SATO et al., 1978).

Aplasmomycin, despite the fact that it is a salt, is very lipophilic, hardly soluble in water and gives good mass spectra even upon electron-impact ionization. Aplasmomycin and aplasmomycin B, but not aplasmomycin C and deboroaplasmomycin, show ionophoric properties, mediating net K^+ transport across a bulk phase. Transport activity correlates with antibiotic activity of these four compounds, aplasmomycin B having about equal antibiotic activity as 7, whereas the other two are inactive. The metal ion specificity is rather pronounced for monovalent cations, with a preference for K^+, Rb^+ and Cs^+ (SATO et al., 1978).

B. NMR Spectral Assignments of Aplasmomycin

Because of the symmetry of the molecule, the ^{13}C-NMR spectrum of aplasmomycin shows only 20 signals (Fig. 2). Their complete assignment (CHEN et al., unpublished results) is based on chemical shift theory, multiplicity analysis, a complete analysis of the 360 MHz proton NMR spectrum of 7 (Fig. 3) followed by single frequency proton decoupling experiments, comparison with several derivatives and model compounds, specific deuterium exchange, and the analysis of one bond carbon-carbon coupling constants measured on a sample of 7

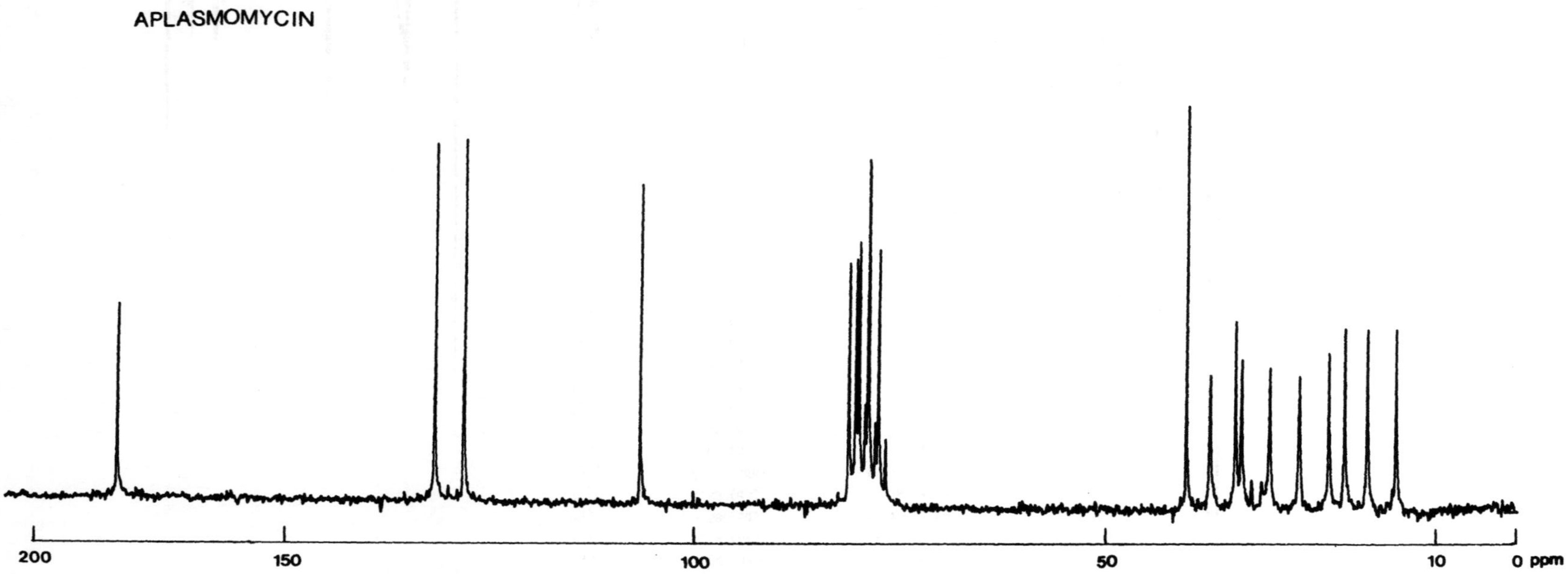

Fig. 2. Proton-noise decoupled natural abundance ^{13}C-NMR spectrum of aplasmomycin

Assignment	Chemical Shift (ppm)	Coupling Constant (Hz)
H_2	4.44 (s)	
H_4	2.04 (m)	
H_5	1.60 (m)	
H_{6S}	1.51 (bd)	12.5
H_{6R}	1.32 (qd)	12.5, 10.65, 6.5
H_7	3.84 (d)	10.65
H_9	3.75 (d)	10.97
H_{10R}	1.92 (ddd)	13.57, 10.97, 5.90
H_{10S}	2.04 (dd)	13.57, 5.90
H_{11}	5.74 (dt)	15.79, 5.90
H_{12}	5.58 (dd)	15.79, 4.25
H_{13}	4.69 (dd)	9.26, 4.54
H_{14R}	2.45 (ddd)	14.31, 9.26, 4.94
H_{14S}	2.03 (d)	14.31
H_{15}	5.06 (d)	4.94
H_{16}	4.68 (q)	6.69
H_{17}	1.18 (d)	6.69
H_{18}	0.98 (d)	6.59
H_{19}	0.68 (s)	
H_{20}	0.73 (s)	

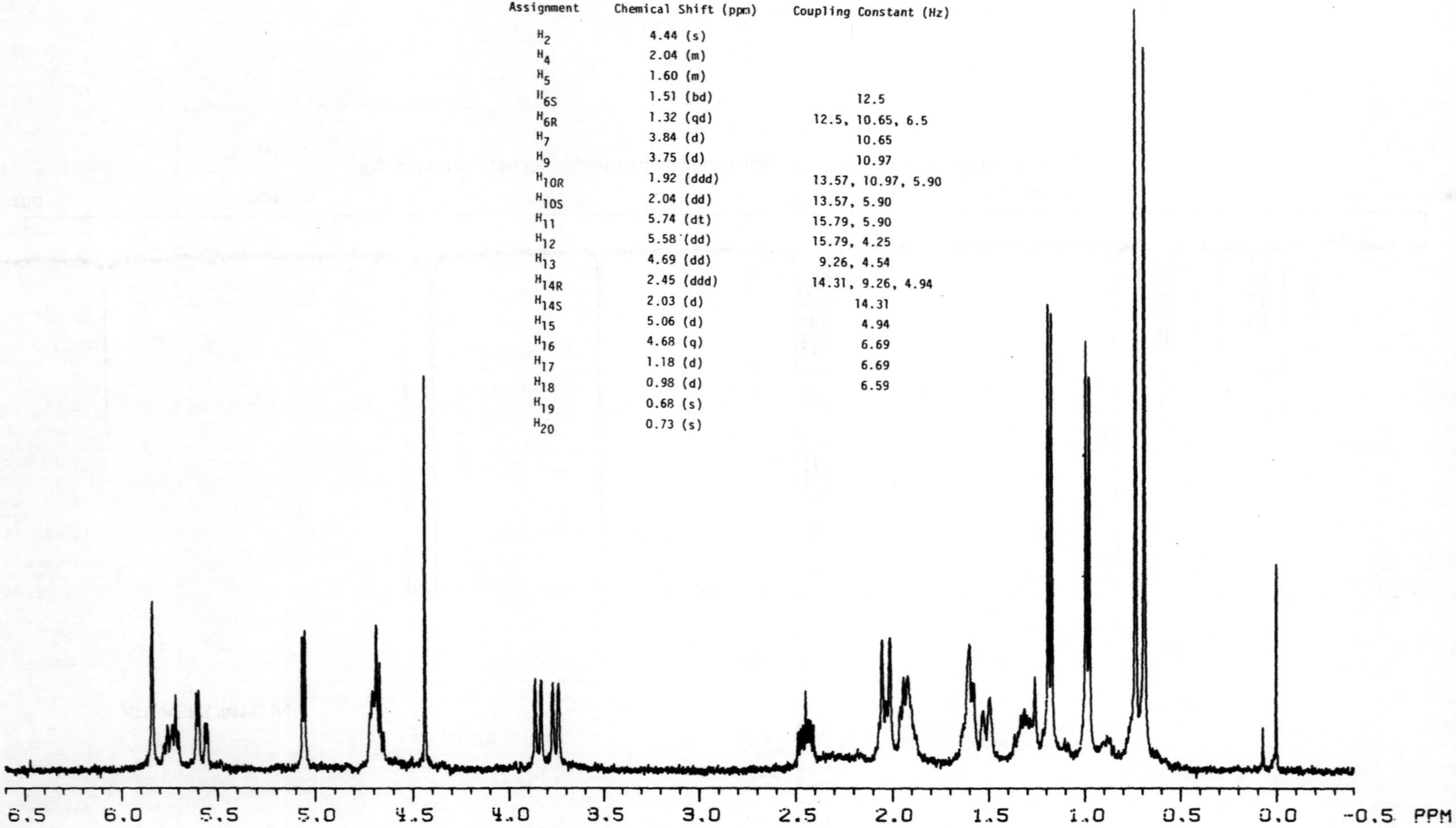

Fig. 3. 360 MHz proton NMR spectrum of aplasmomycin in deuterochloroform solution

biosynthesized from [1,2-$^{13}C_2$]acetate. The distinction of the two stereoheterotopic methyl groups is based on nuclear Overhauser effect measurements. All the assignments, which are listed in Table 6, have been derived without resorting to any assumptions on the biosynthesis of the compound.

C. Biosynthetic Experiments

In analogy to the formation of other macrolide antibiotics one might expect aplasmomycin to be of a mixed acetate/propionate origin, i.e., each half of the molecule would be made up of five acetate and three propionate units in a sequence (Me)P–A–A–A–P–A–P–A(COOH), with an additional C-methylation at the central propionate unit to give the gem-dimethyl structure. As an alternative, the gem-dimethyl portion might result from use of an isobutyryl moiety as chain extension unit. On the other hand, methyl branches might arise entirely by C-methylation of acetate units.

To distinguish between these possibilities we fed a number of ^{14}C-labeled precursors to the aplasmomycin-producing strain SS-20 of *S. griseus* (Chen et al., unpublished results). As shown in Table 5, the specific incorporation values for acetate and methyl-labeled methionine, as well as for several other compounds, are remarkably high. These figures are often greater than 100%, reflecting the very low dilution encountered, the incorporation of multiple units of a precursor, and the fact that the molecule is a dimer. The exceedingly low dilution of these precursors enabled us to proceed immediately to feeding experiments with ^{13}C-labeled acetate and methionine, with the results shown in Table 6. Clearly, carbons 1 through 14 are acetate-derived and show the alternating labeling pattern of a polyketide. An experiment with [1,2-$^{13}C_2$]acetate showed that the seven molecules of acetate making up each chain are indeed incorporated as intact acetate units, i.e., in the spectrum of *7* derived from this experiment the signals for carbons 1–14 each were accompanied by a doublet due to coupling to a neighboring ^{13}C nucleus from the same acetate unit.

Table 5. Incorporation of radioactive precursors into aplasmomycin

Precursor fed	Specific incorporation in *7* (%)
Sodium[1-^{14}C]acetate	40–185
[Methyl-^{14}C]methionine	170
Sodium[1-^{14}C]propionate	2
Sodium[2-^{14}C]propionate	75
Sodium[3-^{14}C]propionate	80
Sodium[1-^{14}C]pyruvate	1.93
Sodium[1-^{14}C]lactate	0.03
[1,4-^{14}C]Succinic acid	4.3
[1,3-^{14}C]Glycerol	18 ~ 170
[2-^{14}C]Glycerol	85

Table 6. ^{13}C Chemical shifts of aplasmomycin and relative ^{13}C abundance in *7* derived from ^{13}C-labeled acetate and methionine

Carbon No.	Chemical shift[a]	% Relative ^{13}C abundance per carbon in *7* biosynthesized from[d]		
		Acetate[b]		[methyl-^{13}C] methionine[c]
		[1-^{13}C]	[2-^{13}C]	
1,1′	170.4	12.3		
2,2′	78.2		9.4	
3,3′	106.0	9.4		
4,4′	32.9		8.6	
5,5′	28.6	9.6		
6,6′	25.0		8.1	
7,7′	79.5	10.8		
8,8′	39.0		7.5	
9,9′	79.3	11.0		
10,10′	32.1		8.1	
11,11′	128.0	7.6		
12,12′	131.8		7.4	
13,13′	76.4	8.6		
14,14′	36.0		8.7	
15,15′	80.4			
16,16′	78.2			
17,17′	19.4			
18,18′	16.5			29.4
19,19′	12.9			29.4
20,20′	21.6			29.4

[a] In ppm downfield from TMS.
[b] Relative to methyl carbons = 1.1
[c] Calculated on the basis of the dilution of [methyl-^{14}C]methionine fed with the ^{13}C material: specific incorporation/6 + 1.1 [%]
[d] Carbons for which no data are listed were not significantly enriched

Three methyl groups in each chain are derived from the methyl group of methionine, and these were identified as carbons 18,18′, 19,19′, and 20,20′. Hence the methyl branches in the chain are derived by C-methylation rather than by incorporation of propionate units into the chain. This is rather unusual in the biosynthesis of macrolide antibiotics.

These results thus establish the origin of the molecule, except for three carbon atoms in each half, carbons 15,15′, 16,16′, and 17,17′, which presumably represent the starter units of the two polyketide chains. Propionate would appear to be a logical precursor of these three-carbon units. Indeed, as shown in Table 5, [2-^{14}C]- and [3-^{14}C]propionate were very efficiently incorporated into *7*. However, very little ^{14}C from the carboxyl group of propionate was incorporated into *7*, and in agreement with this, feeding of [1-^{13}C]propionate did not lead to enrichment of any specific positions in the antibiotic. To check whether C-2 and C-3 of propionate are specifically incorporated into *7*, we carried out Kuhn-Roth oxidations of the antibiotic samples derived from [2-^{14}C]- and

[3-^{14}C]propionate. The acetic acid obtained contained 13.3% and 13.8%, respectively, of the radioactivity of the antibiotic. This suggests that the most likely, although not the only possible explanation is that propionate is converted with loss of C-1 to acetate via symmetrical intermediates, i.e., via succinate and the Krebs cycle. Clearly, propionate is not incorporated intact into the three-carbon starter unit.

Several other three- and four-carbon compounds likewise are not likely to be specific precursors of the starter unit based on their relatively low incorporation into *7* (Table 5). A remarkably efficient precursor of aplasmomycin, however, is glycerol, which gave specific incorporation values of up to 170%. To check whether glycerol is incorporated via conversion to acetate or to the methyl group of methionine, we determined whether an excess of acetate (four-fold) or methionine (two-fold) fed together with [1,3-^{14}C]glycerol would decrease the incorporation of ^{14}C. This was not the case; in fact an increase in the specific incorporation of glycerol was seen in both cases. Kuhn-Roth oxidation of *7* from [1,3-^{14}C]glycerol gave acetic acid containing 31% of the radioactivity of *7*, most of it in the methyl group. This radioactivity could either be located in the methionine-derived C-methyl groups of *7* or in C-17. If glycerol were a specific precursor of the three-carbon starter unit, C-17 and C-15 should each be rabeled up to 50%. Also in this case, a higher percentage of the label from [2-^{14}C]glycerol, up to 100%, should be located at C-16 and should be recovered as acetic acid upon Kuhn-Roth oxidation. This degradation was carried out and gave 54% recovery of the radioactivity of *7* in the acetic acid. The results favor the possibility that glycerol may be a proximate precursor of the three-carbon starter units of the polyketide chains of aplasmomycin. However, further experiments with stable isotope-labeled glycerol, now underway, are necessary to explore this possibility further. If glycerol is a specific precursor, its conversion to *7* probably does not proceed via lactate or pyruvate, since these are poorly incorporated. It is conceivable that glycerol is converted via dihydroxyacetone phosphate to methylglyoxal (SUMMERS and ROSE, 1977), which then may be converted to a suitable thioester for initiation of the polyketide chain.

The biosynthetic origin of aplasmomycin can be summarized as follows:

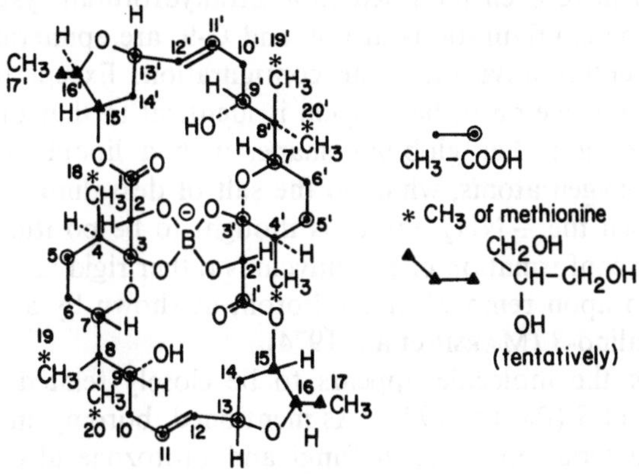

III. Boromycin

A. Background

Isolated from *Streptomyces antibioticus* strain ETH 28 829 (Hütter et al., 1967), boromycin (*8*) was the first defined boron-containing natural product. It has antibiotic activity in vitro against gram-positive organisms and, like aplasmomycin, is active in vivo against *Plasmodium berghei*. The compound was isolated independently from *Streptomyces spec.* MA 4423 at Merck Sharp and Dohme and its use as a coccidiostat has been patented (Miller and Burg, 1975). The structure of boromycin was elucidated by a combination of chemical and crystallographic techniques and follows largely from a single-crystal X-ray analysis of the rubidium salt of the anion (desvalino-boromycin) obtained from *8* by hydrolytic removal of the D-valine moiety with RbOH (Dunitz et al., 1971):

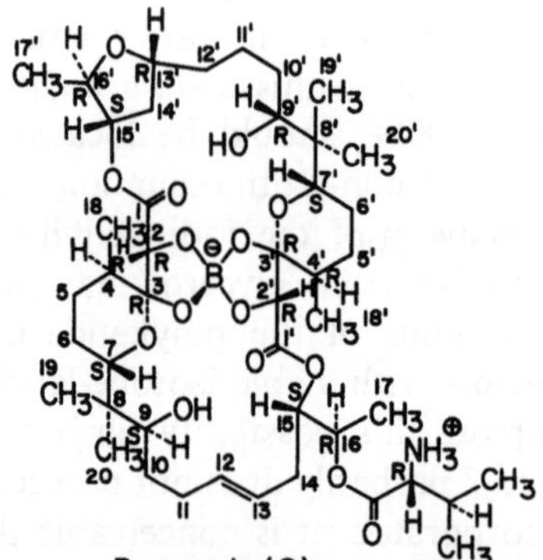

Boromycin (8)

The molecule consists of two almost identical halves which differ only in two aspects. A cis double bond at C-12/C-13 and an esterified hydroxyl at C-16 in one half have been modified to a tetrahydrofuran system in the other half. Secondly, the configurations at C-9 and C-9′ are epimeric while all other pairs of chiral centers have the same configuration. Except for the D-valine moiety the carbon skeleton of boromycin is identical to that of aplasmomycin. The molecule has a rather globular shape, with a lipophilic outside and a cleft lined with oxygen atoms, which in the salt of desvalino-*8* bind the cation. In boromycin itself the $-NH_3^+$ group is thought to be positioned in this cleft. Remarkably, the conformation of boromycin is rather rigid and does not change significantly even upon removal of the boron, as shown by an X-ray structure of desboro-desvalino-*8* (Marsh et al., 1974).

The shape of the molecule appears to be closely related to the mode of antibiotic action of *8* (Pache, 1975). As mentioned, boromycin is active against gram-positive bacteria, and certain fungi and protozoae also, but is inactive against most gram-negative bacteria having a complex cell envelope which seems to impede access (HÜTTER et al., 1967; PACHE, 1975). In *B. subtilis,* the effect of the antibiotic, immediate growth inhibition and cell lysis, is prevented or reversed by lipids, lipoproteins, and by addition of KCl. Boromycin seems to interact with the cytoplasmic membrane, resulting in a breakdown of the potassium barrier. Transport of ions across artificial membranes has been demonstrated for boromycin as well as the desvalino-*8,* although the specificity for potassium was rather low (PACHE and ZÄHNER, 1969).

B. Biosynthetic Work

Biosynthetic studies on boromycin are being pursued in at least two laboratories, that of Prof. PAPE at the University of Münster, Germany, (KIRK and PAPE, paper presented at International Meeting on Medicinal Plant Research, Münster, 1978) and in our own (CHEN et al., unpublished results). Progress has been hampered by three factors: (1) the low yields of the boromycin fermentation (typically 20 mg/l, although PAPE's group has been able to improve upon this yield); (2) the low incorporations obtained with a number of precursors; and (3) the complexity of the ^{13}C-NMR spectrum of *8* (Fig. 4).

The results from the two laboratories are in good agreement and are compatible with a biosynthetic origin of *8* similar to that of aplasmomycin. Using the ETH strain of *S. antibioticus,* KIRK and PAPE fed various ^{14}C-labeled precursors and obtained the following incorporation data: [methyl-^{14}C]methionine, 11% incorporation (dilution 171); D,L-[4-^{14}C]valine, 26.6% incorporation (dilution 243); sodium [1-^{14}C]acetate, 0.4% incorporation (dilution 990); sodium[1-^{14}C]propionate, 0.04% incorporation. Degradation of *8* from [4-^{14}C]valine gave desvalino-*8* containing only 0.3% of the radioactivity, indicating that only the valine moiety was labeled. This renders involvement of an isobutyryl moiety in boromycin biosynthesis unlikely, since this unit would presumably be labeled by [4-^{14}C]valine. A feeding experiment with [methyl-^{13}C]methionine was carried out and the ^{13}C-NMR spectrum of the resulting *8* suggested the incorporation of six methyl groups from methionine.

Parallel and complementary results were obtained in our laboratory. As shown in Table 7, valine and methyl-labeled methionine are very good precursors. The substantially better utilization of D,L-valine compared to the L isomer may suggest that D-valine is the more immediate precursor, but a direct comparison of the D and the L isomer is necessary to be certain of this conclusion. It is interesting to note that desvalino-boromycin binds D amino acids selectively (V. PRELOG, personal communication). The highly efficient utilization of methionine allowed a feeding experiment with [methyl-^{13}C]methionine which gave rather highly ^{13}C-enriched *8*. The spectrum of this sample, shown in Figure 4, clearly displays 6 enriched peaks in the methyl region. However, no assignment of these signals to specific methyl carbons has so far been made. The utilization of most other precursors, including acetate is comparatively low, possibly reflecting the metabolic and nutritional state of the organism. Unlike KIRK and PAPE's experiment with [1-^{14}C]propionate, the specific incorporation of [2-^{14}C]propion-

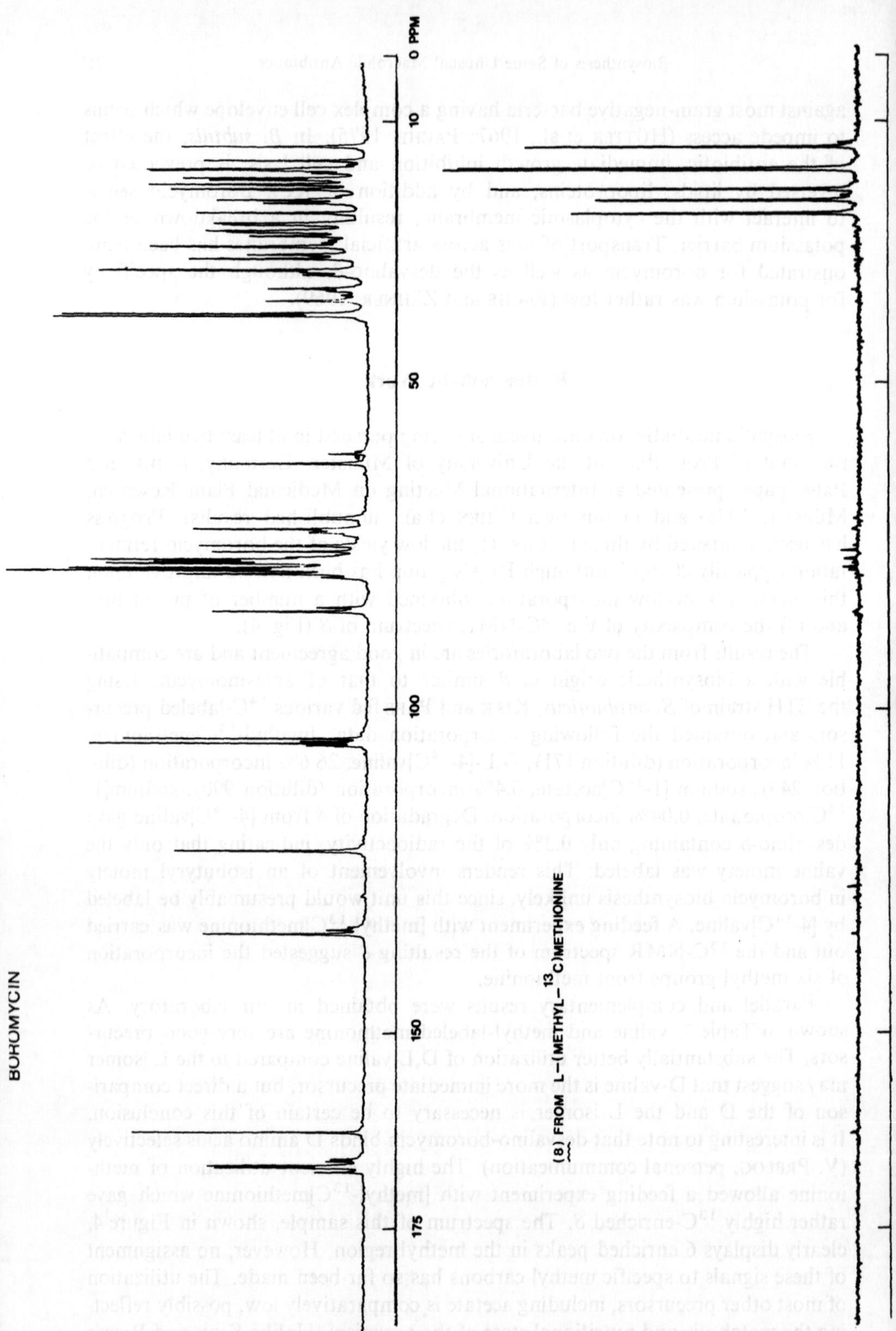

Fig. 4. Proton-noise decoupled ^{13}C-NMR spectra of boromycin. **Top:** natural abundance. **Bottom:** Boromycin derived biosynthetically from L-[methyl-^{13}C]methionine

Table 7. Incorporation of radioactive precursors into boromycin

Precursor fed	Amount added mmole/l	Specific incorporation percent
Sodium[1-^{14}C]acetate	1.64	4
Sodium[2-^{14}C]propionate	2.03	3.5
D,L-[1-^{14}C]valine	1.9	50.8
L-[1-^{14}C]valine	1.36	13.1
Sodium[2-^{14}C]malonate	3.88	14
[methyl-^{14}C]Methionine	4.13	339
[1,3-^{14}C]Glycerol	1.32	2.2

ate is comparable to that of acetate. This again parallels the findings with aplasmomycin. Also unlike the biosynthesis of 7, [1,3-^{14}C]glycerol is not very efficiently utilized, but its specific incorporation is on the same order of magnitude as that of acetate.

Obviously, considerably more work will be necessary to unravel the biosynthetic origin of boromycin, but the results so far indicate that its mode of formation resembles that of aplasmomycin. It will be interesting to examine to what extent the details of the modes of assembly of these two antibiotics are parallel and particularly, how and at what stage the boron is introduced into the carbon skeleton.

Acknowledgments. Work from the author's laboratory was supported by the U.S. Public Health Service through NIH Research Grant AI 11728. This investigation was also supported (in part) by National Institutes of Health Research Grant No. RR 01077 from the Division of Research Resources. We would like to acknowledge the Purdue University Biochemical Magnetic Resonance Laboratory for the 360 MHz proton spectra.

References

Bentley R, Bhate DS, Keil JG (1962) Formation of carlosic and carolic acids in *Penicillium charlesii.* J Biol Chem 237:859–866

Brufani M, Cerrius S, Fedeli W, Mazza F, Muntwyler R (1972) Kristallstrukturanalyse des Chlorothricolid-methylesters. Helv Chim Acta 55:2094–2102

Dunitz JD, Hawley DM, Miklos D, White DNJ, Berlin Yu, Marusic R, Prelog V (1971) Structure of boromycin. Helv Chim Acta 54:1709–1713

Floss HG, Chang C-J, Mascaretti O, Shimada K (1978) Studies on the biosynthesis of antibiotics. Planta Med 34:345–380

Gabriel O (1973) Biological mechanisms involved in the formation of deoxy sugars: Enzymatic hydrogen mediation. A possible example for the evolutionary process of enzyme catalysis. In: Gould R (ed) Carbohydrates in solution, Advances in chemistry series, No 117, pp 387–410. American Chemical Society, Washington DC

Gerhard A, Muntwyler R, Keller-Schierlein W (1975) Über eine unerwartete Umwandlung in der Chlorothricin-Reihe, Helv Chim Acta 58:1323–1338

Holzbach R, Pape H, Hook D, Kreutzer EF, Chang C-J, Floss HG (1978) Biosynthesis of the macrolide antibiotic chlorothricin: Basic building blocks. Biochemistry 17:556–560

Hütter R, Keller-Schierlein W, Knüsel F, Prelog V, Rodgers GC, Suter P, Vogel G, Voser W, Zähner H (1967) Stoffwechselprodukte von Mikroorganismen. 57. Mitteilung. Boromycin. Helv Chim Acta 50:1533–1539

Keller-Schierlein W, Muntwyler R, Pache W, Zähner H (1969a) Chlorothricin und Deschlorothricin. Helv Chim Acta 52:127–142

Keller-Schierlein W, Muntwyler R, Zähner H (1969b) Bromothricin. Experientia 25:786

Lybing S, Reio L (1958) Degradation of ^{14}C-labelled carolic and carlosic acids from *Penicillium charlesii* G. Smith. Acta Chem Scand 12:1575–1584

Marsh W, Dunitz JD, White DNJ (1974) Structure of a boron-free hydrolysis product from boromycin. Helv Chim Acta 57:10–17

Mascaretti O, Chang C-J, Floss HG (1979) Biosynthesis of the antibiotic chlorothricin: Assignment of the carbon-13 magnetic resonance spectrum. J Nat Prod 42:455–460

Miller BM, Burg RW (1975) Boromycin as a coccidiostat. US Patent 3,864,479

Muntwyler R, Keller-Schierlein W (1972) Die Struktur des Chlorothricins, eines neuartigen Makrolid-Antibioticums. Helv Chim Acta 55:2071–2094

Muntwyler R, Widmer J, Keller-Schierlein W (1970) Synthese des 5-Chlor-6-methyl-salicylsäuremethyläthers, eines Abbauproduktes des Chlorothricins. Helv Chim Acta 53:1544–1547

Nakamura H, Titaka Y, Kitahara T, Okazaki T, Okami Y (1977) Structure of aplasmomycin. J Antibiot 30:714–719

Okami Y, Okazoki T, Kitahara T, Umezawa H (1976) Studies of marine microorganisms. V. A new antibiotic, aplasmomycin, produced by a streptomycete isolated from shallow sea mud. J Antibiot 29:1019–1025

Pache W (1975) Boromycin. In: Corcoran JW, Hahn F (eds) Antibiotics. III. Mechanism of action of antimicrobial and antitumor agents, pp 585–587. Springer, Berlin Heidelberg New York

Pache W, Chapman D (1972) Interaction of antibiotics with membranes: Chlorothricin. Biochim Biophys Acta 255:348–357

Pache W, Zähner H (1969) Studies on the mechanism of action of boromycin. Arch Mikrobiol 67:156–165

Sato K, Okazaki T, Maeda K, Okami Y (1978) New antibiotics, aplasmomycins B and C. J Antibiot 31:632–635

Schindler PW (1975) Chlorothricin, an inhibitor of porcine-heart malate dehydrogenases, discriminating between the mitochondrial and cytoplasmic isoenzyme. Eur J Biochem 51:579–585

Schindler PW, Scrutton MC (1975) Mode of action of the macrolide-type antibiotic, chlorothricin. Effect of the antibiotic on the catalytic activity and some structural parameters of pyruvate carboxylases from rat and chicken liver. Eur J Biochem 55:543–553

Schindler PW, Zähner H (1972) Wirkungsweise des Makrolid-Antibioticums, Chlorothricin. I. Hemmer der Pyruvat-Carboxylase aus *Bacillus subtilis*. Arch Mikrobiol 82:66–75

Schindler PW, Zähner H (1973) Mode of action of the macrolide-type antibiotic, chlorothricin. Kinetic study of the inhibition of pyruvate carboxylase from *Bacillus* stearothermophilus. Eur J Biochem 39:591–600

Snipes CE, Chang C-J, Floss HG (1979) The biosynthesis of the antibiotic granaticin. J Am Chem Soc 101:701–706

Summers MC, Rose TA (1977) Proton Transfer Reactions of Methylglyoxal Synthase. J Am Chem Soc 99:4475–4478

Biosynthesis of Isochromanequinone Antibiotics

HEINZ G. FLOSS

I. Structures and Some Properties of Isochromanequinones

A. Introduction

In 1947, a brief note (BROCKMANN and PINI, 1947) reported the isolation from cultures of an actinomycete of a red crystalline pigment, named actinorhodin, which exhibited antibiotic activity against *Staphylococcus aureus*. The compound was subsequently shown to be the first member of a new class of natural products obtained from various streptomycetes, which are termed isochromanequinones (ZEECK et al., 1974) and are characterized by the presence of a benzoisochromane skeleton and a quinone function in one of the aromatic rings:

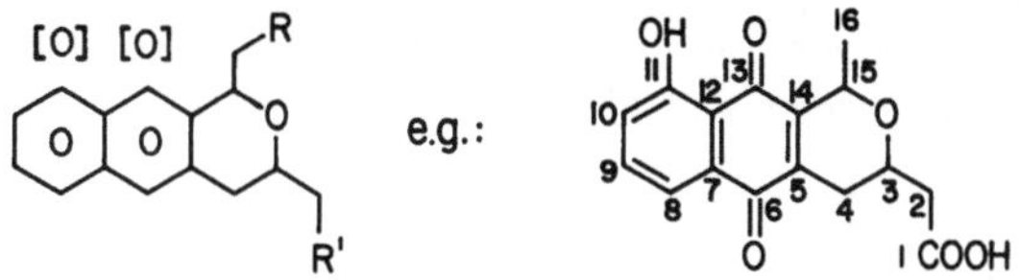

Invariably, the aromatic system carries oxygens in the two positions indicated, in addition to other positions. This substituted benzo-isochromane skeleton represents a biosynthetic unit common to all members of this class, which, as discussed below, is derived from acetate/malonate units via the polyketide pathway. In light of this common origin we use a biosynthetically based numbering system for all these compounds, which differs from numberings used in the literature, but emphasizes the biosynthetic relationships among the compounds in this class.

B. Monomeric Prototypes

The first compound isolated which represents the minimally modified prototype of this class is kalafungin. Obtained from *Streptomyces tanashiensis* (BERGY, 1968) it exhibits antifungal activity and was shown to have structure (*1*) (DUCHAMP, 1968; HOEKSEMA and KRUEGER, 1976). A few years later OMURA's labora-

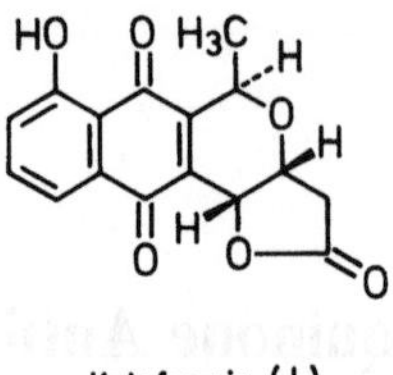

Kalafungin (1)

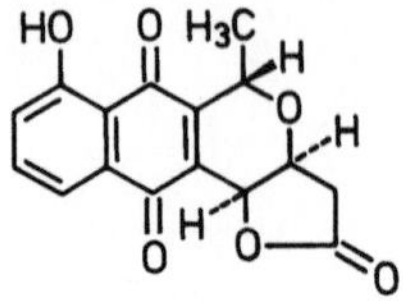

Nanaomycin D (2)

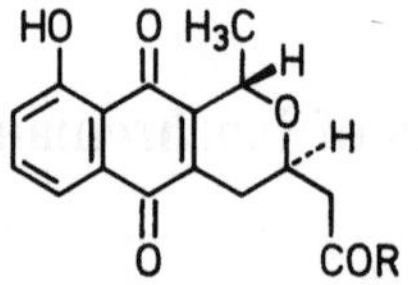

R= OH, Nanaomycin A (3)
R=NH_2, Nanaomycin C (4)

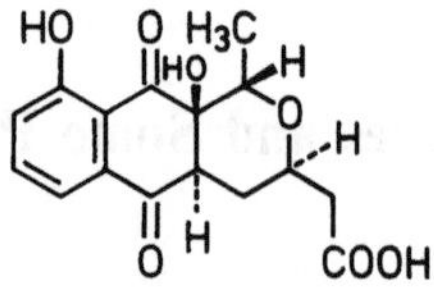

Nanaomycin B (5)

tory reported the isolation of nanaomycins A (*3*) and B (*5*) (Omura et al., 1974, Tanaka et al., 1975a, 1975b) and subsequently also of nanaomycins C (*4*) (Tanaka et al., 1975c) and D (*2*) (Omura et al., 1976) from *Streptomyces rosa* var. *notoensis*. These compounds, particularly *3*, showed activity against many gram-positive bacteria and against mycoplasmas, as well as pronounced antifungal activity (Tanaka et al., 1975a). Nanaomycin B *per se* seems to have little activity, but is slowly converted to *3*. Nanaomycin D is the enantiomer of kalafungin; interconversion of the nanaomycins has shown that they all have the same stereochemistry at C-3 and C-15.

C. Monomers with Modified Carbon Skeleton

In addition to kalafungin and the nanaomycins, which contain the regular octaketide carbon skeleton, a number of compounds are found in nature which represent modified versions of this basic monomeric framework. Frenolicin, a weak antibiotic isolated at the Lederle Laboratories from *Streptomyces fradiae* (Van Meter et al., 1961) was shown to have structure *6* (Ellestad et al., 1968) with an n-propyl side chain instead of the methyl group at C-15. Although *6* has only weak antibiotic activity, it was observed that deoxyfrenolicin (*7*)

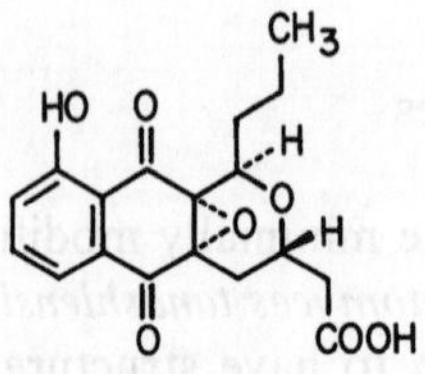

Frenolicin (6)

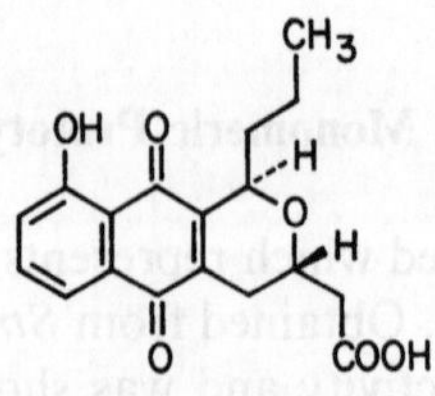

Deoxyfrenolicin (7)

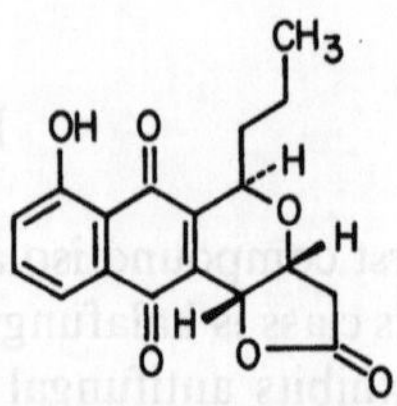

Frenolicin B (8)

derived from it chemically is a potent antifungal agent (ELLESTAD et al., 1968). Recently, OMURA and co-workers showed that deoxyfrenolicin is also a natural product, which is produced together with frenolicin B (*8*) by *Streptomyces roseofulvus* (IWAI et al., 1978). An even more extensive modification of the side chain at C-15 is seen in the griseusins, two closely related compounds isolated from *S. griseus* (TSUJI et al., 1976a, 1976b). The griseusins have antibacterial

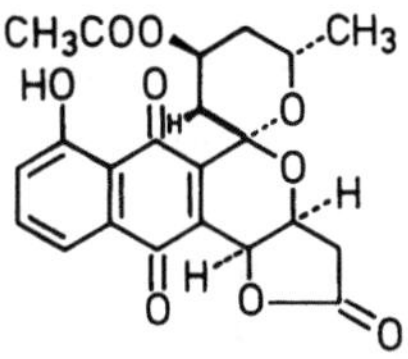

Griseusin A (9)

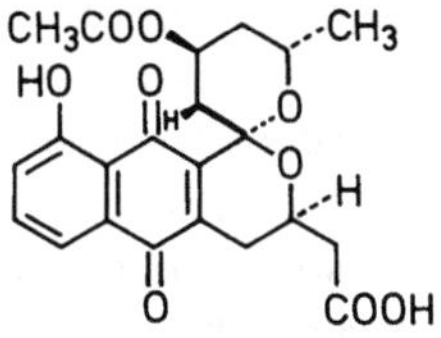

Griseusin B (10)

activity against gram-positive organisms in vitro, but are ineffective in vivo (TSUJI et al., 1976a).

By far the most unique and extensive modification of the basic prototype is seen in the antibiotic granaticin and its relatives. This compound was first isolated from *Streptomyces olivaceus* (CORBAZ et al., 1957), but has also been obtained from various other *Streptomyces species* (BARCZA et al., 1966, CHANG et al., 1975, PYREK et al., 1977). Its structure (*11*) was determined by spectroscop-

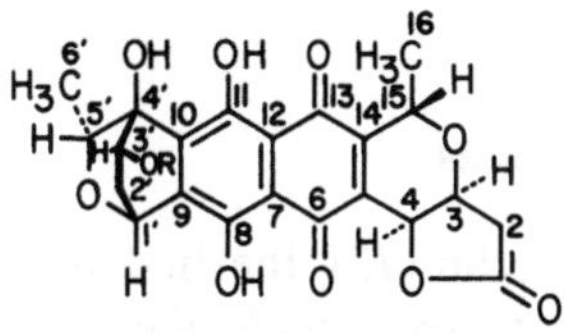

Granaticin (R=H) (11)

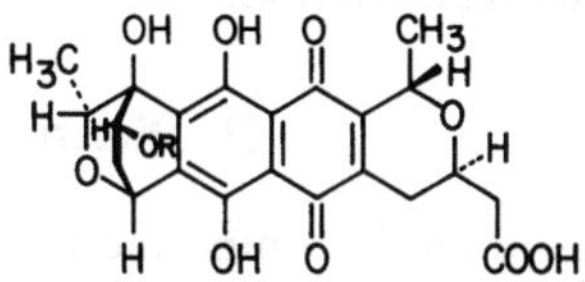

Dihydrogranaticin (R=H) (12)

Granaticin B (R = 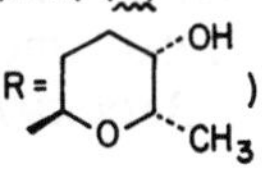)

Dihydrogranaticin B (R = 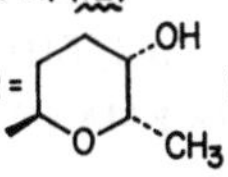)

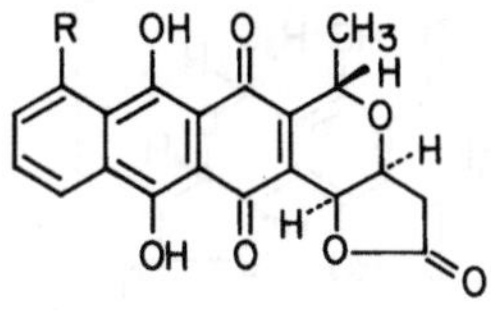

(13) : R = $COCH_3$

(14) : R = $CH(OH)-CH_3$

ic methods (KELLER-SCHIERLEIN et al., 1968) and by a single crystal X-ray analysis of a heavy atom derivative (BRUFANI and DOBLER, 1968). The basic skeleton is modified by the attachment of a six-carbon moiety to the aromatic system in an unusual, rigid [2.2.2] arrangement. Granaticin co-occurs with a glycoside, called granaticin B (BARCZA et al., 1966), the α-L-rhodinoside at the C-3′ hydroxyl group (KELLER-SCHIERLEIN et al., 1968; BRUFANI and DOBLER, 1968) and both compounds are also found in the form of the corresponding ring open dihydro analogs dihydrogranaticin (PYREK et al., 1977) (*12*) and dihydrogranaticin B (SNIPES et al., 1979a). Two unique co-metabolites of granaticin found in *S. thermoviolaceus* were identified as the anthraquinones *13* and *14* (PYREK et al., 1977), which can be thought to have arisen from *11* by opening of the ether bridge between C-1′ and C-5′. Granaticin is active against gram-positive bacteria and protozoa, but not against gram-negative bacteria, mycobacteria, fungi, or yeasts (cf. SNIPES et al., 1979a) and shows modest antitumor activity. Its mode of action in *B. subtilis* involves blocking of the charging of leucyl-tRNA by interference with leucyl-tRNA synthetase, leading to inhibition of protein synthesis and, in stringently controlled strains, but not relaxed mutants, of RNA synthesis (OGILVIE et al., 1975a, b).

The compounds so far mentioned are all metabolites of various streptomycetes. They are structurally, and possibly biogenetically, related to two plant constituents, eleutherin (*15*) and isoeleutherin (*16*), which had been isolated

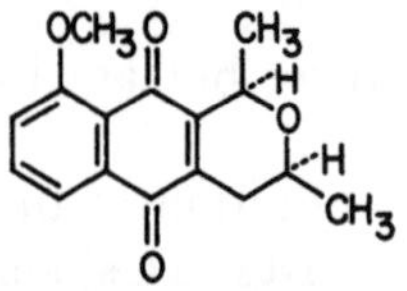

Eleutherin (15)

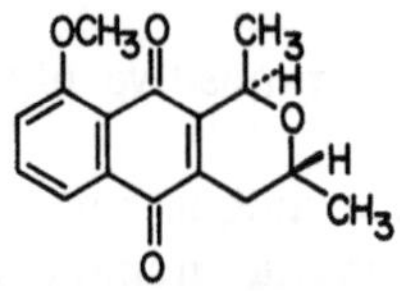

Isoeleutherin (16)

from the tubers of *Eleutherine bulbosa* (SCHMID et al., 1950; SCHMID and EBNÖTHER, 1951a, b). The parent carbon skeleton in this case has apparently undergone a decarboxylation.

D. Dimeric Compounds

The simplest dimeric compound is actinorhodin (*17*), the first isochromanequinone to be isolated. Its isolation from *Streptomyces coelicolor,* its properties and structure elucidation are described in a series of papers from BROCKMANN's laboratory in Göttingen (BROCKMANN et al., 1950; BROCKMANN and LOESCHKE, 1955; BROCKMANN and HIERONYMUS, 1955; BROCKMANN et al., 1966; ZEECK

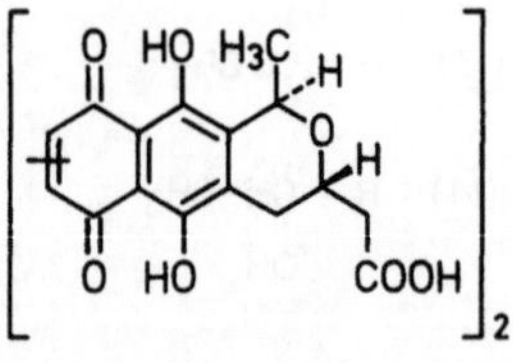

Actinorhodin (17)

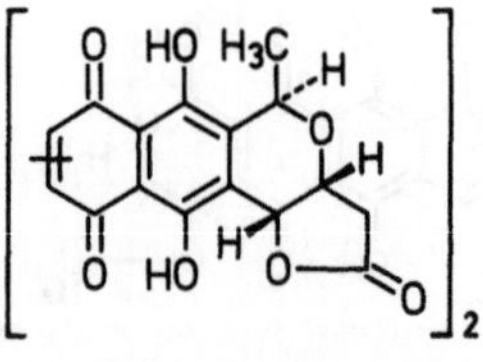

γ-Actinorhodin (18)

and CHRISTIANSEN, 1969). Actinorhodin is present in the mycelium largely as the almost colorless hydroquinone, proto-actinorhodin, which is readily air-oxidized to *17* in alkaline solution (BROCKMANN and LOESCHKE, 1955). In addition the lactone corresponding to *17*, γ-actinorhodin (*18*), has also been isolated (CHRISTIANSEN, Ph.D. dissertation, Göttingen 1970). A slightly more complex dimer, phenocyclinone (*19*), also isolated from *S. coelicolor*, contains an extra three carbon atoms (BROCKMANN and CHRISTIANSEN, 1970). Its absolute stereochemistry is undetermined and the choice between the four possible directions

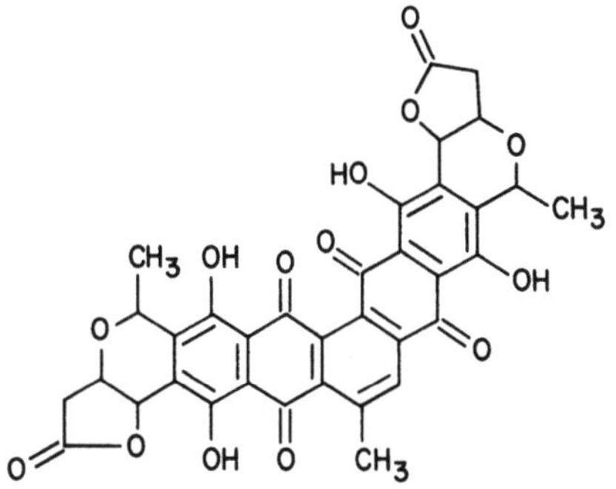

Phenocyclinone (19)

of annellation of the two dihydropyran rings is a tenuous one, based on some less than compelling biosynthetic arguments.

A series of yet more complex dimers are the naphthocyclinones, which were obtained from a strain of *Streptomyces arenae* (ZEECK and MARDIN, 1974; ZEECK et al., 1974). In these compounds the dimerization has led to the modification of one of the benzoisochromane units to an arylketone moiety. The second unit in the case of α-naphthocyclinone (*20*) has only 14 carbon atoms, whereas

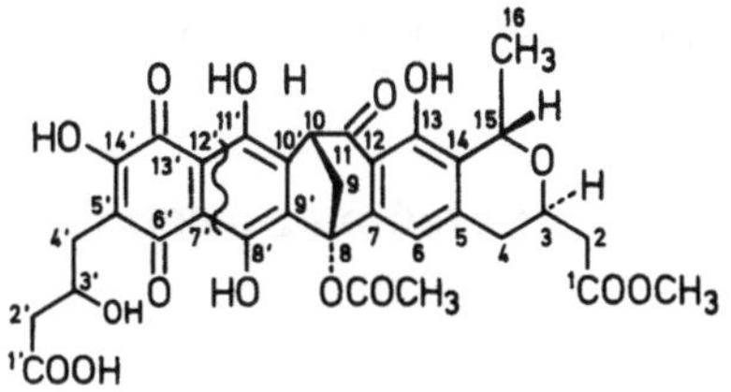

α-Naphthocyclinone (20)

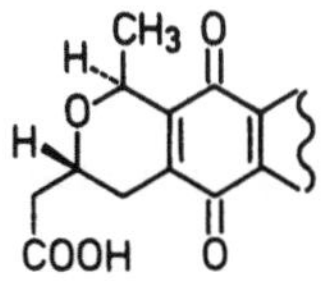

β-Naphthocyclinone (21)

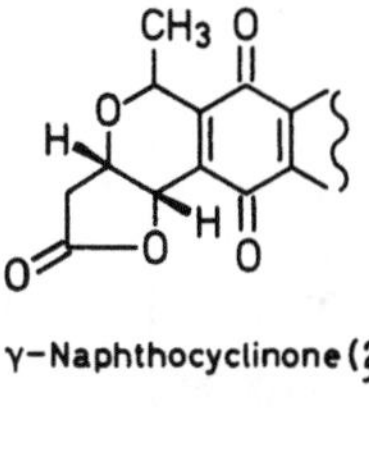

γ-Naphthocyclinone (22)

β- and γ-naphthocyclinone contain as the second unit the open chain and lactone versions, respectively, of the normal benzoisochromane quinone moiety. Interestingly, both *21* and *22* have antibiotic activity, whereas *20* is inactive, leading ZEECK et al. (1974) to suggest that the simple isochromane system represents the minimum structural requirement for antibacterial activity.

Finally, it is worthy of note that the same structural element found in these dimeric streptomycete metabolites, the benzoisochromane quinone system, is also found in a series of dimeric pigments isolated from aphids, the protoaphins and erythroaphins (Cameron et al., 1964; and earlier papers in this series).

E. Stereochemistry of Isochromanequinones

The relative stereochemistry of the compounds obtained from streptomycetes is invariably such that the hydrogens at C-3 and C-15 are trans. In compounds containing the five-membered lactone ring, the latter is, of necessity, always cis-fused. The absolute configurations of several compounds were established by degradation to chiral compounds of known configuration (eleutherin: Schmid and Ebnöther, 1951b; actinorhodin: Zeeck and Christiansen, 1969) or X-ray crystallography (granaticin: Brufani and Dobler, 1968) and further correlations were established by ORD/CD comparisons (Zeeck et al., 1974; Hoeksema and Krueger, 1976). As it turns out, streptomycetes produce compounds of both enantiomeric series, i.e., those with 15R configuration (A-series, actinorhodin, γ-actinorhodin, kalafungin, the frenolicins) and those with 15S configuration (G-series, granaticin, the nanaomycins, and the naphthocyclinones). Based on their configuration at C-3 the griseusins also belong to the G-series. It appears that not only can streptomycetes produce enantiomeric compounds, but that compounds belonging to opposite stereochemical series can even be produced by the same species. It is believed (Rudd, 1978) that the actinorhodin producing *S. coelicolor* is misclassified and in reality belongs to the species *S. violaceoruber*, which is known (Barcza et al., 1966) to produce also granaticin.

II. Biosynthetic Hypotheses Based on Structural and Chemical Arguments

Inspection of all the structures produced by streptomycetes strongly suggests that the basic 16-carbon skeleton of the isochromanequinones is built up entirely from acetate/malonate units via the polyketide pathway:

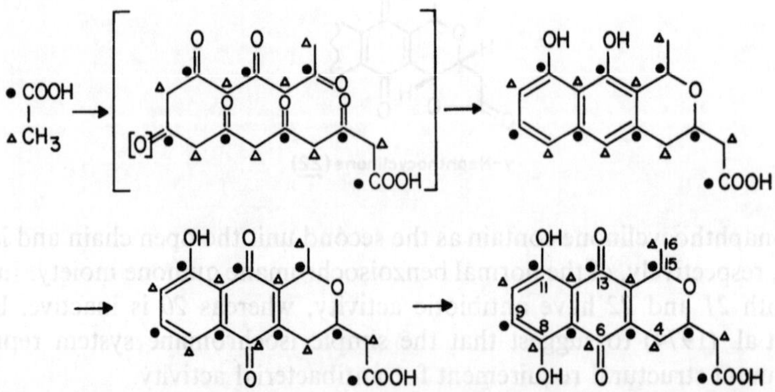

As discussed below, the correctness of this assumption is born out by experiment in all cases examined. The starter unit of the polyketide chain would be a molecule of acetyl-coenzyme A which gives rise to C-16 and C-15; chain extension would occur through stepwise addition of units of malonyl-coenzyme A with simultaneous decarboxylation. As discussed below, a possible alternative is that malonyl-Co A serves both as a starter and chain extension unit. The frenolicins and the griseusins represent variants in which the polyketide chain is elongated by one or two units, respectively, at the starter end. This mode of formation also suggests that the oxygens at C-11 and C-13 should be present early on in the biosynthesis, whereas oxygens at C-4, C-6, or C-8 must be introduced at later stages. None of the streptomycete metabolites, nor for that matter the eleutherins, carry an oxygen function at C-9, a carbon derived from the carboxyl group of acetate. Hence the oxygen at this position must have been eliminated, presumably at the prearomatic stage by reduction of the carbonyl group to a secondary alcohol. From synthetic model experiments (HARRIS and HARRIS, 1977), it seems quite possible that reduction of C-9 to an sp^3 carbon is important for the proper folding of the polyketide chain to favor cyclization to the benzoisochromane ring system.

The dimeric compounds are presumably formed by generation of the monomers followed by some oxidative coupling process. One can also formulate a biosynthesis for phenocyclinone involving condensation of two polyketide chains, one an octaketide and the other a C_{19} nonaketide containing one propionate instead of an acetate unit (BROCKMANN and CHRISTIANSEN, 1970). However, in view of the co-occurrence of *19* with actinorhodin, the formation of a dimer from 2 C_{16} units and insertion of a three-carbon moiety seems much more plausible.

The consistent co-occurrence of the 5-membered lactone ring structures (e.g., nanaomycin D) with the corresponding open-chain dihydro acids (e.g., nanaomycin A) suggests a close biogenetic relationship. As discussed below, some experimental evidence on this point has been obtained in the case of granaticin. It is important to note in this connection that the dihydro acids containing a quinone function adjacent to the dihydropyran ring (e.g., *3, 7, 10, 12*) readily cyclize to the corresponding lactones (e.g., *2, 8, 9, 11*) upon exposure to air (OMURA et al., 1976; TSUJI et al., 1976b; PYREK et al., 1977; IWAI et al., 1978). The reaction is slow, but occurs under very mild conditions, e.g., standing at room temperature in methanol or pyridine, and is completely stereospecific. A plausible mechanism is as follows:

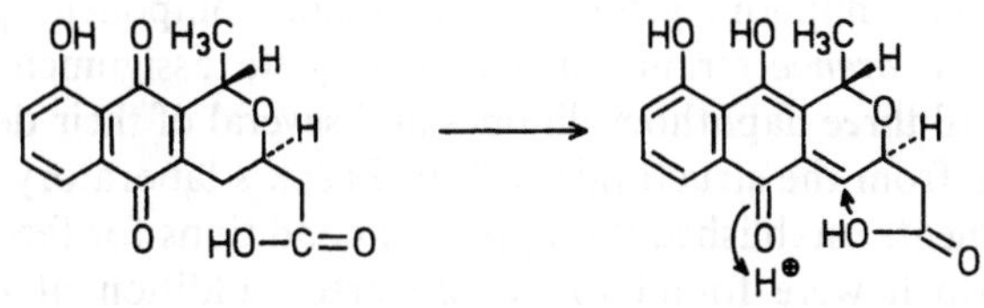

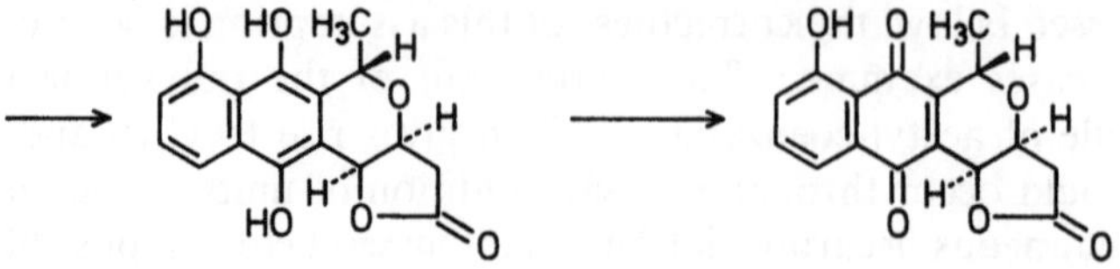

The reverse reaction, reductive opening of the lactone ring by benzylic cleavage, e.g., conversion of *11* to *12,* can be conveniently achieved by catalytic hydrogenation over platinum (PYREK et al., 1977).

III. Experimental Investigations of Isochromanequinone Biosynthesis

A. Nanaomycin

The first tracer study on isochromanequinone biosynthesis was published by OMURA's group (TANAKA et al., 1975b). It was carried out in connection with the structure elucidation of the nanaomycins and it allowed a distinction to be made between two alternative positions of the phenolic hydroxyl group, either at C-8 or at C-11. The study involved feeding sodium[1-^{13}C]acetate to 24-h-old cultures of *S. rosa* var. *notoensis* and isolation of nanaomycin A 3 days later. Analysis of the proton noise decoupled ^{13}C-NMR spectrum of this sample showed the presence of eight enhanced signals, which were assigned to carbons 1, 3, 5, 7, 9, 11, 13, and 15. The assignment of the ^{13}C-NMR spectrum of nanaomycin A is based on off-resonance decoupling, comparison with the spectra of nanaomycin B and related compounds and, to a certain extent, on the assumption that *3* is biosynthesized by the polyketide pathway. The labeling pattern is in accord with and supports this assumption, indicating that *3* is derived from acetate in the following manner:

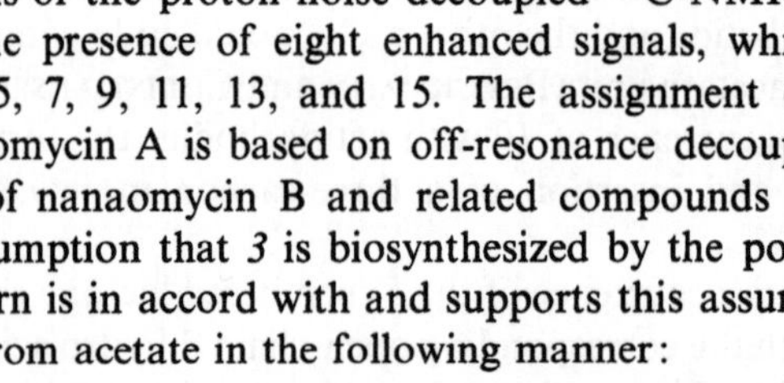

(3)

B. Naphthocyclinones

Similar experiments on the biosynthesis of the naphthocyclinones were carried out in our laboratory (SCHRÖDER and FLOSS, 1978). We used similar methodology and focused on α-naphthocyclinone, the major component produced by shake cultures of *S. arenae* strain Tü 495. Complete assignments of the ^{13}C-NMR spectra of all three naphthocyclinones and several of their derivatives were already available from the structural work in ZEECK's laboratory. A series of preliminary experiments established the optimum conditions for feeding ^{13}C-labeled precursors, which were found to be precursor addition at 48 h and harvest 24 h later. Sodium [1-^{13}C]acetate and [2-^{13}C]acetate were used as precursors; the α-naphthocyclinone was combined with a small amount of the corresponding diacid which was also formed and the mixture was converted to the 14′-methyl-α-naphthocyclinone methyl ester for ^{13}C-NMR analysis. The results, as summarized in Table 1, indicate that *20* is labeled from acetate in the following manner:

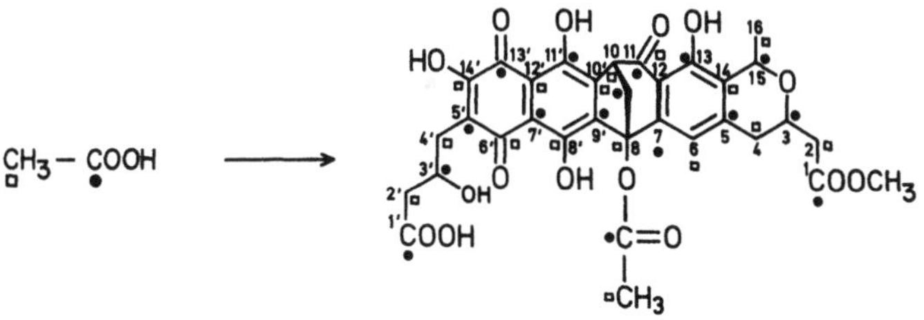

(20)

The compound shows the labeling of alternate carbons from C-1 and C-2 of acetate predicted for a polyketide-derived product. In addition, the acetoxy group, which should also originate from acetyl-coenzyme A, shows indeed the same degree of labeling as the carbon framework of the molecule. The fact that two carbons derived from C-2 of acetate, C-10 and C-10′ are directly connected by a carbon-carbon bond supports the notion that *20* is formed by linkage of two monomeric units. A possible mechanism for the dimerization of two monomers to give the naphthocyclinone system has been proposed by ZEECK et al. (1974). Arguing that unsymmetrical quinone dimers are less common than symmetrical ones they suggest that the condensation of two monomeric units occurs at an early stage and leads to a symmetrical, non-quinoid dimer which is then modified differently in the two halves of the molecule. If this leads to an intermediate *23*, reduction of one of the quinone moieties followed by phenol/carbonyl addition could give rise to the arylketone structure of the naphthocyclinones:

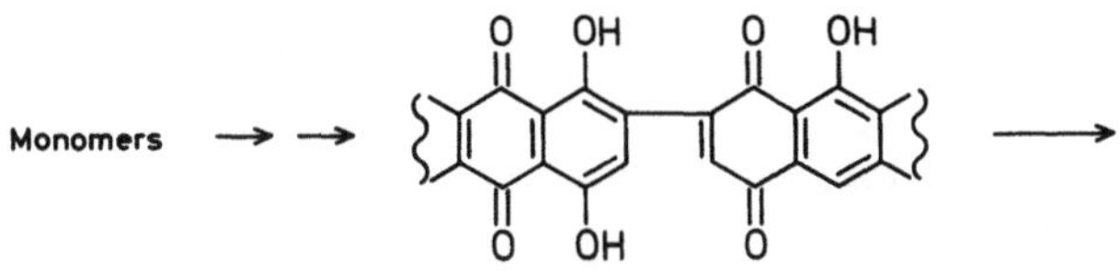

(23)

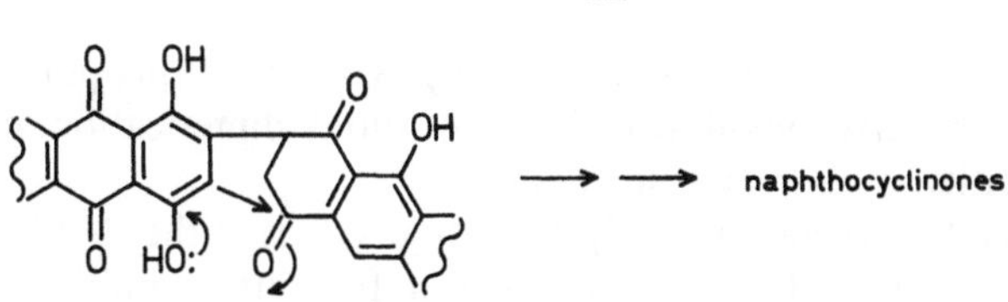

Table 1. ^{13}C Distribution in the α-naphthocyclinone ring system biosynthesized from [^{13}C]acetate and [^{13}C]malonate

Carbon atom number	14′-Methyl-α-naphthocyclinone methyl ester			11′, 14′-Dimethyl-α-naphthocyclinone methyl ester	
	Chemical shift, ppm	^{13}C Abundance[a] from		Chemical shift, ppm	^{13}C Abundance[a] from diethyl [2-^{13}C]malonate
		[1-^{13}C]Acetate	[2-^{13}C]Acetate		
1	171.1	4.2	1.2	171.1	0.9
2	40.6	1.2	2.6	40.5	2.6
3	63.2	3.5	1.3	63.2	1.2
4	34.5	1.0	2.6	34.5	2.6
5	142.1	4.1	1.2	142.3	1.1
6	113.1	1.2	3.3	113.0	3.1
7	140.2	4.1	1.2	140.6	1.5
8	84.8	1.1	2.8	84.7	2.9
9	49.5	4.0	1.1	49.5	1.1
10	51.0	1.2	2.4	51.9	2.5
11	198.6	3.7	1.0	199.5	1.2
12	107.9	1.0	2.5	108.0	3.0
13	159.6	4.0	1.1	159.5	1.1
14	128.8	1.0	2.3	128.6	3.0
15	67.9	3.9	1.1	67.9	1.1
16	18.6	1.1	2.6	18.6	2.8
1′	172.5	4.4	1.2	172.5	1.0
2′	40.9	1.0	3.0	40.8	2.6
3′	66.9	4.2	1.3	66.9	1.1
4′	30.0	1.2	2.6	29.6	3.1
5′	131.8	4.4	1.2		
6′	188.7	1.2	2.8	190.9	2.8
7′	111.9	3.5	1.2		
8′	152.3	1.2	2.8	153.0	3.0
9′	146.1	4.3	1.2		
10′	134.8	1.0	2.6	122.6[b]	2.6
11′	154.6	4.3	1.1	151.0	1.2
12′	112.3	1.2	2.8		
13′	183.5	4.0	1.1	178.9	1.3
14′	158.9	1.2	2.6	159.9	2.5
Acetyl CO	169.5	4.3	1.0	169.3	1.1
Acetyl CH_3	21.1	1.1	2.3	21.1	1.3
Ester OCH_3	51.6	1.2	1.2	51.6	1.3
11′ OCH_3	–	–	–	62.2	1.1
14′ OCH_3	61.8[c]	1.1	1.1	61.3[c]	1.1

[a] Natural abundance = 1.1; values are subject to an error of approximately ±15%
[b] Tentative assignment
[c] Reference signal used for normalization of peak heights

The labeling data are in accord with this proposal, but at this point one cannot rule out the alternative possibility that the initial dimerization involves two differently modified monomeric precursors.

α-Naphthocyclinone contains only *14* carbon atoms in the 'left hand' portion of the molecule and might thus have arisen from two different monomers, one a normal C_{16} unit and one a polyketide of only 14 carbon atoms. The co-occurrence of *20* with β- and γ-naphthocyclinone, on the other hand, suggests that all three are derived by dimerization of two C_{16} units, followed in the case of *20* by loss of two carbon atoms. The two carbons lost would have to be the starter unit of the polyketide chain of that monomer; the ring system of *20* derived in this manner should thus contain only one starter unit, making up carbons 14 and 16, derived directly from acetyl-Co A, in addition to 14 chain extension units derived directly from malonyl-Co A. On the other hand, if the 'left hand' portion of *20* is derived from a C_{14} polyketide then either C-6′ and C-7′ or C-14′ and C-13′ must represent another starter unit which is derived from acetyl-Co A directly rather than via malonyl-Co A. We attempted to distinguish between these two possibilities by feeding [2-^{13}C]malonate, for permeability reasons as its diethyl ester, which we hoped would label preferentially the malonyl-Co A-derived chain extension units. The acetyl-Co A-derived acetoxy group of *20* would serve as an internal reference to indicate the degree of labeling of the acetyl-Co A pool. The ^{13}C-labeled product was in this case converted (by accident) into the 11′,14′-α-naphthocyclinone methyl ester for ^{13}C-NMR analysis, for which only a partial assignment of the ^{13}C-NMR spectrum could be made. The results, as listed in Table 1, nevertheless clearly indicate that *all* the [2-^{13}C]acetate-derived carbons of the ring system are also labeled by [2-^{13}C]malonate, but that the acetoxy group shows no significant enrichment. This rather unexpected finding does not enable us to decide the original question posed and may be interpreted in at least two ways. One possibility would be that at the time of the assembly of the polyketide the acetyl-Co A and malonyl-Co A pools are in complete equilibrium, leading to equal labeling of the starter and the chain extension units and that the acetoxy group is attached at a later time when the added labeled precursor has been depleted. The obvious counter argument, of course, is that acetate, which should be metabolized at least as rapidly as malonate, labels both the ring system and the acetoxy group. The second possibility would be that malonyl-Co A serves not only for chain extension, but also as a starter, leading to a symmetrical C_{17}-polyketide which is subsequently decarboxylated:

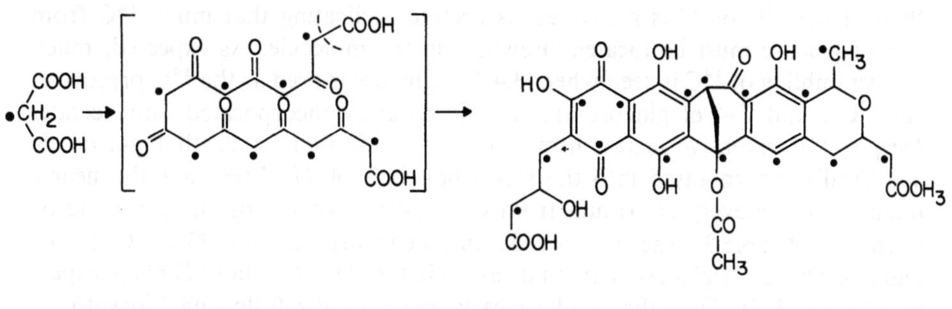

This interpretation is obviously rather unprecedented and further experiments are necessary for its evaluation.

C. Granaticin

KELLER-SCHIERLEIN et al. (1968) had suggested that granaticin is derived from a C_{16} polyketide by attachment of a 6-carbon unit which might either also be derived from acetate or might originate from a hexose. The questions whether *11* is derived entirely from acetate or has a mixed acetate/carbohydrate origin was investigated in two laboratories using the ^{13}C methodology (SNIPES et al., 1979a; ARNONE et al., 1979). For the fermentation, the European group (ARNONE et al., 1979) used *S. olivaceus*, whereas we (SNIPES et al., 1979a) employed shake cultures of *S. violaceoruber* Tü 22, to which precursors were added at 24 h followed by harvesting 24 h later. Both groups independently made complete assignments of the ^{13}C spectra using chemical shift theory, off-resonance and single-frequency decoupling and comparison of a series of analogs and derivatives. Since granaticin and its tetra acetate gave unsatisfactory spectra, the ^{13}C-NMR analysis was carried out on dihydrogranaticin methyl ester prepared from *11* by the method of PYREK et al. (1977). In our assignments (SNIPES et al., 1979b) the critical distinctions of pairs of carbons in the naphthazarin moiety, i.e., C-5/C-14, C-6/C-13, C-7/C-12, C-8/C-11, and C-9/C-10 were largely made on the basis of long-range coupling analysis and spectral comparison of dihydrogranaticin methyl ester with its 3′-keto and 11-*O*-methyl derivatives. The assignments are summarized in Table 2, which also lists the enrichment data for the labeled granaticin biosynthesized from [1-^{13}C]- and [2-^{13}C]acetate (analyzed as dihydrogranaticin methyl ester). It is evident that only carbons 1–16, but not C-1′–C-6′, are labeled by acetate and that they show the alternating labeling pattern characteristic of the polyketide pathway. Results paralleling ours with [1-^{13}C]acetate were obtained by the European group. Both studies thus agree in indicating a mixed biosynthesis of granaticin.

The origin of the remaining 6-carbon unit was further studied in our laboratory (SNIPES et al., 1979a). As indicated in Table 3, feeding of glucose labeled with ^{14}C and tritium in various positions gave results which were complicated by extensive metabolic conversion of glucose to acetate. This is evident, for example, from the comparison of the $^{3}H/^{14}C$ ratios of glucose, granaticin and the acetic acid obtained by Kuhn-Roth oxidation of *11* (representing C-15+C-16 and C-5′ C-6′) in experiments 1 and 2. A much higher percentage of the tritium than of the ^{14}C of *11* is recovered as acetate, indicating that much ^{14}C from C-6 of glucose must be located elsewhere in the molecule. As expected, much less scrambling of ^{14}C is seen when [3,4-^{14}C]glucose is used as the ^{14}C precursor, since C-3 and C-4 of glucose are not significantly incorporated into acetate. Despite this extensive metabolism, there are clear indications that glucose is specifically incorporated into the six-carbon unit of *11*. These are the nearly quantitative recovery of tritium from C-4 and C-6 of glucose in C-6′ (and/or C-16) of *11* (Table 3, experiments 1–3), and the incorporation of [3,4-^{14}C, 1-^{3}H]- and [3,4-^{14}C, 2-^{3}H]glucose without decrease in the $^{3}H/^{14}C$ ratios (Table 3, experiments 4 and 5). Thus the results clearly point to the following biosynthetic origin of granaticin:

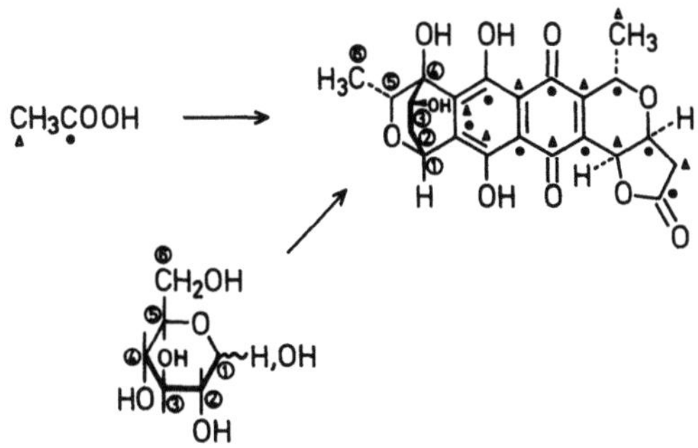

Table 2. ^{13}C-Distribution in granaticin biosynthesized from [^{13}C] acetate

Carbon atoms	Chemical shift δ, ppm	Atom % ^{13}C present in dihydrogranaticin methyl ester obtained from sodium	
		[1-^{13}C]Acetate	[2-^{13}C]Acetate
6	174.9	1.1[a]	2.4
13	174.8	2.2[a]	1.1
1	170.8	2.8	1.0
11	168.5	2.7	1.0
8	162.5	0.8	4.3
14	144.7	0.9	4.2
9	142.0	2.9	1.0
5	140.3	3.2	1.0
10	136.1	1.1	3.5
12	110.3	1.1[a]	2.2
7	110.1	2.0[a]	1.1
4′	80.4	1.1	1.0
5′	72.6	1.2	1.2
3′	70.7	1.3	1.0
15	67.4	3.5	1.1
3	63.1	3.5	1.1
1′	61.8	1.3	1.1
O-Me	51.8	1.1[b]	1.1[b]
2	40.3	1.1	4.6
2′	35.7	1.1	1.1
4	27.6	1.1	4.8
16	19.1	1.1	4.8
6′	16.4	1.2	1.1

[a] The signals for C-6+C-13 and C-7+C-12 were poorly resolved in this spectrum; C-13 and C-7 clearly were enriched. The ^{13}C abundance in C-13 and C-7 is calculated assuming that C-6 and C-12 are unlabeled

[b] The O-methyl carbon was chosen as reference signal; all other signal intensities are given as percentage abundance relative to $O\text{-}CH_3 = 1.10\%$ natural abundance. Signal intensities were determined by integration of the area under each peak using the step height of the integration curves recorded on scale-expanded spectra

Table 3. Incorporation of ^{14}C- and tritium-labeled glucoses into granaticin

Experiment number	Positions of label in glucose fed	$^3H/^{14}C$ of precursor	Incorporation rate into granaticin [%]		Isotope ratio of granaticin $^3H/^{14}C$	Acetate from Kuhn-Roth oxidation of granaticin		Percentage of radioactivity of granaticin isolated as acetate	
			^3H	^{14}C		Yield [%]	$^3H/^{14}C$	^3H	^{14}C
1	[6-^{14}C, 6-^3H]	3.43	0.15	0.76	0.62	70	2.57	82	24
2	[6-^{14}C, 4-^3H]	5.96	0.16	0.76	1.19	96	3.29	90	33
3	[3,4-^{14}C, 4-^3H]	7.3	0.14	0.33	3.09	86		89	4.6
4	[3,4-^{14}C, 1-^3H]	2.33	0.46	0.45	2.39	88		7.7	2.7
5	[3,4-^{14}C, 2-^3H]	12.6	4.06	0.73	15.8	90		3.8	3.2
6	[3,4-^{14}C, 3-^3H]	7.81	0.01	0.12	0.76	66		2.6	3.0
7	[3,4-^{14}C, 5-^3H]	3.52	0.01	0.14	0.29				

The demonstration that glucose is the precursor of the extra 6-carbon unit leads to the realization that this moiety is a 2,6-dideoxyhexose attached to the aromatic system twice, through its C-1 and C-4. In the conversion of glucose to this dideoxyhexose the hydroxyl groups at C-2 and C-6 must be replaced by hydrogen. The data in Table 3 indicate that in the overall process the hydrogens at C-3 and C-5 of glucose are lost, whereas those at C-1, C-2, C-4, and C-6 are retained. Furthermore, tritium, from both C-4 and C-6 of glucose is located at C-6′ of granaticin. These results, exchange of H-5 and migration of H-4 to C-6 (mediated by an enzyme-bound pyridine-nucleotide), are characteristic of the dTDP-glucose oxidoreductase reaction (GABRIEL, 1973) and implicate this reaction as the first specific step in the conversion of the glucose into the 2,6-dideoxyhexose moiety. To obtain further evidence on the involvement of this reaction, we decided to investigate the steric course of the replacement of the hydroxyl group at C-6 of glucose by H-4 and to compare it to that determined for the *in vitro* reaction catalyzed by dTDP-glucose oxidoreductase isolated from *E. coli*. For the earlier work on the *E. coli* enzyme we (SNIPES et al., 1977) had synthesized (6R)- and (6S)-[4-^2H, 6-^3H]glucose-6-phosphate containing deuterium in every tritiated molecule. Samples of these two compounds were hydrolyzed with alkaline phosphatase and the resulting glucose samples were fed to cultures of *S. violaceoruber*. The labeled granaticin samples obtained were subjected to Kuhn-Roth oxidation to give acetic acid from C-5′ and C-6′ (and achiral acetic acid from C-15 and C-16), which was analyzed for the chirality of the methyl group by the method of CORNFORTH et al. (1970) and LÜTHY et al. (1969). In this analysis procedure, which involves sequentially conversion of the acetate into acetyl-Co A and malate followed by equilibration with fumarase, a chirally pure acetate of R configuration will show 79% tritium retention in the fumarase reaction whereas the pure S isomer will show 21% tritium retention (cf. FLOSS and TSAI, 1979). The results from these experiments, 37% tritium retention in the sample from 6R glucose and 78% tritium retention in the material from 6S glucose (SNIPES et al., 1979a) parallel completely those obtained with the isolated *E. coli* enzyme (SNIPES et al., 1977) and indicate the following steric course for the reaction:

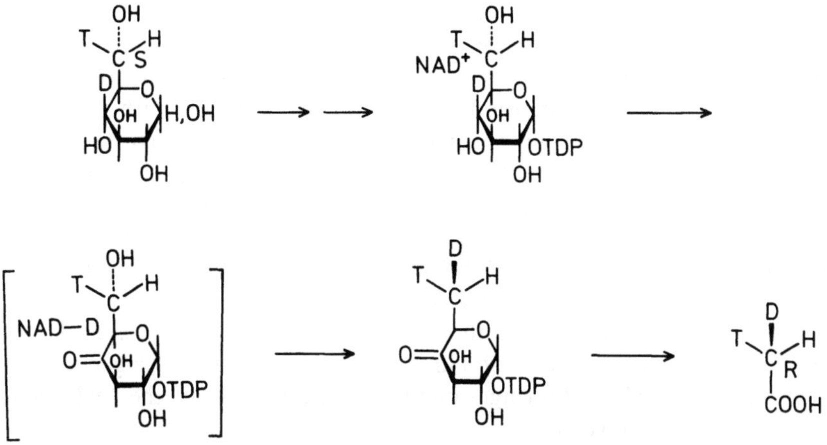

In addition to showing that the reaction is stereospecific, involving replacement of OH by H in an inversion mode, they also indicate that the transfer of H from C-4 to C-6 must be intramolecular. This follows since the glucose samples during the biosynthetic process were heavily diluted (>100 fold) by endogenous, non-labeled glucose; intermolecular crossover of H-4 would thus have produced predominantly tritiated methyl groups not containing deuterium, which would be achiral. Since the transfer is intramolecular, it is most probably suprafacial, which in turn defines the conformation around the C-5/C-6 bond of the substrate in the enzyme active site: OH and H-5 must be *syn* oriented. Consequently, the reaction is unlikely to involve a concerted elimination of water between C-5 and C-6; rather, such a process, if it occurs, should be stepwise. All these results and interpretations taken together lead to a very compelling model for the active site of dTDP-glucose oxidoreductase:

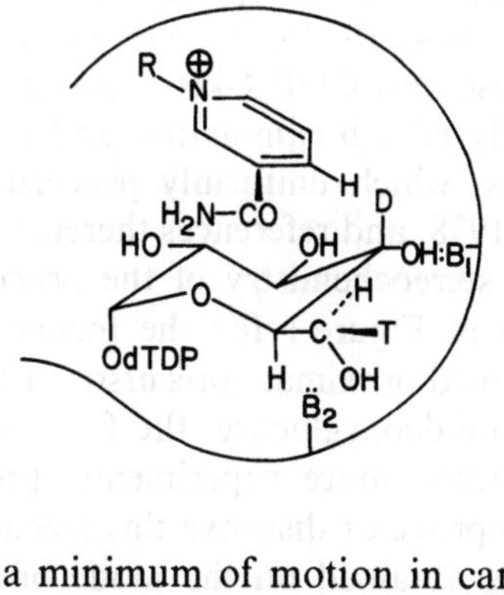

This model allows for a minimum of motion in carrying out the individual steps of this reaction: 1. transfer of H-4 to NAD^+ and OH proton to B_1, 2. enolization between C-4 and C-5, H-5 to B_2, 3. elimination of OH from C-6 to give 4-keto-5,6-ene derivative, 4. transfer of H-4 from NADH to give 4,5-enol (or steps 3. + 4. concerted without a 4-keto-5,6-ene intermediate), and 5. tautomerization to give 4-keto-6-deoxy derivative.

Formation of the 2-deoxy function appears to proceed with loss of H-3 but retention of the original hydrogen from C-2 of glucose. This enabled us to examine the stereochemistry of this process. [2-^{2}H]-Glucose (68 atom % D) was prepared by equilibration of fructose-6-phosphate with D_2O in the presence of glucose-6-phosphate isomerase, followed by cleavage with alkaline phosphatase and chromatographic separation of the resulting glucose and fructose. This glucose was incorporated into granaticin, which was analyzed by proton NMR for the location of the deuterium. Comparison of the coupling pattern for H-3′ with that of unlabeled granaticin and with simulated spectra for the species deuterated in the *pro*-2′R and the *pro*-2′S position indicated that the deuterium was located in the *pro*-2′S position. Hence, replacement of the hydroxyl group at C-2 of glucose by an external hydrogen occurs in a retention mode. The following summarizes the fate of all the hydrogens of glucose during the conversion to *11*:

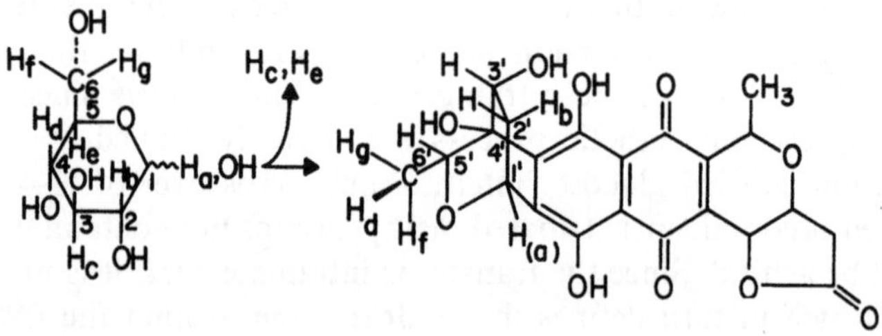

The mechanistic interpretation of this last finding is not as clear-cut as in the case of the formation of the 6-deoxy function. Little is known about the mechanism of generating the 2-deoxy function; however, the analogous formation of a 3-deoxyhexose function in bacteria has been shown to require an adjacent keto function and to involve pyridoxamine phosphate as a cofactor (RUBENSTEIN and STROMINGER, 1974a, b). Mechanistically, this conversion of CDP-4-keto-6-deoxyglucose into CDP-4-keto-3,6-dideoxyglucose resembles the pyridoxal phosphate-catalyzed α,β-elimination and β-replacement reactions of β-substituted amino acids, which uniformly proceed in a retention mode at the β carbon (TSAI et al., 1978, and references therein). The loss of the hydrogen at C-3 and the observed stereochemistry of the process would agree with the reaction sequence shown in Figure 1 for the formation of dTDP-4-keto-2,6-dideoxyglucose, the presumed proximate precursor of the dideoxyhexose moiety of *11*, from dTDP-4-keto-6-deoxyglucose, the first pathway-specific precursor in the biosynthesis. However, more experiments, probably at the enzymatic level, will be necessary to prove or disprove this mechanism.

Some information was obtained on the mode of formation of the lactone ring. PYREK et al. (1977) had noted that the appearance of dihydrogranaticin in the fermentation preceded that of *11*. In following up this observation we found (SNIPES et al., 1979a) that a cell-free extract of *S. violaceoruber* catalyzed the conversion of *12* to *11* at rates significantly above the background of non-enzymatic conversion in boiled controls. The same system also catalyzed the

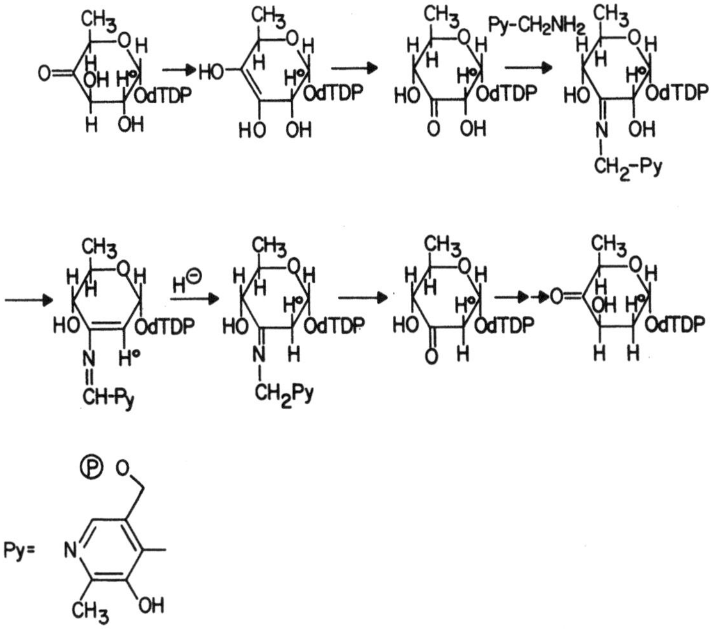

Fig. 1. Proposed mechanism for the conversion of dTDP-4-keto-6-deoxyglucose into dTDP-4-keto-2,6-dideoxyglucose

conversion of dihydrogranaticin B to granaticin B. Incubation under argon instead of air followed by aerobic workup resulted in greatly reduced formation of *11* from *12* and noticeable bleaching of the solutions, indicating a requirement for oxygen and the probable presence of quinone reductases. To check whether the enzymatic process proceeds by a direct cyclization mechanism, as discussed earlier for the non-enzymatic cyclization, or by hydroxylation followed by ring closure with loss of water, we carried out an incubation under an $^{18}O_2$ atmosphere. Mass spectral analysis of the resulting *11* indicated that no ^{18}O had been incorporated in the process. This favors a direct cyclization mechanism analogous to the non-enzymatic process. The above results suggest that oxidative cyclization to give the five-membered lactone ring is a late, possibly the last step in the biosynthesis of *11*.

One can at the moment only speculate on the mode of attachment of the carbohydrate moiety to the aromatic system. One possibility is that it may involve C-glycoside formation with an aromatic moiety at the oxidation state of the quinone-hydroquinone, followed by an aldol-type condensation between C-10 and the keto group in the boat form of the sugar. Regiospecificity of the annelation of the sugar must in this case be a consequence of recognition of the substitution pattern of the aromatic system by the enzyme. Alternatively, the regiospecificity may be due to condensation between C-4 of the sugar and C-10 of an aromatic precursor not yet oxidized at C-8, followed by hydroxylation at C-8 and bond formation between C-9 and C-1′. These two possibilities are outlined in Figure 2. In an attempt to probe the specificity of the sugar annelation

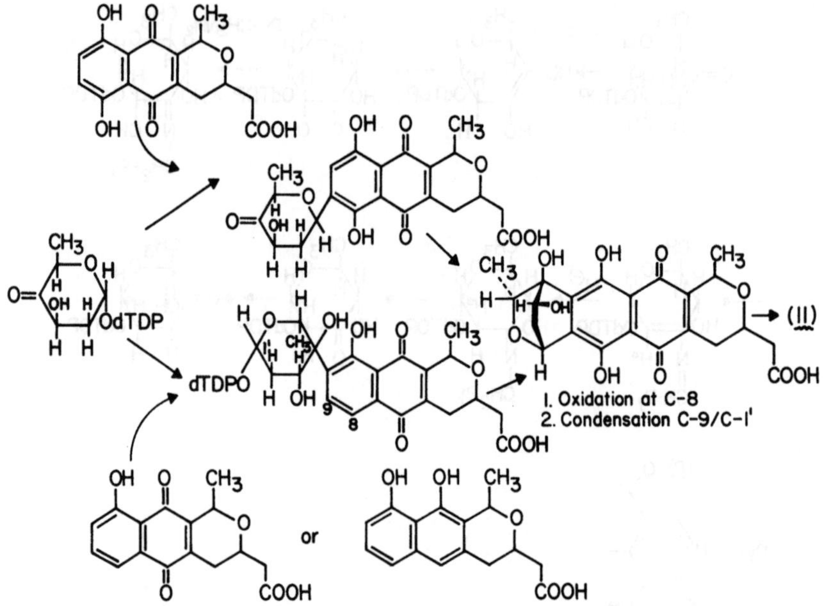

Fig. 2. Two possible modes of attachment of the dideoxyhexose moiety to the aromatic system in the biosynthesis of granaticin

we fed ^{14}C-labeled kalafungin and nanaomycin D, but observed no incorporation into granaticin-like products (H. Hermann, H.G. Floss, unpublished observations). Obviously, however, many other possible precursors need to be explored.

D. Actinorhodin

No tracer studies on the formation of this compound have so far been reported, although from the above-quoted evidence on the various related compounds a polyketide origin via two monomeric units, as proposed by Brockmann et al. (1966), seems a virtual certainty. Unlike that of the other compounds, however, the biosynthesis of actinorhodin has been extensively studied by genetic techniques in Hopwood's laboratory. As the genetically best characterized member of the genus *Streptomyces* (Hopwood et al., 1973), the actinorhodin-producing *S. coelicolor* A3(2) is an ideal object in which to study the basic principles of the genetics of antibiotic formation. Wright and Hopwood (1976) showed that actinorhodin is chromosomally determined.

Using the acid-base indicator properties of actinorhodin as the selection criterium, the antibiotic is red and non-diffusible at the neutral pH of the growth medium, but turns deep blue and becomes diffusible upon exposure to ammonia vapors, they isolated several mutants of *S. coelicolor* A3(2) blocked in the biosynthesis of actinorhodin and they showed that these all mapped in a narrow region of the chromosome. Further extensive work (Rudd, 1978;

Table 4. Classes of mutants blocked in actinorhodin biosynthesis (*act*)

Mutant class	No. of mutants in class	Diffusible pigment formed	Antibiotic activity against *S. aureus*	Cosynthetic reactions	
				As converter	As secretor
I	13	–	–	IV, V, VI, VII	–
II	26	–	–	–	–
III	7	Red	–	IV, V, VI, VII	–
VII[a]	2	Light golden brown	(+)	?, IV, V, VI	I, III
IV	5	Reddish brown	–	V, VI	I, III
VI	2	Light brown	–	V	I, III, IV
V	21	Brown	+	–	I, III, IV, VI

[a] Mutants of class VII produced small quantities of actinorhodin, presumed to be responsible for the limited inhibition of *S. aureus*. This also made the polarity of some cosynthetic reactions doubtful, but class VII mutants probably acted as converter to mutants of classes IV, V, and VI

RUDD and HOPWOOD, 1979) led to the isolation of 76 *act* mutants which fell into seven classes based on two criteria: pigment accumulation and cosynthesis of actinorhodin. These are listed in Table 4. All mutant classes were extensively characterized phenotypically and genetically. They all map between the closely linked markers *his D* and *gua A* on the linkage map. No further sub-groups could be discerned within these classes by experiments involving heterokaryon formation. As shown in Table 4, five mutant classes accumulate pigments of various kinds, probably actinorhodin precursors or shunt products, five classes serve as converters in the cosynthesis of actinorhodin and four as secretors. The latter obviously must accumulate intermediates in the biosynthesis of actinorhodin. Based on the cosynthesis data, it is possible to arrange the classes in a linear sequence in terms of the order of their metabolic blocks in the biosynthesis of actinorhodin:

$$\xrightarrow{\text{III, I}} \xrightarrow{\text{VII(?)}} \xrightarrow{\text{IV}} \xrightarrow{\text{VI}} \xrightarrow{\text{V}} \text{actinorhodin}$$

It is not possible, by cosynthesis, to determine the relative positions of mutants of classes I and III in this sequence, although it might be speculated that class III mutants represent a later block since they presumably produce a precursor or shunt product. The class II mutants cannot be assigned a position in the sequence, since they showed no cosynthesis with any other mutants.

Attempts are now underway in our laboratory to isolate the compounds accumulated by these mutants and to determine their structures and their role in the biosynthesis.

Acknowledgment. Work from the author's laboratory was supported by the US Public Health Service through NIH Research Grant AI 11728.

References

Arnone A, Camarda L, Cardillo R, Fronza G, Merlini L, Mondelli R, Nasini G, Pyrek JS (1979) ^{13}C NMR analysis of dihydrogranaticin methyl ester. A case of mixed biogenesis. Helv Chim Acta 62:30–33

Barcza S, Brufani M, Keller-Schierlein W, Zähner H (1966) Stoffwechselprodukte von Actimoyceten. 52. Mitteilung. Granaticin B. Helv Chim Acta 49:1736–1740
Bergy ME (1968) Kalafungin, a new broad spectrum antibiotic. Isolation and characterization. J Antibiot 21:454–457
Brockmann H, Christiansen P (1970) Actinomycetenfarbstoffe. XI. Phenocyclinon. Chem Ber 103:708–717
Brockmann H, Hieronymus E (1955) Über Actinomycetenfarbstoffe. V. Mitteil.: Zur Konstitution des Actinorhodins. III. Mitteilung. Chem Ber 88:1379–1390
Brockmann H, Loeschke V (1955) Actinomycetenfarbstoffe. IV. Mitteilung. Über die Konstitution des Actinorhodins und die Isolierung des Proto-actinorhodins. Chem Ber 88:778–788
Brockmann H, Pini H (1947) Actinorhodin, ein roter Farbstoff aus Actinomyceten. Naturwissenschaften 34:190
Brockmann H, Pini H, Plotho v O (1950) Über Actinomycetenfarbstoffe. I. Mitteil.: Actinorhodin, ein roter, antibiotisch wirksamer Farbstoff aus Actinomyceten. Chem Ber 83:161–167
Brockmann H, Zeeck A, van der Merwe K, Müller W (1966) Über Actinomycetenfarbstoffe. VIII. Die Konstitution des Actinorhodins. Liebigs Ann Chem 698:209–229
Brufani M, Dobler M (1968) Stoffwechselprodukte von Mikroorganismen. 67. Mitteilung. Die Struktur des Granaticins und des Granaticins B. 2. Teil: Die Kristallstruktur des Tri-O-acetyl-O-jodacetyl-granaticins Helv Chim Acta 51:1269–1275
Cameron DW, Kingston DGI, Sheppard N, Todd L (1964) Coloring matters of the aphididae. XXII. Nuclear magnetic resonance evidence for the structures and conformations of the naphthoquinone dimethyl ethers derived from the protaphins and of the erythroaphins. J Chem Soc 98–104
Chang C-J, Floss HG, Soong P, Chang C-T (1975) Identity of the antitumor antibiotic litmomycin with granaticin A. J Antibiot 28:156
Corbaz R, Ettlinger L, Gäumann E, Kalvoda J, Keller-Schierlein W, Kradolfer F, Manukian BK, Neipp L, Prelog V, Reusser F, Zähner H (1957) Stoffwechselprodukte von Actinomyceten. 9. Mitteilung. Granaticin. Helv Chim Acta 40:1262–1269
Cornforth JW, Redmond JW, Eggerer H, Buckel W, Gutschow C (1970) Synthesis and configurational assay of asymmetric methyl groups. Eur J Biochem 14:1–13
Duchamp DJ (1968) The crystal and molecular structure of kalafungin. Am Cryst Assoc Summer Meet Abstr Pap 82
Ellestad GA, Kunstmann MP, Whaley HA, Patterson EL (1968) The structure of frenolicin. J Am Chem Soc 90:1325–1332
Floss HG, Tsai M-D (1979) Chiral Methyl Groups. Adv Enzymol 50:243–302
Gabriel O (1973) Biological mechanisms involved in the formation of deoxy sugars: Enzymatic hydrogen mediation. A possible example for the evolutionary process of enzyme catalysis. In: Gould R (ed) Carbohydrates in solution, Advances in chemistry series No 117, pp 387–410. American Chemical Society, Washington DC
Harris TM, Harris CM (1977) Synthesis of polyketide-type aromatic natural products by biogenetically modeled routes. Tetrahedron 33:2159–2185
Hoeksema H, Krueger WC (1976) Kalafungin. II. Chemical transformations and the absolute configuration. J Antibiot 29:704–709
Hopwood DA, Chater KF, Dowding JE, Vivian A (1973) Advances in *Streptomyces coelicolor* genetics. Bacteriol Rev 37:371–405
Iwai Y, Kora A, Takahashi Y, Hayashi T, Awaya J, Masuma R, Oiwa R, Omura S (1978) Production of deoxyfrenolicin and a new antibiotic, frenolicin B, by *Streptomyces roseofulvus* strain AM-3867. J Antibiot 31:959–965
Keller-Schierlein W, Brufani M, Barcza W (1968) Stoffwechselprodukte von Mikroorganismen. 66. Mitteilung. Die Struktur des Granaticins und des Granaticins B. 1. Teil: Spektroskopische Eigenschaften und chemischer Abbau. Helv Chim Acta 51:1257–1268
Lüthy J, Retey J, Arigoni D (1969) Preparation and detection of chiral methyl groups. Nature (London) 221:1213–1215
Ogilvie A, Wiebauer K, Kersten W (1975a) Inhibition of leucyl-transfer ribonucleic acid synthetase in *Bacillus subtilis* by granaticin. Biochem J 152:511–515
Ogilvie A, Wiebauer K, Kersten W (1975b) Stringent control of ribonucleic acid synthesis in *Bacillus subtilis* treated with granaticin. Biochem J 152:517–522

Omura S, Tanaka H, Koyama Y, Oiwa R, Katagiri M, Hata T (1974) Nanaomycins A and B, new antibiotics produced by a strain of *Streptomyces*. J Antibiot 27:363–365

Omura S, Tanaka H, Okada Y, Marumo H (1976) Isolation and structure of nanaomycin D, an enantiomer of the antibiotic kalafungin. J Chem Soc Chem Commun 1976:320–321

Pyrek JSt, Achmatowicz O, Zamojski A (1977) Naphtho- and anthraquinones of *Streptomyces thermoviolaceus* WR-141. Structures and model syntheses. Tetrahedron 33:673–680

Rubenstein PA, Strominger JL (1974a) Enzymatic synthesis of cytidine diphosphate 3,6-dideoxyhexoses. VII. Mechanistic roles of enzyme E1 and pyridoxamine 5′-phosphate in the formation of cytidine diphosphate-4-keto-3,6-dideoxy-D-glucose from cytidine diphosphate-4-keto-6-deoxy-D-glucose. J Biol Chem 249:3776–3781

Rubenstein PA, Strominger JL (1974b) Enzymatic synthesis of cytidine diphosphate 3,6-dideoxyhexoses. VIII. Studies of the properties of E3 and its role in the formation of cytidine diphosphate-4-keto-3,6-dideoxyglucose. J Biol Chem 249:3782–3788

Rudd BAM (1978) Genetics of pigmented secondary metabolites in *Streptomyces coelicolor*. PhD Thesis, University of East Anglia

Rudd BAM, Hopwood DA (1979) Genetics of actinorhodin biosynthesis by *Streptomyces coelicolor*. J Gen Microbiol 114:35–43

Schmid H, Ebnöther A (1951a) Isolierung und Konstitution des Isoeleutherins. Allo- und Alloisoeleutherin. Helv Chim Acta 34:561–576

Schmid H, Ebnöther A (1951b) Die Konfiguration der Eleutherinchinone. Helv Chim Acta 34:1041–1049

Schmid H, Ebnöther A, Meijer TM (1950) Über die Konstitution des Eleutherins. Helv Chim Acta 33:1751–1770

Schröder K, Floss HG (1978) Biosynthesis of α-naphthocyclinone. J Org Chem 43:1438–1441

Snipes CE, Brillinger G-U, Sellers L, Mascaro L, Floss HG (1977) Stereochemistry of the dTDP-glucose oxidoreductase reaction. J Biol Chem 252:8113–8117

Snipes CE, Chang C-J, Floss HG (1979a) The biosynthesis of the antibiotic granaticin. J Am Chem Soc 101:701–706

Snipes CE, Chang C-J, Floss HG (1979b) Biosynthesis of the antibiotic granaticin: Assignment of the carbon-13 magnetic resonance spectrum of granaticin and some of its derivatives. J. Nat. Prod. 42:627–632

Tanaka H, Koyama Y, Awaya J, Oiwa R, Katagiri M, Nagai T, Omura S (1975a) Nanaomycins, new antibiotics produced by a strain of *Streptomyces*. I. Taxonomy, isolation, characterization and biological properties. J Antibiot 28:860–867

Tanaka H, Koyama Y, Nagai T, Marumo H, Omura S (1975b) Nanaomycins, new antibiotics produced by a strain of *Streptomyces*. II. Structure and biosynthesis. J Antibiot 28:868–875

Tanaka H, Marumo H, Nagai T, Okada M, Taniguchi K, Omura S (1975c) Nanaomycins, new antibiotics produced by a strain of *Streptomyces*. III. A new component, nanaomycin C, and biological activities of nanaomycin derivatives. J Antibiot 28:925–930

Tsai M-D, Weaver J, Floss HG, Conn EE, Creveling RK, Mazelis M (1978) Stereochemistry of the β-cyanoalanine synthetase and S-alkylcysteine lyase reactions. Arch Biochem Biophys 190:553–559

Tsuji N, Kobayashi M, Wakisaka Y, Kawamura Y, Mayama M, Matsumoto K (1976a) New antibiotics, griseusins A and B. Isolation and characterization. J Antibiot 29:7–9

Tsuji N, Kobayashi M, Terui Y, Tori K (1976b) The structures of griseusins A and B, new isochromanequinone antibiotics. Tetrahedron 32:2207–2210

Van Meter JC, Dann M, Bohonos N (1961) Isolation and characteristics of frenolicin. Antibacterial. Agents annual – 1960, pp 77–80. Plenum Press, New York

Wright LF, Hopwood DA (1976) Actinorhodin is a chromosomally determined antibiotic in *Streptomyces coelicolor* A3(2). J Gen Microbiol 96:289–297

Zeeck A, Christiansen P (1969) Über Actinomycetenfarbstoffe. IX. Konformation und absolute Konfiguration des Actinorhodins. Liebigs Ann Chem 724:172–182

Zeeck A, Mardin M (1974) Isolierung und Konstitution von α-Naphthocyclinon. Liebigs Ann Chem 1063–1099

Zeeck A, Zähner H, Mardin M (1974) Isolierung und Konstitution der Isochromanchinon-Antibiotica β- und γ-Naphthocyclinon. Liebigs Ann Chem 1100–1125

Biosynthesis of Some Aromatic Antibiotics

HEINZ G. FLOSS

Our laboratory has a long-standing interest in the shikimate pathway of aromatic biosynthesis (FLOSS, 1978) and in the metabolic conversions of tryptophan and related indoles (FLOSS, 1976). This led us to investigate the biosynthesis of several related antibiotics and these will be discussed in the following: dihydrophenylalanine formation represents an interesting new variant of the shikimate pathway, pyrrolnitrin arises by an unusual rearrangement of tryptophan, and indolmycin represented one of the first cases of the C-methylation of an amino acid-derived side chain in the *β*-position and led us to study the stereochemistry of biological methyl transfer reactions.

I. Indolmycin

A. Background

Indolmycin (*1*) was first isolated at the Pfizer laboratories (RAO, 1960; MARSH et al., 1960) from a strain of *Streptomyces albus*, later reclassified as *S. griseus* (ROUTIEN, 1966), as an antibiotic with good activity against staphylococci resistant to most commercial antibiotics. The compound is active against gram-positive and gram-negative bacteria and *Mycobacterium tuberculosis* (PADEISKAYA et al., 1972). It was recently isolated again from *S. griseus*, together with N-demethyl-C-demethylindolmycin (*2*) as an active agent in a screen for L-tryptophan antagonists in *E. coli* (HIROTA et al., 1978). Consistent with this antimetabolite activity, mode of action studies have shown (WERNER et al., 1976) that indolmycin prevents formation of tryptophanyl-tRNA in prokaryotes, but not eukaryotic cells, by inhibiting, competitively with tryptophan, the prokaryotic tryptophanyl-tRNA ligase.

The structure of indolmycin was determined (SCHACH V. WITTENAU and ELS, 1961, 1963) largely by chemical means, particularly by degradation to *α*-indolmycenic acid (*3*):

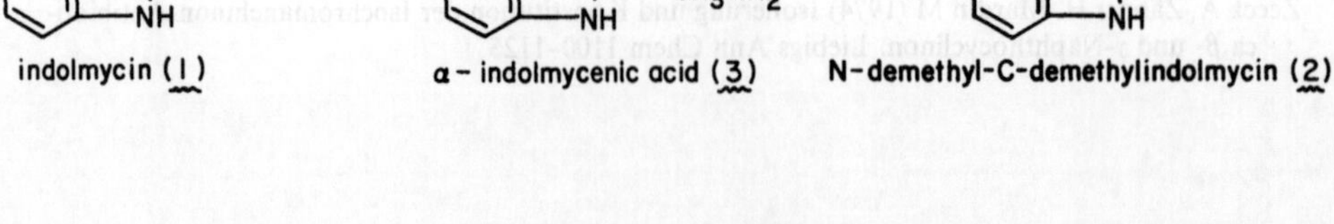

indolmycin (*1*) α-indolmycenic acid (*3*) N-demethyl-C-demethylindolmycin (*2*)

The structural assignment is supported by NMR and mass spectroscopy and was confirmed by two independent total syntheses (SCHACH V. WITTENAU and ELS, 1963; PREOBRAZHENSKAYA et al., 1968). NMR spectroscopy also established the relative configuration of *1*. The absolute configuration of indolmycin was determined by CHAN and HILL (1970) by synthesis from (-)-trans-2,3-epoxybutyric acid of the enantiomer of the α-indolmycenic acid isolated from the degradation of *1*. The configuration established by this unequivocal procedure, 5S, 6R-*1*, is in agreement with that deduced by our laboratory (HORNEMANN, et al., 1971) by a correlation with R-(−)-indole-2-propionic acid, whose configurational assignment, in turn, is based on the quasi-racemate method (SJÖBERG, 1958). α-Indolmycenic acid of the same configuration as that obtained from *1* has also been isolated as a natural metabolite from the indolmycin-producing strain of *S. griseus* (HORNEMANN et al., 1970a, 1971).

A substantial number of analogs and stereoisomers of *1* have been synthesized and tested for biological activity (PREOBRASHENSKAYA et al., 1968; HARNDEN and WRIGHT, 1977). Particularly interesting is the thio analog containing a sulfur atom instead of the oxygen in the oxazoline ring (HARNDEN et al., 1978), which shows very promising antiviral and antibacterial activity.

B. Biosynthetic Origin and Pathway

Inspection of the structure of indolmycin suggests a biosynthetic origin of the main carbon skeleton from tryptophan, which would have to undergo a

Table 1. Incorporation of labeled substrates into indolmycin by *S. griseus*

Precursor	Quantity fed, μmol	Radioactivity fed, dpm	Incorporation into indolmycin, percent
[G-^{3}H]Anthranilic acid	4	5.90×10^{7}	11.6
[1-^{14}C]Acetic acid sodium salt	7	2.07×10^{7}	<0.05
(S)-[U-^{14}C]Alanine	11	1.50×10^{7}	<0.07
(S)-[guanido-^{14}C]Arginine	5	1.40×10^{7}	2.1
(S)-[guanido-^{14}C]Arginine	8	1.32×10^{7}	4.9
(S)-[guanido-^{14}C]Arginine	8	2.20×10^{7}	1.0
[^{14}C]Formic acid sodium salt	14	2.50×10^{7}	<0.05
(R)-[U-^{14}C]Glucose	3	2.20×10^{7}	<0.05
[2-^{14}C]Indole	2	2.66×10^{7}	6.7
(S)-[methyl-^{14}C]Methionine	7	2.61×10^{7}	8.7
(S)-[methyl-^{14}C]Methionine	7	1.06×10^{7}	3.7
(S)-[methyl-^{14}C]Methionine	7	1.75×10^{7}	1.3
(S)-[indole-^{3}H]Tryptophan	2	3.80×10^{7}	18.5
(S)-[alanine-3-^{14}C]Tryptophan	10	1.09×10^{7}	7.2
(R,S)-[alanine-1-^{14}C]Tryptophan	5	6.20×10^{6}	9.6
(R,S)-[alanine-1-^{14}C]Tryptophan	5	1.07×10^{7}	17.6
(R,S)-[alanine-2-^{14}C]Tryptophan	20	2.03×10^{7}	4.6
(R,S)-[alanine-3-^{14}C]Tryptophan	18	2.97×10^{7}	5.0
(R,S)-[alanine-3-^{14}C]Tryptophan	10	5.52×10^{6}	9.0
(S)-[U-^{14}C]Threonine	8	2.40×10^{7}	<0.04
[^{14}C]Urea	20	3.00×10^{7}	<0.03

C-methylation at the β-position of the side chain. As a plausible alternative, the methylated side chain could arise by condensation of indole, possibly generated from indolglycerol-phosphate, with threonine in analogy to the tryptophan synthetase reaction. The remainder of the molecule could be derived from the guanido group of arginine and another methyl group from methionine. To clarify the biosynthesis of *1*, feeding experiments were carried out with *S. griseus* ATCC 12648, which in our hands produces about 20 mg/l of *1* (HORNEMANN et al., 1971). The results with a number of radioactive substrates, summarized in Table 1, indicate good incorporation of ring-labeled anthranilic acid, [guanido-^{14}C]arginine, indole, [methyl-^{14}C]methionine and ring or side-chain labeled tryptophan, but not of acetate, alanine, formate, glucose, L-threonine, or urea. Degradation of several of the indolmycin samples showed that all the radioactivity incorporated from the guanido group of arginine was recovered in the CO_2 produced by alkaline hydrolysis of *1*, [alanine-3-^{14}C]tryptophan had predominantly labeled C-6, and label from the methyl group of methionine was distributed between the C-methyl group (31% recovered) and the N-methyl group (55% recovered). These findings thus established the building block of *1* as follows:

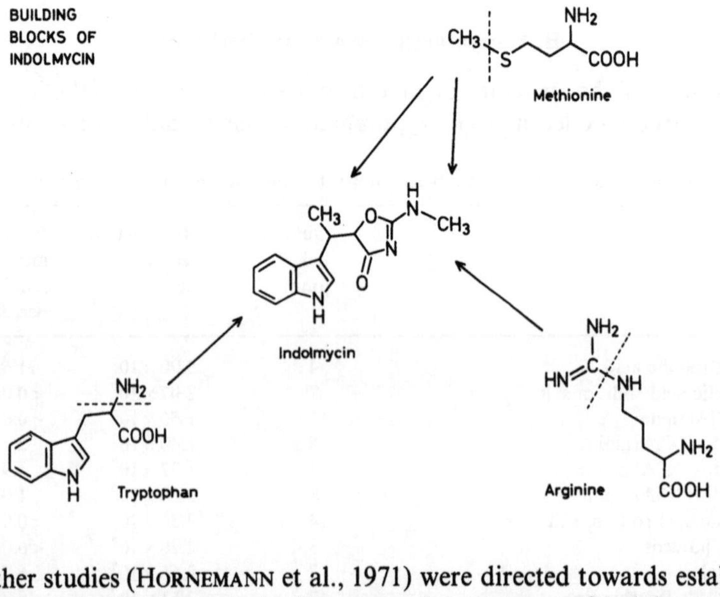

Further studies (HORNEMANN et al., 1971) were directed towards establishing the pathway of this biosynthesis. The natural occurrence of indolmycenic acid in this fermentation suggested that *3* might be a precursor of *1*. This notion was confirmed by experiments which showed that natural indolmycenic acid was efficiently incorporated into *1*. Furthermore all four stereoisomers of indolmycenic acid were prepared in labeled form and fed in separate experiments. Only the isomer of the same configuration as natural *3* (2S, 3R) was efficiently utilized (17% incorporation), whereas the three other stereoisomers gave negligible incorporations (Table 2). Hence, C-methylation must precede elaboration of the oxazolinone ring. Methylation of the side chain may occur before or after replacement of the amino nitrogen by an oxygen function, i.e., at the

Table 2. Incorporation of labeled potential precursors into indolmycin by *S. griseus*

Precursor	Quantity fed, μmol	Radioactivity fed, dpm	Incorporation into indolmycin percent
(S)-3-[ring-^{3}H]Methylindolepyruvate	1.5	1.70×10^7	<0.3
(R)-3-[ring-^{3}H]Methylindolepyruvate	1.0	3.60×10^6	9.0
(R,S)-[alanine-3-^{14}C]Tryptophan	5.0	1.30×10^7	10.0
(2RS,3SR)-3-[ring-^{3}H]Methyltryptophan	5.0	4.02×10^7	5.5
(2RS,3RS)-3-[ring-^{3}H]Methyltryptophan	5.0	2.26×10^7	<0.3
(S)-[alanine-3-^{14}C]Tryptophan	10.0	1.09×10^7	5.8
Natural [3-^{14}C]Indolmycenic acid	1.0	4.16×10^5	28.0
[3-^{14}C]Indolmycenic acid from hydrolysis of indolmycin	1.0	2.30×10^6	12.0
(2S,3R)-[3-^{14}C]Indolmycenic acid	1.0	3.60×10^5	17.0
(2R,3R)-[3-^{14}C]Indolmycenic acid	1.0	1.27×10^5	<0.1
(2S,3S)-[ring-^{3}H]Indolmycenic acid	1.0	8.00×10^5	<0.1
(2R,3S)[ring-^{3}H]Indolmycenic acid	1.0	8.40×10^5	<0.1
(R,S)-[alanine-3-^{14}C]Tryptophan	5.0	1.13×10^6	6.6

tryptophan stage or at the stage of indolepyruvate or indolelactate. The latter possibility is mechanistically less plausible than the other two. Several experiments with precursors double labeled with ^{14}C and tritium did not allow a distinction between these possibilities, but showed that the α-hydrogen of the tryptophan side chain is completely lost in the conversion to *1* (98.4% loss relative to ^{14}C) and *3* (99.5% loss). They also showed retention of almost exactly half of the tritium from the β-position of the tryptophan side chain in *1* (52% retention) and *3* (54% retention), as well as complete retention of tritium from the methyl group of methionine during the conversion into *1* (100% retention) and *3* (96% retention). Direct comparison of the utilization of the C-methylated keto acid and amino acid for *1*-biosynthesis also did not answer this question since both (R)-[ring-^{3}H]-3-methylindolepyruvate, but not the S isomer, and (2RS, 3SR)-[ring-^{3}H]-3-methyltryptophan, but not the (2RS, 3RS) diastereomer, were incorporated into *1* (Table 2). A final distinction in favor of methylation at the indolepyruvate stage could only be made by enzymatic experiments (see below), which demonstrated the presence in the organism of an L-tryptophan transaminase and a C-methylase which accepts indolepyruvate, but not tryptophan as a substrate. The sequence therefore must be (1) transamination, (2) C-methylation, and (3) reduction to give *3*.

The later steps in the pathway, i.e., those leading from *3* to *1* are not entirely elucidated. In the formation of the oxazolinone ring an intact amidino group from arginine is transferred. This follows from two pieces of evidence (ZEE et al., 1975). Firstly, the dione *4* was prepared in labeled form, tritium in the methyl group and ^{14}C at C-2, by acid hydrolysis of indolmycin (SCHACH v. WITTENAU and ELS, 1963) and fed to *S. griseus*. No significant incorporation into *1* was seen. A second and more conclusive piece of evidence is the fact that L-arginine labeled with ^{14}C in the amidino carbon and with ^{15}N in the two amidino nitrogens is incorporated without significant change in the ^{15}N/^{14}C

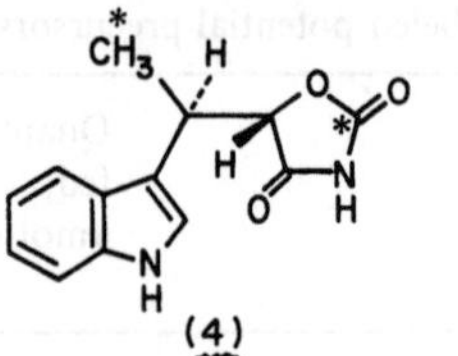

(4)

ratio (Table 3). Furthermore, the intramolecular ^{15}N distribution in the product, as analyzed by mass spectrometry, closely matches that predicted for intact transfer of the amidino group and is quite different from that which would result upon statistical recombination between the two nitrogens if they were separated at any stage in the biosynthesis. Therefore the amidino group of arginine must be transferred to *3* as an intact unit. Whether this process occurs in two stages, with an open chain intermediate carrying the amidino group either on the hydroxyl or the carboxyl group, or leads directly from *3* to an oxazolinone, is still an open question. Likewise it is not clear whether the nitrogen is methylated before or after transfer of the amidino group, although the natural occurrence of *2* would perhaps suggest the latter. The pathway of indolmycin formation can thus be summarized as follows:

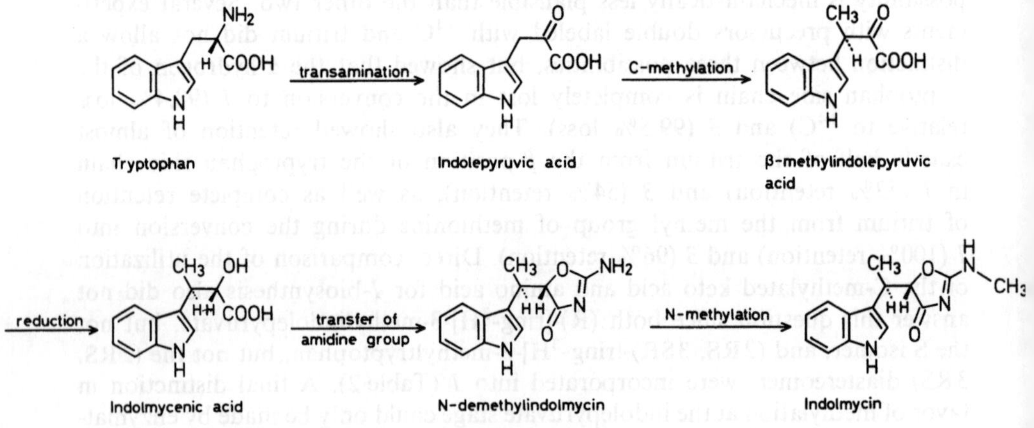

Pathway of Indolmycin Biosynthesis

C. Stereochemical Aspects of Indolmycin Biosynthesis

As already mentioned, the enzymes in the biosynthetic pathway exhibit complete stereospecificity in their utilization of the chiral intermediates 3-methylindolepyruvate and indolmycenic acid, incorporating only those stereoisomers which correspond to natural *1* in their absolute configuration. These also seem to be the only stereoisomers formed in the reactions generating these intermediates. The C-methylation reaction produces only the R isomer of 3-methylindolepyruvate (HORNEMANN et al., 1970b, 1971) and natural *3* consists of only the 2S, 3R isomer (HORNEMANN et al., 1970a, 1971).

Table 3. Incorporation of L-[^{14}C, ^{15}N]arginine into indolmycin

Precursor fed	L-[amidino-^{14}C, ^{15}N]arginine · HCl
Amount fed	25 mg
Specific radioactivity	$2.13 \cdot 10^8$ dpm/mmole
^{15}N enrichment	99.5 atom % excess
Intramolecular ^{15}N distribution	25.7% N_0/47.8% N_1/26% N_2
Product isolated	**Indolmycin**
Specific radioactivity	$1.25 \pm 1 \cdot 0.10^8$ dpm/mmole
^{15}N enrichment	61 atom % excess
^{14}C dilution	1.70
^{15}N dilution	1.63
^{15}N retention	96%
Intramolecular ^{15}N distribution found	52.6% N_0/33.5% N_1/13.8% N_2
Calc. for intact amidino group transfer	54.3% N_0/30.6% N_1/15.1% N_2
Calc. for separation and statistical recombination of the two labeled nitrogens	48.1% N_0/42.5% N_1/9.4% N_2

There are additional stereochemical aspects of this biosynthesis, many of which are cryptic, because they relate to reactions involving centers which are not chiral. These reactions nevertheless can be expected to be stereospecific and their steric course can be deduced by experiments using suitable stereospecifically isotope-labeled precursors. In indolmycin biosynthesis the stereochemical aspects of the two methylation reactions were of particular interest and we decided to investigate these.

In the C-methylation of indolepyruvate we examined two stereochemical questions. The first was whether the replacement of a hydrogen of the methylene group of indolepyruvate by the methyl group proceeds in a retention or in an inversion mode. Since the configuration of the product was already known, this only required determination whether the *pro*-R or the *pro*-S hydrogen from the methylene group is eliminated in the process. L-Tryptophan labeled stereospecifically with tritium in the *pro*-3R or in the *pro*-3S position, available from another project (SKYE et al., 1974; TSAI et al., 1978) was mixed with ^{14}C-labeled material and fed to the cultures of *S. griseus*. The $^3H/^{14}C$ ratios of the precursors and the resulting indolmycin samples were analyzed, with the following results:

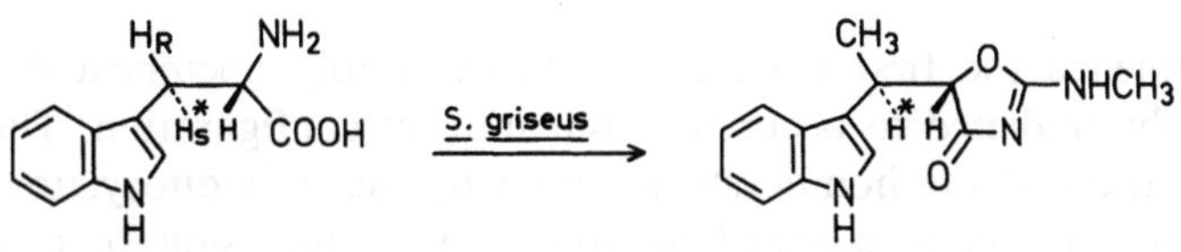

Tryptophan-3-T		Indolmycin	
3R: T/^{14}C	3.47	T/^{14}C 0.25	(7%)
	3.85	0.086	(2%)
3S: T/^{14}C	2.67	T/^{14}C 2.60	(97%)
	2.52	2.62	(104%)

The reaction clearly proceeds with loss of the *pro*-3R and retention of the *pro*-3S hydrogen and thus the replacement of a hydrogen by the methyl group occurs in a retention mode. This finding is rather interesting, because it implies that the two steps, removal of a proton presumably to generate an enol and addition of a methyl group to the double bond of this enol must occur on the same face of the molecule. Unless these two reaction steps occur on separate enzymes or active sites or by the equivalent of a ping-pong mechanism, S-adenosylmethionine binds only after the enol has been generated, the positively charged sulfonium center of S-adenosylmethionine must be situated very close to the unprotonated base group in the active site of the enzyme, which mediates the proton abstraction to generate the enol. One would have to wonder, then, why this base group does not interact with the sulfonium group of S-adenosylmethionine, serving as an alternate acceptor of the methyl group. Obviously, detailed studies on the active site of this enzyme would be of considerable interest.

The second stereochemical question was more difficult to answer; it dealt with the steric course of the reaction at the methyl group (MASCARO et al., 1977). The experimental approach here required use of the chiral methyl group methodology developed by the laboratories of CORNFORTH and ARIGONI (cf. FLOSS and TSAI, 1979), i.e., the use of both tritium and deuterium to generate a methyl group which is chiral by virtue of isotope substitution. The main task was to synthesize methionine carrying a chiral methyl group of known configuration. This was solved by the following sequence of reactions starting from chiral acetate which could be prepared by previously described reactions (ROSE, 1970):

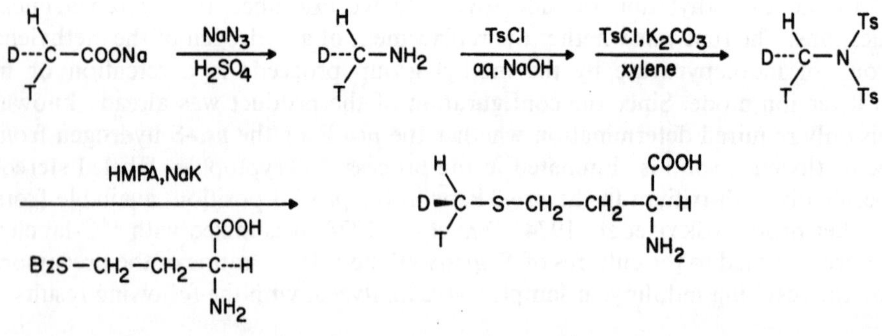

In this sequence the first reaction, based on amply documented precedent, can be safely predicted to occur with retention of configuration. The key step is the alkylation of the homocysteine anion by the N,N-ditosylate of methylamine. This reaction is expected to proceed with inversion of configuration at the methyl group, the only alternative being racemization, in case the reaction proceeds by an SN1 mechanism. Thus, if the methyl group in methionine is chiral, its absolute configuration follows from that of the starting acetate. Feeding of the methionine samples carrying a methyl group of R- or S-configuration followed by Kuhn-Roth oxidation of the resulting indolmycin gave acetate from the C-methyl group of the antibiotic, which was analyzed for its chirality by the method of ARIGONI and CORNFORTH and their co-workers. In this analysis procedure (cf. FLOSS and TSAI, 1979) acetate is converted to acetyl-Co A which is condensed with glyoxylate in a reaction catalyzed by malate synthase to give malate. Because of a substantial deuterium isotope effect in the latter reaction the malate will show an unequal distribution of tritium between the two methylene positions if the acetate was chiral. This tritium distribution can be analyzed by incubation of the malate with fumarase, which equilibrates the *pro*-3R hydrogen of malate with solvent protons. Calibration of the system has shown that R-acetate gives malate which retains >50% of its tritium in the fumarase reaction (F-value of 79 for chirally pure R-acetate), whereas pure S-acetate has an F-value of 21 (21% of tritium of malate retained in the fumarase reaction). The analyses of the acetate samples from the C-methylation reaction are summarized in Table 4. It is clear that the chemical synthesis had produced methionine carrying a chiral methyl group, albeit apparently with some loss of chiral purity, and that the enzymatic transfer of the methyl group from S-adenosylmethionine to carbon 3 of indolepyruvate occurs with inversion of the configuration of the methyl group. Since it is likely that any one transfer of the methyl group from a donor to an acceptor in the enzymatic process proceeds with inversion of configuration, this result suggests that the overall reaction involves a direct transfer of the methyl group from the sulphur of S-adenosylmethionine to the acceptor carbon without any intermediate alkylation of a functional group of the enzyme.

The same stereochemical choices exist in the N-methylation reaction later in the biosynthetic pathway. The steric course of the reaction at the acceptor position can in this case obviously not be determined experimentally. Elucidation of the steric course of the reaction at the methyl group requires recovery of the N-methyl group and conversion into acetate for chirality analysis. This was accomplished using the following sequence of stereospecific reactions:

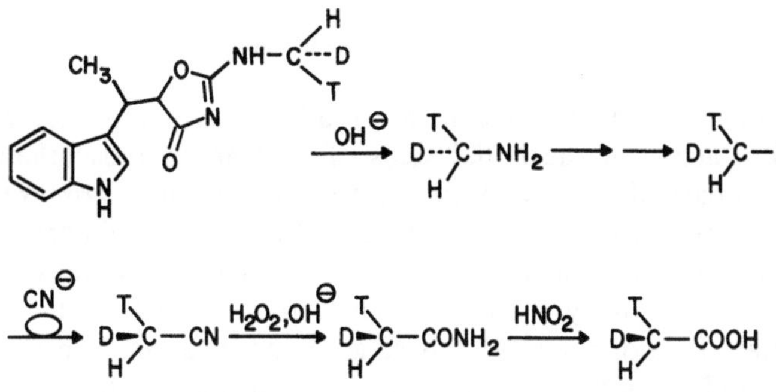

The degradation sequence involves one inversion of configuration in the cyanide displacement step. Since the chemical synthesis of methionine also involves one inversion of configuration, it follows that the starting acetate and that resulting from the degradation will have opposite configurations if the enzymatic methyl transfer occurs with inversion or the same configurations if it occurs

Table 4. Steric course of the S-adenosylmethionine: indolepyruvate methyl transferase reaction

	Starting acetate	Methionine	Acetate from indolmycin	Indolmycin C-methyl group
F-value	31%	–	39%	–
Methyl group configuration	S	R	S	S
F-value	71%	–	63%	–
Methyl group configuration	R	S	R	R

with retention. The results, starting acetates of F=28 and F=68 gave acetates from the degradation of F=64 and F=35, respectively, clearly show that the enzymatic process involves inversion of configuration. It thus presumably also proceeds as a direct transfer of the methyl group from the sulfur to the nitrogen (WOODARD, MASCARO and FLOSS, unpublished results). The stereochemical results on the two methyl transfer reactions in the biosynthesis of *1* can be summarized as follows:

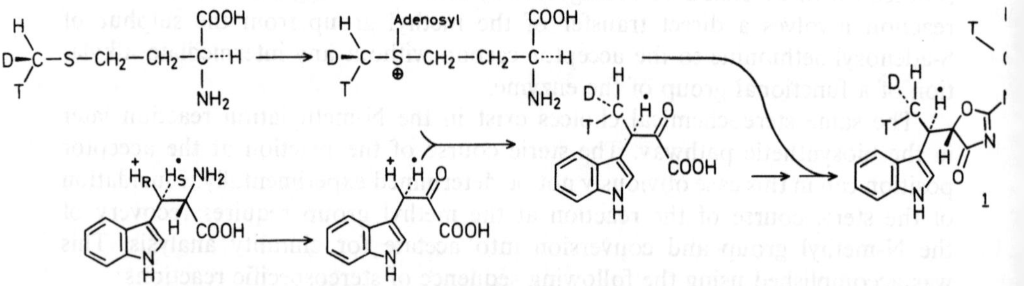

1

D. Enzymology and Regulation

Two enzymes, a tryptophan transaminase and indolepyruvate C-methyltransferase, which are active in the initial steps of indolmycin biosynthesis, have been detected and partially purified from cell-free extracts of *S. griseus* (SPEEDIE et al., 1975). The transaminase is assayed either by using a radioactive amino acid as substrate or by using unlabeled substrate and measuring the absorbance of the enol form of indolepyruvate at 305 nm. It was purified three-fold by ammonium sulfate fractionation. At this stage of purification, it catalyzes the α-keto-glutarate and pyridoxal phosphate-dependent transamination of L-tryptophan, both diastereomers of L-3-methyltryptophan, L-phenylalanine, and L-tyrosine, but not of D-tryptophan.

The C-methyltransferase catalyzes the transfer of a methyl group from S-adenosylmethionine to position 3 of the aliphatic side chain of indolepyruvate. No cofactors are required for the reaction. The enzyme is assayed by using methyl-tritiated S-adenosylmethionine and following the formation of radioactive material which can be extracted into butyl acetate from the acidified incubation mixture. The C-methyltransferase was purified 110-fold by ammonium sulfate fractionation, Sephadex G-150 gel filtration, DEAE-Sephadex column chromatography, and Bio-Gel A-5 m gel filtration. The enzyme has a broad pH optimum of 7.5 to 8.5. A molecular weight of 55,000 ± 5,000 was determined by Sephadex G-200 gel filtration and a value of 58,500 ± 8,000 by sucrose density gradient centrifugation. The enzyme is relatively stable at temperatures of 0–5° C but is destroyed by freezing or by heating. The C-methyltransferase is inhibited strongly by the thiol reagents p-chloromercuribenzoate and N-ethylmaleimide. The Zn^{2+} and Fe^{2+} chelators, 1,10-phenanthroline and 2,2′-bipyridine also inhibit the enzyme activity, but EDTA does not. Michaelis-Menten constants have been determined for the 110-fold purified enzyme as 1.2×10^{-5} M for S-adenosylmethionine and 4.8×10^{-6} M for indolepyruvate. The enzyme activity in the crude extract is inhibited competitively by indolmycin ($K_i = 2.3$ mM) and L-tryptophan ($K_i = 0.17$ mM), but these effects are not observed after the enzyme has been passed through the Sephadex G-150 column during purification. The crude extract is capable of methylating phenylpyruvate and p-hydroxyphenylpyruvate but this capability is lost upon purification of the indolepyruvate C-methyltransferase activity. No methylation of L-tryptophan occurs under the conditions used.

Some studies have been carried out on the regulation of indolmycin formation. HURLEY and BIALEK (1974) have shown that the production of indolmycin is inhibited by glucose at a concentration of 0.5%, whereas lower concentrations of glucose, i.e., 0.005 and 0.01%, were stimulatory. Of a number of sugars tested, only glucose and to a lesser extent mannose were inhibitory, whereas sucrose, galactose, and particularly fructose were stimulatory. It thus appears that the indolmycin fermentation is sensitive to catabolic inhibition or repression.

II. Pyrrolnitrin

A. Background

The antifungal antibiotic pyrrolnitrin (*5*) is produced by various species of *Pseudomonas* (IMANAKA et al., 1965a; ELANDER et al., 1968) and was discovered independently by ARIMA et al. (1965) and at the Lilly Research Laboratories (LIVELY et al., 1966). A number of naturally occurring analogs of the antibiotic have since been isolated from pyrrolnitrin-producing *Pseudomonas* cultures and these include isopyrrolnitrin (*6*) (HASHIMOTO and HATTORI, 1966a), oxypyrrolnitrin (*7*) (HASHIMOTO and HATTORI, 1966b), 2-chloropyrrolnitrin (*8*) (HAMILL et al., 1967), deschloropyrrolnitrin (*9*) (HASHIMOTO and HATTORI, 1968), and aminopyrrolnitrin (*10*) (HAMILL et al., 1967). In a synthetic medium containing ammonium bromide the organism produces bromo analogs of pyrrolnitrin, three of which have been isolated and identified as (*11–13*) (AJISAKA et al., 1969).

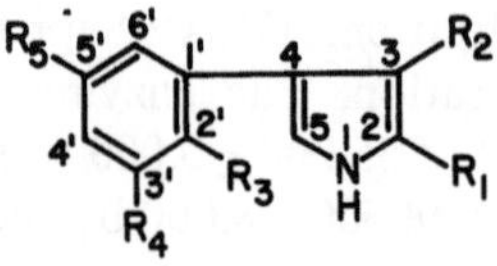

	R_1	R_2	R_3	R_4	R_5
5:	-H	-Cl	$-NO_2$	-Cl	-H
6:	-Cl	-Cl	$-NO_2$	-H	-H
7:	-H	-Cl	$-NO_2$	-Cl	-OH
8:	-Cl	-Cl	$-NO_2$	-Cl	-H
9:	-H	-Cl	$-NO_2$	-H	-H
10:	-H	-Cl	$-NH_2$	-Cl	-H
11:	-H	-Br	$-NO_2$	-Br	-H
12:	-Br	-Br	$-NO_2$	-Br	-H
13:	-Br	-Br	$-NO_2$	-H	-Br

The structure of pyrrolnitrin was elucidated by ARIMA's group (IMANAKA et al., 1965b) and has been confirmed by syntheses (NAKANO et al., 1966; TANAKA et al., 1969; GOSTELI, 1972) and by an X-ray analysis (MORIMOTO et al., 1968). Pyrrolnitrin is considerably less active against bacteria than against most fungi tested and it shows particularly good fungistatic activity against a number of dermatophytes, e.g., *Trychophyton* species (NISHIDA et al., 1965; GORDEE and MATTHEWS, 1969). It is suitable for topical applications, e.g., treatment of athlete's foot, etc., for which purpose it is marketed in Japan, whereas its usefulness as a systemic antifungal agent was judged to be limited (GORDEE and MATTHEWS, 1969). The mechanism of action of pyrrolnitrin was first studied by NOSE and ARIMA (NOSE and ARIMA, 1969), who noted that it inhibits respiration but felt that this was not the primary target site. Rather they suggested that the primary effect was some damage in the cell membrane due to interaction of the antibiotic with phospholipids. Other workers, however, came to the conclusion that inhibition of the respiratory electron transport system is the primary mechanism of action (TRIPATHI and GOTTLIEB, 1969; WONG and AIRALL, 1970; WONG et al., 1971; and LAMBOWITZ and SLAYMAN, 1972). Numerous patents and publications have appeared on the preparation of pyrrolnitrin analogs, both synthetically (e.g., TANAKA et al., 1969; UMIO et al., 1970; FILACCHIONI et al., 1978) and biosynthetically (GORMAN et al., 1968; HAMILL et al., 1970) and structure-activity relationships have been studied (UMIO et al., 1970; HAMILL et al., 1970).

B. Biosynthetic Origin

The biosynthesis of pyrrolnitrin was studied at Eli Lilly and Company and later also in our laboratory using *Pseudomonas aureofaciens*. Early investigations (ELANDER et al., 1968) showed that of a number of compounds tested only labeled tryptophan was efficiently incorporated into pyrrolnitrin and that both D- and L-tryptophan-^{14}C gave radioactive antibiotic. Addition of tryptophan to the cultures also increased pyrrolnitrin production, but only the D isomer was active in this respect. In following up the role of D- and L-tryptophan in pyrrolnitrin biosynthesis it was found that D-tryptophan-^{14}C was incorporated more efficiently than the L isomer (HAMILL et al., 1967). To account for the transformation of tryptophan into pyrrolnitrin GORMAN and LIVELY (1967) proposed the following pathway:

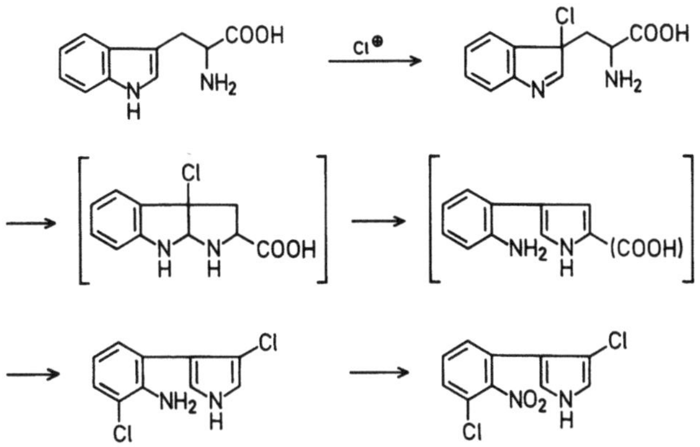

The first step was thought to be catalyzed by a chloroperoxidase. Circumstantial evidence supporting this pathway is (a) the natural occurrence of such pyrrolo[2,3-b] indoles as physostigmine, folicanthine, and the sporidesmin-type antibiotics, (b) the demonstration of the chemical feasibility of the initial cyclization (OHNO et al., 1970), and (c) the isolation of 3-chloroindole from tryptophan-supplemented cultures of the pyrrolnitrin-producing *Pseudomonas* strains (ELANDER et al., 1968), which could readily arise from the postulated first intermediate.

Work in our laboratory, in collaboration with investigators at the Lilly Research Laboratories, was directed towards further examining the mode of tryptophan conversion into pyrrolnitrin (FLOSS et al., 1971). Specific incorporation of tryptophan in a way consistent with the proposed scheme was shown in experiments with D,L-[indole-^{15}N-2-^{14}C]tryptophan which gave pyrrolnitrin of unchanged isotope ratio containing all the ^{15}N in the nitro group and in an experiment with D,L-[alanine-^{15}N-3-^{14}C]tryptophan. The pyrrolnitrin obtained from the latter according to mass spectrometry contained all the ^{15}N in the pyrrole nitrogen, but the ^{15}N/^{14}C ratio had decreased to 19% of that of the precursor. Since another experiment showed 26% tritium retention (relative to ^{14}C) from D,L-[alanine-3-^{14}C-2-T]tryptophan it was felt that the loss of both tritium and ^{15}N was probably due to reversible transamination and, reasoning that D-tryptophan as the closer precursor should show less of this exchange, the experiment was repeated with a sample of D-[alanine-3-^{14}C-3-T-^{15}N]tryptophan. The surprising result was complete loss of the tritium (2% retention) and only 10% retention of the ^{15}N. By extrapolation, the tritium retention from the L isomer has to be higher than from the D,L-form and this was confirmed in a series of experiments which gave tritium retentions of 3.3%, 30.2%, and 71.3% from D-, D,L-, and L-[alanine-3-^{14}C-2-T]tryptophan. Thus D-tryptophan is incorporated with loss and L-tryptophan with retention of the α-hydrogen, a finding which is completely analogous to that observed in the biosynthesis of ergot alkaloids (FLOSS et al., 1964). However, in ergot, L-tryptophan is a three times more efficient precursor than D-tryptophan and the results were interpreted as indicating conversion of D- into L-tryptophan prior to incorporation into the alkaloids.

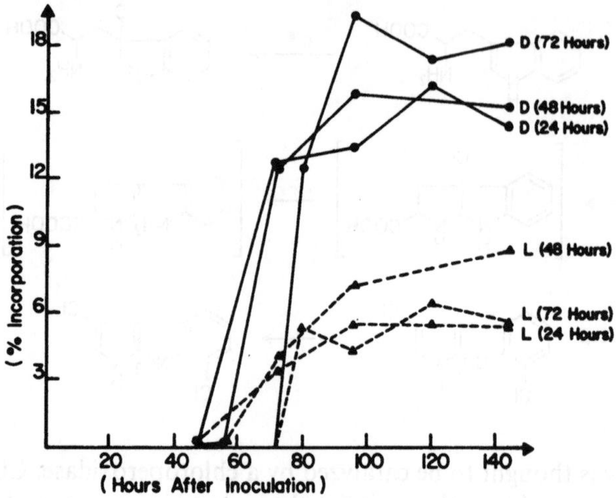

Fig. 1

There is an apparent conflict between the various results bearing on the question, which isomer is the immediate precursor. The conclusion that pyrrolnitrin is probably derived from D- rather than L-tryptophan was further supported by the results of experiments in which radioactive D- or L-tryptophan was fed in the presence of a large nonlabeled pool of either isomer. It was also shown that permeability differences cannot account for the better incorporation of D-tryptophan; if anything, these would favor the L isomer (HAMILL et al., 1967). As another possibility, it was thought that the better incorporation of D-compared to L-tryptophan might be a kinetic phenomenon, i.e., D-tryptophan added early in the fermentation might be used up slowly and more would be available later during antibiotic formation, as compared to the more rapidly metabolized L-isomer. However, the time course experiments shown in Figure 1 clearly indicate that at any time during the culture period the D-isomer is used more efficiently than the L-form (FLOSS et al., 1971). On the other hand it is equally clear from the experiments with α-tritiated tryptophan that the L-isomer must be converted directly to pyrrolnitrin without going through D-tryptophan as an intermediate.

Two explanations offer themselves for this apparent paradox. One would be that D- and L-tryptophan are converted to *5* separately by two independent pathways. The one from D-tryptophan would proceed with loss and that from L-tryptophan with retention of the α-hydrogen. For example, both isomers might be stereospecifically decarboxylated to generate from the α-carbon a methylene group in which the α-hydrogens from D- and L-tryptophan occupy opposite heterotopic positions, followed by stereospecific loss of the methylene hydrogen originating from the α-position of D-tryptophan. This does, however, not account for the difference in the retention of the amino nitrogen from D- and L-tryptophan. As an alternative and perhaps more likely explanation, L-tryptophan may be the more immediate precursor, and the D-isomer is incorporated via L-tryptophan, but, because of regulatory effects, the addition of D isomer gives higher fermentation yields and incorporations than addition of the L isomer. Some recent results from LINGENS' laboratory on tryptophan metabolism in *Pseudomonas aureofaciens* suggest a possible basis for this explanation. These workers reported the isolation of 3-chloroanthranilic acid and 7-chloroindoleacetic acid from pyrrolnitrin-producing cultures incubated in the presence of D-tryptophan (SALCHER and LINGENS, 1978). They noted the operation of two major pathways of tryptophan metabolism in this organism, in addition to the conversion into *5*. One is the indoleacetic acid pathway; both D- and L-tryptophan are apparently converted to indoleacetic acid, but this pathway is quantitatively of minor significance. The second is the kynurenine/anthranilate pathway, which is initiated by the enzyme tryptophan-2, 3-dioxygenase. This enzyme is induced by L-tryptophan, but not by the D isomer, and the product of the pathway, anthranilic acid, effectively inhibits pyrrolnitrin formation (O. SALCHER, F. LINGENS, personal communication). This combination of circumstances could account for the differences seen with D-compared to L-tryptophan. Added L-tryptophan would result in induction of the dioxygenase, production of anthranilate, and hence inhibition of pyrrolnitrin formation. The D isomer would only be converted to L-tryptophan slowly and, therefore, would not lead to build-up of L-tryptophan levels which induce the dioxygenase. Therefore the production of *5* is not inhibited and the incorporation of precursor increased. While this explanation is quite compelling, its validity obviously needs to be examined experimentally.

In summary, there is strong evidence that the biosynthesis of pyrrolnitrin represents a novel pathway of tryptophan metabolism, the details of which remain to be elucidated. However, this conclusion is not entirely uncontested, because a paper by IMANAKA et al. (1972) reports specific incorporation of δ-[^{14}C]aminolevulinic acid into the pyrrole ring of pyrrolnitrin by *Pseudomonas* sp., although only in the presence of phosphate buffer or iron ion in the reaction mixture. Yet the wealth of evidence already discussed and ample data presented below leave little doubt that the normal biosynthesis of *5* proceeds through tryptophan.

C. Biosynthetic Pathway

Of significance for the later stages of pyrrolnitrin formation is the finding (HAMILL et al., 1968) that the amino analog of *5*, aminopyrrolnitrin *14* is a naturally occurring metabolite in the fermentation, that *14* increases the yield of *5* when added to the cultures and that addition of ^{14}C-labeled *14* gives labeled *5*. On this basis, aminopyrrolnitrin is considered to be an intermediate and the oxidation of the amino to the nitro group is assumed to be the last step of the biosynthesis of *5*. Since the presence of halogen substituents in microbial metabolites is often incidental to the biosynthesis it is assumed that the introduction of the chlorine atoms probably occurs after the completion of the ring system. However, it should be noted that this requires introducing chlorine in the 3-position of the pyrrole ring, whereas the normal patterns

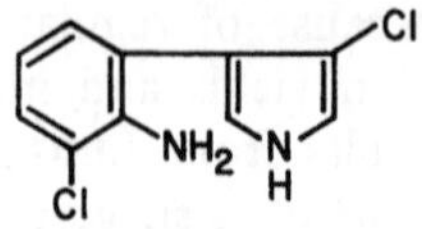

(14)

of electrophilic substitution of pyrroles predict that chlorination occurs in the 2- or 5-position. Furthermore, among all the pyrrolnitrin analogs isolated there is none without halogen in the 3-position. This would be plausible if the chlorine were actually carried over from an earlier stage in the biosynthesis. A way in which this could take place is by a 1,2-aryl shift following the ring opening of the hypothetical chlorinated pyrrolo-indole intermediate, followed by aromatization by dehydrogenation rather than by elimination of HCl. This would lead to a different labeling pattern in *5* than the normal pathway and could thus be examined by an experiment with D,L-[alanine-3-^{13}C]tryptophan. In the normal pathway the ^{13}C would end up at C-3, whereas an aryl shift would give *5* labeled at C-4. The ^{13}C-NMR spectrum of *5* was assigned and the crucial distinction between the signals for C-3 and C-4 was confirmed by comparing the spectra of *5* and *14*. Analysis of the spectrum of the ^{13}C-labeled *5* obtained by feeding D,L-[alanine-3-^{13}C]tryptophan then showed that the signal for C-3 was the only one that was enhanced; hence the normal pathway is operative (MARTIN et al., 1972). The location of the ^{13}C in this sample could also be determined by proton-NMR spectroscopy (CHANG et al., 1976).

That the chlorine in the 3-position of *5* is not a remnant from an earlier step in the biosynthesis agrees with the results of subsequent experiments, in which the compounds *15* and *16* were synthesized carrying a tritium label in

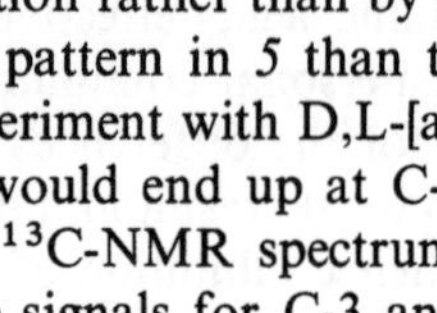

(15): R = NH_2

(16): R = NO_2

positions 2 and 5 of the pyrrole ring. Both compounds were fed to cultures of *P. aeruginosa; 15* gave 6.6% incorporation into *5*, whereas the figure for *16* was only 0.36% (SCHRÖDER, MABE, CHANG and FLOSS, unpublished results). This supports the notion that oxidation of the nitro group is the terminal step in the biosynthesis and that it is immediately preceded by the introduction of the halogens.

Going backwards in the biosynthetic sequence we have to consider the fact that tritium from the α-position of the side chain of L-tryptophan is incorporated into *5*. A chemical degradation of such a sample of *5* showed unequivocally that the tritium is located at C-2 (MARTIN et al., 1972). Therefore, removal of the carboxyl group must precede or must be concerted with the generation of the 2,3-double bond of the pyrrole ring; a pyrrole-2-carboxylic acid as intermediate is incompatible with this finding on the conversion of L-tryptophan to

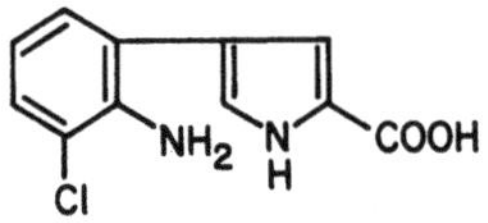

(17)

5. However, just such a compound has recently been isolated from cultures of pyrrolnitrin-producing *P. aureofaciens* (SALCHER et al., 1978). The authors propose that *17* is an intermediate in pyrrolnitrin biosynthesis and that it may be formed from 7-chlorotryptophan as an earlier pathway intermediate. However, based on our data *17* cannot be on the pathway from L-tryptophan to *5*. It could be on a direct pathway from D-tryptophan to *5*, if such a direct pathway not proceeding through the L isomer exists, or it could be a dead-end product formed parallel to *5*.

One weakness of the proposed scheme of pyrrolnitrin biosynthesis via pyrrolo-[2,3-b]indoles is the fact that all such systems so far investigated undergo initial ring cleavage exclusively between C-8a and N-1, not between C-8a and N-8. This suggests the alternative that the skeletal rearrangement may rather proceed via an oxindole intermediate which can undergo transacylation:

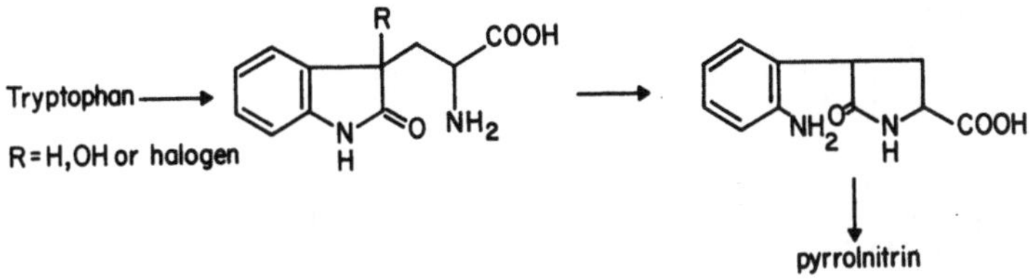

To probe this possibility, we synthesized D,L-tryptophan deuterated in the 2-position of the indole ring and fed this material to *P. aeruginosa*. Very efficient conversion into *5* with retention of the deuterium (44% specific incorporation) indicated that such a pathway can be excluded (MABE, CHANG, SHIEH, FLOSS, unpublished results). Finally, while the postulated pyrroloindole intermediate carrying chlorine in the molecule has not yet been prepared, the corresponding hydroxy analog, *18*, can be obtained from tryptophan as described by SAVIGE

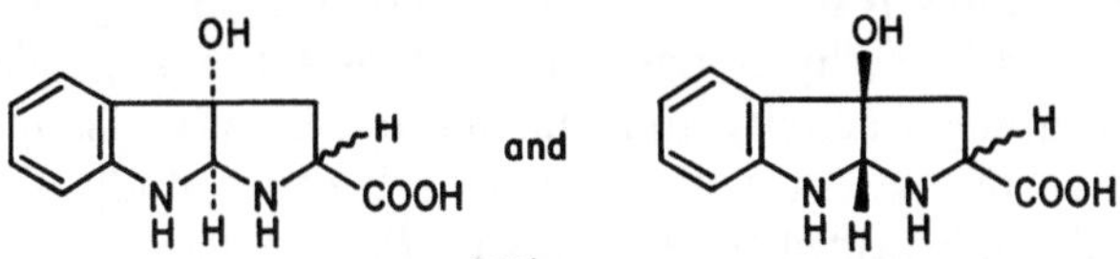

(18)

(1975). We prepared the diastereomeric mixture *18* in labeled form from D,L-[3-^{14}C]tryptophan and fed it to the pyrrolnitrin-producing cultures. No significant incorporation of radioactivity into *5* was observed, whereas tryptophan in a parallel culture gave good incorporation (MABE, CHANG, SHIEH, FLOSS, unpublished results).

The above result does, of course, not rule out the intermediacy of the originally postulated chlorinated pyrroloindole. The mechanistic difficulty with this intermediate, alluded to before, however, suggests that one should consider other possibilities. A plausible alternative is suggested by findings on the mechanism of the reaction catalyzed by indolyl-3-alkane α-hydroxylase, an enzyme recently isolated from *Pseudomonas* species (ROBERTS and ROSENFELD, 1977; TAKAI et al., 1977). Studies by ROSENFELD's group (ROSENFELD et al., 1977) and in our laboratory (TSAI et al., 1979) have shown that the initial reaction catalyzed by this enzyme is a 1,4-dehydrogenation of 3-substituted indoles to give 3-alkylidene indolenines, which then undergo secondary reactions, e.g., addition of water to side chain α-hydroxylated indoles. A similar 3-alkylidene indolenine derived from tryptophan, held on the enzyme in an orientation conducive to cyclization to the amidine, would be an attractive intermediate in pyrrolnitrin biosynthesis. We thus propose the following simple reaction sequence for the biosynthesis of *5*:

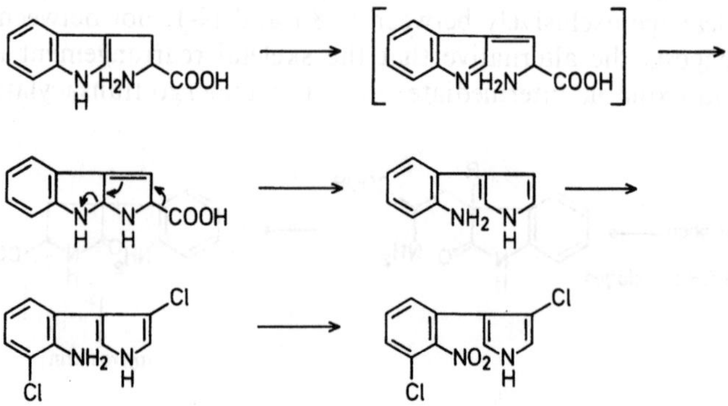

D. Other Aspects

The pyrrolnitrin fermentation represents one of the examples in which manipulation of a microbial system has been used successfully to produce structural analogs of a natural product or to improve the conditions for metabolite formation. Addition of tryptophan analogs, e.g., 6-fluorotryptophan and 7-methyltryptophan, to the cultures resulted in the production of analogs of pyrrolnitrin, e.g., 4′-fluoro-*5* and 3′-methyl-3′-deschloro-*5* (GORMAN et al., 1968). Both these analogs have antifungal activity and the fluoro derivative is, in fact, slightly more potent than the parent compound. In a broader study, the metabolism of 4-, 5-, 6-, and 7-substituted tryptophans by *P. aureofaciens* was investigated. The formation of three types of metabolites was observed: ring-substituted 3-chloroindoles (arising from 4-halogenated tryptophans), benzene-ring substituted pyrrolnitrin analogs, and benzene-ring substituted aminopyrrolnitrin analogs (HAMILL et al., 1970). As mentioned earlier, addition of D-tryptophan to cultures of *P. aeruginosa* increases the production of pyrrolnitrin (ELANDER et al., 1968); i.e., the normal fermentation depends on added D-tryptophan for maximum production of *5*. By selection of mutants resistant to tryptophan analogs, 5- and 6-fluorotryptophan, it was possible to obtain strains which no longer required addition of D-tryptophan for high antibiotic titers (ELANDER et al., 1971).

III. Dihydrophenylalanine

A. Background

L-2,5-Dihydrophenylalanine (*19*) is an almost ubiquitous constituent of Actinomycetes, which has been isolated from a variety of *Streptomyces* species

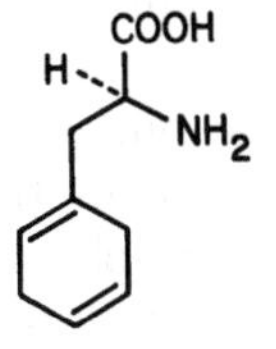

2,5 Dihydrophenylalanine (19)

by several groups (YAMASHITA et al., 1970; SCANNELL et al., 1970; FICKENSCHER et al., 1971). This antibiotic had actually been prepared synthetically before it was recognized as a natural product (SNOW et al., 1968 and SHOULDERS et al., 1968) and some of its biological properties had been studied (SNOW et al., 1968; SHOULDERS et al., 1968; GENGHOF, 1970). Dihydrophenylalanine is an antagonist of phenylalanine both in the rat (SNOW et al., 1968) and in microorganisms (YAMASHITA et al., 1970; SCANNELL et al., 1970; FICKENSCHER et al., 1971; SNOW et al., 1968; SHOULDERS et al., 1968 and GENGHOF, 1970), a finding which is plausible in light of the demonstrated planar conformation of the 1,4-cyclohexadiene ring (SHOULDERS et al., 1968). It inhibits a variety of bacteria but also shows moderate activity against some plant pathogenic fungi (YAMASHITA et al., 1970). In addition, one group reported activity against sarcoma-180 in the mouse (SCANNELL et al., 1970). The antibacterial effect of dihydrophenylalanine is overcome by phenylalanine and while one group reported that this reversal is competitive (SNOW et al., 1968), another laboratory reported noncompetitive reversal by phenylalanine but competitive reversal by tyrosine (FICKENSCHER et al., 1971; FICKENSCHER and ZÄHNER, 1971). The antibacterial activity in *E. coli* is the result of false feedback inhibition of prephenate dehydratase and the phenylalanine-sensitive DAHP synthetase by dihydrophenylalanine (FICKENSCHER and ZÄHNER, 1971). The amino acid is incorporated into the cellular protein in phenylalanine-requiring mutants of *E. coli* and sarcoma 180 (PINE, 1975). Dihydrophenylalanine was recently also isolated from a streptomycete as an inhibitor of tryptophan hydroxylase (OKABAYASHI et al., 1977).

B. Biosynthesis

SCANNELL et al. (1970) carried out two experiments on the biosynthesis of dihydrophenylalanine. Lack of incorporation of [U-^{14}C]phenylalanine

(<0.02%) but good incorporation of [U-^{14}C]shikimic acid (2.5%) indicated that the biosynthesis does not involve reduction of phenylalanine, but presumably a new variant of the shikimic acid pathway. In our studies (SHIMADA et al., 1978) we confirmed the results of SCANNELL et al. and further defined the mode of incorporation of shikimate into dihydrophenylalanine. The experiments were carried out using 100-ml shake cultures of *S. arenae* strain Tü 109, to which labeled precursors were added 24 h after inoculation. The cultures were harvested 48 h later and *19* was isolated by ion-exchange chromatography and purified by recrystallization. Degradation of *19* derived from [U-^{14}C]shikimate to benzoic acid followed by Schmidt degradation of the latter gave essentially non-radioactive CO_2, indicating that only the six ring carbons of shikimate, but not the carboxyl carbon, are incorporated into *19*. In another experiment it was shown that L-[3-^{14}C]serine is not significantly incorporated into *19*. These two pieces of evidence rule out condensation of a C_6C_1 unit with a C_2 unit (e.g., from acetate) and condensation of a C_6 unit with serine or O-acetylserine (in analogy to the tryptophan synthetase reaction) as the mode of biosynthesis of *19* and suggest, by process of elimination, its formation via chorismate.

Two modes of rearrangement of chorismate, or a derivative thereof, are known in nature which lead to attachment of the enol-pyruvyl side chain at different positions of the ring. In the normal mode of aromatic biosynthesis chorismate rearranges to prephenate with attachment of the side chain at C-1. In an alternate pathway, operating in the biosynthesis of the plant amino acids m-carboxyphenylalanine and m-carboxytyrosine (LARSEN et al., 1975), chorismate is converted to isochorismate which then rearranges to a hypothetical isoprephenate with attachment of the side chain at C-5 of chorismate (C-3 of shikimate). The two pathways have different consequences in terms of the fate of specific labels in the shikimate molecule during the conversion to *19*:

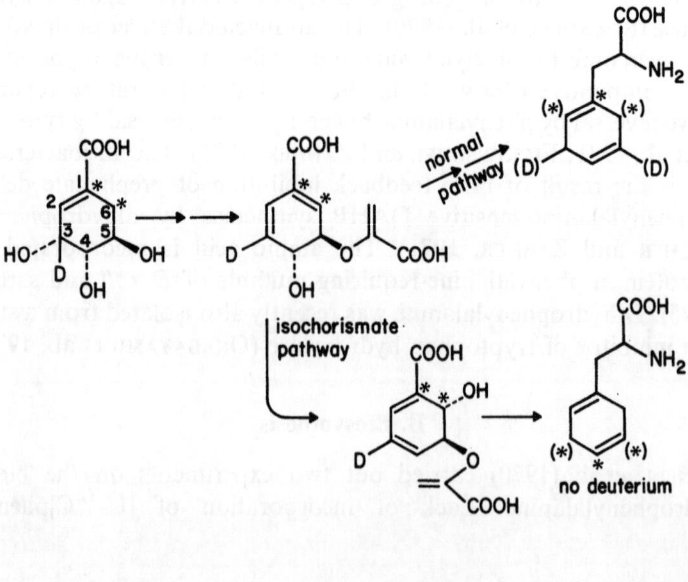

Table 5. Incorporation of chorismate and prephenate into *19*

Radioactive precursor[a]	Specific activity of starting material (μCi/mmol)	Specific activity of product (μCi/mmol)	Specific incorporation rate (%)
DL-[1,6-^{14}C]Shikimic acid[b]	16.41	0.064	0.39
[G-^{14}C]Chorismic acid	7.98	0.116	1.45
Sodium [G-^{14}C]prephenate	7.17	0.029	0.40

[a] In each experiment 0.37 mmol of precursor was fed to four 100-ml cultures; all 12 cultures were inoculated with the same inoculum

[b] DL-[1,6-^{14}C]Shikimic acid (13.9 mCi/mmol) was diluted with carrier D-shikimic acid; the data in the table refer to the D-shikimic acid only

Experimental evaluation showed that [3-^{2}H]shikimate (90% D_1, prepared by reduction of 3-dehydroshikimate with $NaBD_4$) gave *19* containing 13.8% deuterium, and degradation of *19*, biosynthesized from D,L-[1,6-^{14}C]shikimate, via phenylalanine indicated the presence of almost half of the ^{14}C (46%) in the position(s) ortho to the side chain and virtually no ^{14}C (<5%) in the para position. It is therefore concluded that the biosynthesis of *19* proceeds by the normal pathway via prephenate. This conclusion was confirmed by preparing biosynthetically generally ^{14}C-labeled chorismate and prephenate and demonstrating their incorporation into *19* (Table 5). The poorer utilization of prephenate compared to chorismate is probably due to its instability.

The finding that prephenate is a likely intermediate in the biosynthesis of *19* raises an interesting stereochemical question. Both in shikimate and in *19* the two 'halves' of the six-membered ring (assuming the ring is bisected along the C-1/C-4 axis) are not identical, whereas prephenate is a symmetrical compound. However, in the latter the two 'halves' of the ring are in an enantiotopic relationship and should therefore be distinguishable to an enzyme. The mode of conversion of shikimate into prephenate is known, and one can therefore ask the question which side of the ring of prephenate gives rise to which side of the ring of *19*:

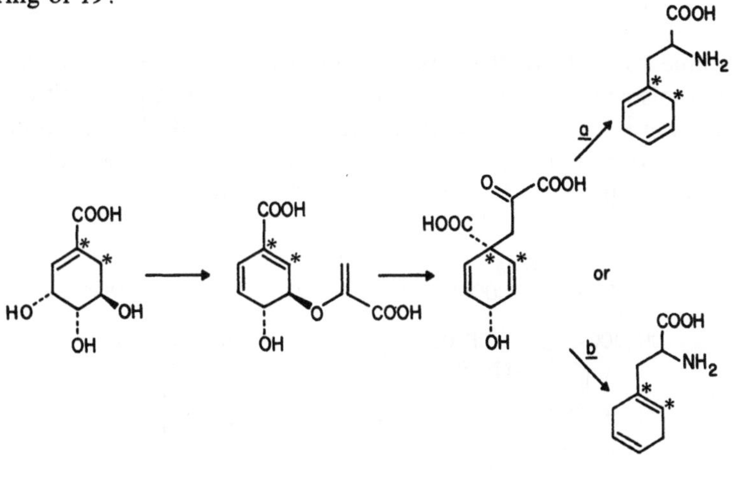

To answer this question a degradation of *19* biosynthesized from D,L-[1,6-^{14}C]shikimate was carried out which preserves the asymmetry of the substituted cyclohexadiene ring. Conversion of *19* to dihydrophenylacetic acid by incubation with L-amino acid oxidase, reduction to the corresponding alcohol followed by ozonolysis, and decomposition of the ozonide gave a mixture of 1,3-propanediol and 1,3,5-pentanetriol, which were separated and isolated as their p-nitro-

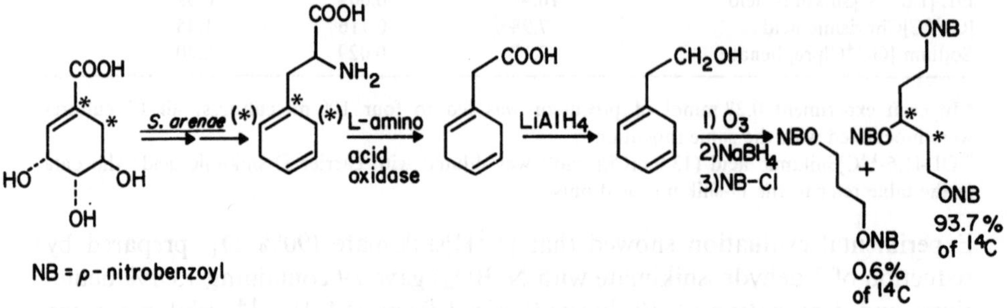

benzoyl derivatives. The results of the degradation, exclusive labeling of the pentanetriol, clearly indicate that the utilization of prephenate is stereospecific and that half of the label from [1,6-^{14}C]shikimate resides at C-6′ of *19*.

The conversion of prephenate to *19* requires a reduction as well as elimination steps, which must occur in such a way that they do not lead to the ultimate formation of a conjugated diene. One plausible reaction sequence would be initiated by reduction of one of the double bonds in the ring of prephenate, followed by an allylic decarboxylation and loss of water:

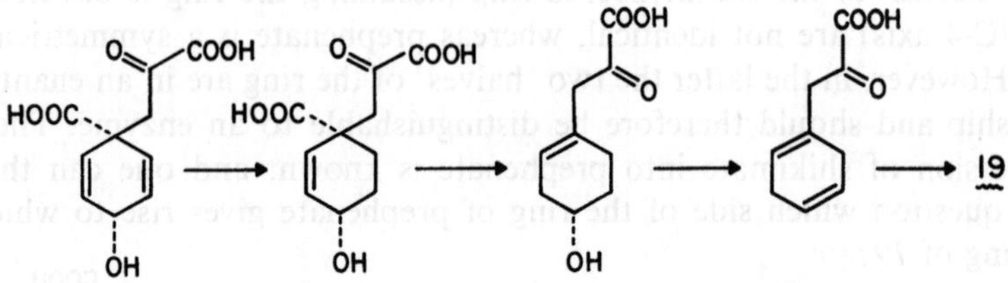

We were able to evaluate this route by preparing and feeding a mixture of all four stereoisomers of dihydroprephenate tritiated in the 4-position of the ring. These were obtained by tritiated sodium borohydride reduction of the dimethyl ester dimethyl ketal of the corresponding α, β-unsaturated ketone, which was kindly provided by Prof. DANISHEFSKY, Pittsburgh:

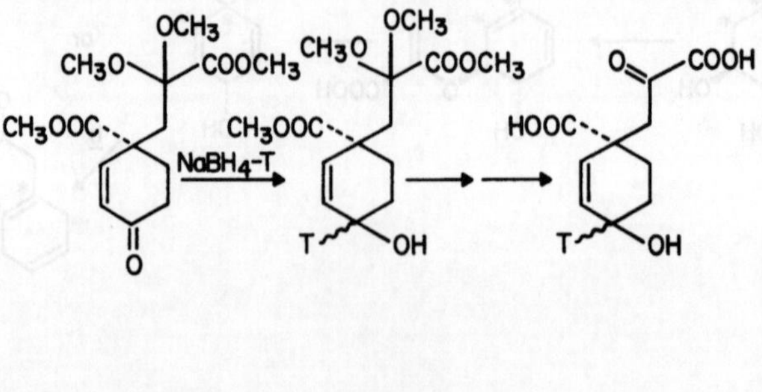

Table 6. Comparison of the incorporation of dihydroprephenate, prephenate, and shikimate into *19*

Radioactive precursor	Specific activity of starting material (µCi/mmol)	Specific activity of product (µCi/mmol)	Radio-activity of starting material (µCi)	Radio-activity of product (µCi)	Specific incorpo-ration rate (%)	Incorpo-ration rate (%)
DL-[1,6-^{14}C]Shikimic acid	⩾1,000		10.7	1.76×10^{-1}		1.64
[4-^{3}H]Dihydroprephenic acid dimethyl ester	⩾1,000		29.5	4.19×10^{-3}		0.01
[4-^{3}H]Dihydroprephenic acid	⩾1,000		19.8	8.59×10^{-3}		0.04
DL-[1,6-^{14}C]Shikimic acid, 0.38 mmol	31.42	1.04×10^{-1}			0.33	
Sodium [G-^{14}C]prephenate, 0.38 mmol	6.29	2.59×10^{-2}			0.41	

Both the free acid form of the compound and the dimethyl ester were fed to the cultures in order to compare their incorporation to that of prephenate. Because of large differences in the specific activities and the lack of carrier material a direct comparison was not possible; instead, under two different sets of identical conditions, dihydroprephenate and prephenate were each compared to shikimate. As the results summarized in Table 6 indicate, there was no significant incorporation of dihydroprephenate into *19*, while both shikimate and prephenate were well utilized.

The elimination of a biosynthetic route to *19* via dihydroprephenate suggests as an alternative the following reaction sequence, which would constitute a plausible pathway:

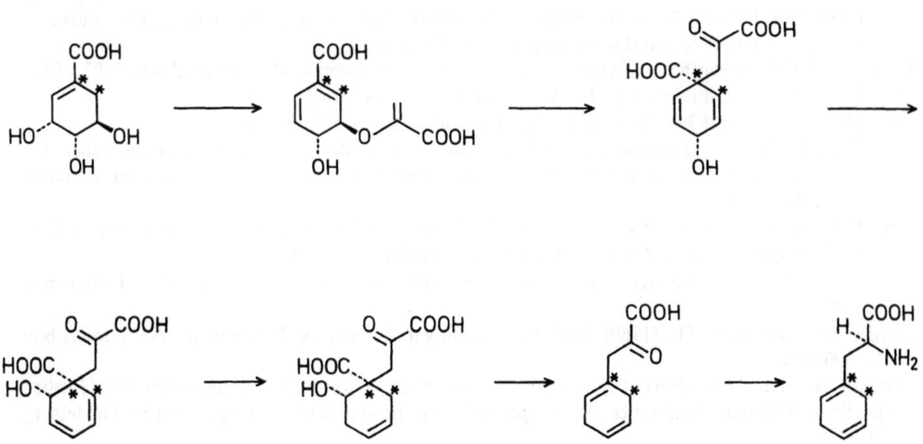

The proposed mechanism for the conversion of prephenate to the keto acid corresponding to *19* consists of two reaction steps which combined would constitute the normal prephenate dehydratase reaction, and interposed between them the 1,4-reduction of an intermediate diene system. The proposed intermediates in this sequence are obviously compounds which are very hard to synthesize, making it difficult to prove or disprove this proposal. We are therefore embarking on a program to obtain mutants of *S. arenae* Tü 109, which are blocked in the conversion of prephenate to tyrosine and phenylalanine, in order to study the formation of *19 in vitro*.

Acknowledgments. Work from the author's laboratory was supported by the U.S. Public Health Service through NIH Research Grants AI 11728 and GM 18852. This chapter was written during a visit to the University of Riyad; the author wishes to thank Dean Ibrahim A. Al-Sowaygh of the Faculty of Pharmacy for his kind hospitality.

References

Ajisaka M, Kariyone K, Fomon K, Yazawa H, Arima K (1969) Isolation of the bromo analog of pyrrolnitrin from *Pseudomonas pyrrolnitrica*. Agric Biol Chem 33:294–295

Arima K, Imanaka H, Konsaka M, Fukuda A, Tamura G (1965) Studies on pyrrolnitrin, a new antibiotic. I. Isolation and properties of pyrrolnitrin. J Antibiot Ser A 18:201–204

Chan TM, Hill RK (1970) The absolute configuration of indolmycin. J Org Chem 35:3519–3521

Chang C-J, Floss HG, Hurley LH, Zmijewski M (1976) Application of long-range spin-spin couplings in biosynthetic studies. J Org Chem 41:2932–2934

Elander RP, Mabe JH, Hamill RH, Gorman M (1968) Metabolism of tryptophan by *Pseudomonas aureofaciens*. VI. Production of pyrrolnitrin by selected *Pseudomonas* species. Appl Microbiol 16:753–758

Elander RP, Hamill RL, Gorman M, Mabe J (1971) Biosynthesis of pyrrolnitrin by analogue-resistant mutants of *Pseudomonas fluorescens*. Folia Microbiol 16:156

Fickenscher U, Zähner H (1971) Zur Wirkungsweise des L-2,5-Dihydrophenylalanins, eines Phenylalaninantagonisten. Arch Mikrobiol 76:28–46

Fickenscher U, Keller-Schierlein W, Zähner H (1971) L-2,5-Dihydrophenylalanin. Arch Microbiol 75:346–352

Filacchioni G, Artico M, Brosio E, Conti F (1978) Pyrrolnitrin analogues. V. Knorr's pyrrole condensation between N-(4-nitrophenacyl)-3,5-dimethylaniline and ethyl acetoacetate. Farmaco Ed Sci 33:48–63 (1978); and 4 earlier papers in this series

Floss HG (1976) Biosynthesis of ergot alkaloids and related compounds. Tetrahedron 32:873–912

Floss HG (1978) The shikimate pathway. Recent Adv Phytochem 12:59–89

Floss HG, Tsai MD (1979) Chiral methyl groups. Adv Enzymol 50:243–302

Floss HG, Mothes U, Guenther H (1964) Zur Biosynthese der Mutterkornalkaloide. Über den Einbau der Tryptophan-Seitenkette und den Mechanismus der Reaktion am α-C-Atom. Z Naturforsch 19b:784–788

Floss HG, Manni PE, Hamill RL, Mabe JA (1971) Further studies on the biosynthesis of pyrrolnitrin from tryptophan by *Pseudomonas*. Biochem Biophys Res Commun 45:781–787

Genghof DS (1970) 2,5-Dihydrophenylalanine as an inhibitor of microbial growth. Can J Microbiol 16:545–547

Gordee RS, Matthews TR (1969) Systemic Antifungal Activity of Pyrrolnitrin. Appl Microbiol 17:690–694

Gorman M, Lively DH (1967) Pyrrolnitrin: A new mode of tryptophan metabolism. In: Gottlieb D, Shaw PD (ed) Antibiotics vol II, pp 433–438. Biosynthesis, Springer, Berlin Heidelberg New York

Gorman M, Hamill RL, Elander RP, Mabe J (1968) Preparation of substituted phenyl pyrroles through the metabolism of tryptophan analogues. Biochem Biophys Res Commun 31: 294–298

Gosteli J (1972) Eine neue Synthese des Antibioticums Pyrrolnitrin. Helv Chim Acta 55:451–460

Hamill R, Elander R, Mabe J, Gorman M (1968) Metabolism of tryptophans by *Pseudomonas aureofaciens*. V. Conversion of tryptophan to pyrrolnitrin. Antimicrob Agents Chemother-1967, 388–396

Hamill RL, Elander RP, Mabe JA, Gorman M (1970) Metabolism of tryptophan by *Pseudomonas aureofaciens*. III. Production of substituted pyrrolnitrins from tryptophan analogues. Appl Microbiol 19:721–725

Harnden MR, Wright ND (1977) Total synthesis of thiazolinone analogues of indolmycin. J Chem Soc Perkin I:1012–1018

Harnden MR, Bailey S, Boyd MR, Taylor DR, Wright ND (1978) Thiazolinone analogues of indolmycin with antiviral and antibacterial activity. J Med Chem 21:82–87

Hashimoto M, Hattori K (1966a) Isopyrrolnitrin, a metabolite from *Pseudomonas*. Bull Chem Soc 39:410

Hashimoto M, Hattori K (1966b) Oxypyrrolnitrin: A metabolite of *Pseudomonas*. Chem Pharm Bull 14:1314–1316

Hashimoto M, Hattori K (1968) A new metabolite from *Pseudomonas pyrrolnitrica*. Chem Pharm Bull 16:1144

Hirota A, Higashinaka Y, Sakai H (1978) Isolation of indolmycin and its derivative as antagonists of L-tryptophan. Agric Biol Chem 42:147–151

Hornemann U, Hurley LH, Speedie MK, Floss HG (1970a) Isolation and absolute configuration of indolmycenic acid, an intermediate in the biosynthesis of indolmycin by *Streptomyces griseus*. Tetrahedron Lett 2255–2258

Hornemann U, Speedie MK, Hurley LH, Floss HG (1970b) Demonstration of a C-methylating enzyme in cell free extracts of indolmycin-producing *Streptomyces griseus*. Biochem Biophys Res Commun 39:594–599

Hornemann U, Hurley LH, Speedie MK, Floss HG (1971) The biosynthesis of indolmycin. J Am Chem Soc 93:3028–3035

Hurley LH, Bialek D (1974) Regulation of antibiotic production: Catabolite inhibition and the dualistic effect of glucose on indolmycin production. J Antibiot 27:49–56

Imanaka H, Kousaka M, Tamura A, Arima K (1965a) Studies on pyrrolnitrin, a new antibiotic. II. Taxonomic studies on pyrrolnitrin-producing strain. J Antibiot Ser A 18:205–206

Imanaka H, Kousaka M, Tamura G, Arima K (1965b) Studies on pyrrolnitrin, a new antibiotic. III. Structure of pyrrolnitrin. J Antibiot Ser A 18:207–210

Imanaka H, Ajisaka M, Hattori K, Tamura G, Arima K (1972) Studies on pyrrolnitrin fermentation. In: Terui G (ed) Fermentation Technology Today, pp 619–621. Proc 4th Int Ferment Symp, Kyoto

Lambowitz AM, Slayman CW (1972) Effect of pyrrolnitrin on electron transport and oxidative phosphorylation in mitochondria isolated from *Neurospora crassa*. J Bacteriol 112:1020–1022

Larsen PO, Onderka D, Floss HG (1975) Biosynthesis of phenylalanine, tyrosine, 3-(3-carboxyphenyl)alanine and 3-(3-carboxy-4-hydroxyphenyl)alanine in higher plants. Biochem Biophys Acta 381:397–408

Lively DH, Gorman M, Haney ME, Mabe JA (1966) Metabolism of tryptophans by *Pseudomonas aureofaciens*. I. Biosynthesis of pyrrolnitrin. Antimicrob Agents Chemother 462–469

Marsh WS, Garretson AL, Wesel EM (1960) PA 155A, B and X. Antibiotics produced by a strain of *Streptomyces albus*. Antibiot Chemother 10:316–320

Martin LL, Chang C-J, Floss HG, Mabe JA, Hagaman EW, Wenkert E (1972) A ^{13}C nuclear magnetic resonance study on the biosynthesis of pyrrolnitrin from tryptophan by *Pseudomonas*. J Am Chem Soc 94:8942–8944

Mascaro L, Hörhammer R, Eisenstein S, Sellers LK, Mascaro K, Floss HG (1977) Synthesis of methionine carrying a chiral methyl group and its use in determining the steric course of the enzymatic C-methylation of indolepyruvate during indolmycin biosynthesis. J Am Chem Soc 99:273–274

Morimoto Y, Hashimoto M, Hattori K (1968) The crystal structure of pyrrolnitrin. Tetrahedron Lett 209–211

Nakano H, Umio S, Kariyone K, Tanaka K, Kishimoto T, Noguchi H, Ueda J, Nakamura H, Morimoto Y (1966) Total synthesis of pyrrolnitrin, a new antibiotic. Tetrahedron Lett 737–740

Nishida M, Matsubara T, Watanabe N (1965) Pyrrolnitrin, a new antifungal antibiotic. Microbiological and toxicological observations. J Antibiot Ser A 18:211–219

Nose M, Arima K (1969) On the mode of action of a new antifungal antibiotic, pyrrolnitrin. J Antibiot 22:135–143

Ohno M, Spande TF, Witkop B (1970) Cyclization of tryptophan and tryptamine derivatives to 2,3-dihydropyrrolo[2,3-b]indoles. J Am Chem Soc 92:343–348

Okabayashi K, Morishima H, Hamada M, Takeuchi T, Umezawa H (1977) A tryptophan hydroxylase inhibitor produced by a Streptomycete: 2,5-Dihydro-L-phenylalanine. J Antibiot 30:675–677

Padeiskaya E, Pershin GN, Kutchak SN, Gerchikov LN, Egorova EF, Preobrazhenskaya MN, Suvorov NN (1972) Experimental studies on indolmycin. Antibiotiki 17:927–932

Pine MJ (1975) Incorporation of L-2,5-dihydrophenylalanine into cell proteins of *Escherichia coli* and Sarcoma 180. Antimicrob Agents Chemother 7:601–605

Preobrazhenskaya MN, Balashova EG, Turchin KF, Padeiskaya EN, Uvarova NY, Pershin GN, Suvorov NN (1968) Total synthesis of antibiotic indolmycin and its stereoisomers. Tetrahedron 24:6131–6143

Rao KV (1960) PA 155H: A new antibiotic. Antibiot Chemother 10:312–315

Roberts J, Rosenfeld HJ (1977) Isolation, crystallization, and properties of indolyl-3-alkane α-hydroxylase. J Biol Chem 252:2640–2647

Rose JA (1970) Stereochemistry of pyruvate kinase, pyruvate carboxylase, and malate enzyme reactions. J Biol Chem 245:6052–6056

Rosenfeld HJ, Watanabe N, Roberts J (1977) Mechanism of action of indolyl-3-alkane α-hydroxylase. J Biol Chem 252:6970–6973

Routien JB (1966) Identity of Streptomycete producing antibiotic PA 155A. J Bacteriol 91:1663

Salcher O, Lingens F (1978) Biosynthese von Pyrrolnitrin. Nachweis von 3-chloranthranilsäure and 7-chlorindolessigsäure im Kulturmedium von *Pseudomonas aureofaciens*. Tetrahedron Lett 3101–3102

Salcher O, Lingens F, Fischer P (1978) Biosynthese von Pyrrolnitrin. Nachweis von 4-(2′-amino-3′-chlorphenyl)pyrrol-2-carbonsäure. Tetrahedron Lett 3097–3100

Savige WE (1975) New oxidation products of tryptophan. Aust J Chem 28:2275–2287

Scannell JP, Pruess DL, Demney TC, Williams T, Stempel A (1970) L-3-(2,5-Dihydrophenyl)alanine, an antimetabolite of L-phenylalanine produced by a streptomycete. J Antibiot 23:618–619

Schach v Wittenau M, Els H (1961) The structure of indolmycin. J Am Chem Soc 83:4678–4679

Schach v Wittenau M, Els H (1963) Chemistry of indolmycin. J Am Chem Soc 85:3425–3431

Shimada K, Hook DJ, Warner GF, Floss HG (1978) Biosynthesis of the antibiotic 2,5-dihydrophenylalanine by *Streptomyces arenae*. Biochemistry 17:3054–3058

Shoulders BA, Gipson RM, Jandacek RF, Simonsen SH, Shive W (1968) Conformation and biological activity of 1,4-cyclohexadiene derivatives. J Am Chem Soc 90:2992–2993

Sjöberg B (1958) Stereochemical studies. VI. Steric relations of some α-arylpropionic acids. Ark Kemi 13:1–10

Skye GE, Potts R, Floss HG (1974) Stereochemistry of the tryptophan synthetase reaction. J Am Chem Soc 96:1593–1595

Snow ML, Lauinger C, Ressler C (1968) 1,4-Cyclohexadiene-1-alanine (2,5-dihydrophenylalanine), a new inhibitor of phenylalanine for the rat and *Leuconostoc dextranicum* 8086. J Org Chem 33:1774–1780

Speedie MK, Hornemann U, Floss HG (1975) Isolation and characterization of tryptophan transaminase and indolepyruvate C-methyltransferase. Enzymes involved in indolmycin biosynthesis in *Streptomyces griseus*. J Biol Chem 250:7819–7825

Takai K, Ushiro H, Noada Y, Navomiya S, Tokuyama T, Hayaishi O (1977) Crystalline hemoprotein from *Pseudomonas* that catalyzes oxidation of side chain of tryptophan and other indole derivatives. J Biol Chem 252:2648–2656

Tanaka K, Kariyone K, Umio S (1969) Total synthesis of pyrrolnitrin. X. Synthesis of pyrrolnitrin. Chem Pharm Bull 17:622–628 and nine earlier papers in this series

Tripathi RK, Gottlieb D (1969) Mechanism of action of the antifungal antibiotic pyrrolnitrin. J Bacteriol 100:310–318

Tsai MD, Schleicher E, Potts R, Skye GE, Floss HG (1978) Stereochemistry and mechanism of reactions catalyzed by tryptophan synthetase and its B_2 subunit. J Biol Chem 253:5344–5349
Tsai MD, Floss HG, Rosenfeld HJ, Roberts J (1979) Stereochemistry and mechanism of reactions catalyzed by indolyl-3-alkane α-hydroxylase. J Biol Chem 254:6437–6443
Umio S, Kariyone K, Tanaka K, Kishimoto T, Nakamura H, Nishida M (1970) Structure activity studies of pyrrolnitrin analogues. Chem Pharm Bull 18:1414–1425
Werner RG, Thorpe LF, Reuter W, Nierhaus KH (1976) Indolmycin inhibits prokaryotic tryptophanyl-tRNA ligase. Eur J Biochem 68:1–3
Wong DT, Airall JM (1970) The mode of action of antifungal agents: Effect of pyrrolnitrin on mitochondrial electron transport. J Antibiot 23:55–62
Wong DT, Horng J-S, Gordee RS (1971) Respiratory chain of a pathogenic fungus; *Microsporum gypseum:* Effect of the antifungal agent pyrrolnitrin. J Bacteriol 106:168–173
Yamashita T, Miyairi N, Kumugita K, Shimizu K, Sakai H (1970) L-1,4-cyclohexadiene-1-alanine, an antagonist of phenylalanine, from Streptomyces. J Antibiot 23:537–541
Zee L, Hornemann U, Floss HG (1975) Further studies on the biosynthesis of the antibiotic indolmycin in *Streptomyces griseus.* Biochem Physiol Pflanz 168:19–25

Pyrrolo(1,4)benzodiazepine Antibiotics: Anthramycin, Tomaymycin, and Sibiromycin

LAURENCE H. HURLEY and MARILYN K. SPEEDIE

I. Introduction

The pyrrolo(1,4)benzodiazepine antibiotics are a group of structurally closely related antitumor agents that include anthramycin, tomaymycin, sibiromycin, and the neothramycins A and B (Fig. 1). Biosynthetic studies have been carried out primarily on anthramycin, tomaymycin, and sibiromycin (L.H. Hurley, 1977). The purpose of this review is to present a comprehensive, up-to-date account of both the published work and more recent studies aimed at elucidating the general biosynthetic pathways which lead to these antibiotics. A more general review on the chemistry, biosynthesis, mechanism of action, biological effects, and toxicities of these antibiotics has appeared (L.H. HURLEY, 1977).

Although the therapeutic potential of anthramycin and related compounds as antitumor agents has not as yet been proven in clinical practice, these agents are of potential interest in chemotherapy since the manner in which these compounds interact with DNA is unusual (L.H. HURLEY et al., 1977; K.W. KOHN et al., 1974).

Structurally, the pyrrolo(1,4)benzodiazepine antibiotics are unique in nature and upon inspection of their structures for possible biosynthetic correlates it is only immediately obvious that the anthranilic acid moieties are probably derived from tryptophan via the kynurenine pathway. The C_2 and C_3-proline units of anthramycin, tomaymycin, and sibiromycin would appear to be most rationally derived from either proline or condensation of two molecules of δ-aminolevulinic acid or conceivably an acetate/propionate pathway (Scheme 1). Early biosynthetic experiments, however, quickly eliminated these as viable possibilities. A clue to their biosynthetic origin can be found in some earlier work carried out by WITZ and co-workers at Upjohn Company (D.F. WITZ et al., 1971). In this case the propylhygric acid moiety of lincomycin A was found to be derived from tyroisine and involved a 'meta cleavage' of the aromatic ring. Subsequent work at Kentucky revealed that the C_2 and C_3-proline units of anthramycin, tomaymycin, and sibiromycin were biosynthetically derived in an essentially similar way from tyrosine via dopa and a ring cleavage product (Scheme 1).

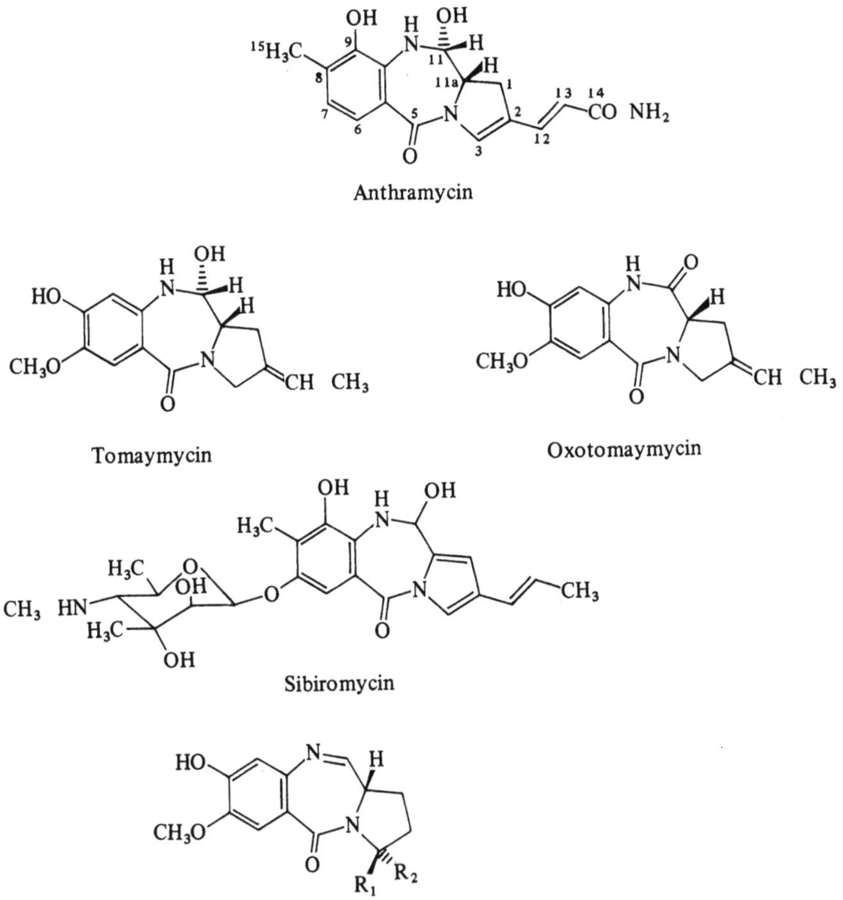

Neothramycin A $R_1 = H$ $R_2 = OH$
Neothramycin B $R_1 = OH$ $R_2 = H$

Fig. 1. Structures of the pyrrolo(1,4)benzodiazepine antitumor antibiotics

II. Physiological Studies

A. Anthramycin

1. Growth and Production

Conditions for optimal growth and production on complex media were first described by BERGER et al. (1971). As is expressed in the name, *Streptomyces refuineus* var *thermotolerans* is a thermophilic organism and optimal growth and production occur when the organism is grown in the range from 40° to about 50° C (J. BERGER et al., 1971). Most of the physiological and biosynthetic studies have been performed using the organism grown at 46° C. Agitation

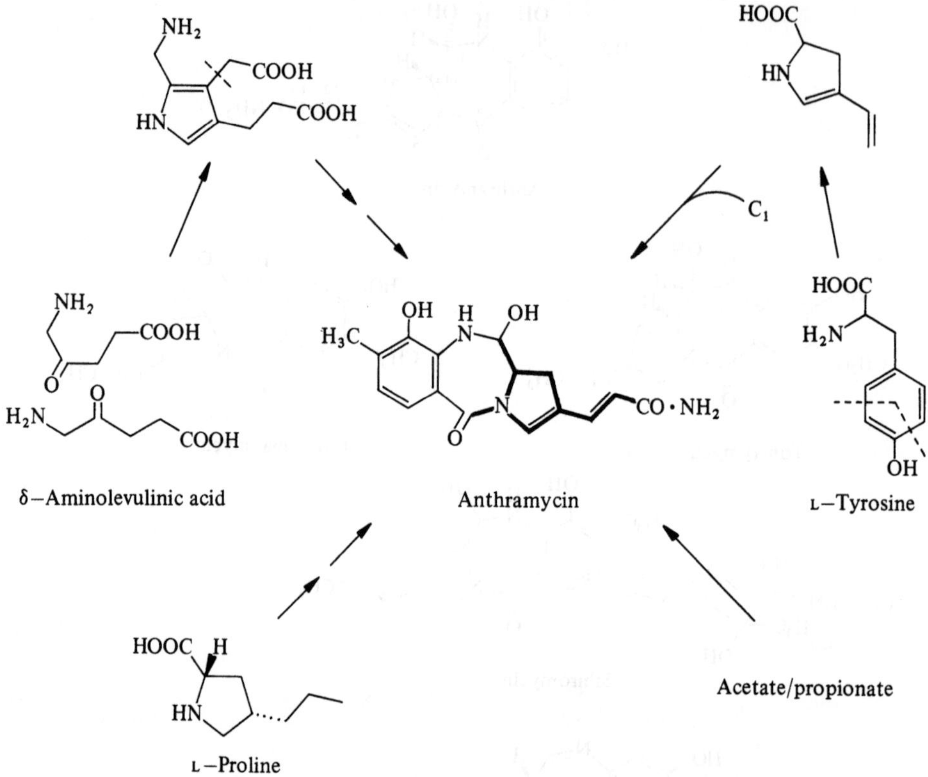

Scheme 1. Possible biosynthetic precursors for the C_3-proline unit of anthramycin

and adequate aeration are important to production. When shake flask fermentation is desired, adequate aeration can be achieved by employing baffled flasks and a rotatory shaker speed of 250 r.p.m. A variety of complex and defined media have been used for the biosynthetic and physiological regulation studies. Typically, a seed medium of trypticase-soy broth (DIFCO) or a complex medium composed of cornstarch, peptonized milk, and dried yeast (L.H. HURLEY et al., 1975) inoculated with spores from agar slants and grown for 24 h. Cells are centrifuged and rinsed and used to inoculate complex or defined production media. The complex medium usually employed is that previously described as the 'seed medium.' The defined media used include one composed of lysine HCl (0.15%), potato starch (1.0%), KH_2PO_4 (0.01%), and $CaCO_3$ (0.01%), and one modified from HOPWOOD (1977) in that glucose 1.0% is substituted for the mannitol, glycerol and sucrose and an amino acid mixture (50 μg/ml) is added. An alternative procedure employed to achieve production of anthramycin is to inoculate the complex medium with cells from the seed culture and after 16-h growth, centrifuge, wash, and resuspend the cells with a two- to threefold increase in cell concentration in 0.05 M phosphate buffer, pH 6.8. Anthramycin production starts promptly when the flasks are shaken at 46° C at 250 r.p.m. and continues for 6 h (C. GAIROLA and L.H. HURLEY, 1976).

2. Time Course

In all media studies as described above, anthramycin is produced during the growth phase or trophophase although the time course of production varies somewhat from medium to medium (Fig. 2a–d). In the defined media employed, production starts promptly upon inoculation and proceeds throughout the growth phase, usually reaching maximum with or slightly preceding the peak in growth as measured by mycelial weight. However, in a complex medium (the 'seed' medium described above) there is a lag in production followed by a spurt of synthesis in the late growth phase. In another complex medium consisting of 2% peptone, 0.2% yeast, and trace elements, production occurs during growth phase but continues into the idiophase and peaks after growth has stopped. While secondary metabolite formation by microorganisms if frequently reported to occur principally during the stationary phase (idiophase), the formation of anthramycin during the growth phase is not a unique situation.

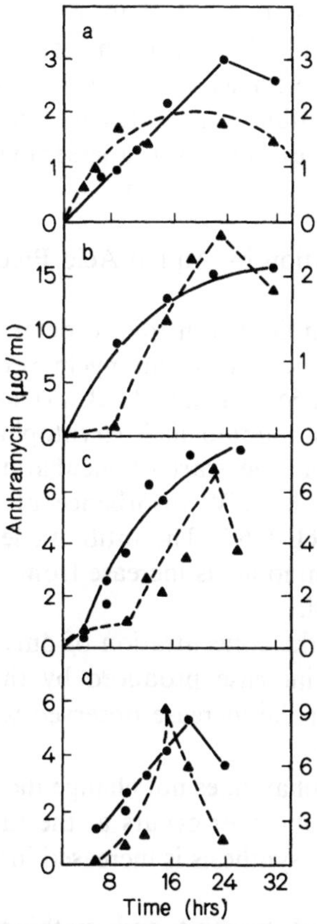

Fig. 2a–d. Time course patterns for anthramycin production in four different culture media. Mycelial dry weight (–●–); anthramycin (–▲–). **a** $NaNO_3$/mannitol-sucrose-glycerol/salts (defined) medium; **b** Lysine/potato starch medium (defined); **c** Peptone/yeast extract medium (complex); **d** Peptonized milk/cornstarch/yeast extract medium (complex)

Numerous examples of antibiotic synthesis occurring simultaneously with the cells' growth have been reported (T.K. AUDHYA and D.W. RUSSELL, 1975; D. HENDLIN, 1949). The production of actinomycin (V.K. WILLIAMS and E. KATZ, 1977) and the production of chloramphenicol (V.S. MALIK, 1972) both have been reported to occur during the idiophase in complex medium and during the exponential growth phase in defined medium. The time course pattern of biosynthesis appears to depend somewhat on environmental and nutritional factors in these examples and anthramycin biosynthesis is apparently similarly controlled.

In all media used in these studies the levels of anthramycin peak after 12- to 23-h incubation, depending upon the medium, and then decrease. It is possible the fall is due to pH factors as it is known that anthramycin is unstable in aqueous solution outside a narrow pH range near neutrality (J. BERGER et al., 1971). Incubation of added anthramycin with the filtered medium after various periods of fermentation indicates that the rate of decomposition of the antibiotic increases substantially in the period following the normal peak of anthramycin production (M.K. SPEEDIE, unpublished results). GAIROLA and HURLEY (1976) reported that the addition of exogenous methionine reduces anthramycin yields presumably by the formation of methionine metabolites which interact with anthramycin as it is formed. They also reported a loss of anthramycin when the antibiotic is added to filtered broths of the control cultures (no added methionine), though to a lesser extent.

3. Regulation by Amino Acid Precursors

Experiments performed in defined media to determine the effects of varying levels of precursor amino acids on anthramycin production have resulted in the following findings (M.K. SPEEDIE and M.B. FORBES, 1977).

1. When the three precursor amino acids (tryptophan, tyrosine, and methionine) are added to a media at the start of incubation there is an increase in antibiotic titer as measured by UV absorbance at 335 nm and by bioassay against *Bacillus subtilis* (NRRL 3167). The antibiotic level progressively increases as the levels of exogenous amino acids increase from 0.1 mM to 0.5 mM, where a three-fold increase is found.

2. Experiments in which the concentration of only one precursor was varied at a time showed that the increase produced by the addition of tryptophan alone could fully account for the increase observed when all three amino acids were added at 0.5 mM levels.

3. The addition of tryptophan does not change the time course of the biosynthesis. The maximum antibiotic titer occurs at the same time as in the control flask but the *rate* of antibiotic synthesis is increased in the tryptophan-containing fermentation.

4. Addition of exogenous tyrosine and methionine at concentrations of 0.5 mM and higher decrease the stimulatory effect caused by the addition of tryptophan. Methionine causes a 67% and a 74% decrease in antibiotic levels at 0.5 mM and 2.5 mM of methionine respectively. Tyrosine, on the other hand,

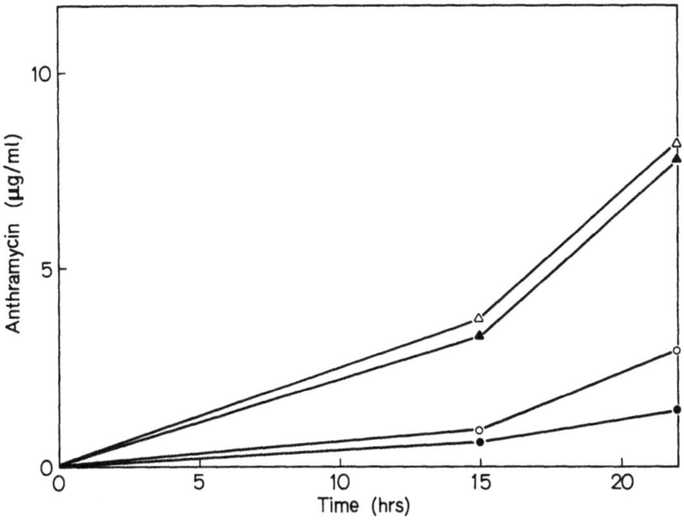

Fig. 3. Effect of late additions of tryptophan on anthramycin production. L-tryptophan was added to cultures as follows: none added (-●-); none at start, 1 mM after 15 h (-○-); 1 mM at start only (-▲-); 1 mM at start, additional 204 μg/ml (-△-) added after 15 h of incubation

has no significant effect at 0.5 mM but causes a 43% decrease at 2.5 mM. The effect of methionine is congruent with the findings of GAIROLA and HURLEY (1976) in an experiment performed in the system which employs cells suspended in phosphate buffer.

5. Addition of tryptophan later in the fermentative course (at 15 h in a system in which production peaks at 24 h) has a lesser stimulatory effect upon the rate of antibiotic production than the addition of tryptophan at the start of incubation. No additional stimulation is observed when cultures which contain tryptophan at the start of incubation receive additional tryptophan after 15 h (M.K. SPEEDIE, unpublished results) (see Fig. 3). This suggests that the rate of production is not strictly proportional to tryptophan concentration at any given time although uptake of the added tryptophan may be an interfering factor.

The question arises whether the observed effect of tryptophan represents an induction of an enzyme or enzymes in the biosynthetic pathway such as is seen with ergot alkaloid biosynthesis (V.M. KRUPINSKI et al., 1976) or simply a substrate effect involving saturation of existing enzyme at the rate-limiting step of the biosynthetic pathway. Tryptophan analogs have proved very useful in the study of ergot alkaloid biosynthesis because the analogs will sometimes replicate the regulatory aspects of tryptophan without themselves being incorporated into the product. This permits differentiation between increases due to the role of the precursor as an inducer of an enzyme and the increases due simply to increased availability of substrate. The requirements for such an analog are 1. that the analog is not itself incorporated into product and 2. that the analog does not inhibit growth of the organism.

To test this approach with the anthramycin producer, tryptophan analogs including D,L-thiotryptophan, D,L-5-methyltryptophan, L-5-hydroxytryptophan, and D,L-7-azatryptophan were added to the fermentation broth at the start of incubation. Only the extract from the culture incubated with 5-methyltryptophan gave UV absorbances at 335 nm comparable to those obtained when L-tryptophan is added to the medium (M.K. SPEEDIE and M.B. FORBES, 1977). All the other analogs resulted in a reduction in mycelial weights and anthramycin production, as indicated by UV absorbance of the butanol extract. While these results suggest that 5-methyltryptophan may be causing enzyme induction, a bioassay of the extracts from cultures exposed to 5-methyltryptophan indicated that there was less antibiotic activity present than even the control cultures, suggesting that the observed UV absorbance is not entirely due to anthramycin. This was confirmed by experiments in which the radioactive precursor of the non-tryptophan moiety, L-(1-^{14}C)tyrosine, was fed to the cultures along with nonradioactive 5-methyltryptophan. A scan of the thin-layer chromatograph of the resulting extract shows a peak which runs at a slightly lower Rf than anthramycin methylether and a calculation of tyrosine incorporation into the peak corresponding to anthramycin methylether shows incorporation about 70% of control, thus substantiating the bioassay results (M.K. SPEEDIE, unpublished results). Experiments are currently underway to determine the identity of the tyrosine-incorporating substance that appears in the 5-methyltryptophan supplemented cultures.

The negative results of the tryptophan analog studies do not exclude the possibility that inducation by tryptophan does occur so experiments are currently underway to determine levels of enzymes early in the branch of the pathway leading from tryptophan to 3-hydroxy-4-methylanthranilic acid. Specifically, the first enzyme in the pathway, tryptophan oxygenase, is a likely candidate as a site of regulation. This enzyme has been detected in cell-free extracts of *S. refuineus* using a well-established assay for tryptophan oxygenase activity (G. SCHULTZ and P. FEIGELSON, 1972) and work is in progress toward characterizing it and studying its regulatory properties (M.K. SPEEDIE, unpublished results).

B. Tomaymycin

Tomaymycin is a Japanese antibiotic which is produced alongside its biologically inactive metabolite oxotomymycin by *Streptomyces achromogenes* var. *tomaymyceticus* (K. ARIMA et al., 1972; L.H. HURLEY et al., 1976a). Tomaymycin is produced in a complex media at 32°, antibiotic production occurring at 72 h at the end of the growth phase (L.H. HURLEY et al., 1976a) (Fig. 4).

C. Sibiromycin

Sibiromycin, a Russian antibiotic, is produced by the actinomycete *Streptosporangium sibiricum* sp. *nov* and was isolated by GAUSE and workers at the Moscow Institute for New Antibiotics (G.F. GAUSE et al., 1969). This antibiotic is produced in a complex media at 28° C (L.H. HURLEY et al., 1979b) (Fig. 5).

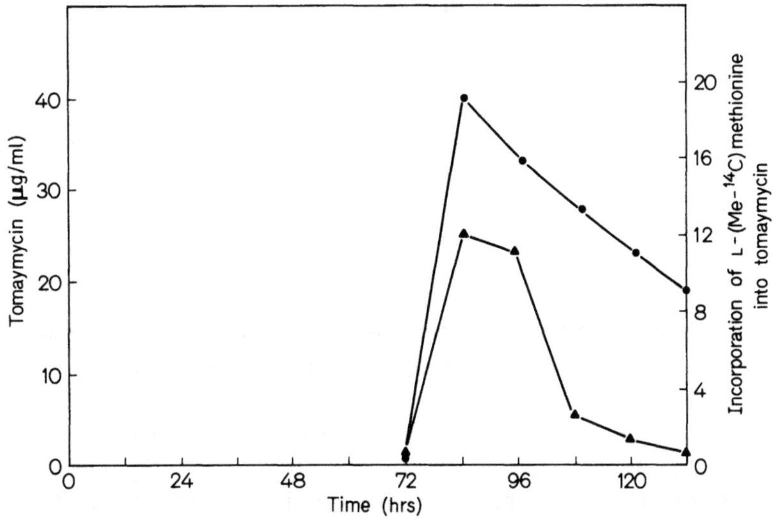

Fig. 4. Time course production of tomaymycin and incorporation of L-(CH_3-^{14}C)methionine into tomaymycin. At the times indicated flasks were harvested and L-(CH_3-^{14}C)methionine was added 12 h prior to harvesting. (-●-) µg/ml tomaymycin; (-▲-) % incorporation into tomaymycin (HURLEY et al., 1976a)

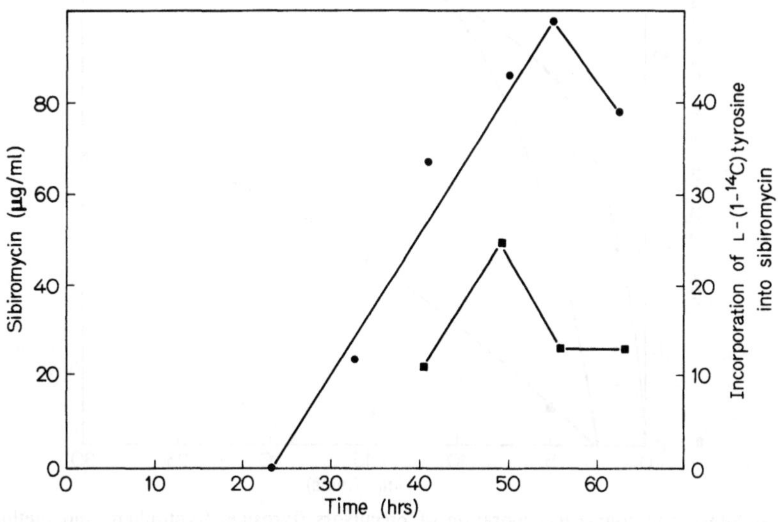

Fig. 5. Time course production of sibiromycin and incorporation of L-(1′-^{14}C)tyrosine into sibiromycin. At the times indicated flasks were harvested and L-(1′-^{14}C)tyrosine was added 12 h prior to harvesting. (-●-) µg/ml sibiromycin; (-■-) % incorporation into sibiromycin (HURLEY et al., 1979b)

D. Neothramycins A and B

The most recent additions to the naturally occurring pyrrolo(1,4)-benzodiazepine antibiotics are the neothramycins A and B (T. TAKEUCHI et al., 1976). These compounds are isomers and are interconvertible in aqueous solution (M. MIYAMOTO et al., 1977). Conditions for production and isolation of these antibiotics from cultures of *Streptomyces* No. MC916-C4 have been described (T. TAKEUCHI et al., 1976).

III. Tryptophan, Tyrosine, and Methionine as Precursors of the Pyrrolo(1,4)benzodiazepine Antibiotics

Conclusive evidence for the precursor roles of tryptophan, tyrosine, and methionine in anthramycin, tomaymycin, and sibiromycin biosynthesis has been obtained through radioisotope and stable isotope experiments (L.H. HURLEY

a

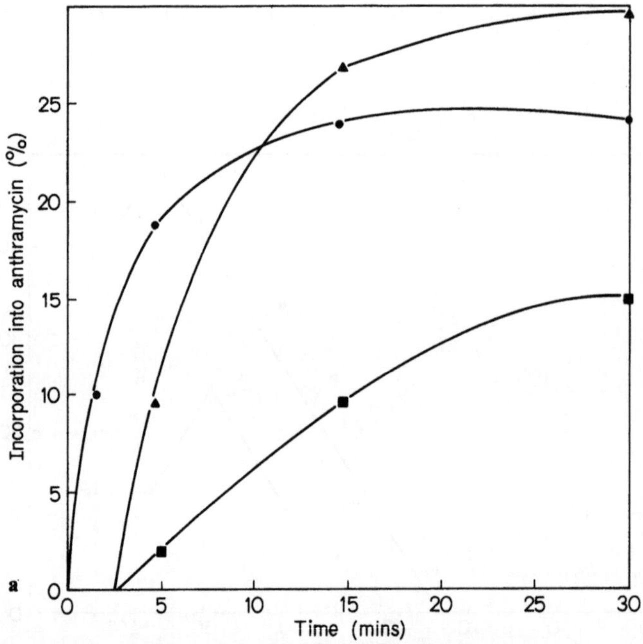

Fig. 6a–c. Short-term course incorporation of precursors (tyrosine, tryptophan, and methionine) into anthramycin, tomaymycin, and sibiromycin. (-●-) % incorporation of L-(1′-^{14}C)tyrosine; (-■-) % incorporation of L(methyl-^{14}C)methionine; (-▲-) % incorporation of DL-(7a-^{14}C)tryptophan. **a** 1.1×10^7 dpm tyrosine, 5.1×10^6 dpm of methionine, and 1.2×10^7 dpm of tryptophan was added to 50 ml of a 9-h culture of *S. refuineus* and 5 ml aliquots were taken at the times indicated (L.H. HURLEY and C. GAIROLA, unpublished results); **b** 2.14×10^7 dpm of tyrosine was added to 95 ml of a 8-h culture of *S. achromogenes* and 5 ml aliquots were taken at the times indicated (L.H. HURLEY et al., 1976a); **c** 1.1×10^7 dpm of tyrosine, 4.1×10^6 dpm of methionine and 4.9×10^6 dpm of tryptophan was added to 95 ml of a 42-h culture of *S. sibiricum* and 5 ml aliquots were taken at the times indicated (L.H. HURLEY et al., 1979a)

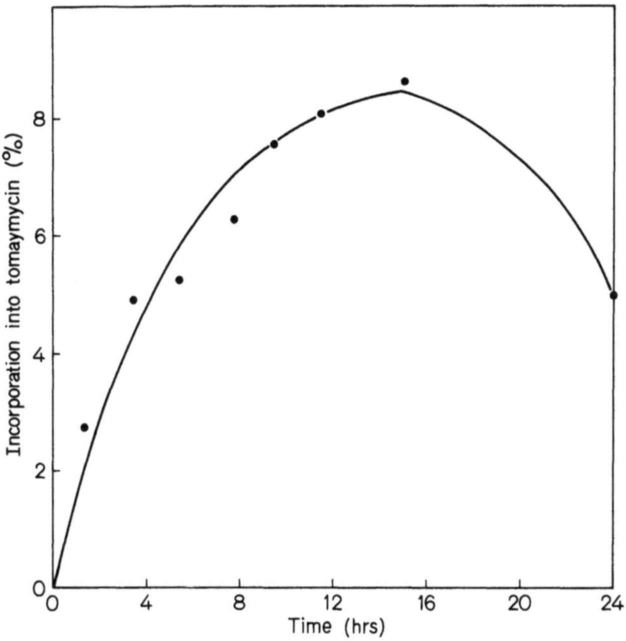
Incorporation into tomaymycin (%)
0
2
4
6
8
0
4
8
12
16
20
24
Time (hrs)

Fig. 6b

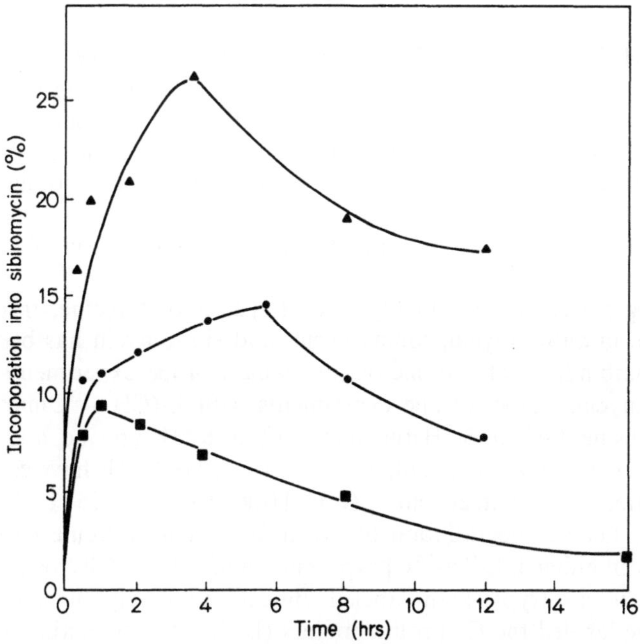
Incorporation into sibiromycin (%)
0
5
10
15
20
25
0
2
4
6
8
10
12
14
16
Time (hrs)

Fig. 6c

Table 1. Incorporation of labeled substrates into anthramycin, tomaymycin, and sibiromycin (L.H. HURLEY et al., 1975; L.H. HURLEY et al., 1976b; L.H. HURLEY et al., 1979a)

Precursor fed	% Incorporation		
	Anthramycin	Tomaymycin	Sibiromycin
L-(1'-^{14}C)Dihydroxyphenylalanine	22.1	6.9	18.4
L-(CH_3-^{14}C)Methionine	16.4	17.8	35.2
DL-(7a-^{14}C)Tryptophan	13.7	6.1	8.1
L-(1'-^{14}C)Tyrosine	10.4	10.1	15.4
L-(U-^{14}C)Tyrosine	11.7	7.6	9.9
D-(6-^{14}C)Glucose	0.2	n.e.	2.1
(1-^{14}C)Acetic acid	0.1	n.e.	n.e.
L-(U-^{14}C)Phenylalanine	0.1	n.e.	n.e.
L-(U-^{14}C)Proline	0.1	n.e.	n.e.
L-(Ala-3'-^{14}C)Tryptophan	0.3	n.e.	n.e.
(4-^{14}C)-δ-Aminolevulinic acid	0.1	n.e.	n.e.
(2-^{14}C)-3-hydroxy-4-methylanthranilic acid	0.1[a]	n.e.	14.1
(COOH-^{14}C)Anthranilic acid	0.1[a]	10.4[c]	0.1
(COOH-^{14}C)Anthranilic acid + trp	n.e.[b]	1.9[c]	n.e.

[a] Radiolabeled substrate failed to be taken up to significantly by the *S. refuinius* cells in these experiments
[b] n.e. not examined
[c] Parallel feeding experiments in which a 100-ml culture of *S. achromogenes* was divided into equal halves prior to additions of the (COOH-^{14}C)anthranilic acid (4.42×10^6 dpm) to each flask and 16.5 μmoles of DL-tryptophan to one of the two flasks

et al., 1975; L.H. HURLEY et al., 1976a; L.H. HURLEY et al., 1979a). A comparison of the incorporation values from radioisotope tracer feeding experiments in each of the antibiotics is shown in Table 1. The results of short-term time course experiments for the incorporation of tryptophan, tyrosine, and methionine into the three antibiotics are shown in Figs. 6a–c. The extremely rapid incorporation of the three amino acids into anthramycin relative to tomaymycin and sibiromycin agrees with the more rapid time course production of anthramycin.

The labeling pattern of specifically labeled species of tyrosine, tryptophan, and methionine in anthramycin, tomaymycin, and sibiromycin has been determined by a combination of radioactive or stable isotope experiments. In the case of anthramycin, stable isotope experiments with L-(CH_3-^{13}C)methionine, DL-(1'-^{13}C)tyrosine, L-(3- or 5-^{2}H)tyrosine, L-(2- or 6-^{2}H)tyrosine, and L-(3',3'-$^2H_2$)tyrosine in combination with either ^{13}C-NMR or ^{1}H-NMR have established the labeling patterns shown in Scheme 2 (L.H. HURLEY et al., 1975; L.H. HURLEY et al., 1979b). Chemical degradation of the anthramycin molecule biosynthetically labeled from either DL-[7a-^{14}C]tryptophan and L-[U-^{14}C]tyrosine demonstrated that, whereas tryptophan labeled almost exclusively the anthranilate moiety, tyrosine labeled the C_3-proline moiety (L.H. HURLEY et al., 1975). The labeling pattern of L-(CH_3-^{14}C)methionine and L-(3- or 5-^{3}H)tyrosine in tomaymycin was determined by chemical degradation of the appropriately labeled species and is as shown in Scheme 2 (L.H. HURLEY et al., 1976a). In the case

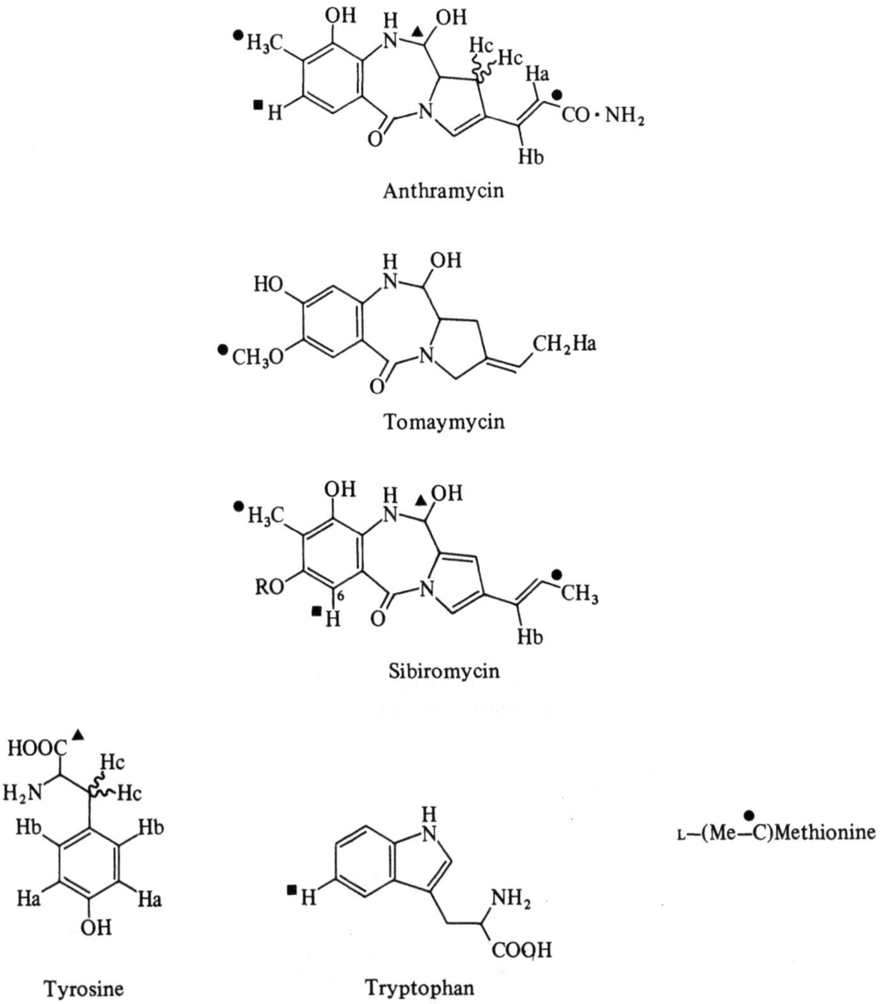

Scheme 2. Confirmed biosynthetic labeling patterns of tyrosine, tryptophan, and methionine in anthramycin, tomaymycin, and sibiromycin (L.H. HURLEY et al., 1975; L.H. HURLEY et al., 1976a; L.H. HURLEY et al., 1979a)

of sibiromycin, stable isotope experiments with L-(CH_3-^{13}C)-methionine, DL-(1-^{13}C)tyrosine, and L-(2- or 6-^2H)tyrosine in combination with ^{13}C-NMR or ^1H-NMR established the the labeling pattern shown in Scheme 2 (L.H. HURLEY et al., 1979a). Chemical degradation of a sample of sibiromycin biosynthetically labeled from DL-(5-^3H)tryptophan demonstrated that the tritium undergoes an NIH shift during its conversion to sibiromycin such that the tritium is found at C-6 of the antibiotic (L.H. HURLEY et al., 1979a).

These determined labeling patterns of tryptophan, tyrosine, and methionine in the three pyrrolo(1,4)benzodiazepine antibiotics led us to speculate that; 1. tryptophan is degraded via the kynurenine pathway to the anthranilic acid

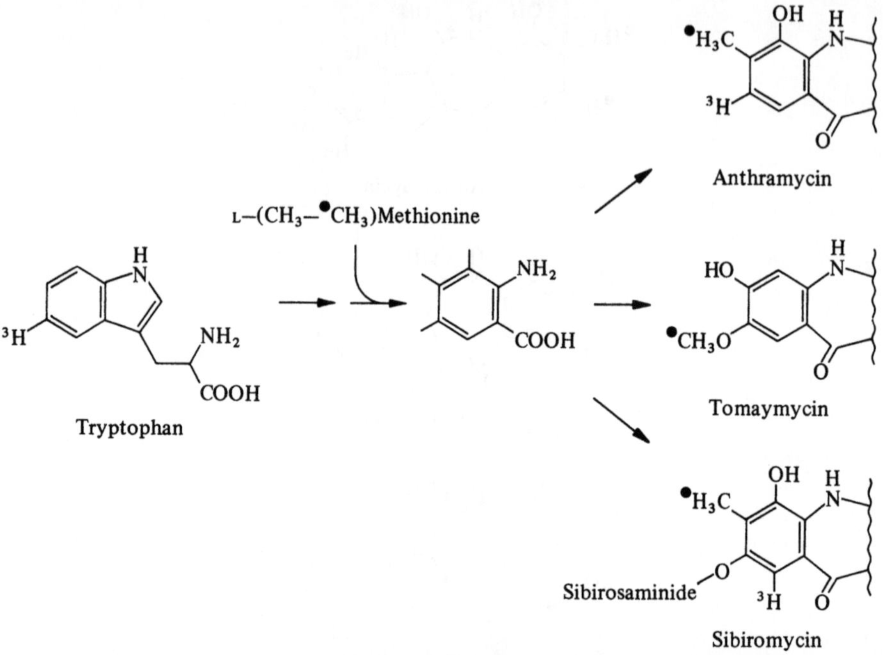

Scheme 3. Proposed biosynthetic conversion of tryptophan to the anthranilic acid moieties of anthramycin, tomaymycin, and sibiromycin

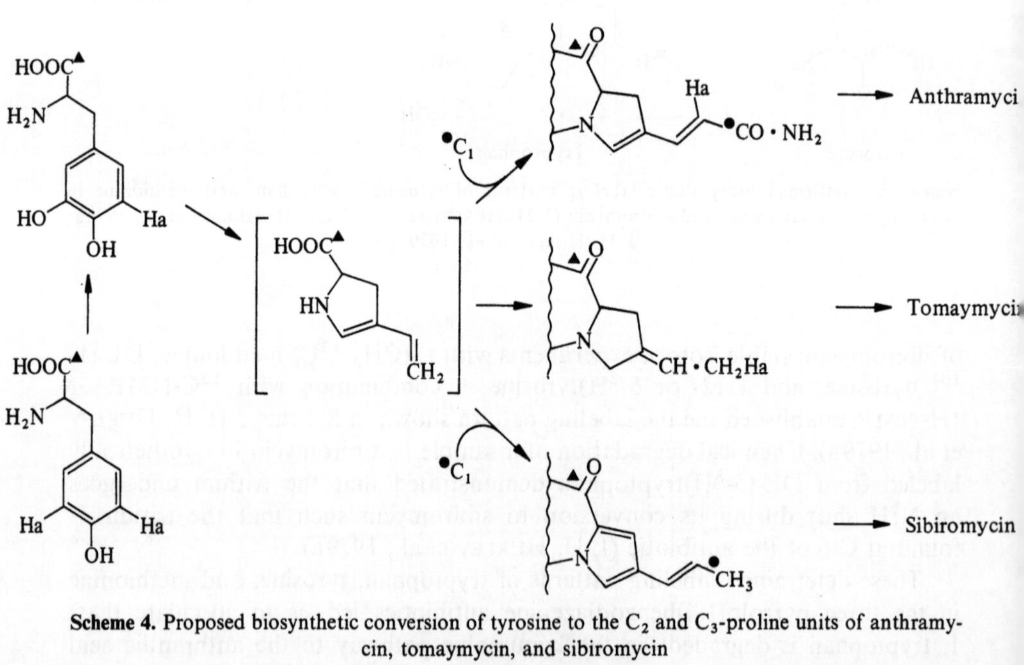

Scheme 4. Proposed biosynthetic conversion of tyrosine to the C_2 and C_3-proline units of anthramycin, tomaymycin, and sibiromycin

moieties, and 2. tyrosine is degraded via dopa and a ring cleavage product ultimately to give rise to the C_2-proline unit of tomaymycin and the C_3-proline moieties of anthramycin and sibiromycin in which case a C-1 unit is added from methionine (Schemes 3 and 4).

IV. Biosynthetic Conversion of Tryptophan to the Anthranilic Acid Units of Anthramycin, Tomaymycin, and Sibiromycin

Of the three antibiotics the intermediates in the biosynthetic pathway from tryptophan to the anthranilic acid moiety of sibiromycin have been most thoroughly examined (L.H. HURLEY and GAIROLA, 1979). In this case competition experiments between DL-(7a-^{14}C)tryptophan and the suspected unlabeled intermediates have been carried out, together with incorporation experiments using radiolabeled compounds. The results of the competition experiments (Fig. 7) in which the effect of increasing amounts of unlabeled compounds on the specific activity of sibiromycin labeled from DL-(7a-^{14}C)tryptophan was followed, showed that 3-hydroxy-4-methylanthranilic acid, 3-hydroxy-4-methylkynurenine, 3-hydroxykynurenine and less significantly anthranilic acid are effective competitors in the conversion of tryptophan to the anthranilic acid moiety of sibiromycin. The effect of anthranilic acid is probably due to its precursor role in tryptophan biosynthesis rather than its intermediacy in the conversion of tryptophan to sibiromycin. This therefore suggests that the aromatic ring is modified at the kynurenine stage except for the 7-hydroxylation which may take place

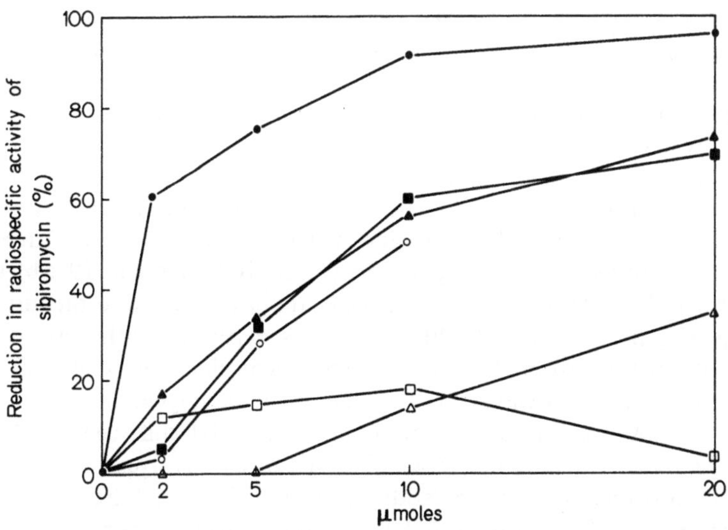

Fig. 7. Effect of various compounds on the specific activity of sibiromycin labeled from DL-(7a-^{14}C) tryptophan. 2.5×10^6 dpm of DL-(7a-^{14}C)tryptophan was added to 100 ml aliquots of a 30-h culture of *S. sibiricum*, 3-hydroxy-4-methylanthranilic acid (-●-); kynurenine (-■-); 3-hydroxykynurenine (-▲-); 3-hydroxy-4-methylkynurenine (-○-); 3-hydroxyanthranilic acid (-□-); anthranilic acid (-△-) (L.H. HURLEY and C. GAIROLA, 1979)

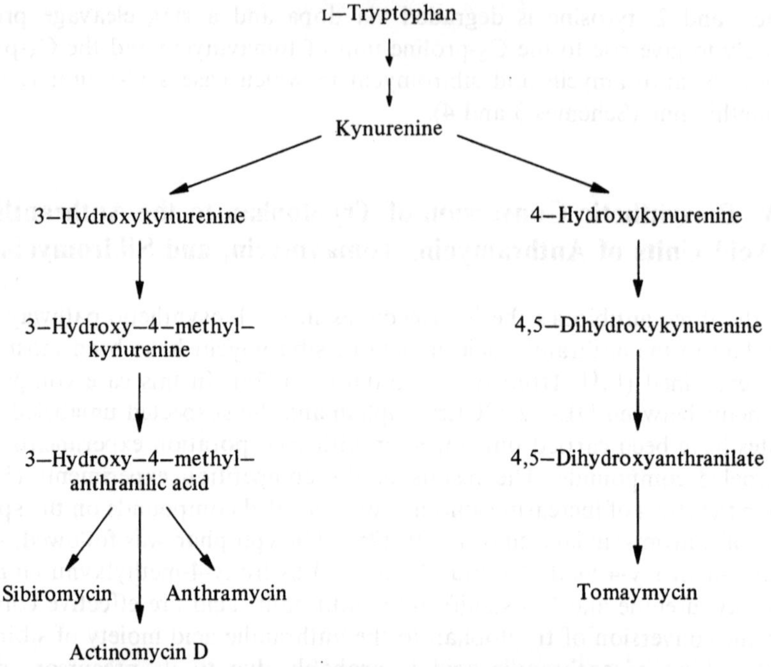

Scheme 5. Proposed general pathway for the conversion of tryptophan to the anthranilate moieties of various antibiotics (L.H. HURLEY and C. GAIROLA, 1979)

at a later stage. This supposition is further substantiated by the efficient incorporation of 3-hydroxy-4-(2-^{14}C)-methylanthranilic acid and non-incorporation of (COOH-^{14}C)anthranilic acid into sibiromycin (Table 1). While (COOH-^{14}C) anthranilic acid was incorporated into tomaymycin this was almost certainly via tryptophan, since this incorporation into tomaymycin was reduced by greater than 80% when cold tryptophan was added in a parallel experiment (Table 1). Parallel experiments with the anthramycin producing organism were not carried out due to the impermeability of these cells to many of these substrates.

Experiments utilizing DL-(5-^{3}H)(7a-^{14}C)tryptophan have been carried out with all three antibiotic-producing strains (L.H. HURLEY et al., 1976b) to shed some light on the order in which substituents are introduced into the anthranilic acid ring of tomaymycin and sibiromycin. As expected, anthramycin retains 100% of the tritium from this feeding experiment since an NIH shift in this case is not possible. However, in the case of tomaymycin in which a 17% retention of tritium was found, a consideration of NIH shift rules (J.W. DALY et al., 1972) indicates that the most likely pathway involves insertion of the 8-hydroxy substituent prior to the addition of the 7-hydroxyl group (Scheme 5). The same species of tryptophan fed to the sibiromycin culture led to a 93% retention of tritium in sibiromycin (L.H. HURLEY et al., 1976b; L.H. HURLEY et al., 1979a). The step at which hydroxylation of the aromatic ring occurs resulting in an NIH shift is indicated by the following facts. 3-Hydroxy-4-(1-^{14}C) methylanthranilic acid (L.H. HURLEY and C. GAIROLA, 1979) is efficiently incor-

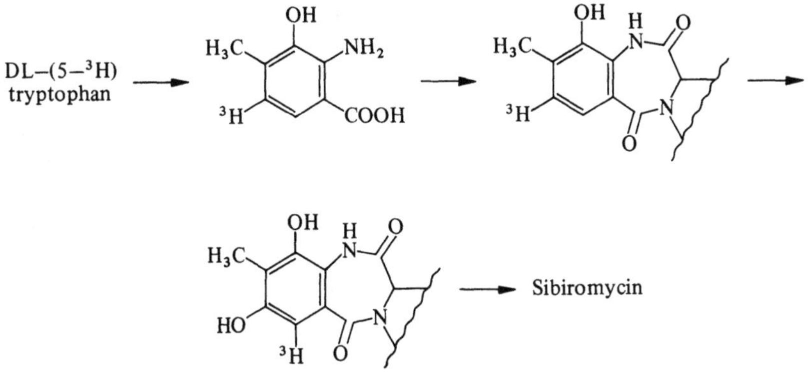

Scheme 6. Proposed step in the biosynthetic pathway at which hydroxylation at C-7 of sibiromycin occurs (L.H. HURLEY et al., 1979a)

porated into sibiromycin (Table 1). An almost complete retention of tritium from DL-(5-^{3}H)tryptophan takes place in sibiromycin at C-6. The empirical rule that enzymatic hydroxylation para to a highly activating group such as $-NH_2$ results in virtually complete loss of isotopic hydrogen from the product (J.W. DALY et al., 1972, p. 1139) leads us to suspect that the hydroxylation may take place on a compound possessing a less activating para substituent such as that shown in Scheme 6. All these results taken together led us to suggest the general scheme shown in Scheme 5 for the biosynthesis of the anthranilic acid moieties of anthramycin, tomaymycin, and sibiromycin.

V. Origin of the C-1 Units in Anthramycin, Tomaymycin, and Sibiromycin

The biosynthetic labeling pattern of L-(CH_3-^{14}C)methionine or L-(CH_3-^{13}C) methionine in each antibiotic is illustrated in Scheme 2. This labeling pattern has been determined by either chemical degradation (anthramycin and tomaymycin) or by stable isotope studies with carbon-13 (anthramycin and sibiromycin). The enrichment positions in anthramycin were determined by both direct examination of the ^{13}C-NMR spectra and an indirect examination using ^{1}H-NMR and observation of long-range ^{1}H-^{13}C spin-spin coupling (C.J. CHANG et al., 1976). Experiments utilizing L-(CH_3-$^{14}C^3H_3$)methionine have demonstrated that the C-1 units in tomaymycin and sibiromycin are transferred as intact methyl groups, as is also the case for the aromatic methyl of anthramycin (L.H. HURLEY et al., 1975; L.H. HURLEY et al., 1976a; L.H. HURLEY et al., 1979a). The amide carbonyl in anthramycin which is derived from the C-1 pool is probably transferred as an intact methyl group and then subsequently oxidized and aminated since (^{14}C) formic acid was not incorporated into anthramycin (L.H. HURLEY, unpublished results) and the equivalent C-1 unit in sibiromycin is transferred as an intact CH_3 group (L.H. HURLEY et al., 1979a).

VI. Biosynthetic Origin of the Benzodiazepine Nitrogen Atoms of Anthramycin

The biosynthetic fate of the α-NH_2 of tyrosine in anthramycin was explored using L-(1′-^{14}C, ^{15}N)tyrosine. Mass spectral analysis of the recovered anthramycin from this experiment showed species of D, D_1, and D_2 in the ratio of 88, 12, and 0. The enrichment in anthramycin as estimated by the dilution of L-(1-^{14}C)tyrosine in the antibiotic was 25%. This therefore confirms that the α-NH_2 group is transferred to anthramycin partially intact with the carbon skeleton of tyrosine. In order to determine whether the L or D isomer of tyrosine is the more immediate precursor of anthramycin, parallel experiments were carried out with DL-(1′-^{14}C), L-(2- or 6-^{3}H)tyrosine and DL-(1-^{14}C), D-(2-or 6-^{3}H)tyrosine. The results (Table 2) reveal that the L isomer is the more immediate precursor (L.H. HURLEY et al, 1979b).

To determine the biosynthetic fate of the tryptophan indole nitrogen an experiment was carried out in which species of L-(5-^{3}H), (Indole-^{15}N)tryptophan and DL-(1′-^{13}C)tyrosine were fed in the same experiment. Sufficiently high enrichment of both labels (^{15}N and ^{13}C) were obtained such that the location of the nitrogen-15 was determined in anthramycin by examination of the result-

Table 2. Comparison of the incorporation of L-(2- or 6-^{3}H)tyrosine with D-(2- or 6-^{3}H)tyrosine using DL-(1′-^{14}C)tyrosine as a reference label (L.H. HURLEY and J. OSTRANDER, 1978)

Species of tyrosine	^{3}H/^{14}C ratio of tyrosine	^{3}H/^{14}C ratio of anthramycin	% Tritium [a] Retention
L-(2- or 6-^{3}H), DL-(1′-^{14}C)	18.0	17.7	98.3
D-(2- or 6-^{3}H), DL-(1′-^{14}C)	11.9	0.54	4.5
L-(2- or 6-^{3}H), L-(1′-^{14}C)	8.16	4.25	52.6

[a] Taking into account the retention of only approximately 50% of the tritium from L-(2- or 6-^{3}H) tyrosine during its conversion into anthramycin, then the experiments with L-(2- or 6-^{3}H), DL-(1′-^{14}C)tyrosine and D-(2- or 6-^{3}H), DL-(1′-^{14}C)tyrosine have relative retentions of: $98.3 \times 2 = 196.6\%$ and $4.5 \times 2 = 9\%$ respectively, i.e., the L isomer is incorporated twice as efficiently as the DL isomer and conversely the D isomer is incorporated insignificantly compared to the DL isomer

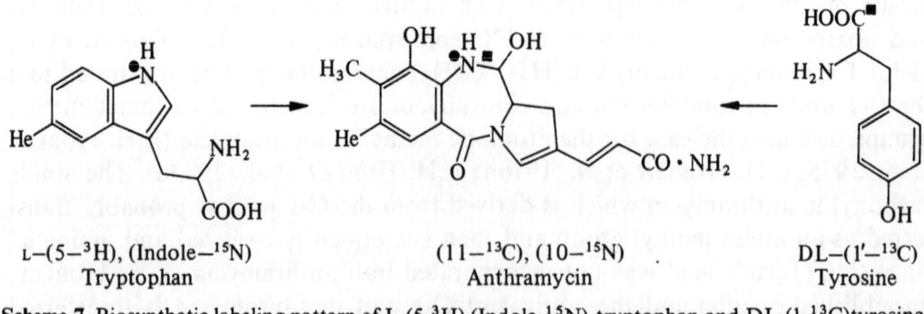

Scheme 7. Biosynthetic labeling pattern of L-(5-^{3}H) (Indole-^{15}N)-tryptophan and DL-(1-^{13}C)tyrosine in anthramycin

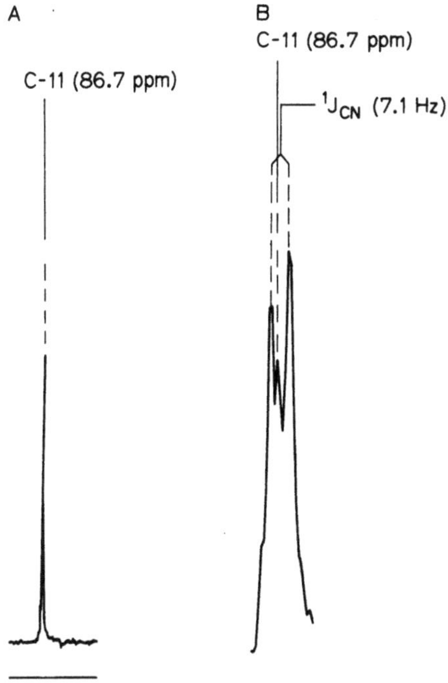

Fig. 8 A, B. Proton noise-decoupled Fourier transform carbon magnetic resonance spectra of anthramycin methyl ether (AME). **A** Carbon-11 of AME biosynthetically enriched with DL-(1-^{13}C)tyrosine and **B** carbon-11 of AME biosynthetically enriched from L-(Indole-^{15}N)tryptophan (95%) and DL-(1-^{13}C)-tyrosine (90%) (see Scheme 7). Spectra were recorded on a Varian CFT-20 in 8-mm spinning tubes. Deuteriodimethyl sulfoxide was used as solvent and chemical shifts are given relative to TMS (L.H. HURLEY and J.M. OSTRANDER, 1978)

ing ^{15}N splitting of the adjacent ^{13}C-enriched carbon (see Scheme 7 and Fig. 8). The clear ^{15}N-^{13}C coupling shown in Figure 12 together with an analysis of the isotopic abundancies for D_0, D_1, D_2, and D_3 (27, 45, 25, 2.7) and the enrichment of L-(5-^{3}H)tryptophan in the same experiment (49%) confirm that the indole nitrogen of tryptophan is transferred intact with the aromatic ring (L.H. HURLEY and J. OSTRANDER, 1978).

VII. Biosynthetic Conversion of Tyrosine to the C_2 and C_3-Proline Units of Anthramycin, Tomaymycin, and Sibiromycin

Recent biosynthetic studies on the pyrrolo(1,4)benzodiazepine antibiotics have centered around the fate of the various carbon, hydrogen, and nitrogen atoms of tyrosine in all three antibiotics, with the overall aim of rationally formulating a general biosynthetic pathway which will lead to the C_2 and C_3-proline units. This section, therefore, summarizes the results of biosynthetic experiments which narrow down the choice of possible intermediates which are probably candidates for future biosynthetic experiments.

The first question deals with the biosynthetic origin of the carbon atoms in the C_2 and C_3-proline units. A comparison of the incorporation of L-(U-^{14}C) tyrosine and L-(1′-^{14}C)tyrosine using L-(3- or 5-^{3}H)tyrosine or L-(2- or 6-^{3}H) tyrosine as internal reference labels demonstrated that this amino acid contributed seven of its nine carbon atoms to each of these antibiotics (L.H. HURLEY et al., 1975; L.H. HURLEY et al., 1976a; L.H. HURLEY et al., 1979b). This then accounted for seven of the eight carbons of the C_3-proline units of anthramycin and sibiromycin and all seven carbon atoms of the C_2-proline unit of tomaymycin. The labeling pattern from L-(1′-^{13}C)tyrosine (Scheme 2) predicted that the non-tyrosine-derived carbon atoms of anthramycin and sibiromycin should be in each case the terminal side chain carbon (C-14). This was confirmed from experiments in which L-(CH_3-^{13}C)methionine was found to serve as the source of this carbon in both antibiotics (Scheme 2).

Questions relating to the type of ring cleavage (ortho vs. meta), the timing of the cyclization reaction to form the pyrrolo ring and the biosynthetic fate of the side chain hydrogens of tyrosine were answered using a combination of double-labeling experiments (^{3}H and ^{14}C) and/or stable isotope experiments (^{2}H in combination with ^{1}H-NMR) (L.H. HURLEY et al., 1979c). Each question will be considered in turn and the results rationalized in a suggested biosynthetic scheme leading to these antibiotics.

A. What Routes are Possible via Aromatic Ring Cleavage and Cyclization to Form the Five-membered Ring?

During the conversion of tyrosine through dopa to the C_2 and C_3-proline moieties of the pyrrolo(1,4)benzodiazepine antibiotics cleavage of the aromatic ring must take place. This in turn will be followed by condensation with the 2 or 6 position of tyrosine to form the pyrrolo ring. The alternative pathways for ring cleavage and condensation are shown in Scheme 8. Biosynthetic pathways leading to structures of the type I, III, or V in Scheme 8 would necessarily require elimination of both tritium atoms from L-(3- or 5-^{3}H)tyrosine, whereas, pathways leading to II, IV, or VI only require loss of one of the two tritium atoms from this substrate. The results in Table 3 (experiments 1, 2, and 3) exclude pathways leading to I, III, or V as possible alternatives in the cases of anthramycin and tomaymycin. However, the almost complete loss of tritium in diacetylanhydrosibiromycinone (Scheme 9) would be in agreement with any of the pathways in Scheme 8. The position of the retained tritium from L-(3- or 5-^{3}H)tyrosine in anthramycin (L.H. HURLEY et al., 1975) and tomaymycin (L.H. HURLEY et al., 1976a) was at C-13 of these antibiotics as expected. Since the meta cleavage pathway is implicated not only for anthramycin and tomaymycin but also in the case of the lincomycin antibiotics (J.P. ROLLS et al., 1976), which contain similar C_3 and C_2-proline units to the pyrrolo(1,4)benzodiazepine antibiotics, we suspect that the almost complete loss of tritium from L-(3- or 5-^{3}H)-tyrosine in sibiromycin is due to a later biosynthetic transformation. A plausible hypothesis for this loss, peculiar to sibiromycin, is presented later.

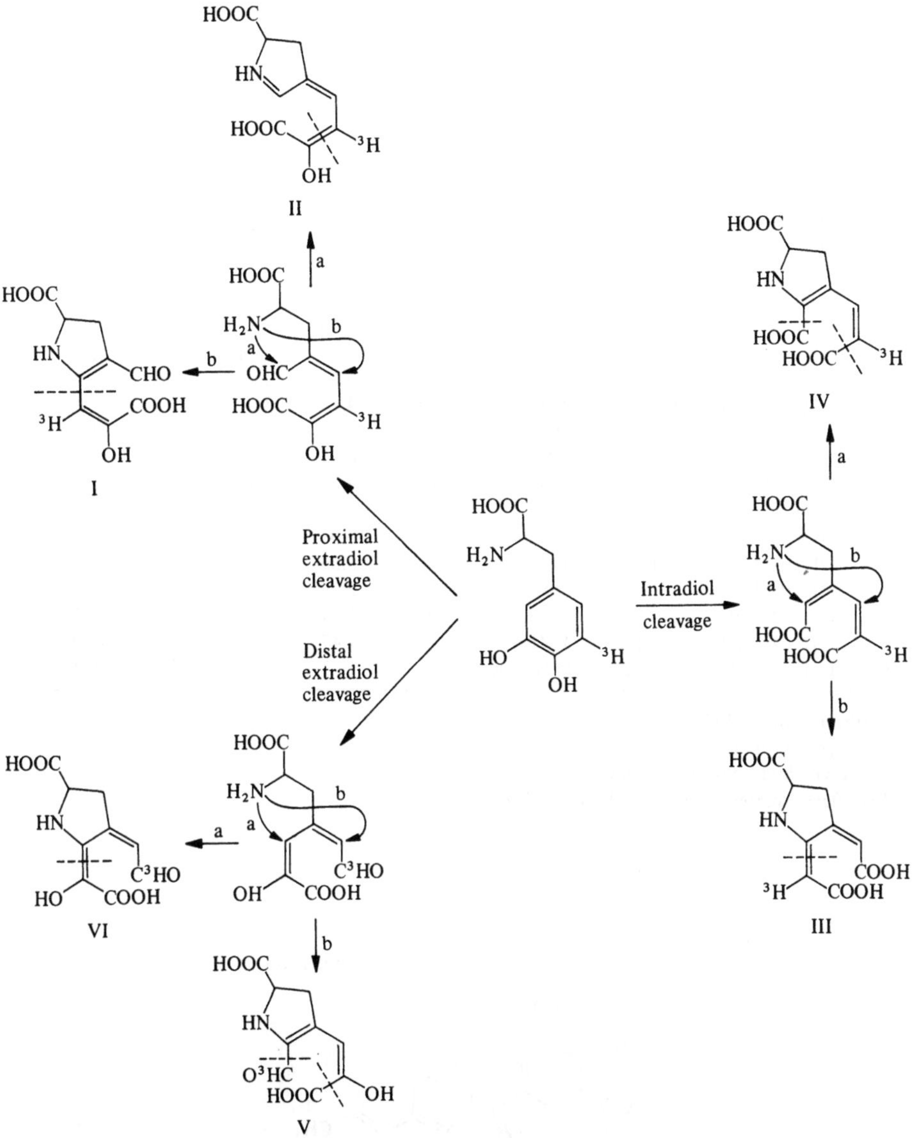

Scheme 8. Alternative pathways for the conversion of L-(3- or 5-^{3}H)-tyrosine into the C_2 and C_3-proline moieties of anthramycin, tomaymycin, and sibiromycin involving various cleavage pathways (L.H. HURLEY, 1979b)

B. Does Ring Cleavage of the Aromatic Ring to Form the Five-membered Ring Take Place Before or After Cyclization?

Just as L-(3- or 5-^{3}H)tyrosine can be used to differentiate between alternative methods for ring cleavage of dopa, species of L-(2- or 6-^{3}H)tyrosine can be utilized to shed some information on the stage at which cyclization to form

Table 3. Results of co-crystallization of AME[a], TME[b], and DAS-one[c] from feeding experiments with various double-labeled tyrosine molecules (L.H. HURLEY et al., 1979b)

Number	Species of tyrosine	Product	$^3H/^{14}C$ ratio of tyrosine	$^3H/^{14}C$ ratio of crystallization 1st	2nd	3rd	Final tritium retention (%)
1	L[1′-^{14}C, 3- or 5-^{3}H]	AME[a]	9.17	4.74	4.68	4.68	51
2	L[1′-^{14}C, 3- or 5-^{3}H]	TME[b]	6.45	3.25	3.16	3.07	48.9
3	L[1′-^{14}C, 3- or 5-^{3}H]	DAS-one[c]	8.91	0.32	0.26	0.47	3.9
4	L[1′-^{14}C, 2- or 6-^{3}H]	AME	8.16	4.31	4.31	4.25	52.6
5	L[1′-^{14}C, 2- or 6-^{3}H]	TME	8.75	7.22	6.83	6.82	78.0
6	L[1′-^{14}C, 2- or 6-^{3}H]	DAS-one	8.33	2.77	2.74	2.65	32.7
7	DL[1′-^{14}C, 3′RS(3′-^{3}H)]	AME	3.19	2.97	3.06	3.06	95.0
8	DL[1′-^{14}C, 3′RS(3′-^{3}H)]	TME	3.18	3.18	3.31	–[d]	102.0
9	DL[1′-^{14}C, 3′RS(3′-^{3}H)]	DAS-one	4.87	2.84	3.00	3.07	61.0
10	DL-[1′-^{14}C, 3′R(3′-^{3}H)]	AME	11.04	10.81	9.03	9.12	87.4
11	DL-[1′-^{14}C, 3′R(3′-^{3}H)]	TME	4.86	4.29	4.49	–[d]	90.3
12	DL-[1′-^{14}C, 3′R(3′-^{3}H)]	DAS-one	9.70	9.68	9.37	9.40	97.8
13	DL-[1′-^{14}C, 3′S(3′-^{3}H)]	AME	9.85	10.03	8.12	7.81	80.9
14	DL-[1′-^{14}C, 3′S(3′-^{3}H)]	TME	3.94	3.59	3.75	–[d]	92.4
15	DL-[1′-^{14}C, 3′S(3′-^{3}H)]	DAS-one	6.92	2.29	2.36	–[d]	33.7
16	L-[1′-^{14}C, Ala-2′,-3′-^{3}H]	AME	3.30	1.64	1.64	–[d]	49.7
17	L-[1′-^{14}C, Ala-2′,-3′-^{3}H]	TME	3.30	1.47	1.69	–[d]	47.9
18	L-[1′-^{14}C, Ala-2′,-3′-^{3}H]	DAS-one	9.12	1.71	1.62	–[d]	19.3

[a] Anthramycin methylether
[b] Tomaymycin methylether
[c] Diacetylanhydrosibiromycinone
[d] Insufficient material for a third recrystallization

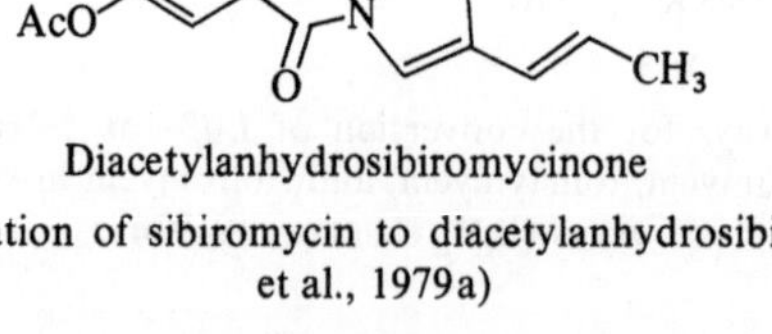

Scheme 9. Chemical degradation of sibiromycin to diacetylanhydrosibiromycinone (L.H. HURLEY et al., 1979a)

the five-membered ring of anthramycin, tomaymycin, and sibiromycin takes place. The intermediacy of cyclodopa (Scheme 10, pathway a) would require the loss of at least 50% of the tritium from L-(2- or 6-^{3}H)tyrosine in these antibiotics. Pathway b in Scheme 10, in which ring cleavage occurs prior to formation of the five-membered ring, would not, however, require loss of either

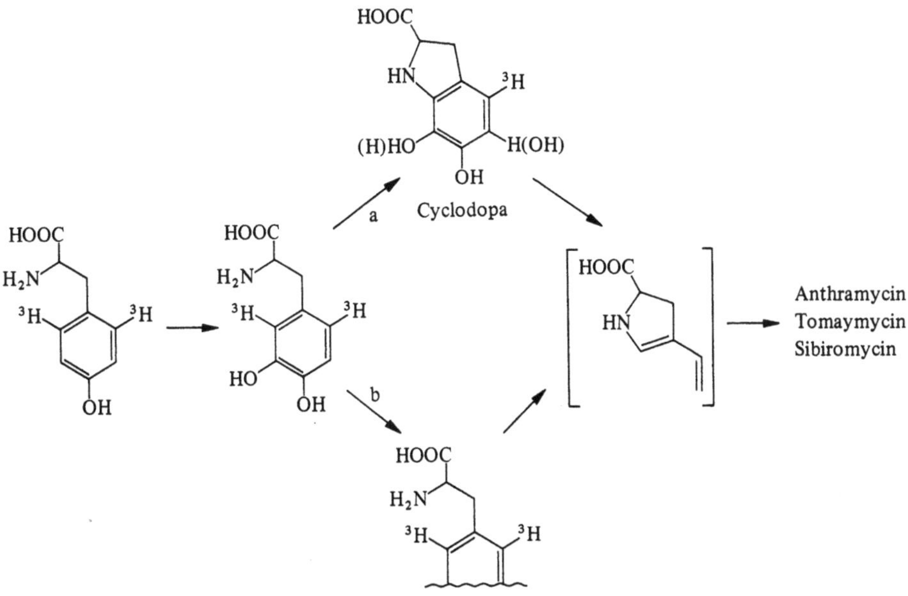

Scheme 10. Alternative pathways leading to the C_2 and C_3-proline moieties of anthramycin, tomaymycin, and sibiromycin involving ring cleavage either before or after cyclization of the proline ring (L.H. HURLEY et al., 1979b)

of the tritium atoms from L-(2-or 6-^{3}H)-tyrosine in these antibiotics. The results in Table 3 (experiments 4, 5, and 6) show considerable variation in retention of tritium from one antibiotic to another. The 78% retention of tritium in tomaymycin would appear to rule out cyclodopa as a plausible intermediate in this case. However, the 52% and 33% retentions in the cases of anthramycin and diacetylanhydrosibiromycinone agree with either pathway.

Information on the labeling pattern of these species of tyrosine in anthramycin and sibiromycin was obtained by feeding the corresponding deuterated tyrosine molecules. L-(2- and 6-$^2H_2$)-tyrosine (97% $^2H_2$) was fed to anthramycin- and sibiromycin-producing cultures. The anthramycin isolated was crystallized as anthramycin methyl ether and subjected to mass spectra and ^{1}H-NMR analysis. Mass spectral analysis of anthramycin methyl ether showed only species of D_0 and D_1 in the ratio of 48.15 to 51.85, confirming that one deuterium atom was lost during the conversion of L-(2- and 6-$^2H_2$)tyrosine to anthramycin. The ^{1}H-NMR analysis of the same sample showed a clear reduction of the doublet due to substitution of deuterium for the proton at C-12 of anthramycin methyl ether (Fig. 9a). Significantly no reduction in the intensity of the proton signal at C-3 was found. The sibiromycin isolated from a similar feeding experiment in which L-(2- and 6-$^2H_2$)tyrosine was added was converted to diacetylanhydrosibiromycinone (L.H. HURLEY et al., 1979b). Mass spectral analysis on this sample showed only species of D_0 and D_1 in the ratio of 72.5 to 27.5. The ^{1}H-NMR analysis revealed that the remaining deuterium atom was located

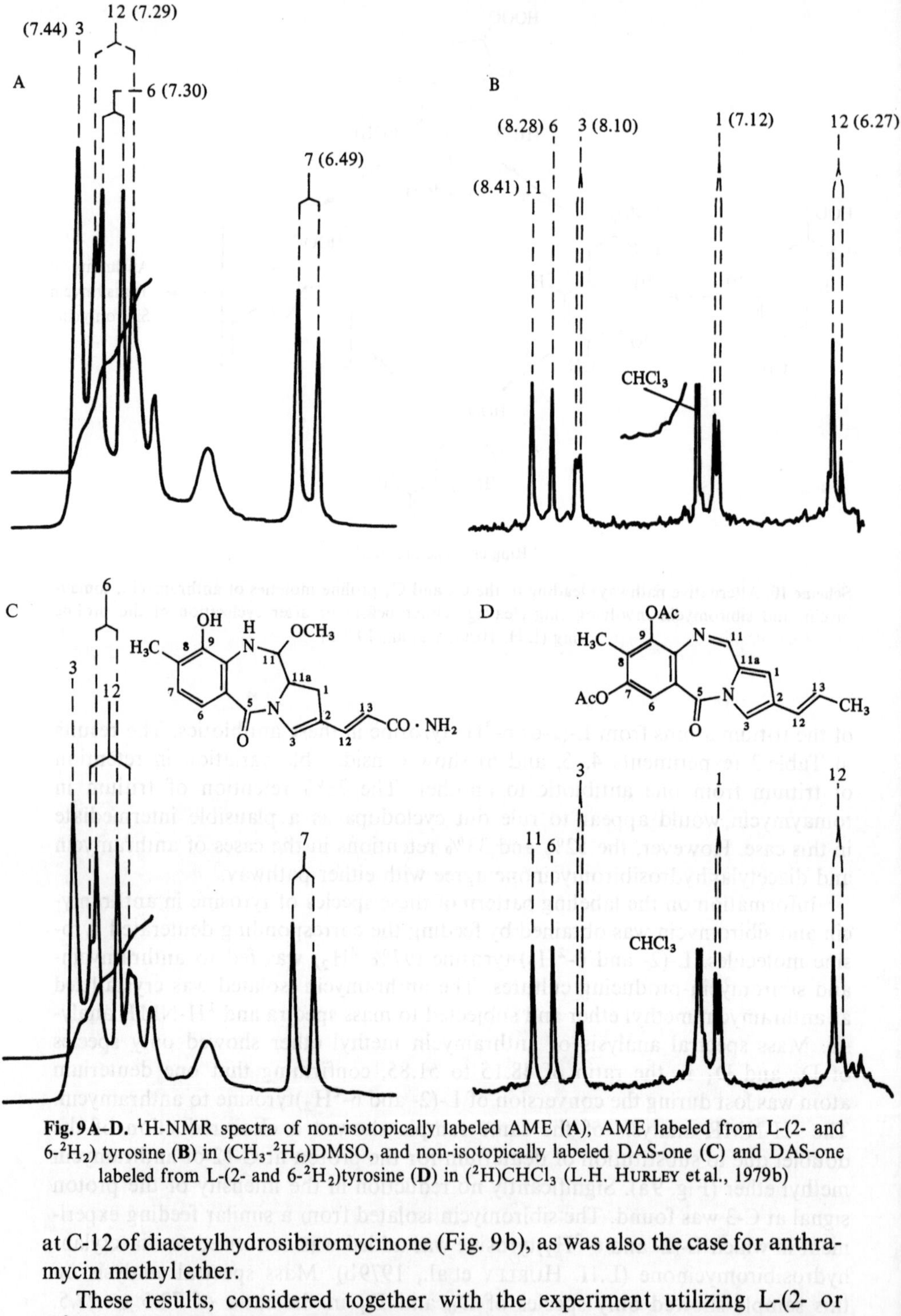

Fig. 9A–D. ^{1}H-NMR spectra of non-isotopically labeled AME (**A**), AME labeled from L-(2- and 6-$^2H_2$) tyrosine (**B**) in (CH_3-$^2H_6$)DMSO, and non-isotopically labeled DAS-one (**C**) and DAS-one labeled from L-(2- and 6-$^2H_2$)tyrosine (**D**) in (^{2}H)$CHCl_3$ (L.H. HURLEY et al., 1979b)

at C-12 of diacetylhydrosibiromycinone (Fig. 9b), as was also the case for anthramycin methyl ether.

These results, considered together with the experiment utilizing L-(2- or 6-^{3}H)tyrosine lead to the conclusion that the 67% loss of tritium in diacetylanhydrosibiromycinone is due to complete loss of the tritium that will reside at C-6 of dopa and a partial loss of tritium (17%) that ultimately labeled C-12 of diacetylanhydrosibiromycinone.

Stable-isotope analysis of tomaymycin samples labeled from L-(2- and 6-$^2H_2$)tyrosine are lacking, due to the low antibiotic-producing ability of the available culture. Our double-labeling experiment with L-(1′-^{14}C, 2- or 6-^3H) tyrosine in which we found a retention of 78% of tritium is, however, only compatible with a pathway involving ring cleavage of dopa prior to formation of the five-membered ring.

C. What is the Biosynthetic Fate of the Side-Chain Hydrogens of Tyrosine in Anthramycin, Tomaymycin, and Sibiromycin?

From our previous biosynthetic results with the pyrrolo-(1,4)benzodiazepine antibiotics, the 2′ and 3′ side-chain hydrogens of tyrosine should reside at carbon atoms 1 and 11a of these antibiotics respectively (see Scheme 11). Inspection of the appropriate carbon atoms in tyrosine (side chain) and the three antibiotics (carbon atoms 11a and 1) reveals that, whereas in anthramycin and tomaymycin the oxidation states of the corresponding carbon atoms are similar, in sibiromycin an additional double bond exists. This would therefore suggest that, whereas, in anthramycin and tomaymycin all three side-chain hydrogens might be retained, in sibiromycin the 2′-hydrogen and one of the two diastereotopic 3′-hydrogens must be lost. Double-labeled species of tyrosine labeled with tritium either at the 3′-carbon DL-[1′-^{14}C, 3′RS-(3′-^3H)], DL-[1′-

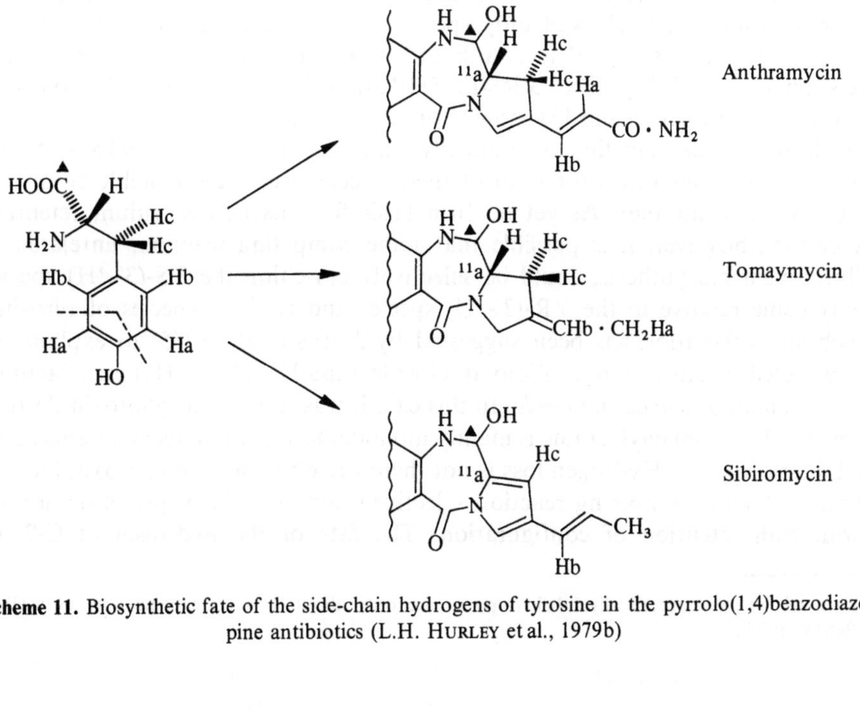

Scheme 11. Biosynthetic fate of the side-chain hydrogens of tyrosine in the pyrrolo(1,4)benzodiazepine antibiotics (L.H. Hurley et al., 1979b)

^{14}C, 3′R-(3′-^3H)], DL-[1-^{14}C, 3′S-(3′-^3H)], or at both the 2′ and 3′ carbons L-(1′-^{14}C, Ala-2′ or -3′-^3H) were fed to all three antibiotic producing strains, the antibiotics isolated and the tritium to carbon-14 ratios used to determine the fate of these hydrogens in anthramycin, tomaymycin, and sibiromycin.

Conclusive evidence for the biosynthetic origin of C-1 of anthramycin as C-3′ of tyrosine was obtained, when it was found that species of anthramycin methyl ether biosynthetically labeled from DL-(3′3′-$^2H_2$)tyrosine when examined by ^{2}H-NMR showed only deuterium at C-1 of anthramycin methyl ether (J. WRIGHT and L.H. HURLEY, unpublished results).

The results of feeding experiments with tyrosine non-specifically labeled at C-3′ and the two largely stereospecifically labeled tyrosine molecules, [DL-(3′S)-(3′-^3H) and DL-(3′R)-(3′-^3H)] with the anthramycin- and tomaymycin-producing cultures (Table 3, experiments 7, 10, 13, and 8, and 11 and 14) not unexpectedly failed to show any significant loss of tritium. Therefore any intermediate requiring loss of either one of these diastereotopic hydrogens can be eliminated from consideration. The equivalent experiments utilizing the same specifically labeled substrates, but with the sibiromycin producing organism showed that appreciable loss of tritium occurred from the DL-[1′-^{14}C, 3′RS-(3′-^3H)] and DL-[1′-^{14}C, 3′S-(3′-^3H)]-tyrosine in diacetylanhydrosibiromycinone (Table 3, experiments 9 and 15). Very little loss occurred from DL-[1′-^{14}C, 3′R-(3′-^3H)]tyrosine (Table 3, experiment 12) in accord with the stereospecific loss of the 3′S proton from tyrosine. The predominant loss of the 3′S hydrogen from tyrosine is analogous to that found in secrurinine, mycelianamide, cryptoschiculine A, and in the ammonium-lyase reaction (R.J. PARRY, 1978). The loss of one of the two diastereotopic 3′ hydrogens from tyrosine during its conversion to sibiromycin is further substantiated by an experiment in which L-(3′3′-$^2H_2$)tyrosine was fed to a culture of *S. sibiricum*. The isolated diacetylanhydrosibiromycinone showed only species of D_0 and D_1 in the ratio of 89.2 to 10.8. Our results with diacetylanhydrosibiromycinone isolated from feeding experiments with DL-[1′-^{14}C, 3′RS-(3′-^3H)] and DL-[1′-^{14}C, 3′S-(3′-^3H)]tyrosine (Table 3, experiment 9 and 15) show tritium retentions (61 and 34% respectively) which are higher than that theoretically expected (3′RS-50%, 3′S-15%).* The excess tritium retentions for both of these species were reproducible from one experiment to another. As yet no firm basis for this excess tritium retention is known; however, it is possible that some competing reaction, unrelated to sibiromycin biosynthesis, could be selectively enriching the 3′S-(3′-^3H) species of tyrosine relative to the 3′R-(3′-^3H) species and (1′-^{14}C) species of tyrosine. Such an explanation has been suggested by JOHNS et al. (1975) to explain the unexpected results found in gliotoxin after feeding DL-(3′-3′-$^2H_2$)phenylalanine to the fungus *Trichoderma viride*. In this case it was found that gliotoxin derived from (3′,3′-$^2H_2$)phenylalanine is mainly monodeuteriated but also contains some dideuterio species. Hydrogen loss is not therefore obligatory in gliotoxin biosynthesis but some competing reaction selectively removes the 3′-pro-R-deuterium atom with retention of configuration. The fate of the hydrogen at C-2′ of

* Each of the stereospecifically labeled species are only about 85% stereochemically pure (R.J. PARRY, 1975).

tyrosine in the three antibiotics was determined using L-(1′-^{14}C, Ala-2′-, or 3′-^{3}H)tyrosine since the tritium labeling pattern in this amino acid is known (G.W. KIRBY et al., 1975). Firstly, the tritium is distributed equally between position 2′ and 3′ of tyrosine. Secondly, the tritium at C-3′ of tyrosine is predominantly in the pro-S position (41.5±0.5%) relative to 8.5±0.5% in the pro-R position. Since we had demonstrated using the C-3 labeled species of tyrosine that complete retention of this tritium is found in anthramycin and tomaymycin, then any loss of tritium in these antibiotics from feeding experiments using L-(Ala-2′ or 3′-$^{3}H_2$)tyrosine would necessarily have to be from the C-2′ position. The results in Table 3 (experiments 16 and 17) show an approximate 50% retention of tritium in both anthramycin and tomaymycin showing that complete loss of the tritium from C-2′ of tyrosine occurs during its conversion of these antibiotics. Whether the loss of tritium from C-2′ of tyrosine during its conversion to anthramycin and tomaymycin is an obligatory event or only the result of a rapid transaminase is as yet unknown.

The result of the feeding experiment with L-(1′-^{14}C, Ala-2′, or 3′-^{3}H)tyrosine with the sibiromycin-producing organism revealed a retention of 19.3% of tritium in diacetylanhydrosibiromycinone (Table 3, experiment 18). This is again larger than the expected 8.5% based upon the relative distribution of tritium in this species of tyrosine. However, this agrees with our finding in experiments 9 and 15 shown in Table 3. As expected the result with L-(Ala-2′ or 3′-^{3}H) predicts the loss of the 3′R hydrogen and the 2′ hydrogen of tyrosine.

VIII. Formulation of a General Biosynthetic Pathway Leading to the C_2 and C_3-Proline Moieties

The results of these experiments with the variously labeled tyrosine species suggest that there are inconsistencies between the pathways leading to these antibiotics. For example, whereas pathways leading to I, III, and V in Scheme 8 can be eliminated for anthramycin and tomaymycin, they are compatible with the sibiromycin result in which almost complete loss of tritium from L-(3- or 5-^{3}H)tyrosine was found in diacetylanhydrosibiromycinone. Likewise, the results from experiments with L-(2- or 6-^{3}H)tyrosine appear to show reproducible but differing retention of tritium from one antibiotic to another. In this instance a cyclodopa intermediate can probably only be eliminated for tomaymycin.

We felt that it was unlikely that the biosynthetic pathways to these structurally, and more importantly, biosynthetically related antibiotics were as dissimilar as suggested by a cursory examination of our results. An attempt was therefore made to consolidate the general results into a biosynthetic scheme that would accomodate some if not all of these apparent inconsistencies. The biosynthetic pathway shown in Scheme 12 was proposed based upon the following assumptions:

1. Proximal extradiol cleavage of dopa is involved as the common ring cleavage reaction. Neither the distal extradiol cleavage nor the ortho cleavage

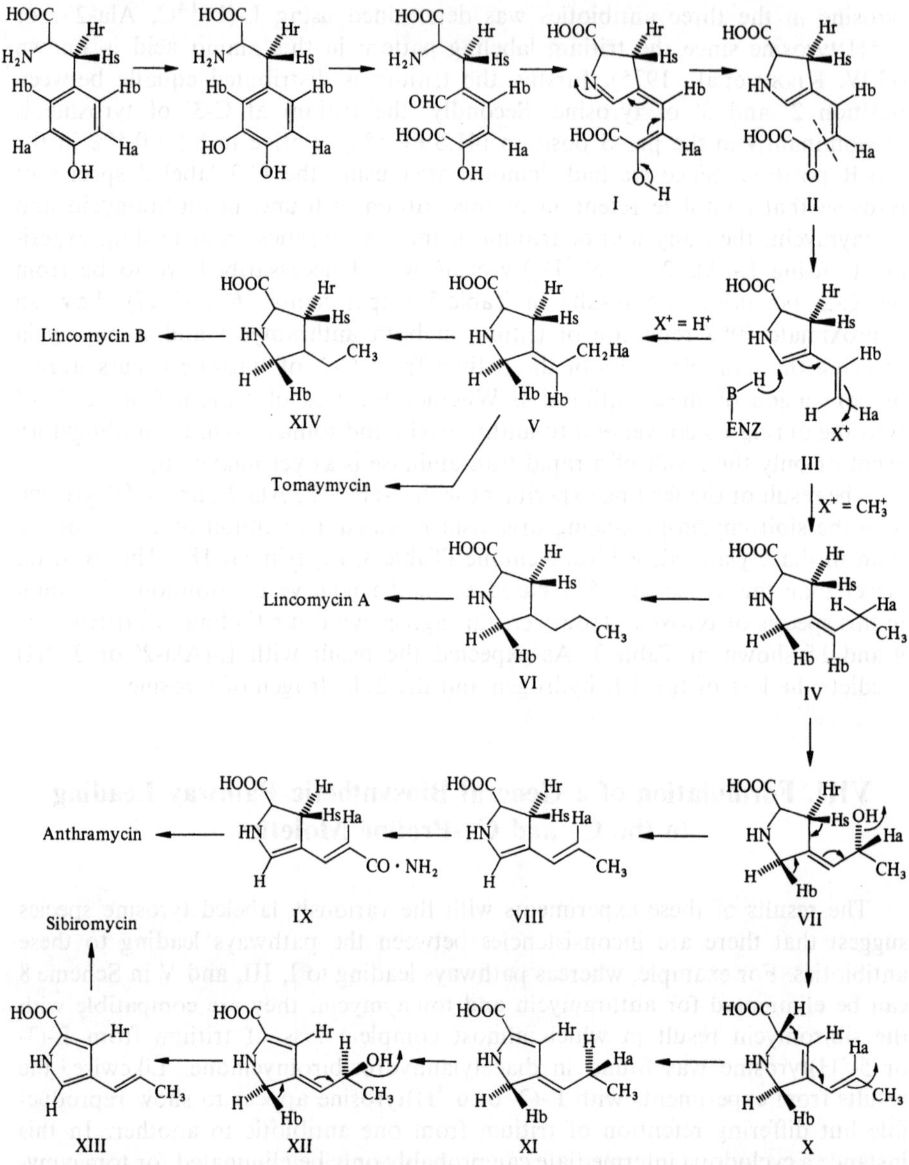

Scheme 12. Proposed parallel biosynthetic pathways for the conversion of tyrosine into the C_2 and C_3 proline moieties of anthramycin, tomaymycin, sibiromycin, and lincomycins A and B (L.H. HURLEY et al., 1979b)

(pathways b and c in Scheme 8) can be completely eliminated from consideration at this time; however, these were considered to be less likely than the proximal extradiol cleavage for the following reasons.

a) When substituted catechol derivatives are used as substrates for metapyrocatechase they are cleaved exclusively at this proximal site by the action of this enzyme (M. NOZAKI et al., 1970).

b) Mechanistically the formation of a Schiff base (I in Scheme 12) and its subsequent conversion to the diene (III in Scheme 12) are attractive.

c) The presence of a similar yellow compound derived from tyrosine in the acid extract of the broths of all three antibiotic fermentations with spectral properties similar to products of extradiol ring fission of aromatic compounds is supportive evidence for a pathway involving a metapyrocatechase (L.H. HURLEY, unpublished results).

2. Cyclodopa is unlikely to be a common intermediate in the pathway.

3. Divergence of the pathways occurs at the step at which addition of either a CH_3^+ group or a H^+ to a common C_2-proline unit takes place.

4. Formation of the ethylidene methyl group of tomaymycin, the conjugated acrylamide side chain of anthramycin and the unsaturation in the side chain and pyrrolo ring of sibiromycin are cosmetic after events which occur subsequent to the main pathway.

The important features of the main and branch pathways leading to the C_2 and C_3-proline units of the pyrrolo(1,4)benzodiazepine antibiotics and the lincomycins shown in Scheme 12 are as follows:

1. Following 2,3 extradiol cleavage of the aromatic ring of dopa, a condensation reaction to form a Schiff base between the α-amino group and the aldehydic group takes place.

2. The conjugated enol (I) then undergoes enolization to yield the α-keto acid (II) which itself then loses two carbon atoms (carbon atoms 4 and 5 of dopa) in a stepwise manner to form the diene (III).

3. The diene (III) is considered to be the branch point compound for which a 1,4 addition of H-X results in divergent pathways dependent upon the nature of X^+. If X^+ is H^+, then the pathway leads to the C_2-proline moieties of tomaymycin and lincomycin B, whereas if X^+ is S^+-CH_3 then the pathway leads to the C_3-proline moieties of anthramycin, sibiromycin, and lincomycin A.

4. Subsequent modification of the first intermediates past the branch point leads to the propyl proline unit of lincomycin A (IV → VI), the acrylamide proline unit of anthramycin (IV → IX), the propylidene proline unit of sibiromycin (IV → XIII), and the ethyl proline unit of lincomycin B (V → XIV). The ethylidene proline unit of tomaymycin is formed directly from the branch point compounds (III → V). Where modifications are required, these would be considered as 'cosmetic or after events' which occur subsequent to the main pathway. The cosmetic modifications leading to the lincomycins are straight-forward and do not require further comment. For the branch pathways leading to the C_3-proline units of anthramycin and sibiromycin, hydroxylation at the allylic carbon in a stereospecific manner leads to VII. This compound can then undergo 1,4 elimination reactions in two analogous but different ways (VII → VIII and VII → X). These reactions result in the stereospecific loss of hydrogen that was originally at C-2 or 6 of tyrosine (anthramycin pathway) or the 3′S position of tyrosine (sibiromycin pathway). The conversion of VIII to IX requires oxidation and amination to produce the acrylamide proline moiety of anthramycin. In the case of the sibiromycin branch X undergoes an allylic rearrangement to produce XI which is then hydroxylated at the allylic carbon thereby eliminat-

ing in a stereospecific manner the hydrogen that was originally located at C-3 or 5 of tyrosine. The product of this reaction XII is then able to undergo a second 1,4 stereospecific elimination of HOY which leads to loss of the hydrogen originally located at C-2 or C-6 of tyrosine and concomitantly the formation of the desired propylidene side chain of sibiromycin.

This proposed biosynthetic pathway for conversion of tyrosine to the C_2 and C_3-proline units of anthramycin, tomaymycin, and sibiromycin can be used to rationalize *all of the apparent inconsistencies* found in this biosynthetic study. Each of the inconsistencies between the results can be related directly to a structural modification peculiar to one or two of the three antibiotics. In each case the structural modification responsible for the apparent inconsistency will be explained.

Anthramycin and sibiromycin differ from tomaymycin in that whereas tomaymycin has a methylene group at C-3, the equivalent position in anthramycin and sibiromycin carries a methine carbon. Assuming ring cleavage prior to formation of the five-membered ring then the intermediacy of compounds such as IV containing a methylene carbon at C-3 (numbering as for antibiotics) which is stereospecifically labeled from L-(2- or 6-^{3}H)tyrosine, would allow the stereospecific removal of the labeled hydrogen in a later step. Such is the case for the anthramycin and sibiromycin branch pathways during the 1,4 elimination reactions (VII → VIII and XI → XII, respectively). Since the tomaymycin branch pathway lacks this reaction, then such removal of tritium would not occur and the tritium at the 3 position of tomaymycin originally located at C-2 or 6 of tyrosine is retained. Based upon this prediction, the theoretical retentions of tritium in tomaymycin, anthramycin, and sibiromycin from feeding experiments which L-(1′-^{14}C, 2- or 6-^{3}H)tyrosine should be 100, 50, and 50% respectively. Examination of the result in Table 3 shows that the retentions of tritium in tomaymycin and diacetylanhydrosibiromycinone are somewhat less than expected (78 and 32.7% for tomaymycin and diacetylanhydrosibiromycinone respectively). A possible explanation for this is the lability of the C-6 hydrogen in dopa. Such a non-enzymatically controlled reaction could lead to washing out of a portion of the tritium originally located at C-6 of dopa and produce a lower than theoretically expected tritium retention in tomaymycin and sibiromycin.

Sibiromycin differs from anthramycin and tomaymycin in that, whereas, sibiromycin has a double bond at the 11a-1 positions, both anthramycin and tomaymycin are saturated at the equivalent positions. Assuming an ‘extradiol cleavage’ pathway for all three antibiotics then the branch point compound (III in Scheme 12) should retain 50% of the tritium from L-(3- or 5-^{3}H)tyrosine. However, the final retention of this tritium at C-13 of the three antibiotics depends upon lack of elimination of this hydrogen in the subsequent cosmetic modifications. In the case of tomaymycin and anthramycin the proposed biosynthetic scheme allows this retention. However, in sibiromycin the introduction of the double bonds at the 11a-1 and 2-3 positions (numbering as for antibiotics) depends on two allylic hydroxylations at C-13. Assuming that the allylic rearrangement (X → XI) and the allylic hydroxylations (VI → VII and XI → XII) are enzymatically controlled and therefore are stereospecific, and if one of the two hydroxylation results in elimination of the hydrogen originally located at C-3 or 5 of tyrosine, then the almost complete loss of tritium in sibiromycin from a feeding experiment with L-(3- or 5-^{3}H)tyrosine can be rationalized.

The occurrence of biosynthetic pathways common to different organisms, together with the accumulating evidence that antibiotic biosynthetic information is carried on plasmids (M. YAGISAWA et al., 1978) and is therefore readily exchangeable between microorganisms within the same family argues strongly against dissimilar general pathways for antibiotic biosynthesis. It is, however, apparent that families of antibiotics produced from common intermediates are found in nature. For example, the erythromycins, tetracyclines, anthracyclines, and peptide antibiotics are a few of the families of antibiotics which contain large numbers of individual members. We would like to suggest that the C_2 and C_3-proline units of anthramycin, tomaymycin, sibiromycin, and lincomycins A and B are derived from similar precursors (tyrosine, with or without C-1 units via methionine) through a general pathway which diverges at the point at which the proline ring is formed and a proton or a methyl group is added. Structural modifications subsequent to this are cosmetic in nature and depend upon the variety of enzymes available to each particular organism. We are, therefore, tempted to suggest that the biosynthetic steps on the main pathway are common to all members of this family of antibiotics. Consequently, if one or more members of this family have residual information in the final antibiotic which eliminates one, two, or more alternative pathways for an early step (e.g., meta vs. ortho cleavage or the point in the pathway at which ring cleavage occurs), then this will be applicable to other members of the family. Using this rationale we have postulated a main biosynthetic pathway leading to a branch point compound, which incorporates information obtained from one or more members of the family for these early steps. The explanations for the anomalous results are then found in the cosmetic after-events which occur in the branch pathways leading to the individual antibiotics. For the examples in this paper, we have been able directly to relate the structural differences between the different antibiotics to a rationale basis for the apparent anomolous results.

Although the proposed biosynthetic pathways shown in Scheme 12 is probably not the only one capable of explaining our results, we feel its development and existence is an important step in our program to establish a general biosynthetic pathway to these interesting antibiotics.

IX. Biosynthetic Relationship Between Tomaymycin and Oxotomaymycin

Oxotomaymycin (Fig. 1) is biologically inactive and is found alongside tomaymycin in the fermentation broth of *S. achromogenes* (K. KARIYONE et al., 1971; L.H. HURLEY et al., 1976a). The biosynthetic relationship between these two compounds has been explored by feeding tomaymycin and oxotomaymycin in parallel flasks. The results indicate that tomaymycin is enzymatically converted to oxotomaymycin by an intracellular enzyme that is present both in the trophophase and idiophase (L.H. HURLEY et al., 1976a). Whether this is a protective response of the tomaymycin culture to the toxic effects of this antibiotic or the enzyme is merely fortuitously present is unknown. It is, however, perhaps significant that oxotomaymycin is the only product produced from tomaymycin by *S. achromogenes* and this compound is biologically inactive.

X. Conclusion

The data thus far obtained on the biosynthesis of anthramycin, tomaymycin, and sibiromycin has established unequivocally the basic biosynthetic building blocks for these antibiotics and the labeling patterns of tyrosine, tryptophan, and methionine in these antibiotics. Some information on possible intermediates in the conversions of tryptophan to the anthranilic acid moieties and tyrosine to the C_2 and C_3-proline moieties of the pyrrolo(1,4)benzodiazepine antibiotics is available from double-labeling experiments ($^3H/^{14}C$) and competition experiments. Little, however, is known about the absolute identity of true intermediates in the biosynthetic pathway and even less concerning the enzymes or the function, if any, of these compounds to the producer organisms. Our continued studies are directed toward these objectives.

Acknowledgments. The work summarized here is that of present and former graduate students and post-doctoral associates. Their names appear in the references cited. The financial support of the National Institutes of Health, Research Grant CA 17047 is gratefully acknowledged. Our thanks to Ms. Laurie West for her patience in preparing this manuscript.

References

Arima K, Kohsaka M, Tamura G, Imanaka H, Sakai H (1972) Studies on tomaymycin, a new antibiotic. I. Isolation and properties of tomaymycin. J Antibiot 24:437–444

Audhya TK, Russell DW (1975) Enniatin production by *Fusarium sambucinum*; primary, secondary, and unitary metabolism. J Gen Microbiol 86:327–331

Berger J, Karr AE, Leimgruber W, Tabenkin B, Schocher AJ, Stefanovic V (1971) Antibiotic production utilizing *Streptomyces refuineus* var. *thermotolerans*. US Patent 3,619,374

Chang C-J, Floss HG, Hurley L, Zmijewski M (1976) Application of long-range spin-spin coupling in biosynthetic studies. J Org Chem 41:2932–2935

Daly JW, Jerina DM, Witkop B (1972) Arene oxides and the NIH shift: The metabolism, toxicity and carcinogenicity of aromatic compounds. Experientia 28:1129–1149

Gairola C, Hurley LH (1976) Mechanism for the methionine mediated reduction of anthramycin yields in *Streptomyces refuineus* fermentations. Eur J Appl Microbiol 2:95–101

Gause GF, Preobrazhenskaya TP, Ivanitskaya LP, Sveshnikova MA (1969) Production of the antibiotic sibiromycin by *Streptosporangium sibiricum* sp. *nov.* Antibiotiki 14:963–969

Hendlin D (1949) The nutritional requirements of a bacitracin producing strain of *Bacillus subtilis*. Arch Biochem 24:435–446

Hopwood DA (1967) Genetic analysis and genome structure in *Streptomyces coelicolor*. Bacteriol Rev 31:373–403

Hurley LH (1977) Pyrrolo(1,4)benzodiazepine antitumor antibiotics. Comparative aspects of anthramycin, tomaymycin and sibiromycin. J Antibiot 30:349–370

Hurley LH, Gairola C (1979) Pyrrolo(1,4)benzodiazepine antitumor antibiotics. Biosynthetic studies on the conversion of tryptophan to the anthranilic acid moieties of sibiromycin and tomaymycin. Antimicrobial Ag. Chemother., *15*:42–46

Hurley LH, Ostrander JM (1978) The biosynthetic origin of the nitrogens in the antitumor antibiotic anthramycin. Abstr Annu Meet Acad Pharm Sci No 9:111

Hurley LH, Zmijewski M, Chang C-J (1975) Biosynthesis of anthramycin. Determination of the labelling pattern by the use of radioactive and stable-isotope techniques. J Am Chem Soc 97:4372–4378

Hurley LH, Gairola C, Das N (1976a) Pyrrolo(1,4)benzodiazepine antibiotics. Biosynthesis of the antitumor antibiotic 11-demethyltomaymycin and its biologically inactive metabolite oxotomaymycin by *Streptomyces achromogenes*. Biochemistry 15:3760–3769

Hurley LH, Gairola C, Das N, Zmijewski M (1976b) Biosynthetic incorporation of DL-(5-^{3}H) tryptophan into anthramycin, sibiromycin and tomaymycin. NIH shift produced by actinomycetes. Tetrahedron Lett 1976:1419–1423

Hurley LH, Gairola C, Zmijewski M (1977) Pyrro(1,4)benzodiazepine antitumor antibiotics. In vitro interaction of anthramycin, sibiromycin and tomaymycin with DNA using specifically radiolabelled molecules. Biochim. Biophys. Acta 475:521–535

Hurley LH, Lasswell WL, Malhotra RK, Das NV (1979a) Pyrrolo(1,4)benzodiazepine antibiotics. Biosynthesis of the antitumor antibiotic sibiromycin by *Streptosporangium sibiricum*. Biochemistry 18:4225–4229

Hurley LH, Lasswell WL,Ostrander J, Parry R (1979b) Pyrrolo(1,4)benzodiazepine antibiotics. Biosynthetic conversion of tyrosine to the C_2 and C_3-proline moieties of anthramycin, tomaymycin and sibiromycin. Biochemistry 18:4230–4237

Johns N, Kirby GW, Bu'Lock JD, Ryles AP (1975) Stereospecific exchange of a β-methylene proton in phenylalanine preceding biosynthetic incorporation into gliotoxin. J Chem Soc Perkin I: 383–386

Kariyone K, Yazawa H, Kohsaka M (1971) The structures of tomaymycin and oxotomaymycin. Chem Pharm Bull 19:2289–2293

Kirby GW, Narayanaswami S, Rao PS (1975) On the preparation of L-(2,3-^{3}H)phenylalanine and L-(2,3-$^3H_2$)tyrosine. J Chem Soc Perkin I:645–647

Kohn KW, Glaubiger D, Spears CL (1974) The reaction of anthramycin with DNA. II. Studies of kinetics and mechanism. Biochim Biophys Acta 361:288–302

Krupinski VM, Robbers JE, Floss HG (1976) Physiological study of ergot: Induction of alkaloid synthesis by tryptophan at the enzymatic level. J Bacteriol 125:158–165

Malik VS (1972) Chloramphenicol. Adv Appl Microbiol 15:297–331

Miyamoto M, Kondo S, Naganawa H, Maeda K, Ohro M, Umezawa H (1977) Structure and synthesis of neothramycin. J Antibiot 30:340–343

Nozaki M, Kotani S, Ono K, Senoh S (1970) Metapyrocatechase. III. Substrate specificity and mode of ring fission. Biochem Biophys Acta 222:213–223

Parry RJ (1975) Biosynthesis of the securinega alkaloids. Stereospecificity of hydrogen loss from C-3 of tyrosine. J Chem Soc Chem Commun 144–145

Parry RJ (1978) The synthesis and metabolism of chirally labelled α-amino acids in bioorganic chemistry. In: Tamelen van EE (ed) Substrate behavior, vol XI, p 4. Academic Press, London New York

Rolls JP, Ruff, BD, Haak WJ, Hessler EJ (1976) Comparison of the biosynthesis of the amino acid moieties of lincomycin. Abstr 76th Annu Meet ASM 027

Schultz G, Feigelson P (1972) Expression of total enzyme activity by means of thermal activation of hepatic tryptophan oxygenase. Anal Biochem 46:149–155

Speedie MK, Forbes MB (1977) Regulation of anthramycin biosynthesis in *Streptomyces refuineus* (abstract). Lloydia 40:612

Takeuchi T, Miyamoto M, Ishizuka M, Naganawa H, Kondo S, Hamada M, Umezawa H (1976) Neothramycins A and B, new antitumor antibiotics. J Antibiot 29:93–96

Williams WK, Katz E (1977) Development of a chemically defined medium for the synthesis of actinomycin D by *Streptomyces parvulus*. Antimicrob Agents Chemother 11:281–290

Witz DF, Hessler EJ, Miller TL (1971) Bioconversion of tyrosine into the propylhygric acid moiety of lincomycin. Biochemistry 10:1128–1131

Yagisawa M, Rossana Huang T-S, Davies JE (1978) Possible involvements of plasmids in biosynthesis of neomycin. J Antibiot 31:809–813

Addendum

Recent studies on the regulation of tyrosine biosynthesis in *S. refuineus* have demonstrated a shuttle mechanism. Phenylalanine was found to feedback-inhibit prephenate dehydratase, resulting in increased prephenate dehydrogenase activity and a channelling of the common precursor, prephenic acid to tyrosine*.

Experiments with plasmid agents have shown that while acridine orange, ethidium bromide and acriflavin did not result in loss of anthramycin production by *S. refuineus*, novobiocin treatment resulted in a 12% cure rate. Using physical and biochemical techniques such as CsCl ethidium bromide density gradient, agarose gel electrophoresis and electron microscopy we have demonstrated that a plasmid is present in both the producer and non-producer. Since other changes occurred in the non-producer such as loss of resistance to anthramycin and change in colony morphology we speculate that novobiocin may produce a deletion mutation which causes pleiotropic effects**.

* M.K. Speedie and M.O. Park. Regulation of Tyrosine Biosynthesis by Phenylalanine in Anthramycin Producing *S. refuineus*. J. Antibiotics **33**, 579–582 (1980)

** J.R. Rokem and L.H. Hurley. Curing of Antibiotic Production and Plasmid DNA in the Anthramycin Producer *Streptomyces refuineus* V. *Thermotolerans*. J. Antibiotics, submitted for publication.

Biosynthesis of the Mitomycins

ULFERT HORNEMANN

I. Introduction

The mitomycins and porfiromycin (Fig. 1) constitute a complex of anticancer antibiotics which are produced by *Streptomyces caespitosus* (HATA et al., 1956), *Streptomyces ardus* sp. n (DEBOER et al., 1960) *Streptomyces verticillatus* (LEFEMINE et al., 1962) and *Streptomyces michiganensis* (WOLF et al., 1975). Their structures have been determined by chemical, physicochemical, and X-ray methods (WEBB et al., 1962a, 1962b; STEVENS et al., 1965; TULINSKY and VAN DEN HENDE, 1967; YAHASHI and MATSUBARA, 1976). Mitomycin A (Ia) (TULINSKY and VAN DEN HENDE, 1967) and Mitomycin B (Ib) (YAHASHI and MATSUBARA, 1976) differ stereochemically at C-9. The structure of mitiromycin (II), a biologically inactive close relative, has been reported (MORTON et al., 1970). The mitomycins and the *Streptomyces* metabolite (S)-2,3-dicarboxyaziridine (III) (NAGANAWA et al., 1975) are unique among naturally occurring metabolites owing to the presence of an aziridine ring. A related ring system, an azirine ring, occurs in the *Streptomyces aureus* antibiotic azirinomycin (IV) (MILLER et al., 1971).

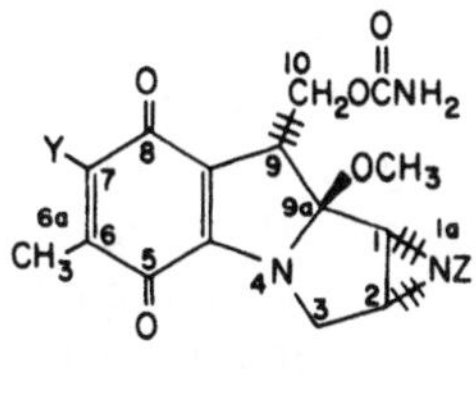

I (a,c,d)

		Y	Z
Ia	Mitomycin A	CH_3O	H
Ic	Mitomycin C	NH_2	H
Id	Porfiromycin	NH_2	CH_3

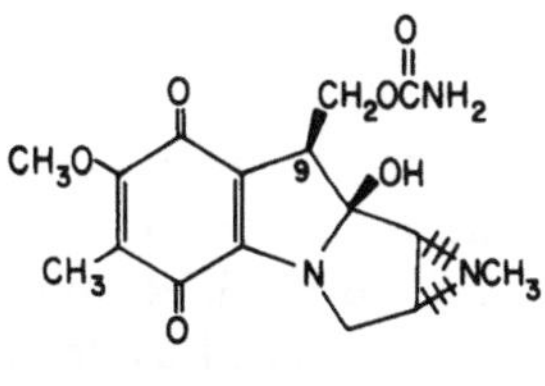

Ib Mitomycin B

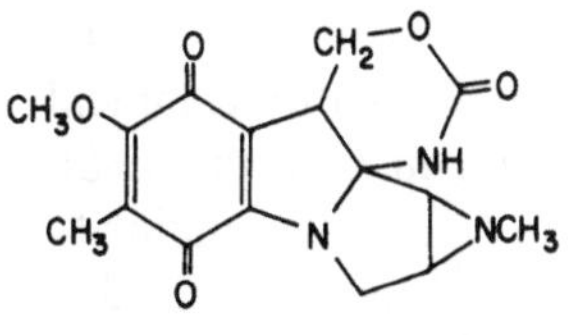

II Mitiromycin

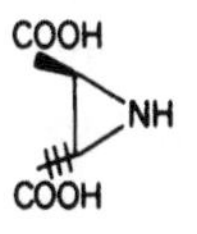

III (S)-2,3-Dicarboxy aziridine

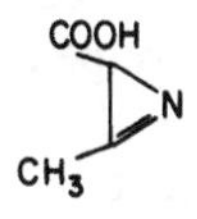

IV Azirinomycin

Fig. 1. Structures of mitomycins and of related compounds

The total synthesis of the mitomycins, with the exception of mitomycin B, has been achieved (NAKATSUBO et al., 1977; FUKUYAMA et al., 1977) and a variety of analogs have been prepared and several of these have been tested as antitumor and antibacterial agents (KINOSHITA et al., 1971; LIN et al., 1974; TAYLOR et al., 1977; AKHTAR et al., 1975). The mode of action of the mitomycins has been reviewed by SZYBALSKI and IYER (1967), and more recently by KERSTEN (1975). It is recognized that they function as mono- and bifunctional alkylating agents of biological macromolecules after they have undergone activation by reduction. DNA is considered to be the essential mitomycin target and cross-linking of the two DNA strands resulting from bifunctional alkylation has been reported. In spite of many investigations (SZYBALSKI and IYER, 1964; LIPSETT and WEISSBACH, 1965; OTSUJI and MURAYAMA, 1972; TOMASZ et al., 1974; LOWN and WEIR, 1978) it is not known with certainty which sites on mitomycin and on DNA are involved in the formation of covalent bonds. Mitomycin C (Ic) (NSC-26980) is an FDA-approved anticancer agent and has been used frequently in clinical trials in cancer chemotherapy (CROOKE and BRADNER, 1976).

Studies on the biosynthesis of the mitomycins have been reported by KIRSCH and co-workers (KIRSCH and KORSHALLA, 1964; KIRSCH, 1967), by BEZANSON and VINING (1971), by NISHIKOHORI and FUKUI (1975), and from this laboratory (HORNEMANN and CLOYD, 1971; HORNEMANN and AIKMAN, 1973; HORNEMANN et al., 1974a, 1974b, 1974c, 1975). KIRSCH et al. showed that among a number of compounds fed to replacement cultures of *S. verticillatus* only L-[$^{14}CH_3$]methionine gave radioactive mitomycin A. The highest incorporation obtained was 1% and the radioactivity was essentially confined to the O-methyl groups. Thus C-methylation does not seem to occur in mitomycin biosynthesis. L-[alanine-3-^{14}C]tryptophan, L-[U-^{14}C]tyrosine, and [1-^{14}C]acetate were not incorporated. The more extensive studies of BEZANSON and VINING yielded results which are in full agreement with those of KIRSCH and KORSHALLA and with many of the results obtained in this laboratory. BEZANSON and VINING observed O-methylation by L-[$^{14}CH_3$]methionine of mitomycin C and no C-methylation. Aromatic amino acids and acetic acid did not label the ring skeleton of the antibiotic nor did mevalonic acid and several other amino acids. Also shikimic acid did not label mitomycin C even though its uptake by the mycelium could be ascertained as demonstrated by the specific labeling of the aromatic amino acids of proteins. The best precursor investigated was D-glucose and it was stated that the distribution of radioactivity in C-6 and the attached methyl group of mitomycin C labeled from D-[1-^{14}C]-, -[2-^{14}C]-, and -[6-^{14}C]glucose was consistent with derivation of the methylbenzoquinone moiety from a seven-carbon intermediate which could originate from glucose by reactions of the nonoxidative pentose phosphate pathway. Specifically it was shown by chemical degradation that label from these glucose samples appeared in C-6 and C-6a to the extent of 4.42, 14.5, and 0.27%, respectively, and that the majority of the label incorporated into C-6 and C-6a from D-[1-^{14}C]glucose resided at C-6a, while the majority of the label incorporated into these two positions from D-[2-^{14}C]glucose was found at C-6. The work reported by NISHIKOHORI and FUKUI was mainly concerned with the later stages of the pathway, specifically with the role of methylation.

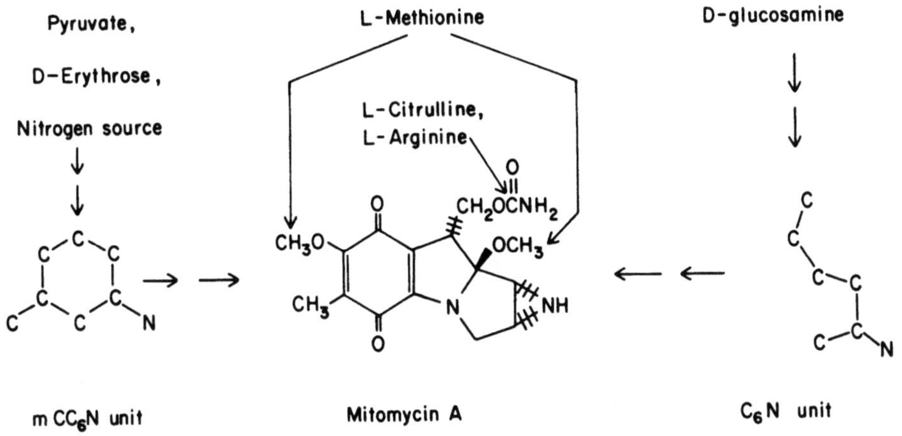

Fig. 2. Building blocks of the mitomycins

The biosynthetic studies conducted in this laboratory have provided strong evidence that the heterocyclic ring system of the mitomycins is elaborated by the joining of two principal moieties: a C_6N unit and an mCC_6N unit (comprising a six-membered ring with meta-disposed carbon and nitrogen substituents). D-glucosamine has been recognized as an efficient progenitor of the C_6N unit. The mCC_6N unit has been shown in recent experiments to be specifically labeled by erythrose and by pyruvate, and it is suggested that a very early intermediate of the shikimic acid pathway may play a role in its formation. The carbamoyl group of the mitomycins has been shown to be efficiently labeled by L-[guanidino-^{14}C]arginine, and by L-[ureido-^{14}C]citrulline, and L-[$^{14}CH_3$]-methionine, as also shown in this laboratory, is the precursor for O and N-methyl groups. These findings are summarized in Figure 2. The feeding experiments which established the origin of the different moieties will be outlined. Attention will be drawn to the occurrence and the biosynthesis of mCC_6N units in other antibiotics which appear to be related to the mCC_6N unit of the mitomycins. Furthermore possible mechanisms for the joining of the C_6N and the mCC_6N unit as well as aspects of the later stages of mitomycin biosynthesis, including a possible precursor role of mitomycin A for mitomycin B and mitiromycin will be discussed.

The biosynthetic studies were carried out with *Streptomyces verticillatus* (ATCC 13495) which was grown on a complex natural medium (KIRSCH and KORSHALLA, 1964) for 4 days. Cells were then replaced into a synthetic medium containing D-mannose instead of D-glucose (KIRSCH and KORSHALLA, 1964) in which a mixture of approximately 4 mg of mainly mitomycin A and B was produced per 100 ml after an additional 4 days. Radioactive precursors were added on day 3 to replaced cells which were harvested by filtration. Stable isotope-labeled precursors were added to replaced mycelia 1 or 2 days before harvest.

The mitomycins were isolated by extraction of the filtered broth with ethyl acetate and purified by thin layer chromatography (HORNEMANN and CLOYD,

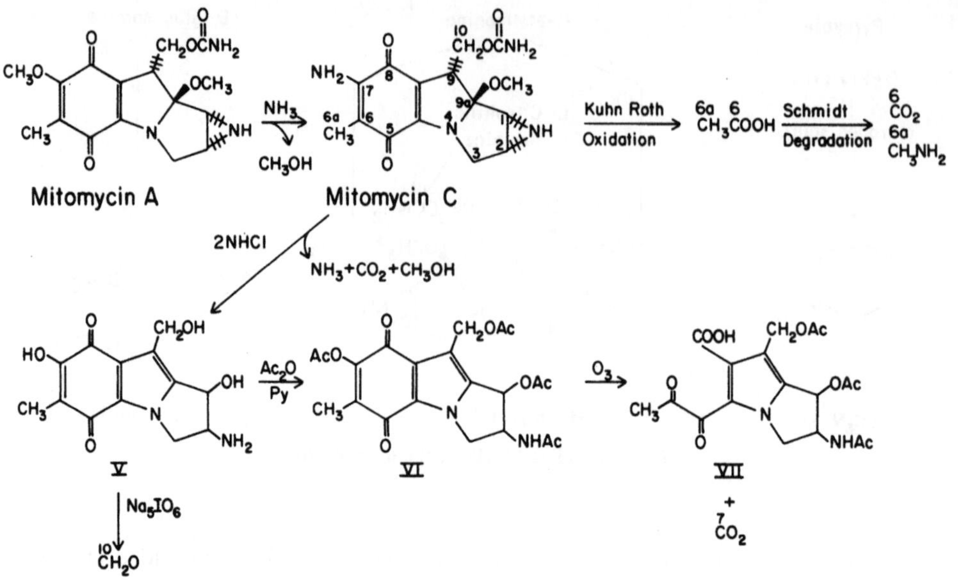

Fig. 3. Chemical degradations of mitomycin A

1971). Radioactive samples of mitomycin A were converted into mitomycin C by treatment with ammonia (HORNEMANN and CLOYD, 1971) followed by recrystallization to constant specific radioactivity with carrier mitomycin C. Samples of mitomycin C were then subjected, as appropriate, to degradation reactions as outlined in Figure 3. The resulting products were recrystallized to constant specific radioactivity where applicable. The incorporation of precursors into the carbamoyl group and/or into the O-methyl group of mitomycin C was investigated by comparing the specific radioactivity of mitomycin C with that of tetraacetylmitomycinone (VI) prepared according to STEVENS et al. (1965). Carbon atom 10 was isolated as formaldehyde from the decarbamoylindicatorquinone (V) in an unspecific periodate oxidation (HORNEMANN et al., 1974a). Radioactivity incorporated into C-7 was determined by comparing the specific radioactivity of VI with that of its derived ozonolysis product (VII). Carbon atom 6 and its attached methyl group were accessible by the Kuhn Roth oxidation, affording acetic acid which was further degraded by the Schmid degradation to yield C-6 as CO_2 and C-6a as methylamine. Detailed analysis of the incorporation of stable isotope-labeled precursors into the carbamoyl group was possible by high-resolution, electron-impact, mass-spectroscopic analysis of the ion $m/e = 44$ and its isotope satellites (HORNEMANN and EGGERT, 1975) and information on the incorporation of precursors into C-1, C-2, C-3 and into the aziridine nitrogen was gained by analysis of the ion $m/e = 70$ and its isotope satellites (HORNEMANN et al., 1974a; VAN LEAR, 1970) using labeled mitomycin B. The relevant fragmentations and the mass spectrum of mitomycin B are shown in Figure 4.

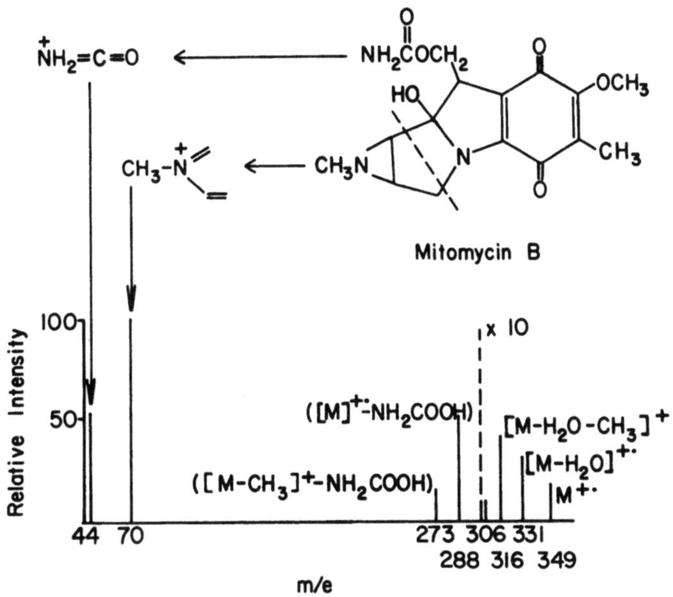

Fig. 4. Mass spectrum of mitomycin B redrawn from van Lear (1970)

II. Origin of the C_6N Unit

At the outset of our biosynthetic studies it appeared attractive to postulate that the highly functionalized, right-hand portion of the mitomycins consisting of carbons 1, 2, 3, 9, 9a, and 10 and the aziridine nitrogen could arise from a hexosamine. Subsequent feeding experiments with various labeled hexosamines and with glucosaminitol listed in Table 1 have shown that D-glucosamine is indeed an efficient precursor of these antibiotics. Since both D-glucosamine and D-galactosamine showed similar incorporation rates competition feeding experiments were carried out. The results obtained showed that D-glucosamine was the more proximal precursor (U. HORNEMANN and J.P. KEHRER, unpublished observations). D-Mannosamine is clearly a less efficient precursor than D-glucosamine, and D-glucosaminitol was practically not incorporated. The results of specific labeling studies indicated that D-glucosamine is utilized, most likely as an intact unit. Chemical degradations (Fig. 3) indicated that at least 72% of the label incorporated into mitomycin A from D[6-^{14}C]glucosamine resides at C-10 (HORNEMANN et al. 1974a), and high-resolution, mass-spectroscopic analysis (Fig. 4) showed that D-[1-^{13}C, ^{15}N]-glucosamine is incorporated into a fragment C_4H_8N comprising C-1, C-2, C-3, N-1a and the attached methyl group of mitomycin B essentially without separation of the labels (HORNEMANN et al., 1974a) (Table 2). The latter result indicates that during the inversion of configuration at C-2 of D-glucosamine, which is required during mitomycin biosynthesis, the nitrogen is not separated and reintroduced into the carbon skeleton. Furthermore, since D-mannosamine, which possesses the correct chira-

Table 1. Incorporation of hexosamines and of D-glucosaminitol into mitomycins

Precursor				Mitomcyins (Ia–d)	
	Quantity fed (µmol)	Radio-activity fed (dpm)	T/C ratio	^{14}C-Incor-poration (%)	T/C ratio of mito-mycin A [T reten-tion (%)]
D-[1-^{14}C]glucosamine	20	$4.3 \cdot 10^6$		3.0	
D-[6-^{14}C]glucosamine	23	$5.6 \cdot 10^6$		5.1	
D-[1-^{13}C, ^{15}N, 1-^{14}C]-glucosamine	230	$1.0 \cdot 10^7$		1.8	
D-[2-^{3}H, 1-^{14}C]glucosamine	20	^{14}C: $1.1 \cdot 10^7$ ^{3}H: $7.2 \cdot 10^7$	6.6	1.0	2.9 [44]
D-[4-^{3}H, 1-^{14}C]glucosamine	12	^{14}C: $2.9 \cdot 10^6$ ^{3}H: $9.5 \cdot 10^6$	3.3	2.5	1.3 [39]
D-[5-^{3}H, 1-^{14}C]glucosamine	14	^{14}C: $2.7 \cdot 10^6$ ^{3}H: $1.3 \cdot 10^7$	4.5	2.5	1.0 [22]
D-[6-^{3}H, 1-^{14}C]Glucosamine	13	^{14}C: $2.7 \cdot 10^6$ ^{3}H: $1.3 \cdot 10^7$	4.8	2.3	3.9 [82]
D-[1-^{14}C]glucosamine	3	$2.1 \cdot 10^7$		2.3	
D-[1-^{14}C]galactosamine	3	$2.1 \cdot 10^7$		1.8	
D-[1-^{14}C]mannosamine	5	$1.8 \cdot 10^7$		0.6	
D-[1-^{14}C]glucosaminitol	5	$1.2 \cdot 10^7$		<0.1	

Table 2. Labeling of ions belonging to the ion cluster C_4H_8N (m/e 70) of mitomycin B isolated after feeding D-glucosamine-[1-^{13}C, ^{15}N] to *S. verticillatus*

Ion	$^{12}C_4H_8{}^{14}N$	$^{12}C_4H_8{}^{15}N$	$^{12}C_3{}^{13}CH_8{}^{14}N$	$^{12}C_3{}^{13}CH_8{}^{15}N$	$^{12}C_2{}^{13}C_2H_8{}^{14}N$
Relative intensity × 100	55.6	8.4	4.9	31.1	<2

lity at C-2 is an inefficient precursor it is very likely that it is not involved as an underivatized compound in this biosynthetic pathway. Its possible participation as a derivatized compound such as a phosphate and/or nucleotide derivative and the possible participation of untested hexosamines in mitomycin biosynthesis requires further studies.

The results of the feeding experiments with the tritium-labeled glucosamines are not fully evaluable in the absence of knowledge on the location of the respective tritium atoms in mitomycin but some conclusions can nevertheless be drawn and some plausible hypotheses can be formulated to guide future studies. Since 44% of the tritium of D-[2-^{3}H]glucosamine is retained in mitomycin A an Amadori-type rearrangement cannot be involved after a possible initial formation of a Schiff's base between the amino group of the mCC_6N unit and D-glucosamine. An Amadori-type rearrangement would require the transfer of the C-2 hydrogen of glucosamine to the nitrogen atom of the mCC_6N unit from which it would be expected to be lost completely by exchange. Partial loss of the C-2 hydrogen, however, may be due to its possible removal, partial exchange, and reintroduction during an enzyme-catalyzed isomerization reaction taking place at C-2. The partial retention of an equivalent hydrogen atom in the reaction catalyzed by uridine diphosphoglucose 4-epimerase has been reported previously (NELSESTUEN and KIRKWOOD, 1971). The retention of 39% of the tritium of D-[4-^{3}H]glucosamine in mitomycin A, which is devoid of hydrogen at C-9a, was unexpected. It is suggested as one possible explanation that this hydrogen is partially transferred to C-3 of mitomycin by a process which would bear some analogy to the transfer of the C-4 hydrogen of D-glucose to C-6 during rhamnose biosynthesis (GABRIEL and LINDQUIST, 1968). It was likewise unexpected to find that most of the tritium of D-[5-^{3}H]glucosamine was excorporated despite the likelihood that C-5 of glucosamine labels C-9 of mitomycins which carries a hydrogen atom. One possible explanation is the transient generation of a carbonyl function at this position and the loss of the tritium in this process. Finally it was curious that tritium of D-[6-^{3}H]glucosamine is not completely retained. It is possible that C-6 of glucosamine may be oxidized to the aldehyde stage to facilitate the joining of C-5 with the mCC_6N unit. Retention of 82% of the tritium would then demand that the respective hydrogen is partially reintroduced. Alternatively the partial loss of the C-6 hydrogen of D-glucosamine may be due to side reactions which may be unrelated to mitomycin biosynthesis and which lead to hydrogen exchange in this position. Future experiments will be designed to shed light on the possibilities discussed above and to elucidate the fate of the hydrogens at C-1 and at C-3 of D-glucosamine. It is anticipated that specifically deuterium-labeled glucosamines will prove to be useful in these studies.

III. Origin of the Carbamoyl Group

Both L-[guanidino-^{14}C]arginine and L-[ureido-^{14}C]citrulline label the mitomycins efficiently (Table 3) and in both cases the label is specifically incorporated into the carbamoyl group (HORNEMANN et al., 1974a; HORNEMANN and EGGERT, 1975). Urea is not a precursor but potassium cyanate, a potential precursor of carbamoyl-phosphate, labels the mitomycin carbamoyl group as do L-[U-^{14}C]aspartic acid and presumably a variety of other precursors which yield CO_2 and hence presumably carbamoyl phosphate (BEZANSON and VINING, 1971). The efficient utilization of both L-arginine and L-citrulline in mitomycin biosynthesis raised the question whether citrulline was incorporated via arginine or vice versa or whether independent pathways were operative. A series of competition feeding experiments such as the ones shown in Table 3 left open the possibility that independent pathways were operative. This follows from the fact that while excess unlabeled L-arginine does not diminish the incorporation of labeled L-citrulline, an excess of unlabeled L-citrulline does not abolish the incorporation of labeled L-arginine as would be expected if L-citrulline were the ultimate

Table 3. Feeding experiments and competition feeding experiments with precursors of the carbamoyl group of mitomycins

Precursor			Mitomycins (Ia–d)
	Quantity fed (μmol)	Radioactivity fed (dpm)	Incorporation (%)
L-[ureido-^{14}C]citrulline	12	$2.4 \cdot 10^7$	11.2
L-[guanidino-^{14}C]arginine	10	$1.2 \cdot 10^7$	9.8
L-[NH_2CO-^{14}C, ^{13}C, ^{15}N]citrulline	86	$9.9 \cdot 10^6$	3.8
[^{14}C]potassium cyanate	11	$1.8 \cdot 10^7$	0.2
[^{14}C]urea	20	$2.2 \cdot 10^7$	<0.1
9 μmol of L-[guanidino-^{14}C]arginine +26 μmol of L-citrulline		$2.2 \cdot 10^7$	5.8
36 μmol of L-[guanidino-^{14}C]arginine (9 μmol labeled, 27 μmol nonlabeled)		$2.2 \cdot 10^7$	5.7
36 μmol of L-[ureido-^{14}C]citrulline (9 μmol labeled, 27 μmol nonlabeled)		$2.2 \cdot 10^7$	8.2
9 μmol of L-[ureido-^{14}C]citrulline +26 μmol of L-arginine		$2.2 \cdot 10^7$	10.6

Table 4. Labeling of ions belonging to the ion cluster NH_2CO (m/e 44) of mitomycin B isolated after feeding L-[NH_2CO-^{13}C, ^{15}N]citrulline to *S. verticillatus*

Ion	NH_2CO	$^{15}NH_2CO$	$NH_2{}^{13}CO$	$^{15}NH_2{}^{13}CO$
Relative intensity × 100	60.8	9.9	<3.3	29.0

precursor, arising obligatorily from L-arginine. To investigate whether the intact carbamoyl group of citrulline was transferred L-[NH_2CO-^{13}C, ^{15}N]citrulline was synthesized (HORNEMANN and EGERT, 1975) and administered together with L-[ureido-^{14}C]citrulline and the isolated mitomycin was analyzed by high-resolution mass spectrometry for species containing both isotopes, or only ^{13}C or ^{15}N. As shown in Table 4 the most abundant labeled peak was seen for the ion $^{15}NH_2$ ^{13}CO, indicating that the intact carbamoyl group of citrulline is utilized in mitomycin biosynthesis. Chemical degradation of the mitomycin sample to the mitomycinone tetraacetate (VI) indicated the complete loss of radioactivity. In preparation of the above feeding experiments favorable conditions had to be established. Upon feeding 50 mg of L-citrulline per 100 ml culture we observed specific incorporation rates of 69% (dilution factors as low as 1.4), suggesting very efficient uptake of citrulline at the time of the feeding experiments, or perhaps the existence of exoenzymes involved in carbamoyl phosphate generation or carbamoyl group transfer to a biosynthetic intermediate from citrulline. This efficient utilization of citrulline is comparable to similar observations made in streptozocin biosynthesis as outlined in Chapter 14. It is interesting that when competition feeding experiments between arginine and citrulline were carried out at the time when the cultures were replaced into

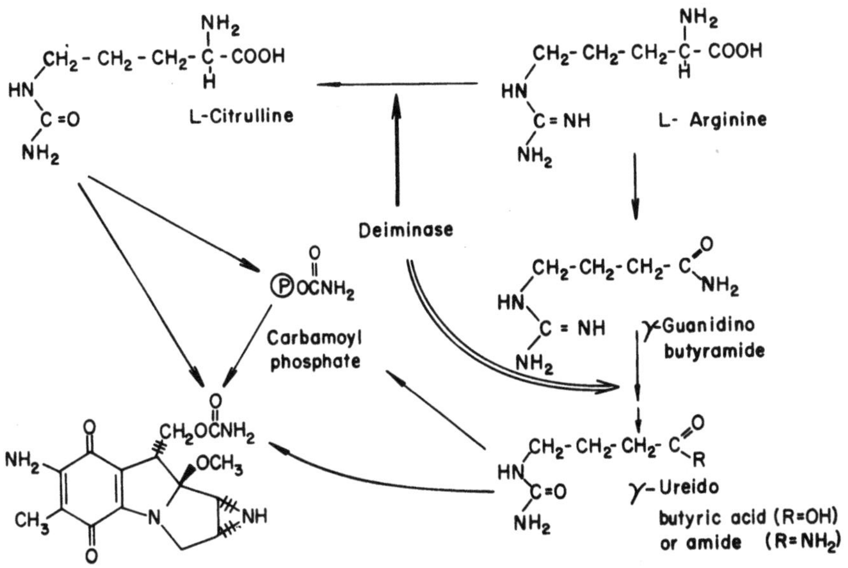

Fig. 5. Hypotheses on the conversion of L-citrulline and L-arginine into the carbamoyl group of mitomycin C

the D-mannose-containing medium, then arginine showed no incorporation into the mitomycins at all, while citrulline showed incorporation comparable to that obtained when citrulline was fed 5 hours before harvest on the fourth day of the fermentation in the D-mannose medium. Presumably citrulline is not utilized for general metabolic reactions in young cultures, perhaps because of a lack of an uptake system. This question deserves further study.

The suggested possibility that L-citrulline and L-arginine label the mitomycin carbamoyl group by independent pathways is supported by unpublished enzymatic evidence which was gathered recently in this laboratory. In searches for the presence of L-arginine deiminase in *S. verticillatus* very little activity was detected and the enzyme was purified 47-fold. When γ-guanidinobutyrate was tested as a possible inhibitor it was unexpectedly found to be a 10-fold better substrate than L-arginine. This finding together with information on arginine catabolism in *Streptomycetes* published by THOAI et al. (1966) suggests that *S. verticillatus* may be able to convert the guanidino group of L-arginine into carbamoylphosphate or into another carbamoyl group donor by the following reaction sequence or one related to it:

L-arginine → γ-guanidinobutyramide → γ-guanidinobutyric acid →
γ-ureidobutyric acid → carbamoylphosphate + γ-aminobutyrate.

The first two enzymes required have not been demonstrated in *S. verticillatus* but further studies are planned to investigate this novel pathway of arginine catabolism. It will be of particular interest to explore the possible participation of γ-ureidobutyric acid and its amide in transcarbamoylation reactions. It should be noted that the above pathway may be of major importance for arginine catabolism in *Streptomycetes* especially since they may be lacking arginase (THOAI et al., 1966), an observation for which we have obtained corroborative evidence in *S. verticillatus* (S. BERNHARD and U. HORNEMANN, unpublished observations). Figure 5 summarizes the possible pathways for the independent generation of the carbamoyl group of mitomycin C from L-citrulline and from L-arginine. It is noteworthy that British workers have reported on the presence in *Streptomyces clavuligerus* of an enzyme capable of transfering the carbamoyl group from carbamoylphosphate to desacetyl-7α-methoxy-cephalosporin C (BREWER et al., 1977).

IV. Origin of the mCC_6N Unit

While the origins of the C_6N unit and of the carbamoyl group of the mitomycins were comparatively readily accessible to theoretical proposals and also to their experimental verification, it has proven to be more difficult to shed light on the origin of the mCC_6N unit. When it was found in this laboratory that glucose could label the mitomycins in the ring skeleton even when a large excess of D-glucosamine was also administered (Table 5) it appeared attractive to suggest the possible involvement of a hepto-2,6-diulose in mitomycin biosynthesis (HORNEMANN et al., 1974b). A similar proposal was also made by BEZANSON and VINING (1971) and the observation that shikimic acid was not a mitomycin precursor (BEZANSON and VINING, 1971; HORNEMANN and CLOYD, 1971) appeared to agree with this idea. However, the results of the degradative studies on mitomycin labeled from glucose samples reported by BEZANSON and VINING (1971) indicated some difficulties with the simple postulate that a C_2-unit comprising C-1 and C-2 of glucose would combine with a pentose to yield a heptulose, because the degree of labeling of C-6a plus C-6 by D-[1-^{14}C]glucose was much lower than expected. We therefore repeated these experiments with the same labeled D-glucose species, but with the modification that an excess of nonlabeled D-glucosamine was administered at the same time. Included in these feeding experiments were D-[3,4-^{14}C]glucose and different labeled pyruvic acids which were also added together with a vast excess of D-glucosamine. It was anticipated that the addition of glucosamine would inhibit the possible incorporation of D-glucose and of pyruvate into the C_6N unit and thus reveal more clearly the fate of the individual labeled atoms. The results presented in Table 5 show an increased discrepancy in the labeling of C-6+C-6a by D-[1-^{14}C]- and -[2-^{14}C]glucose and in conjunction with the mode of incorporation of D-[3,4-^{14}C]glucose and of the pyruvate samples, suggest, that phosphoenolpyruvate may be acting as a common intermediate. This would be most readily possible via the involvement of an early intermediate of the shikimic acid pathway such as 3-deoxy-D-arabino heptulosonic acid-7-phosphate (DAHP), 3-dehydroquinic acid (3 DHQ) or 3-dehydro-shikimic acid (3 DHS). In order for exogenous pyruvate to participate in this pathway it must be converted into phosphoenolpyruvate. This conversion may be carried out by the enzyme pyruvate, phosphate dikinase (WOOD et al., 1977) which was shown to be present and inducible

Table 5. Mode of incorporation of D-glucose and pyruvic acid into mitomycins by *S. verticillatus*

Precursor[a]	Incorporation into mitomycins A, B, C, and porfiromycin (%)	Radioactivity of mitomycin C remaining in tetraacetylmitomycinone derivative (%)	Radioactivity of mitomycin C residing in C-6+C-6a (%)	Radioactivity of C-6+C-6a residing in C-6a (%)	Radioactivity of C-6+C-6a residing in C-6 (%)
D-[1-^{14}C]glucose	0.7	68	4.6	44.0	19.0
D-[2-^{14}C]glucose	0.8	63	28.2	21.0	75.5
D-[3,4-^{14}C]glucose	0.3	74	22.6	61.2	9.9
D-[6-^{14}C]glucose	0.8	76	0.4	–	–
[1-^{14}C]pyruvic acid	0.2	33	27.4	104.7	0
[2-^{14}C]pyruvic acid	0.2	68	40.0	6.5	75.7
[3-^{14}C]pyruvic acid	0.5	61	2.0	35.7	60.3

[a] Adminstered together with 465 µmol of unlabelled D-glucosamine to suppress incorporation into the C_6N unit

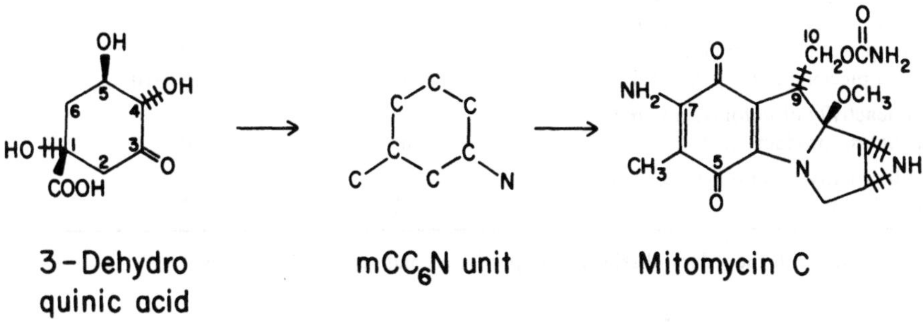

Fig. 6. Possible origin of the mitomycin mCC_6N unit from 3-dehydroquinic acid

by pyruvate in *S. verticillatus* (Redman and Hornemann, 1978). The postulated involvement of an early intermediate of the shikimic acid pathway in the formation of the mCC_6N unit was supported by the finding that D-[4-^{14}C]erythrose was an efficient mitomycin precursor (Table 6). This compound would have to be converted into erythrose-4-phosphate, which is a known precursor of DAHP, however, it is presently not known if the requisite kinase is present in *S. verticillatus*.

3-Dehydroquinic acid or 3-dehydroshikimic acid appear *a priori* to be well suited for the formation of an mCC_6N unit, especially since the nitrogen could conceivably be introduced at position C-3 by transamination (Fig. 6); however, introduction of the amino group at C-5 is not at all excluded. The orientation of pyruvate and of erythrose and hence the orientation of the early shikimate pathway derived precursor in the mCC_6N unit was determined in feeding experiments with sodium[3-^{14}C]pyruvate and D-[4-^{14}C]-erythrose and subsequent degradations (Table 6, Fig. 3). The results obtained indicate that [3-^{14}C]pyruvate, while providing label to peripheral substituents (-$OCONH_2$, -OCH_3), donates

Table 6. Mode of incorporation of [3-^{14}C]pyruvate and D-[4-^{14}C]erythrose into mitomycins by *S. verticillatus*

	Sodium [3-^{14}C]pyruvate	D-[4-^{14}C] erythrose
Quantity fed (mg)	2.2	7.3
Radioactivity fed (dpm)	$4.36 \cdot 10^7$	$4.93 \cdot 10^7$
Incorporation into mitomycins A, B, C, and porfiromycin (%)	0.2	0.8
Specific radioactivity of mitomycin C		
1st recrystallization (dpm/mmole)	$6.9 \cdot 10^4$	$1.91 \cdot 10^5$
2nd recrystallization (dpm/mmole)	$6.9 \cdot 10^4$	$1.83 \cdot 10^5$
Specific radioactivity of tetraacetylmitomycinone derivative		
1st recrystallization (dpm/mmole)	$4.98 \cdot 10^4$	$1.99 \cdot 10^5$
2nd recrystallization (dpm/mmole)	$4.94 \cdot 10^4$	$1.78 \cdot 10^5$
Radioactivity of mitomycin C remaining in tetraacetylmitomycinone derivative (%)[a]	72	97
Specific radioactivity of tetraacetyl-mitomycinone ozonolysis product		
1st precipitation (dpm/mmole)	$4.47 \cdot 10^4$	$1.08 \cdot 10^5$
2nd precipitation (dpm/mmole)	$4.48 \cdot 10^4$	$1.10 \cdot 10^5$
Radioactivity of mitomycin C remaining in ozonolysis product (%)[a]	65	60
Radioactivity of mitomycin C residing at C-7 (%)[a]	7	37

[a] Calculated with the values obtained in respective second repurification step

only very little label to C-7. Thus C-5 is left as the most likely location for the majority of the label if the plausible assumption is made that the carbon skeleton of pyruvate is incorporated as an intact unit without detachment of the methyl group. The results obtained with D-[4-^{14}C]erythrose are of a complementary nature. While there is only weak labeling of peripheral substituents a very significant amount of the label is introduced at C-7. These data define the orientation of pyruvate and of erythrose in the mCC_6N unit as shown in Figure 7. The demonstration of the efficient incorporation of D-erythrose into the mCC_6N unit constitutes the first reported such incorporation into any of several known mCC_6N units (see below). Clearly not all of the label introduced from D-[4-^{14}C]erythrose however resides at C-7 and it is therefore suggested that some of the label may reside at C-10 after conversion of D-erythrose into D-[6-^{14}C]glucosamine via D-glucose and that a certain amount of the label may also reside at C-5 through conversion of D-erythrose labeled D-glucose into [3-^{14}C]phosphoenolpyruvate. It can be concluded from the results with sodium[3-^{14}C]pyruvate and D-[4-^{14}C]erythrose that if 3 DHQ or 3 DHS were actual mitomycin precursors that they would undergo amination at C-5 and not as might have been predicted at C-3 which bears the keto group.

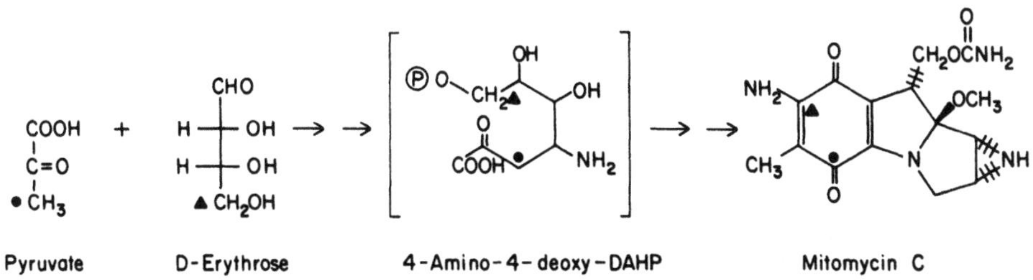

Fig. 7. Mode of incorporation of sodium-[3-^{14}C]pyruvate and of D-[4-^{14}C]erythrose into the mCC_6N unit of mitomycin A via a suggested novel intermediate

Feeding experiments with 3-[7-^{14}C] DHQ and with D-[1,6-$^{14}C_2$]-shikimic acid methyl ester did not reveal any incorporation (D.P. Honor and U. Hornemann, unpublished observations). Failure of labeling by these precursors may mean that they are not true intermediates of the mitomycin biosynthetic pathway or that their uptake is inefficient at the time of feeding. The latter possibility has not been studied in depth. If it is assumed that these compounds are not on the pathway, then only DAHP or perhaps a derivative thereof such as 4-amino-4-deoxy DAHP can be considered as possible intermediates. It is of interest to note that cyclization of 4-amino-4-deoxy-DAHP, which might be generated from the 5-dehydroderivative, a postulated intermediate in the cyclization of DAHP (Maitra and Sprinson, 1978), in a manner similar to normal DAHP cyclization, would appear to be possible and that it would place the amino group into the position demanded by the results of the degradations reported above. Present information on the origin of the mitomycin mCC_6N unit is summarized in Figure 7.

The mitomycins are not the only antibiotics in which an mCC_6N unit can be discerned as a biosynthetic building block. Similar mCC_6N units, often referred to as C_7N units (Haber et al., 1977) are clearly involved in the biosynthesis of the ansamycin antibiotics rifamycin (White and Martinelli, 1974) and geldanamycin (Haber et al., 1977) and presumably in other ansamacrolide antibiotics as well, as outlined by Lancini in Chapter 2. In addition, studies on pactamycin biosynthesis (Weller and Rinehart, 1978) have shown that the acetophenone moiety of this antibiotic is elaborated from a related mCC_6N unit. The mode of incorporation of D-[1-^{13}C]- and/or -[6-^{13}C]glucose samples into the mCC_6N units of the antibiotics rifamycin (White and Martinelli, 1974) and pactamycin (Weller and Rinehart, 1978), respectively, was compared with the mode of D-[1-^{14}C]- and -[6-^{14}C]glucose incorporation into shikimic acid (Srinivasan et al., 1956). These studies assumed that glucose was incorporated after its conversion into phosphoenolpyruvate and into erythrose-4-phosphate. The results obtained suggested in the case of rifamycin biosynthesis that if 3 DHQ were involved in its biosynthesis, amination would occur at C-5, the carbon atom not bearing the carbonyl group, and thus would be similar to mitomycin. In the case of pactamycin biosynthesis, the results obtained suggested the opposite, namely amination at C-3. Similar studies on geldanamycin biosynthesis with D-[6-^{13}C]glucose did not permit a decision to be made concerning the orientation of the presumed precursor, 3 DHQ, in the geldanamycin mCC_6N unit. The proposed involvement of an early intermediate of the shikimic acid pathway in rifamycin biosynthesis has been strengthened by studies with aromatic amino acid auxotrophs (GHISALBA and NÜESCH, 1978). From the published information it appears that mCC_6N units may be generated in two different ways. However, this suggestion should probably not be accepted too easily. All experiments with the labeled glucose species rely on the assumption that the relative intensity of labeling of [3-^{14}C]pyruvate and of D-[4-^{14}C]erythrose-phosphate by glucose is the same in the actinomycetales studied as it was in the experiments by DAVIS et al. with *E. coli* (SRINIVASAN et al., 1956). It is, however, conceivable that the strains have differences of glucose metabolism that could significantly influence the ratio of phosphoenolpyruvate versus erythrose-4-phosphate formation and independent studies, therefore, perhaps through an analysis of the labeling of tryptophan or of NAD^+ would seem to be desirable. It would appear that the orientation of early shikimate pathway intermediates in mCC_6N units may be analyzed with more precision by determining the mode of incorporation of pyruvate and of erythrose directly as was done in the mitomycin biosynthetic studies reported above.

V. Late Stages in Mitomycin Biosynthesis

Since the structures of the mCC_6N unit and the C_6N unit which combine to form the mitomycin skeleton are not known with certainty, detailed proposals for the joining reaction cannot be made. A crucial step will certainly be the attachment of C-5 of glucosamine to the respective carbon atom of DAHP or a DAHP-related precursor. No direct analogy for this process is available; however, a somewhat similar joining of C-5 of a hexose or a hexosamine with a ring system must be accomplished in nogalamycin biosynthesis (WILEY et al., 1978) and the joining of C-4 of glucose with a ring system is known to take place in the biosynthesis of granaticin (SNIPES et al., 1979) as outlined by FLOSS in chapter 9. Both these antibiotics differ from mitomycin in that the sugar-derived carbon which establishes the junction carries an oxygen in the final product, whereas C-9 of mitomycin does not carry an oxygen. This may suggest different mechanisms of the joining reactions or further modifications on the mitomycin skeleton after the joining reaction. SNIPES et al. (1979) have postulated an involvement of a keto function at C-4 of glucose in granaticin biosynthesis. An analogous participation of a keto function at C-5 of glucosamine in mitomycin biosynthesis, as stated above, could explain the loss of most of the C-5 hydrogen.

Very little information is presently available concerning the biosynthetic relationship among the different members of the family of the mitomycin antibiotics. Since mitomycin C can be obtained from mitomycin A simply by treatment of the latter with ammonia, it appears likely that mitomycin A is its natural precursor. As shown in Figure 8, I propose that mitomycin A after its conversion into N-methylmitomycin A is also the precursor of the other mitomycins. N-

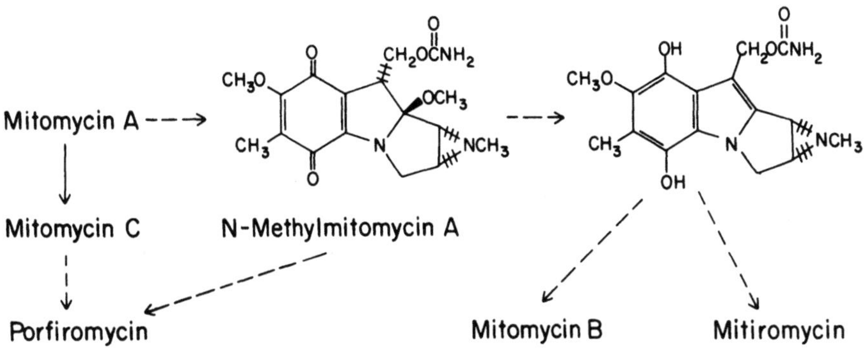

Fig. 8. Known and hypothetical interconversions of mitomycins

Methylmitomycin A has been detected as a minor constituent in the fermentation broth and has been identified by chromatographic comparison with synthetic N-methyl-mitomycin A in three TLC systems and by conversion into porfiromycin by treatment with ammonia followed by chromatographic comparison with authentic material (U. HORNEMANN and M.J. HEINS, unpublished observations). Thus, it is readily conceivable that N-methyl-mitomycin A could be the natural precursor of porfiromycin. Mitomycin B is unique among the mitomycins in that it possesses a hydroxy group at C-9a and R rather than S chirality at C-9. Since the C-9a-OCH_3 group is labile when mitomycins are reduced in nonaqueous (PATRICK et al., 1964) or in aqueous media (HORNEMANN et al., 1976), I propose that reduction of N-methylmitomycin A to the hydroquinone followed by loss of methanol from C-9 and C-9a generates an intermediate which, upon trans addition of water across the C-9-9a double bond, and subsequent oxidation, will generate mitomycin B. It is conceivable that mitiromycin may be generated by an analogous intramolecular addition of the carbamoyl group to the same intermediate and subsequent reoxidation. The stereochemistry of mitiromycin is not known but it seems likely that the substituents at the positions equivalent to C-9 and C-9a might be cis disposed as in mitomycin B. It is not known why mitomycin B is found in large excess over N-methylmitomycin A and it will therefore be of interest to compare the redox potentials of these compounds. A feeding experiment with radioactive N-methyl mitomycin A, prepared from mitomycin A and [$^{14}CH_3$]methyl iodide, afforded only radioactive porfiromycin. It is possible that porfiromycin was formed extra-cellularly and that mitomycin B was not labeled because N-methylmitomycin A was not taken up. Therefore it may be necessary to repeat the experiment with protoplasts or with cell-free systems to explore the possible conversion of N-methylmitomycin A into mitomycin B and into mitiromycin.

Acknowledgment. The scientific contributions of my collaborators, generous gifts of mitomycins from Drs. S. WAKAKI, KYOWA HAKKO KOGYO, Tokyo, Japan and I. PACHTER, Bristol Laboratories, Syracuse, New York, and financial support through research grant CA 14378 from the National Cancer Institute, DHEW are gratefully acknowledged.

References

Akhtar MH, Begleiter A, Johnson D, Lown JW, McLaughlin L, Sim S-K (1975) Studies related to antitumor antibiotics. VI. Correlation of covalent cross-linking of DNA by bifunctional aziridinoquinones with their antineoplastic activity. Can J Chem 53:2891–2905

Bezanson GS, Vining LC (1971) Studies on the biosynthesis of mitomycin C by *Streptomyces verticillatus*. Can J Biochem 49:911–918

Brewer SJ, Boyle TT, Turner MK (1977) The carbamoylation of the 3-hydroxymethyl group of 7α-methoxy-7β-(5-D-aminoadipamido)-3-hydroxymethylceph-3-em-4-carboxcylic acid (desacetyl-7α-methoxycephalosporin C) by homogenates of *Streptomyces clavuligerus*. Biochem Soc Trans 5:1026–1029

Crooke ST, Bradner WT (1976) Mitomycin C: a review. Cancer Treat Rev 3:121–139

DeBoer C, Dietz A, Lummis NE, Savage GM (1960) Porfiromycin, a new antibiotic. I. Discovery and biological activities. Antimicrob Agents Ann 17–22

Fukuyama T, Nakatsubo F, Cocuzza AJ, Kishi Y (1977) Synthetic studies toward mitomycins. III. Total syntheses of mitomycins A and C. Tetrahedron Lett 4295–4298

Gabriel O, Lindquist LC (1968) Biological mechanisms involved in the formation of deoxy sugars. IV. Enzymatic conversion of thymidine diphosphoglucose-4T to thymidine diphospho-4-keto-6-deoxyglucose-6T. J Biol Chem 243:1479–1484

Ghisalba O, Nüesch J (1978) A genetic approach to the biosynthesis of the rifamycin chromophore in *Nocardia mediterranei*. I. Isolation and characterization of a pentose-excreting auxotrophic mutant of *Norcardia mediterranei* with drastically reduced rifamycin production. J Antibiot 31:202–214

Haber A, Johnson RD, Rinehart Jr KL (1977) Biosynthetic origin of the C_2 units of geldanamycin and distribution of label from D-[6-^{13}C]glucose. J Am Chem Soc 99:3541–3544

Hata T, Sano Y, Sugawara R, Matsumae A, Kanamori K, Shima T, Hochi T (1956) Mitomycin, a new antibiotic from Streptomyces. I. J Antibiot 9:141–146

Hornemann U, Aikman MJ (1973) Mitomycin biosynthesis by *Streptomyces verticillatus*. Incorporation of the amino group of D-[^{15}N]glucosamine into the aziridine ring of mitomycin B. Chem Commun 88–89

Hornemann U, Cloyd JC (1971) Studies on the biosynthesis of the mitomycin antibiotics by *Streptomyces verticillatus*. Chem Commun 301–302

Hornemann U, Kehrer JP, Nunez CS, Ranieri RL (1974a) D-Glucosamine and L-citrulline, precursors in mitomycin biosynthesis by *Streptomyces verticillatus*. J Am Chem Soc 96:320–322

Hornemann U, Kehrer JP, Nunez CS, Ranieri RL, Ho YK (1974b) Precursors in mitomycin biosynthesis by *Streptomyces verticillatus*. Dev Ind Microbiol 15:82–92

Hornemann U, Kehrer JP, Eggert JH (1974c) Pyruvic acid and D-glucose as precursors in mitomycin biosynthesis by *Streptomyces verticillatus*. Chem Commun 1045–1046

Hornemann U, Eggert JH (1975) Utilization of the intact carbamoyl group of L-(NH_4CO-^{13}C, ^{15}N]citrulline in mitomycin biosynthesis by *Streptomyces verticillatus*. J Antibiot 28:841–843

Hornemann U, Ho YK, Mackey Jr JK, Srivastava SC (1976) Studies on the mode of action of the mitomycin antibiotics. Reversible conversion of mitomycin C into sodium-7-aminomitosane-9a-sulfonate. J Am Chem Soc 98:7069–7074

Kersten H (1975) Mechanism of action of mitomycins. In: Handb Exp Pharmacol 38:47–64

Kinoshita S, Uzu K, Nakano K, Shimizu M, Takahashi T (1971) Mitomycin derivatives. 1. Preparation of mitosane and mitosene compounds and their biological activities. J Med Chem 14:103–109

Kirsch EJ (1967) Mitomycins. In: Gottlieb D, Shaw PD (ed) Antibiotics, Biosynthesis, vol II, pp 66–76. Springer, Berlin Heidelberg New York

Kirsch EJ, Korshalla JD (1964) Influence of biological methylation on the biosynthesis of mitomycin A. J Bacteriol 87:247–255

Lefemine DV, Dann M, Barbatschi F, Hausmann WK, Zbinovsky V, Monnikendam P, Adam J, Bohonos N (1962) Isolation and characterization of mitiromycin and of other antibiotics produced by *Streptomyces verticillatus*. J Am Chem Soc 84:3184–3185

Lin AJ, Shansky CW, Sartorelli AC (1974) Potential bioreductive alkylating agents. 3. Synthesis and antineoplastic activity of acetoxymethyl and corresponding ethyl carbamate derivatives of benzoquinones. J Med Chem 17:558–561

Lipsett MN, Weissbach A (1965) The site of alkylation of nucleic acids by mitomycin. Biochemistry 4:206–211
Lown JW, Weir G (1978) Studies related to antitumor antibiotics. XIV. Reactions of mitomycin B with DNA. Can J Biochem 56:296–304
Maitra US, Sprinson DB (1978) 5-Dehydro-3-deoxy-D-arabino-heptulosonic acid-7-phosphate. J Biol Chem 253:5426–5430
Miller TW, Tristram EW, Wolf FJ (1971) Azirinomycin. II. Isolation and chemical characterization as 3-methyl-2(2H)-azirine carboxylic acid. J Antibiot 24:48–50
Morton GO, Van Lear GE, Fulmor W (1970) The structure of mitiromycin. J Am Chem Soc 92:2588–2590
Naganawa H, Usui N, Takita T, Hamada M, Umezawa H (1975) S-2,3-dicarboxy-aziridine, a new metabolite from a streptomyces. J Antibiot 28:828–829
Nakatsubo F, Fukuyama T, Cocuzza AJ, Kishi Y (1977) Synthetic studies toward mitomycins. 2. Total synthesis of dl-porfiromycin. J Am Chem Soc 99:8115–8116
Nelsestuen GL, Kirkwood S (1971) The mechanism of action of the enzyme uridine diphosphoglucose 4-epimerase. Proof of an oxidation-reduction mechanism with direct transfer of hydrogen between substrate and the β-position of the enzyme-bound pyridine nucleotide. J Biol Chem 246:7533–7543
Nishikohori K, Fukui S (1975) Biosynthesis of mitomcyin in *Streptomyces caespitosus*. Relation of intracellular vitamin B12 level to mitomycin synthesis and enzymatic methylation of a demethylated derivative of mitomycin. Eur J Appl Microbiol 1:129–145
Otsuji N, Murayama I (1972) Deoxyribonucleic acid damage by monofunctional mitomycins and its repair in *Escherichia coli*. J Bacteriol 109:475–483
Patrick JB, Williams RP, Meyer WE, Fulmor W, Cosulich DB, Broschard RW, Webb JS (1964) Aziridinomitosenes: a new class of antibiotics related to the mitomycins. J Am Chem Soc 86:1889–1890
Redman KL, Hornemann U (1978) Interaction of pyruvate, phosphate dikinase, pyruvate kinase, alanine dehydrogenase and phosphoenolpyruvate carboxylase from *Streptomyces verticillatus* with Cibaron Blue 3G-A-Sepharose. Abstr Joint Central-Great Lakes Reg Meet Am Chem Soc, Indianapolis, Indiana, BIOL-16
Snipes CE, Chang CJ, Floss HG (1979) Biosynthesis of the antibiotic granaticin. J Am Chem Soc 101:701–706
Srinivasan PR, Shigeura HT, Sprecher M, Sprinson DB, Davis BD (1956) The biosynthesis of shikimic acid from D-glucose. J Biol Chem 220:477–497
Stevens CL, Taylor KG, Munk ME, Marshall WS, Noll K, Shah GD, Shah LG, Uzu K (1965) Chemistry and structure of mitomycin C. J Med Chem 8:1–10
Szybalski W, Iyer VN (1964) Crosslinking of DNA by enzymatically or chemically activated mitomycins and porfiromycins, bifunctionally "alkylating" antibiotics. Fed Proc 23:946–957
Szybalski W, Iyer VN (1967) The mitomycins and porfiromycin. In: Gottlieb D, Shaw PD (ed) Antibiotics. Mechanism of Action, Vol I, pp 211–245. Springer, Berlin Heidelberg New York
Taylor WG, Leadbetter G, Fost DL, Remers WA (1977) Mitomycin antibiotics. Synthesis and activity of 1,2-disubstituted mitosenes. J Med Chem 20:138–141
Thoai NV, Thome-Bean F, Olomucki A (1966) Induction et spécificité des enzymes de la nouvelle voie catabolique de l'arginine. Biochim Biophys Acta 115:73–80
Tomasz M, Mercado CM, Olson J, Chatterjie N (1974) The mode of interaction of mitomycin C with deoxyribonucleic acid and other polynucleotides in vitro. Biochemistry 13:4878–4887
Tulinski A, Van den Hende JH (1967) The crystal and molecular structure of N-brosylmitomycin A. J Am Chem Soc 89:2905–2911
Van Lear GE (1970) Mass spectrometric studies of antibiotics. I. Mass spectra of mitomycin antibiotics. Tetrahedron 26:2587–2597
Webb JS, Cosulich DB, Mowat JH, Patrick JB, Broschard RW, Meyer WE, Williams RP, Wolf CF, Fulmor W, Pidacks C, Lancaster JE (1962a) The structures of mitomycins A, B and C and porfiromycin. Part I. J Am Chem Soc 84:3185–3186
Webb JS, Cosulich DB, Mowat JH, Patrick JB, Broschard RW, Meyer WE, Williams RP, Wolf CF, Fulmor W, Pidacks C, Lancaster JE (1962b) The structures of mitomycins A, B and C and poriformycin. Part II. J Am Chem Soc 84:3186–3188

Weller DD, Rinehart Jr KL (1978) Biosynthesis of the antitumor antibiotic pactamycin. A methionine-derived ethyl group and a C_7N unit. J Am Chem Soc 100:6757–6760

White RJ, Martinelli E (1974) Ansamycin biogenesis: Incorporation of [1-^{13}C]glucose and [1-^{13}C]glycerate into the chromophore of rifamycin S. FEBS Lett 49:233–236

Wiley PF, Elrod DW, Marshall VP (1978) Biosynthesis of the anthracycline antibiotics nogalamycin and steffimycin B. J Org Chem 43:3457–3461

Wolf G, Wörth J, Achenbach H (1975) Mitomycin und ein neues Phenoxazon – Pigment aus *Streptomyces michiganensis*. Stoffwechselprodukte von Mikroorganismen. Arch Mikrobiol 106:245–259

Wood HG, O'Brien WE, Michaels G (1977) Properties of carboxytransphosphorylase; pyruvate, phosphate dikinase; pyrophosphate phosphofructokinase and pyrophosphate-acetate kinase and their roles in the metabolism of inorganic pyrophosphate. In: Meister A (ed) Advances in enzymology, pp 85–155. Wiley and Sons, New York

Yahashi R, Matsubara I (1976) The molecular structure of 7-demethoxy-7-p-bromoanilino mitomycin B. J Antibiot 29:104–106 and correction notice published in J Antibiot 31: issue of June 1978 last page

Nitrogen-Nitrogen Bond Containing Antibiotics: Biosynthesis of Streptozocin

ULFERT HORNEMANN

The structures and properties of approximately 20 antibiotics from Streptomycetes as well as other microorganisms and of another 20 metabolites from bacteria, mushrooms, and plants which contain a nitrogen-nitrogen bond were recently reviewed by LARUE (1977). The physiological activities of these compounds comprise antitumor, cytotoxic, carcinogenic, and diabetogenic activities, but, despite the pharmacologic interest in these compounds, only scanty information is available on their biosynthesis and none on the enzymology and genetics of the formation of their nitrogen-nitrogen bonds. Our interest in the biosynthetic capabilities of Streptomycetes in general and a particular interest in the unexplored area of biological nitrogen-nitrogen bond formation prompted us to undertake biosynthetic studies on the antibiotic streptozocin and to initiate such studies with the antibiotic N-acetyl-6-diazo-5-oxo-L-norleucine (N-acetyl DON).

Streptozocin (WILEY et al., 1979; ANDERSON et al., 1956), previously known as streptozotocin (HERR et al., 1967), is produced by *Streptomyces achromogenes* var. *streptozoticus* (NRRL 3125) (VAVRA et al., 1960), and is apparently the only naturally occurring N-methyl-N-nitrosourea. Like other nitrosoureas it acts as an anticancer agent and it is at present the most important clinical agent among all the known compounds containing nitrogen-nitrogen bonds. It is used mainly to treat insulinomas of the pancreas (BEYLOT et al., 1976) and has been shown to be active against L 1210 mouse leukemia (BHUYAN et al., 1972). It causes diabetes in animals (LIKE and ROSSINI, 1976) and it is a carcinogen (KAZUMI et al., 1978). Several total syntheses have been reported

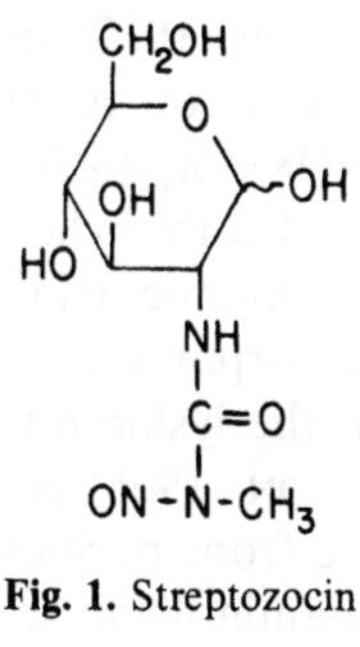

Fig. 1. Streptozocin

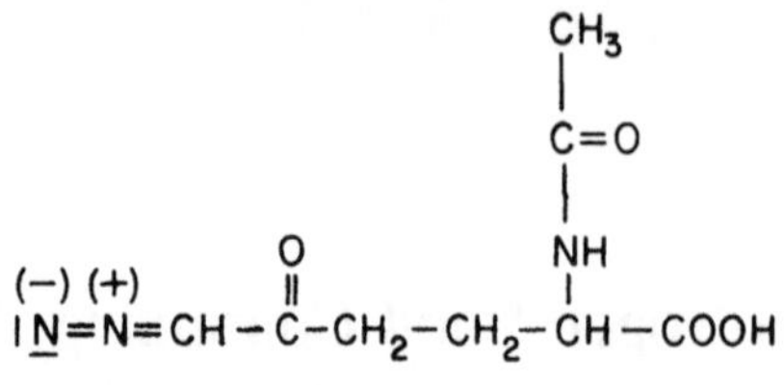

Fig. 2. N-Acetyl-6-diazo-5-oxo-L-norleucine

(HESSLER and JAHNKE, 1970) and many analogs have been prepared (MORUZZI et al., 1978). Alanosine (βN-hydroxy-βN-nitroso, α,β-diaaminopropionic acid (CORONELLI et al., 1966) produced by *Streptomyces alanosinicus* and the *Pseudomonas* metabolites dopastin (INUMA et al., 1972) and fragin (MURAYAMA and TAMURA, 1970) as well as the mushroom constituent p-methylamino-N-nitroso-benzaldehyde (HERRMANN, 1961) are the only other natural products known to contain N-nitroso functions.

N-acetyl-DON, also named duazomycin A (RAO, 1961), is one of the few naturally occurring compounds containing an aliphatic α diazoketo group, and is produced by *Streptomyces ambofaciens* (RAO et al., 1960). N-acetyl-DON is probably a derivative of 6-diazo-5-oxo-L-norleucine (DON) (DION et al., 1956) which was initially isolated from an unidentified *Streptomyces species* and which is produced together with N-acetyl-DON and duazomycin B by *S. ambofaciens* (RAO et al., 1960). Duazomycin B, also named azotomycin (RAO, 1962) is a peptide composed of two moles of DON and one mole of aminoterminal γ-glutamic acid. Diazo groups are also encountered in the duazomycin B-related compound alazopeptin (DEVOE et al., 1957) which contains two moles of DON and one mole of aminoterminal alanine in peptide linkage and which is produced by *Streptomyces griseoplanus* (BACKUS et al., 1957) and by *Streptomyces* strain 05-3256 (HATA et al., 1973), as well as in the antibiotic azaserine (O-diazoacetyl-L-serine (FUSARI et al., 1954) produced by *Streptomyces fragilis* (ANDERSON et al., 1956). The clinical usefulness of these antibiotics which act as glutamine antagonists in cancer chemotherapy has been reviewed (LEPAGE and LOO, 1973).

The few compounds containing nitrogen-nitrogen bonds whose biosynthesis has been investigated include the antibiotics monamycin (HASSALL et al., 1971), formycin (KOYAMA et al., 1966) and 8-azaguanine (ANZAI et al., 1961), which were not mentioned in LARUE's review (1977), as well as the antibiotic toxoflavin (DAVES et al., 1962), the mushroom constituent agaritine (LEVENBERG, 1964), and the alkaloid withasomnine (ONAKA, 1968). It was shown by HASSALL and co-workers that the piperidazine-3-carboxylic acid moiety and its derivatives of monamycin are labeled from glutamic acid (ARROYO et al., 1976). Japanese workers reported that lysine is incorporated into formycin and that the linked nitrogens presumably arise from the lysine nitrogen atoms (OCHI et al., 1976). Toxoflavin (LEVENBERG and LINTON, 1966) and 8-azaguanine (HIRASAWA and ISONO, 1978) were shown to arise from purines by expulsion of C-8. Agaritine was shown to be formed from p-aminobenzoic acid (SCHÜTTE et al., 1972) and

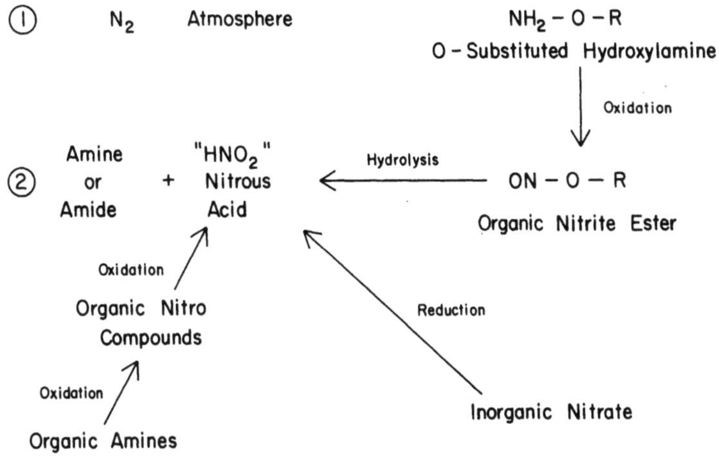

Fig. 3. Hypotheses on the origin of the nitrogen atoms of nitrogen-nitrogen bond containing antibiotics

withasomnine was shown to arise from ornithine and phenylalanine (O'DONOVAN and FORDE, 1970). None of these studies have as yet shed any substantial light on the formation of the nitrogen-nitrogen bonds of these compounds. This lack of specific information makes it necessary to theorize on possible pathways of nitrogen-nitrogen bond formation.

Two different processes can in principle be considered for the biochemical formation of nitrogen-nitrogen bonds: 1. the linked nitrogen atoms may be derived from atomospheric nitrogen which becomes fixed in their structures, or 2. the linked nitrogen atoms may be derived from two fragments each containing one of the nitrogens to be linked which undergo a coupling reaction (Fig. 3). In a recent review (DALTON, 1974) *Streptomyces* were not listed as being capable of fixing dinitrogen by the nitrogenase pathway, although a small number of microorganisms possibly belonging to the genus *Norcardia* were listed as active. An actinomycete has been claimed to be responsible for root nodulation of woody dicotyledonous plants (CALLAHAM et al., 1978) but the taxonomic position of the respective bacterium is considered by many authors to be uncertain. Since *Streptomyces* most probably do not possess nitrogenase any process of antibiotic biosynthesis involving nitrogen fixation would probably proceed by an as yet undiscovered mechanism. Although this possibility cannot be ruled out, it is considered to be unlikely and the following considerations will be based on the assumption that process 2 is operative.

By analogy with well-known reactions in organic chemistry it may be assumed that the nitrogen-nitrogen bonds of streptozocin and of N-acetyl DON are formed directly by the interaction of an amide or an amine with either free nitrous acid, nitrite anion, or a suitable biochemical equivalent such as a nitrite ester (Fig. 3). If nitrous acid were indeed involved in these biosyntheses, then mechanisms would have to exist in the producing organisms to generate it and to assure the suppression of potentially harmful effects that it may have on cells. In the following discussion the possible occurrence and participation of nitrous acid in microbial metabolism will be examined.

Recent studies have indicated that involvement of nitrous acid or a bound form of this acid in N-nitrosation is likely. SANDER (1968) showed that various bacteria, including *E. coli,* that are capable of reducing nitrate to nitrite, can form nitrosamines in vitro when incubated at 37° C at physiological pH on a complex medium containing glucose, secondary amines, and sodium nitrite. It was assumed that a bound form of nitrous acid was involved in these N-nitrosations. Subsequently a number of laboratories reported similar formation of nitrosamines from nitrite and secondary amines by a variety of microorganisms. Some authors suggested non-enzymatic processes (COLLINS-THOMPSON et al., 1972), while others suggested the involvement of enzymes (AYANABA and ALEXANDER, 1973; MILLS and ALEXANDER, 1976). A *Norcardia* species was included in these studies (AYANABA and ALEXANDER, 1973) but this strain was capable neither of nitrate-to-nitrite reduction nor of N-nitrosation under the experimental conditions. Some strains of *Streptomyces* can grow with nitrate as the sole nitrogen source, while others including *S. achromogenes* var. *streptozoticus* (VAVRA et al., 1960) cannot. *S. ambofaciens* was apparently not investigated in this regard. It appears to be unlikely that nitrous acid formation in the strains of interest occurs by nitrate reduction.

Nitrite or nitrous acid may also be generated by oxidation of ammonium salts, rather than by nitrate reduction. Nitrifying bacteria provide examples of such a pathway and also many strains of *Streptomyces* were found to be capable of nitrite production from ammonium salts (VERSTRAETE and ALEXANDER, 1972a). It is not certain whether the oxidation occurs by an inorganic or by an organic pathway (VERSTRAETE and ALEXANDER, 1972b). Nitrite and nitrous acid could conceivably be formed by an oxidative organic pathway starting with amines and involving bound intermediates. Several advantages may be associated with an organic pathway. Firstly, if all intermediates and also the endproduct are held in a bonded form, then regulatory controls can presumably be exerted more readily, and secondly, potential toxicity problems which might be associated with free hydroxylamine, which is an intermediate in an inorganic pathway, or free nitrous acid may be avoided. The nature of bound intermediates in an organic pathway and the compound from which nitrous acid could be generated however, are relatively unexplored.

Aliphatic nitrocompounds may be a source for nitrous acid via oxidative degradation yielding aldehydes or ketones and nitrous acid. KIDO et al. (1975) described many microorganisms capable of oxidizing nitroalkanes to yield this acid. Their report prompted us to study the oxidation of these compounds in *Streptomyces* which were not included by the Japanese workers. All nine strains of *Streptomyces* investigated were able to oxidize primary and secondary nitroalkanes, with concomitant production of nitrous acid. A nitroalkane-oxidizing enzyme from streptozocin-producing *S. achromogenes* var. *streptozoticus* was partially purified and characterized. It catalyzes the oxidative denitrification of 2-nitropropane as follows: $2\,CH_3CH(NO_2)CH_3 + O_2 \rightarrow 2\,CH_3COCH_3 + 2\,HNO_2$ (DHAWALE and HORNEMANN, 1979). This enzyme was enriched up to 35-fold and several of its properties were studied. 3-Nitropropionic acid was shown to be used about 100 times less efficiently than 2-nitropropane. Both the *S. achromogenes* enzyme and a similar enzyme purified by KIDO et al.

(1976) from *H. mrakii* show Km values for 2-nitropropane of approximately 2×10^{-2} M. The role of the nitroalkane-oxidizing activity as a possible provider of nitrous acid for the biosynthesis of nitrogen-nitrogen bond containing antibiotics is presently not clear. Since the enzyme has been encountered in all *Streptomyces* examined, it would seem that one needs to postulate that only those *Streptomyces* strains that produce N-N bond-containing antibiotics actually produce the substrate nitroalkanes. Information on the natural occurrence of aliphatic nitro compounds is very scanty. Only 3-nitropropionic acid and 1-nitro-2-phenylethane have been isolated from living organisms. 3-Nitropropionic acid is known to occur in *Penicillium atrovenetum* (RAISTRICK and STÖSSL, 1958) and to be oxidized to nitrite in this species (GRUNER et al., 1972) and this acid has also been isolated from a *Streptomyces* species and was named bovinocidin (ANZAI and SUZUKI, 1960). The natural occurrence of 1-nitro-2-phenylethane has been reported in the brazilian trees *Ocotea pretiosa* and *Ariba canellilla* (GOTTLIEB and MAGELHAES, 1959) and in the fruits of the Nigerian plant *Dennettia tripetala* g. *Baker* (OKOGUN and EKONG, 1969) and it would be interesting to know if microorganisms can produce this compound or related compounds.

It seems to be highly likely that *Streptomyces* and other microorganisms indeed form higher oxidation levels of nitrogen, which might be employed for nitrous acid formation, by oxidation of organic amines. For instance, it has been shown that the *Streptomyces* antibiotics chloramphenicol and aureothin, both of which contain nitro groups, arise through the intermediate formation of p-aminophenylalanine which undergoes oxidation of the para-amino group to provide the nitro group (CARDILLO et al., 1974). A similar situation appears to exist in the biosynthesis of 3-nitro-propionic acid in *Penicillium atrovenetum* where the nitro group does not originate from nitrate or from ammonium salts, but rather from the bound amino group of aspartic acid (SHAW and DEANGELO, 1969). Information on the biosynthesis of bovinocidin is not available. The enzymatic oxidation of the amino group of p-aminobenzoic acid to p-nitrobenzoic acid was observed with a cell-free extract from *Streptomyces thioluteus,* the producer of aureothin (KAWAI et al., 1965), and it has been reported that chloroperoxidase can catalyze the conversion of 4-chloroaniline with H_2O_2 into 4-chloronitrosobenzene (CORBETT et al., 1978) therefore, more detailed investigations of these conversions appear to be possible.

The general biosynthetic considerations may be summarized as follows. Nitrogen fixation is probably not involved in the biosynthesis of the antibiotics in question and it is considered likely that nitrous acid may be involved which could arise presumably by an organic pathway.

Streptozocin biosynthesis was studied using two methods of cultivation and antibiotic isolation (SINGARAM et al., 1979). In method A *S. achromogenes* var. *streptozoticus* was propagated by flask-to-flask inoculation and grown in a complex natural medium containing cornmeal, potato starch, cerelose, and peptone as well as $(NH_4)_2SO_4$ to stabilize the pH at 4–5. Radioactive precursors were added 24 h before harvest. This medium afforded approximately 3 mg of streptozotocin per 100 ml in 5 days at 27° C. The antibiotic was isolated from the supernatant of an acetone precipitation step and purified by paper chromatography, eluted from the paper with water and recrystallized with 300 mg of nonla-

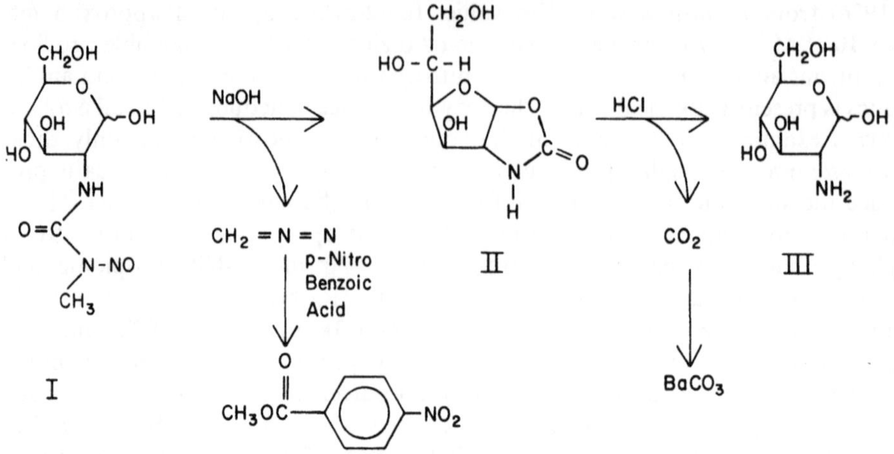

Fig. 4. Chemical degradation of streptozocin. Reproduced with permission of "The Journal of Antibiotics"

beled carrier material prior to chemical degradation. In method B a spore inoculum was used to prepare a seed culture in a cotton seed-cerelose medium at 27° C (VAVRA et al., 1960). Two-day-old mycelium obtained in this seed culture was used to inoculate a medium similar to the corn meal medium given above. Shake cultivation at 27° C yielded streptozocin titers of 25–30 mg/100 ml or 70 mg/100 ml after 5 or 14 days, respectively. After two acetone precipitation steps and chromatography on Sephradex G-10 in acetate buffer at pH 4 the antibiotic was purified by two subsequent paper chromatographic steps and used for chemical degradation upon recrystallization with 300 mg of carrier streptozocin. Radioactive samples of the antibiotic were degraded as shown in Figure 4. Diazomethane generated by base treatment of streptozocin was trapped and counted as methyl-p-nitrobenzoate, while CO_2 liberated from II with acid was trapped and counted as $BaCO_3$ (SINGARAM et al., 1979). Glucosamine (III) was purified by chromatography prior to counting.

The results obtained in feeding experiments with singly and doubly labeled precursors are shown in Tables 1 and 2. It is apparent from the results presented in Table 1 that D-glucosamine, L-arginine, L-citrulline, and L-methionine act as efficient precursors but that the incorporation value varies quite considerably between methods A and B. It can be concluded from the results presented in both Tables that the carbon skeleton of D-glucosamine is utilized as an intact unit in streptozocin biosynthesis, that the urea carbonyl group is labeled specifically by L-[guanidino-^{14}C]-arginine and by L-[ureido-^{14}C]-citrulline, and that the N-methyl group arises from the methyl group of L-methionine. Thus, it appears that, with the exception of the precursor for the nitroso group, the building blocks of streptozotocin are known in broad outline. The finding that L-[$^{14}CH_3$]methionine is an efficient precursor is not surprising in view of the many biochemical N-methylations that have been observed to depend on methionine. Arginine and citrulline were fed since the acidity of the broth precluded the feeding of sodium[^{14}C]carbonate and sodium[^{14}C]cyanate and

Table 1. Incorporation of singly and doubly labeled precursors into streptozocin. Reproduced with permission of "The Journal of Antibiotics"

	Precursor			Streptozocin		
	Quantity fed (mg)	Radioactivity fed (dpm)	T/C Ratio	Method of cultivation and isolation	^{14}C Incorporation (%)	T/C Ratio [T retention]
D-[6-^{3}H]glucosamine	2.2	7.92×10^{6}		A	1.5[a, b]	
D-[1-^{14}C, 6-^{3}H]glucosamine	5.4	$^{14}C = 8.38 \times 10^{6}$ $^{3}H = 7.58 \times 10^{7}$	9.05	B	42.0	9.00 [99.9]
D-[1-^{14}C, 2-^{3}H]glucosamine	7.6	$^{14}C = 2.16 \times 10^{6}$ $^{3}H = 1.92 \times 10^{7}$	8.90	B	34.0	7.16 [80.8]
L-[guanidino-^{14}C]arginine	2.1	2.11×10^{7}		A	1.5[b]	
L-[guanidino-^{14}C]arginine	1.9	1.46×10^{7}		B	33.0	
L-[ureido-^{14}C]citrulline	1.7	2.51×10^{7}		A	5.4	
L-[ureido-^{14}C]citrulline	1.7	4.55×10^{7}		B	38.6[b]	
L-[$^{14}CH_3$]methionine	1.6	2.66×10^{7}		A	6.1[b]	

[a] In this instance the tritium incorporation is given
[b] Subjected to chemical degradation, see Table 2

Table 2. Degradation of streptozocin. Reproduced with permission of "The Journal of Antibiotics"

Precursor	Incorporation into streptozocin (%)	Specific Radioactivity (dpm/mM) [percentage of streptozocin specific radioactivity]			
		Streptozocin	Methyl p-nitro benzoate	$BaCO_3$	Glucosamine
D-[6-^{3}H]glucosamine	1.5	5.32×10^{4}	[a]	[a]	4.73×10^{4} [89.0]
L-[guanidino-^{14}C]arginine	1.5	6.51×10^{4}	[a]	6.46×10^{4} [99.2]	[a]
L-[ureido-^{14}C]citrulline	38.6	3.99×10^{4}	[a]	3.61×10^{4} [90.5]	[a]
L-[$^{14}CH_3$]methionine	6.1	2.43×10^{5}	2.36×10^{5} [97.1]	[a]	[a]

[a] Less than 0.5% of specific radioactivity of streptozocin detected in fragment

since studies reported in Chapter 13 on the origin of the carbamoyl group in mitomycin biosynthesis demonstrated their participation in the establishment of that carbamoyl group (HORNEMANN and EGGERT, 1975). It is possible that L-arginine serves as a donor of the carbamoyl group after its conversion into citrulline. It is of interest in this regard that we have demonstrated the presence

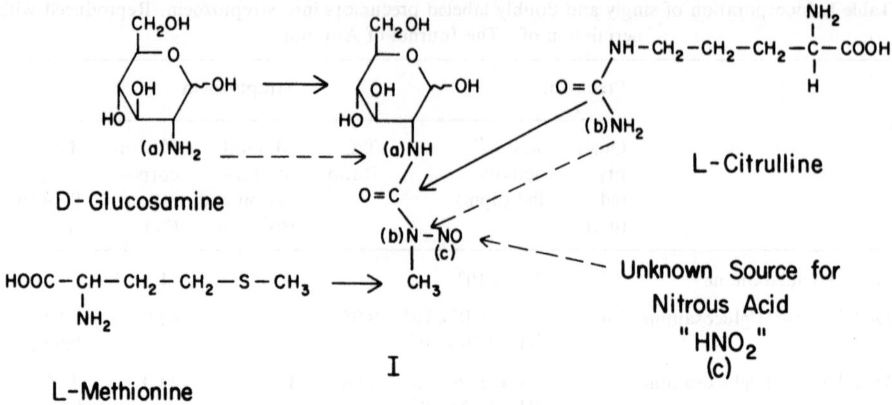

Fig. 5. Biosynthetic building blocks of streptozocin. Reproduced with permission of "The Journal of Antibiotics"

Table 3. Dilution factors of glucosamine and citrulline (method B). Reproduced with permission of "The Journal of Antibiotics"

Precursor		Streptozocin	
Radioactivity fed: 10 μCi	Amount fed (mg)	Yield (mg)	Dilution factor
D-[1-^{14}C]glucosamine	25	14.0	2.3
	50	15.5	2.1
	100	10.4	
	300	7.6	
L-[ureido-^{14}C]citrulline	25	21.5	4.4
	50	10.5	3.3
	100	8.8	2.2
	300	6.3	

in *S. achromogenes* var. *streptozoticus* of arginine deiminase activity. This enzyme has also been detected in mitomycin-producing *Streptomyces verticillatus* and is currently under further investigation.

The demonstration that D-[1-^{14}C, 6-^{3}H]glucosamine and L-[ureido-^{14}C]citrulline are specific precursors of streptozocin suggests that N(a) and N(b), respectively, of the antibiotic may be provided by these precursors, as outlined in Figure 5. However, the partial loss of tritium from D[2-^{3}H, 1-^{14}C]glucosamine suggests that the aminohexose may equilibrate to some extent with D-fructose and that its nitrogen may enter, at least in part, some of the other positions. In preparation for experiments to investigate if indeed D-glucosamine and L-citrulline donate N(a) and N(b), we determined dilution factors for these precursors using the respective ^{14}C-labeled compounds. The results of these experiments which are shown in Table 3 demonstrate that there is extremely efficient utilization of these precursors. Given the fact that dilution factors as low as two are observed and assuming that during the 24-h feeding period approximately 6 mg of streptozocin were synthesized, it is conceivable that the dilution is due entirely to streptozocin that had been produced prior to the addition of the precursors. This would mean that the added precursors were incorporated essentially without dilution from endogenous precursor. Two possible explanations for this efficient utilization may be considered: 1. the existence of very efficient uptake systems for both precursors and 2. the possible existence of membrane-bound enzymes involved in the streptozocin pathway coupled with the active excretion of the antibiotic or even the existence of exoenzymes. If the latter possibility were used by *S. achromogenes* var. *streptozoticus* and if the uptake of the antibiotic were restricted then a facile mechanism would exist to prevent the highly mutagenic streptozocin from damaging the DNA of the producing organism.

Future studies on the streptozocin biosynthetic pathway will aim to analyze the origin of the nitrogen atoms of the antibiotic and, when pathway intermediates that would serve as enzyme substrates have been identified, enzymatic studies will be made. Furthermore, attepts will be made to characterize the pathway genetically using auxotrophic mutants which were isolated and using streptozocin non-producing mutants that will hopefully become available.

Studies initiated to explore the biosynthesis of N-acetyl DON in *Streptomyces ambofaciens* have led to reproducible production of a compound containing an α diazoketone chromophore. However, on chromatographic analysis this compound does not appear to be identical with reference N-acetyl-DON. While *S. ambofaciens* was reported to produce DON, duazomycin B, and the unknown compound duazomycin C in addition to duazomycin A (Rao et al., 1960) the culture in our hands never seemed to produce more than one diazoketone. The compound appears to be readily labeled by either D,L-[1-^{14}C]- or [6-^{14}C]lysine and this may be compatible with the assumption that a DON-related moiety is present. An initial chromatographic comparison of the compound with reference alazopeptin suggests that both compounds may be identical; however, more thorough studies will be required to establish its identity. *S. ambofaciens* in our hands has proven to be highly unstable, producing white and gray colonies on agar plates upon prolonged propagation by transfer of pieces of mycelium. It is conceivable that the capacity of the strain to produce the duazomycin family of antibiotics may also be unstable, perhaps giving rise to alazopeptin production upon occurrence of an event involving the DNA of the strain.

It is hoped that the outcome of the planned future studies will contribute to the understanding of the mechanisms employed by microorganisms to generate the nitrogen-nitrogen bonds of streptozocin and diazoketone-containing antibiotics and that this knowledge may extend our understanding of the formation by intestinal bacteria of carcinogenic nitrosamines and nitrosamides which may be contributing to the development of human cancer (Tannenbaum et al., 1978).

Acknowledgments. The scientific contributions of my collaborators Dr. S. Singaram, Dr. M.R. Dhawale, and R.S. Lucas-Lawrence, the generous gifts of streptozocin from Dr. R.B. Whitfield, Upjohn Company, Kalamazoo, Michigan, of D-[2-^{3}H]glucosamine from Dr. M.A.E. Sallam, Alexandria University Egypt, and of strains NRRL 2697 and 3125 from Dr. T.G. Pridham, Peoria, Illinois, and the financial support through grant CA 18587 from the National Cancer Institute, DHEW, were greatly appreciated.

References

Anderson LE, Ehrlich J, Sun SH, Burkholder PR (1956) Strains of Streptomyces, the sources of azaserine, elaiomycin, griseoviridin and viridogrisein. Antibiot Chemother 6:100–115

Anzai K, Suzuki S (1960) A new antibiotic bovinocidin, identified as β-nitropropionic acid. J Antibiot 13:133–136

Anzai K, Nagatsu J, Suzuki S (1961) Pathocidin, a new antifungal antibiotic. I. Isolation, physical and chemical properties, and biological activities. J Antibiot Ser A 14:340–342

Arroyo V, Hall MJ, Hassall CH, Yamasaki Y (1976) Incorporation of amino acids into the cyclohexadepsipeptide, monamycin. Chem Commun 845–846

Ayanaba A, Alexander M (1973) Microbial formation of nitrosamines in vitro. Appl Microbiol 25:862–868

Backus EJ, Tresner HD, Campbell TH (1957) The nucleocidin and alazopeptin producing organisms: Two new species of *Streptomyces*. Antibiot Chemother 7:532–541

Beylot J, Veyret V, Vallat I, Longy M, Moretti S (1976) Streptozotocine et insulinomes malins. A propos d'un cas. Revue de la literature. Sem Hôp 52:489–496

Bhuyan BK, Fraser TJ, Buskirk HH, Neil GL (1972) Antileukemic activity of streptozotocin (NSC-85998) and its analogs. Cancer Chemother Rep Part 1 56:709–720

Callaham D, Del Tredici P, Torrey JG (1978) Isolation and cultivation in vitro of the actinomycete causing root nodulation in *Camptonia*. Science 199:899–902

Cardillo R, Fuganti C, Ghiringhelli D, Giangrasso D, Graselli P, Santopietro-Amisano A (1974) The biosynthesis of aureothin. Tetrahedron 30:459–461

Collins-Thompson DL, Sen NP, Aris B, Schwinghamer L (1972) Non-enzymic in vitro formation of nitrosamines by bacteria isolated from meat products. Can J Microbiol 18:1968–1971

Corbett MD, Chipko, BR, Baden DG (1978) Chloroperoxidase-catalyzed oxidation of 4-chloroaniline to 4-chloronitrosobenzene. Biochem J 175:353–360

Coronelli C, Pasqualucci CR, Tamoni G, Gallo GG (1966) Isolation and structure of alanosine, a new antibiotic. Farmaco Ed Sci 21:269–277

Dalton H (1974) Fixation of dinitrogen by free-living microorganisms. CRC Crit Rev Microbiol 3:183–220

Daves GD, Robins RK, Cheng CC (1962) Antibiotics. I. Synthesis of 1,6-dimethyl-5,7-dioxo-1,5,6,7-tetrahydro pyrimido[5,4-e]as-triazine (toxoflavin) and related compounds. J Am Chem Soc 84:1724–1729

DeVoe SE, Rigler NE, Shay AJ, Martin JH, Boyd TC, Backus EJ, Mowat JH, Bohonos N (1957) Alazopeptin: production, isolation, and chemical characteristics. Antibiot Ann 1956–1957:730–735

Dhawale MR, Hornemann U (1979) nitroalkane oxidation by Streptomycetes. J Bacteriol 137:916–924

Dion HW, Fusari SA, Jakubowski ZL, Zora JG, Bartz QR (1956) 6-Diazo-5-oxo-L-norleucine, a new tumor-inhibitory substance. II, Isolation and characterization. J Am Chem Soc 78:3075–3076

Fusari GA, Haskell TH, Frohardt RP, Bartz QR (1954) Azaserine, a new tumor-inhibitory substance. Structural studies. J Am Chem Soc 76:2881–2883

Gottlieb OR, Magalhaes MT (1959) Occurrence of 1-nitro-2-phenylethane in *Ocotea pretiosa* and *Ariba canelilla*. J Org Chem 24:2070–2071

Gruner BJ, DeAngelo AB, Shaw PD (1972) The isolation and some properties of an enzyme system which catalyzes the degradation of β-nitropropionic acid. Arch Biochem Biophys 148:107–114

Hassall CH, Morton RB, Ogihara Y, Phillips DAS (1971) Amino-acids and peptides. Part XII. The molecular structures of the monamycins, cyclodepsipeptide antibiotics. J Chem Soc (C): 526–532

Hata T, Umezawa I, Iwai Y, Katagiri M, Awaya J, Komiyama K, Oiwa R, Atsumi K (1973) Studies on the antitumor activity of an alazopeptin isolated from a new strain of *Streptomyces*. J Antibiot 26:181–183

Herr RR, Jahnke HK, Argoudelis AD (1967) The structure of streptozotocin. J Am Chem Soc 89:4808–4809

Herrmann H (1961) Identifizierung eines Stoffwechselproduktes von *Clitocybe suaveolens* als 4-Methylnitrosaminobenzaldehyd. Hoppe-Seylers Z Physiol Chem 326:13–16

Hessler EJ, Jahnke HK (1970) Improved synthesis of streptozotocin, J Org Chem 35:245–246

Hirasawa K, Isono K (1978) Formation of 8-azaguanine from guanine by *Streptomyces albus*. J Antibiot 31:628–629

Hornemann U, Eggert JH (1975) Utilization of the intact carbamoyl group of L-[NH_2CO-^{13}C, ^{15}N]citrulline in mitomycin biosynthesis by *Streptomyces verticillatus*. J Antibiot 28:841–843

Inuma H, Takeuchi T, Kondo S, Matsuzaki M, Umezawa H (1972) Dopastin, an inhibitor of dopamine β-hydroxylase. J Antibiot 25:497–500

Kawai S, Kobayashi K, Oshima T, Egami F (1965) Studies on the oxidation of p-aminobenzoate to p-nitrobenzoate by *Streptomyces thioluteus*. Arch Biochem Biophys 112:537–543

Kazumi T, Yoshino G, Fujii S, Baba S (1978) Tumorigenic action of streptozotocin on the pancreas and kidney in male wistar rats. Cancer Res 38:2144–2147

Kido T, Yamamoto T, Soda K (1975) Microbial assimilation of alkyl nitro compounds and formation of nitrite. Arch Mikrobiol 106:165–169

Kido T, Yamamoto T, Soda K (1976) Purification and properties of nitroalkane oxidizing enzyme from *Hansenula mrakii*. J Bacteriol 126:1261–1265

Koyama G, Maeda K, Umezawa H, Iitaka Y (1966) The structural studies of formycin and formycin B. Tetrahedron Lett 597–602

LaRue TA (1977) Naturally occurring compounds containing a nitrogen-nitrogen bond. Lloydia 40:307–321

LePage GA, Loo TL (1973) Purine antagonists. In: Holland JF, Frei E III (ed) Cancer medicine, p 754. Lea and Febiger, Philadelphia

Levenberg B (1964) Isolation and structure of agaritine, a γ-glutamyl-substituted arylhydrazine derivative from *Agaricaceae*. J Biol Chem 239:2267–2273

Levenberg B, Linton SN (1966) On the biosynthesis of toxoflavin, an azapteridine antibiotic produced by *Pseudomonas cocovenenans*. J Biol Chem 241:846–852

Like AA, Rossini AA (1976) Streptozotocin-induced pancreatic insulinitis: New model of diabetes mellitus. Science 193:415–417

Mills AL, Alexander M (1976) N-Nitrosamine formation by cultures of several microorganisms. Appl Environ Microbiol 31:892–895

Moruzzi A, Montero JL, Oiry J, Imbach JL (1978) Sur de nouveaux analogues de la streptozotocine. Eur J Med Chem 13:421–424

Murayama A, Tamura S (1970) Über Fragin, ein neues biologisches Stoffwechselproduct von *Pseudomonas fragi*. II. Mitt. Zur Struktur und Chemie des Fragins. Agric Biol Chem 34:122–129

Ochi K, Kikuchi S, Yashima S, Eguchi Y (1976) Biosynthesis of formycin. Incorporation and distribution of labeled compounds into formycin. J Antibiot 29:638–645

O'Donovan DG, Forde TJ (1970) Biosynthesis of withasomnine, a unique pyrazole alkaloid. Tetrahedron Lett 3637–3638

Okogun JI, Ekong DEU (1969) The fragrant principle of the fruits of *Dennettia tripetala* S. Baker: a new naturally occurring nitrocompound. Chem Ind 1272

Onaka T (1968) Biogenetic-type three-step synthesis of withasomnine. Tetrahedron Lett 5711–5714

Raistrick H, Stössl A (1958) Studies in the biochemistry of microorganisms. 104. Metabolites of *Penicillium atrovenetum* G. Smith: β-nitropropionic acid, a major metabolite. Biochem J 68:647–653

Rao KV (1961) Chemistry of the duazomycins. I. Duazomycin A. Antimicrob Agents Chemother 178–183

Rao KV (1962) Chemistry of the duazomycins. II. Duazomycin B. Antimicrob Agents Chemother 179–187

Rao KV, Brooks Jr SC, Kugelman M, Romano AA (1960) Diazomycin A, B and C, three antitumor substances. I. Isolation and characterization. Antibiot Ann 1959–1960:943–949

Sander J (1968) Nitrosaminsynthase durch Bacterien. Hoppe-Seylers Z Physiol Chem 349:429–432

Schütte HR, Liebisch HW, Miersch O, Senf L (1972) Untersuchungen zur Biosynthese des Agaritins in *Agaricus bisporus*. Anal Quim 68:899–903

Shaw PD, DeAngelo AB (1969) Role of ammonium ion in the biosynthesis of β-nitropropionic acid. J Bacteriol 99:463–468

Singaram S, Lawrence RS, Hornemann U (1979) Studies on the biosynthesis of the antibiotic streptozotocin by *Streptomyces achromogenes* var *streptozoticus*. Feeding experiments with carbon-14 and tritium labeled precursors. J Antibiot 32:501–507

Tannenbaum SR, Fett D, Young VR, Land PD, Bruce WR (1978) Nitrite and nitrate are formed by endogenous synthesis in the human intestine. Science 200:1487–1489

Vavra JJ, DeBoer C, Dietz A, Hanka LJ, Sokolski WT (1960) Streptozotocin a new antibacterial antibiotic. Antibiot Ann 1959–1960:230–235

Verstraete W, Alexander M (1972a) Heterotrophic nitrification by *Arthrobacter* sp. J Bacteriol 110:955–961

Verstraete W, Alexander M (1972b) Mechanism of nitrification by *Arthrobacter* sp. J Bacteriol 110:962–967

Wiley PF, Herr RR, Jahnke HK, Chidester CG, Mizsak SA, Spaulding LB, Argoudelis AD (1979) Streptozocin: Structure and Chemistry. J Org Chem 44:9–16

Biosynthesis of Peptide Antibiotics

KIYOSHI KURAHASHI

I. Introduction

Elucidation of the biosynthetic mechanisms of gramicidin S (KLEINKAUF and GEVERS, 1969; KLEINKAUF and KOISCHWITZ, 1980; KURAHASHI, 1974; KURAHASHI et al., 1969; LALAND and ZIMMER, 1973; LIPMANN, 1971; LIPMANN et al., 1971; SAITO et al., 1970) and tyrocidines (FRØYSHOV et al., 1978; KURAHASHI, 1974; KURAHASHI et al., 1969; LIPMANN, 1971; LIPMANN et al., 1971) by cell-free enzyme systems revealed a novel feature of the synthesis of peptides of defined sequence, quite distinct from protein and glutathione synthesis. The former involves nucleic acids and ribosomes, and the latter is carried out by phosphoryl activation of glutamic acid and free γ-glutamylcysteine. In gramicidin S and tyrocidine synthesis, the constituent amino acids are first activated as aminoacyl adenylates by the respective subunit of the multienzyme synthetases followed by the transfer of the aminoacyl groups to thiols of the same subunit proteins to form thioesters. The subsequent peptide chain elongation is mediated by 4′-phosphopantetheine which is attached to a small subunit, a carrier protein, of the multienzyme. The specificity and sequence of the amino acids in the peptide antibiotics are determined by the substrate specificity and the spatial arrangement of the thiols on the subunits of the synthetases. LALAND and ZIMMER (1973) called such a mechanism of peptide biosynthesis the 'protein thiotemplate mechanism' and LIPMANN et al. (1971) termed it the 'protein template mechanism'. In a recent review KATZ and DEMAIN (1977) state that the biosynthesis of peptide antibiotics by the genus *Bacillus* is directed by multienzyme thiotemplates. The author considers that it describes best the novel type of peptide biosynthesis and proposes to term it the 'multienzyme thiotemplate mechanism'.

In recent years a number of reviews of the biogenesis of small peptides or antibiotic peptides have appeared (ASSELINEAU and ZALTA, 1973; FRØYSHOV et al., 1978; JOHNE and GRÖGER, 1977; KATZ and DEMAIN, 1977; KLEINKAUF, 1979; KLEINKAUF and KOISCHWITZ, 1978; KURAHASHI, 1974; MAIER and GRÖGER, 1972; PERLMAN and BODANSZKY, 1971). The reader is referred to this literature for thorough bibliography of structural elucidations and biogenetic studies. The review by KATZ and DEMAIN cited above is informative on chemistry, biogenesis, and possible functions of peptide antibiotics. The review presented here gives a brief account of the historical development and the present-day knowledge of the biosynthetic mechanisms of antibiotic peptides obtained by cell-free enzyme systems.

II. Tyrocidines

Although a breakthrough in elucidation of the biosynthetic mechanisms of antibiotic peptides was made by the successful preparation of a cell-free enzyme system that could synthesize gramicidin S (BERG et al., 1965; BHAGAVAN et al., 1966; GEVERS et al., 1968; TOMINO et al., 1967b; YUKIOKA et al., 1965), the better characterized enzyme of tyrocidine synthesis is first illustrated here as a typical example of peptide biosynthesis by the multienzyme thiotemplate mechanism.

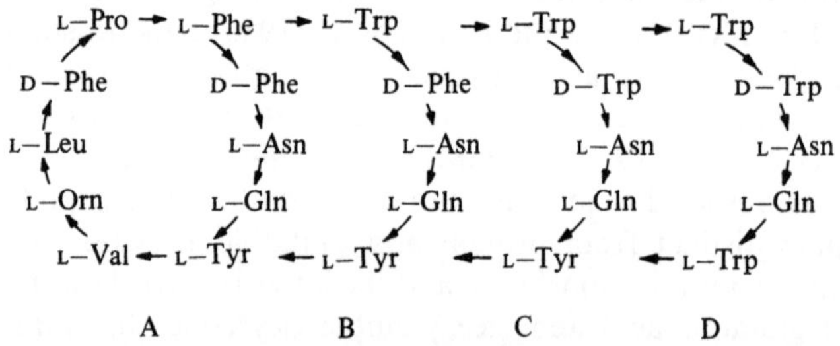

Fig. 1. Structure of tyrocidines

Bacillus brevis ATCC 8185 produces a mixture of tyrocidines as shown in Figure 1. A cell-free enzyme system of tyrocidine synthesis was first developed by FUJIKAWA et al. (1966) and TOMINO et al. (1967a). They resolved the enzyme into two complementary components and showed that tyrocidine synthesis must take place in the enzyme-bound state (FUJIKAWA et al., 1968b). Later the enzyme system was found to consist of three complementary components (KAMBE et al., 1974; LEE et al., 1973; ROSKOSKI et al., 1970a). Table 1 shows the features of the multienzyme. The details of isolation, purification, and properties are found in the references cited in the table.

The first step in the activation of the constituent amino acids is the formation of aminoacyl adenylates similar to that in protein synthesis.

$$\text{Enz}\diagup^{\text{SH}} + \text{AA} + \text{ATP} \rightleftharpoons \text{Enz}\diagup^{\text{SH}}\ldots\text{AA-AMP} + \text{PP}_i \qquad \text{(Reaction 1)}$$

The enzyme can be the light enzyme (LE), which adenylates L- or D-phenylalanine or each subunit of the intermediate enzyme (IE) or the heavy enzyme (HE) (FUJIKAWA et al., 1971; KAMBE et al., 1971; KURAHASHI et al., 1969; LEE et al., 1973; ROSKOSI et al., 1970a). The aminoacyl group is then transferred to a thiol, possibly the thiol of the cysteine residue of the enzyme, forming an acid-stable and alkali-labile aminoacylthioester-enzyme complex as follows (FUJIKAWA et al., 1971; LEE et al., 1973; ROSKOSI et al., 1970a).

Table 1. Features of tyrocidine synthetase

Fraction number	Nomenclature	Amino acid activated	PPan[a] mole/mole of enzyme	Molecular weight	References
I	Light enzyme (LE)	L- and D-Phe	0	100,000	FUJIKAWA et al., 1971; LEE and LIPMANN, 1975; LEE et al., 1973
II	Intermediate enzyme (IE)	Pro, L- and D-Phe (Trp)[b]	1	230,000	KAMBE et al., 1971; LEE and LIPMANN, 1975; LEE et al., 1973
III	Heavy enzyme (HE)	Asn, Gln, Tyr (Trp, Phe), Val, Orn (Lys), Leu (Ile)	1	440,000	FUJIKAWA et al., 1971; KAMBE et al., 1971; KLEINKAUF et al., 1970; LEE and LIPMANN, 1975; LEE et al., 1973

[a] 4′-Phosphopantetheine
[b] The amino acids in parentheses can be activated and incorporated into tyrocidines

$$\text{Enz}\overset{\text{SH}}{\diagup}\ldots\text{AA-AMP} \rightleftharpoons \text{Enz}\overset{\text{S-AA}}{\diagup}+\text{AMP} \qquad \text{(Reaction 2)}$$

The aminoacylthioester-enzyme complex can still activate another molecule of the amino acid and bind it as an aminoacyl adenylate as evidenced by the release of half of the labeled amino acid by an acid treatment and the other half by an alkali or mercuric salts treatment (ROSKOSI et al., 1970a). When a constituent amino acid of the peptide assumes the D-configuration, racemization takes place at this stage, as was proven for phenylalanine bound to LE and IE by LEE (1976) and LEE et al. (1973).

$$\text{Enz}\overset{\text{S-L-AA}}{\diagup} \rightleftharpoons \text{Enz}\overset{\text{S-D-AA}}{\diagup} \qquad \text{(Reaction 3)}$$

As illustrated in Figure 2A, all the constituent amino acids of tyrocidine are activated and bound covalently to LE, IE, and HE. The interaction of LE with IE brings about the transfer of the D-phenylalanine on LE to the proline on IE to form a dipeptide, which is in turn transferred to the 4′-phosphopantetheine arm on the carrier protein (Pan carrier) as illustrated in Figure 2B (KLEINKAUF et al., 1971; LEE et al., 1973; ROSKOSKI et al., 1970b). The LE can now again be charged with L-phenylalanine followed by its conversion to the D-enantiomorph. The dipeptide on Pan carrier is translocated to the phenylalanine at Site 3 of IE (Figure 2C) and by the repetition of the sequence of events a tetrapeptide, D-Phe-Pro-Phe-D-Phe, bound to IE through a thioester linkage is formed as shown in Figure 2D (LEE et al., 1973; ROSKOSKI et al., 1970b). The thiols of the subunits of IE vacated can be recharged by the respective substrate amino acids. The interaction of the tetrapeptide-charged IE with the constituent amino acids-charged HE brings about the transfer of the tetrapeptide to the asparagine on HE to form a pentapeptide, D-Phe-Pro-

Tyrocidine synthetase

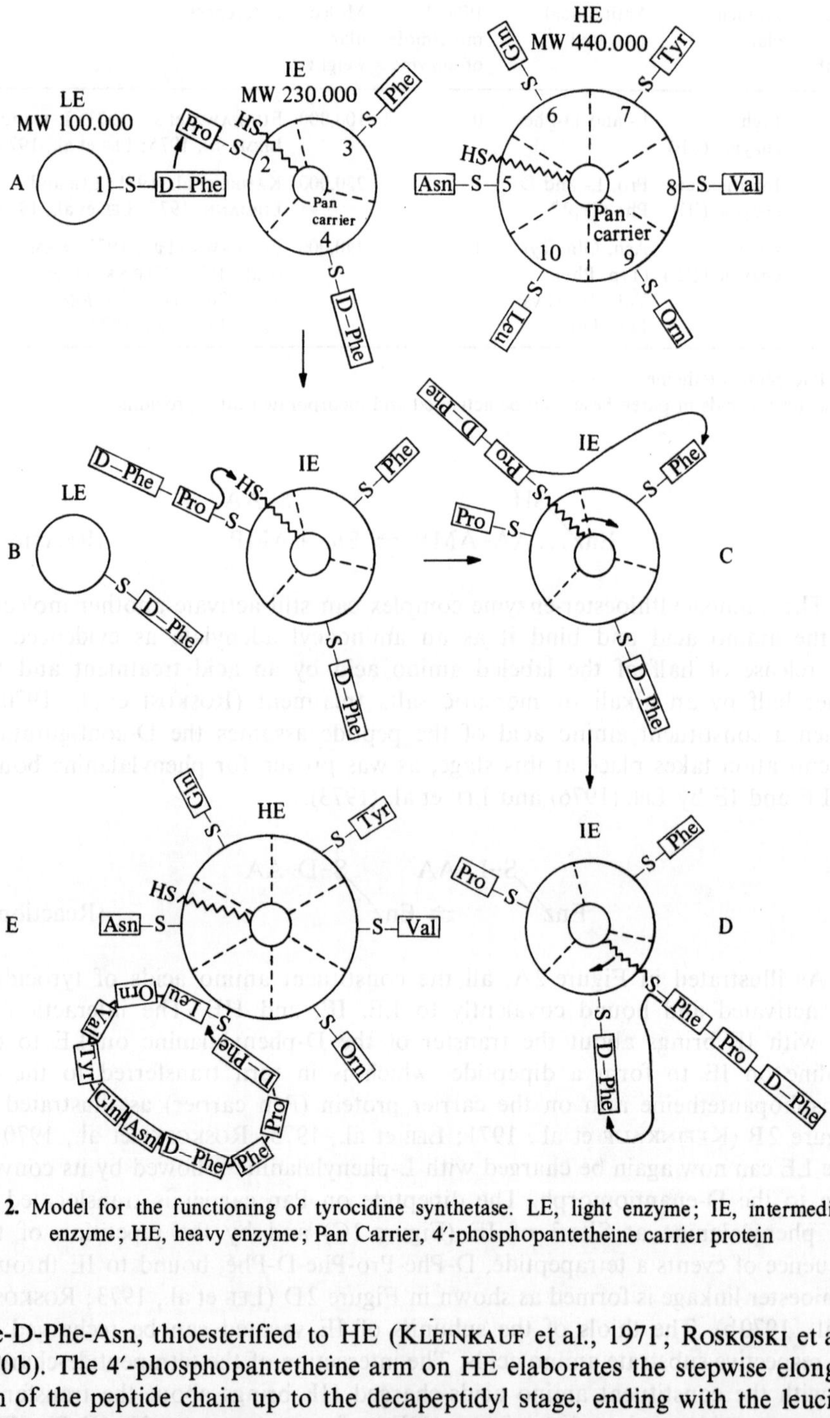

Fig. 2. Model for the functioning of tyrocidine synthetase. LE, light enzyme; IE, intermediate enzyme; HE, heavy enzyme; Pan Carrier, 4′-phosphopantetheine carrier protein

Phe-D-Phe-Asn, thioesterified to HE (KLEINKAUF et al., 1971; ROSKOSKI et al., 1970b). The 4′-phosphopantetheine arm on HE elaborates the stepwise elongation of the peptide chain up to the decapeptidyl stage, ending with the leucine at Site 10 of HE (ROSKOSKI et al., 1970b). Although the detailed mechanism of cyclization is not known, the leucine carboxyl group, activated as a thioester, reacts with the free amino group of D-phenylalanine, causing cyclization and release of the final product. This last step seems to be the rate-limiting step of tyrocidine synthesis, because it is possible to isolate intermediary peptides of various lengths including the linear decapeptide by the treatment of the peptide-charged synthetase with mild alkali (ROSKOSKI et al., 1970b). The stoichiometry of the overall reaction is presented in reaction 4 (FUJIKAWA et al., 1968b).

$$10 \text{ amino acids} + 10 \text{ ATP} \rightarrow \text{tyrocidine} + 10 \text{ AMP} + 10 \text{ PP}_i \qquad \text{(Reaction 4)}$$

LEE et al. (1973) succeeded in disaggregating IE and HE into, respectively, three and six subunits of 70,000-Dalton molecular mass which activated amino acids and also one 4′-phosphopantetheine carrying subunit each with a molecular mass of 17,000–20,000 Daltons. They proved that the nascent peptides are bound to the 4′-phosphopantetheine carrier proteins (KLEINKAUF et al., 1971; LEE and LIPMANN, 1974). More recently they reported isolation of 90,000-Dalton, amino acid activating subunit-4′-phosphopantetheine carrier protein complexes in addition to 70,000-Dalton amino acid activating subunits from IE and HE (LEE and LIPMANN, 1977). By comparing the binding affinity of proline to the 90,000-Dalton complex and to the 70,000-Dalton proline-activating subunit, they showed that the 21,000-Dalton 4′-phosphopantetheine carrier protein has a high-affinity proline-binding site. They postulate that each amino acid on the respective activating subunit of IE and HE of the multienzyme tyrocidine synthetase is first translocated to the amino acid acceptor site on the 4′-phosphopantetheine carrier protein, where polymerization of amino acids takes place by receiving D-phenylalanine from LE or a peptidyl unit from the 4′-phosphopantetheine arm of IE and HE. The newly formed nascent peptide, one amino acid residue longer, is then translocated back to the 4′-phosphopantetheine arm. However, the other constituent amino acids have not been proven to be bound to the 4′-phosphopantetheine carrier protein with a high affinity, and the simultaneous presence of intermediate peptides of various lengths thioesterified to IE and HE (LEE et al., 1973; ROSKOSKI et al., 1970b), as proven by the proportional increase of ^{14}C-phenylalanine incorporation with the stepwise addition of the constituent amino acids in sequence, contradicts the above postulate. The translocation of the D-phenylalanine on LE to the adjacent proline on IE and that of the intermediate peptides on IE and HE to the adjacent amino acids need further study.

MACH and TATUM (1964) obtained tyrocidine D, whose aromatic amino acids were all replaced by tryptophan, except for the D-phenylalanine at position 1, by growing *B. brevis* in a minimal medium supplemented with L-tryptophan. FUJIKAWA et al. (1968a) and RAO et al. (1968) reported the preferential utilization of tryptophan by a cell-free enzyme system. The ambiguity in substrate specificity of tyrocidine synthetase is not restricted to aromatic amino acids, but leucine and ornithine can be replaced by isoleucine and lysine, respectively as shown in Figure 3 (FUJIKAWA et al., 1968a). ROSKOSKI et al. (1970b) reported that even D-phenylalanine at position 1 of tyrocidines and gramicidin S was replaced by tyrosine, giving rise to tyrocidine and gramicidin S with all the

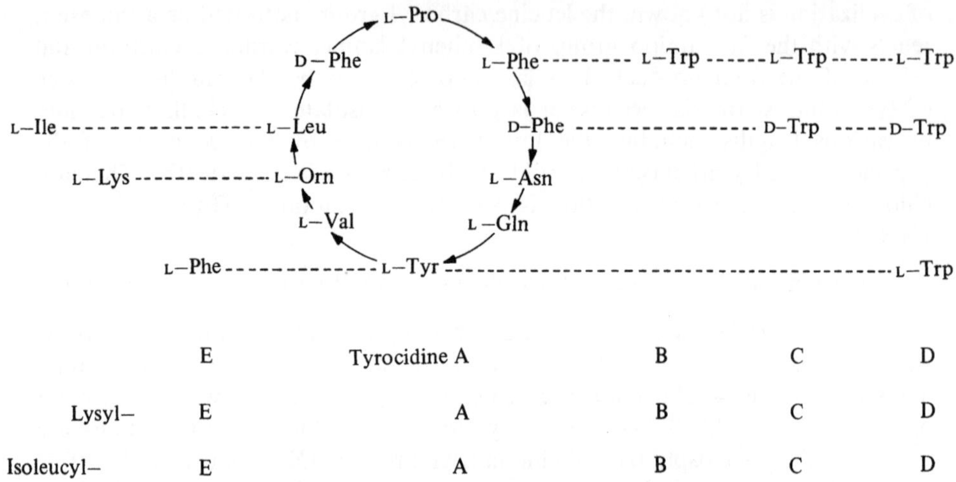

Fig. 3. Formation of tyrocidine analogs by amino acid substitution

aromatic amino acid residues replaced by tyrosine, though their structural analyses were not carried out. The tyrosine dependent ATP-PP_i exchange catalyzed by LE of either synthetase was shown very weak (FUJIKAWA et al., 1971; YAMADA and KURAHASHI, 1969).

III. Gramicidin S

In contrast to tyrocidines, gramicidin S produced by *Bacillus brevis* ATCC 9999 or Nagano consists of two identical pentapeptides as shown in Figure 4. This structure posed a problem in polymerization and cyclization of the antibiotic: whether two pentapeptides are synthesized and cyclized or a linear decapeptide is formed and a head to tail condensation takes place. The early studies by KURAHASHI (1961), TOMINO and KURAHASHI (1964), and HOLM et al. (1966) indicated that the synthesis of the peptide started with D-phenylalanine and a stepwise elongation of the chain towards the C-terminus occurred. However, a tripeptide, D-Phe-Pro-Val, isolated from a reaction mixture was found not to serve as a precursor for gramicidin S synthesis and the presence of all five constituent amino acids in the reaction shifted the

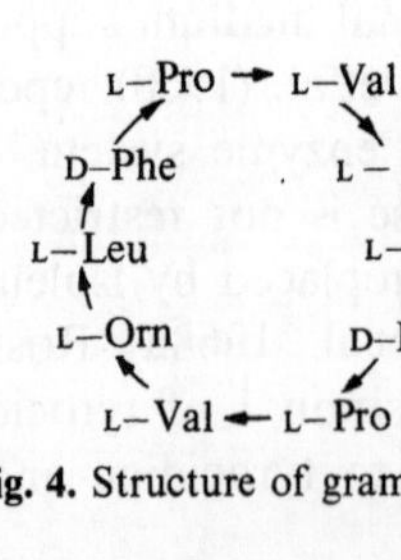

Fig. 4. Structure of gramicidin S

Table 2. Features of gramicidin S synthetase

Fraction number	Nomenclature	Amino acid activated	PPan[a] mole/mole of enzyme	Molecular weight	References
II	Light enzyme (LE)	L- and D-Phe	0	100,000	ITOH et al., 1968; KANDA et al., 1978; KLEINKAUF et al., 1969; TAKAHASHI et al., 1971; VATER and KLEINKAUF, 1976; YAMADA and KURAHASHI, 1969; ZIMMER and LALAND, 1975
I	Heavy enzyme (HE)	Pro, Val (Leu, Ile, AIle[b], NVal[c])[d], Orn, Leu (Ile, AIle[b], NLeu[e])	1	280,000	CHRISTIANSEN et al., 1977; GILHUUS-MOE et al., 1970; HORI et al., 1978; ITOH et al., 1968; KLEINKAUF et al., 1969; KOISCHWITZ and KLEINKAUF, 1976a; KURAHASHI et al., 1969; LIPMANN et al., 1971; ZIMMER and LALAND, 1975

[a] 4′-Phosphopantetheine
[b] Alloisoleucine
[c] Norvaline
[d] The amino acid in parentheses can be activated and incorporated into gramicidin S
[e] Norleucine

synthesis from the tripeptide to gramicidin S (TOMINO and KURAHASHI, 1964). The presence of an ATP-dependent phenylalanine racemase was early detected in the organism by YAMADA et al. (1964). This enzyme was shown later to be identical with the light enzyme (LE) of gramicidin S synthetase (ITOH et al., 1968). YUKIOKA et al. (1965), BERG et al. (1965), BHAGAVAN et al. (1966), and GREVERS et al. (1968) also achieved cell-free synthesis of gramicidin S that was insensitive to inhibitors of protein synthesis.

Gramicidin S synthetase was separated into two complementary fractions by TOMINO et al. (1967b) and both fractions have been purified to a near homogeneous state (CHRISTIANSEN et al., 1977; HORI et al., 1978; ITOH et al., 1968; KANDA et al., 1978; KLEINKAUF et al., 1969; KOISCHWITZ and KLEINKAUF, 1976a; KURAHASHI et al., 1969; TAKAHASHI et al., 1971; VATER and KLEINKAUF, 1976; YAMADA and KURAHASHI, 1969; ZIMMER and LALAND, 1975). The features of the enzyme are shown in Table 2. The discovery of 4′-phosphopantetheine in the heavy enzyme (HE) was first made by GILHUUS-MOE et al. (1970). The activation, thioesterification, and racemization of L-phenylalanine by LE have been extensively studied (GEVERS et al., 1969; KURAHASHI et al., 1969; LIPMANN et al., 1971; TAKAHASHI et al., 1971; YAMADA and KURAHASHI, 1968, 1969). Racemization occurs while phenylalanine is thioesterified to LE (GEVERS et al., 1969; TAKAHASHI et al., 1971). The LE of gramicidin S synthetase and the LE of tyrocidine synthetase are interchangeable in the synthesis of tyrocidine in vitro (FUJIKAWA et al., 1971; KURAHASHI et al., 1969), suggesting the presence of some molecular homology between the two for interaction with the HE of gramicidin S synthetase and the IE of tyrocidine synthetase, in addition to the similarity of their catalytic activities for phenylalanine. The activation (GEVERS et al., 1968; ITOH et al., 1968; KLEINKAUF and GEVERS, 1969; KURAHASHI et al., 1969) and thioesterification of the remaining four constituent amino acids by HE (FRØYSHOV et al., 1970; GEVERS et al., 1968, 1969; KLEINKAUF and GEVERS, 1969; LIPMANN et al., 1971; LJONES et al., 1968), the initiation of the peptide chain elongation by the formation of a dipeptide, D-Phe-Pro (KURAHASHI, 1961; KURAHASHI et al., 1969), thioesterified to HE (FRØYSHOV et al., 1970; GEVERS et al., 1969; KLEINKAUF et al., 1971; LIPMANN et al., 1971), and the subsequent elongation of the chain to the pentapeptide stage by the aid of the 4′-phosphopantetheine arm (FRØYSHOV et al., 1970; GEVERS et al., 1969; LALAND et al., 1972; LIPMANN, 1971) follow the similar sequence of events as illustrated for tyrocidine synthesis.

Since no intermediary peptides larger than pentapeptides thioesterified to HE were found and the addition of leucine to the reaction diminished the amount of the enzyme-bound intermediary peptides, resulting in gramicidin S synthesis, it was concluded that the cyclic decapeptide synthesis took place by a rapid condensation reaction of the two pentapeptides thioesterified to HE (FRØYSHOV et al., 1970; GEVERS et al., 1969). LIPMANN proposed that the condensation was intermolecular, that is, two pentapeptides on two different HEs condense (LIPMANN, 1973; LIPMANN et al., 1971). ROSKOSKI et al. (1971) showed that the incubation of the LE and HE which were precharged with the respective substrate amino acids produced gramicidin S, which supports this postulate. On the other hand, STOLL et al. (1970) provided evidence that intramolecular condensation was the final step of the decapeptide synthesis. LALAND and his associates presented a scheme for cyclization of two pentapeptides as illustrated in Figure 5 (FRØYSHOV et al., 1978; LALAND et al., 1972; LALAND and ZIMMER, 1973). The first pentapeptide completed is supposedly translocated from the leucine site to another thiol site on HE, where it awaits completion of the second pentapeptide. They postulate that the waiting site may be the same site where D-leucine, an inhibitor of gramicidin S synthesis, is bound as a thioester (SAXHOLM et al., 1972).

Using affinity chromatography, PASS et al. (1974) demonstrated that there was an amino acid accepting site for D-phenylalanine on HE which could be either the thiol of the 4′-phosphopantetheine arm or a cysteine of the enzyme protein. To incorporate into gramicidin S the labeled D-phenylalanine translocated from LE to this site in the presence of all five amino acids and ATP, the addition of LE was necessary. These results were also taken to support the intramolecular cyclization of two pentapeptides.

As in the case of tyrocidine synthetase, activation of some analogs of the substrate amino acids by gramicidin S synthetase was reported by ITOH et al. (1968), LEUNG and BAXTER (1972), and YAMADA and KURAHASHI (1969). LIPMANN et al. (1971) showed the incorporation of L-isoleucine, L-alloisoleucine, L-norleucine, L-norvaline, and *p*-fluoro-L-phenylalanine into gramicidin S. Recently ALTMANN et al. (1976) obtained (3,3′-Leu)-gramicidin S which contained four residues of leucine.

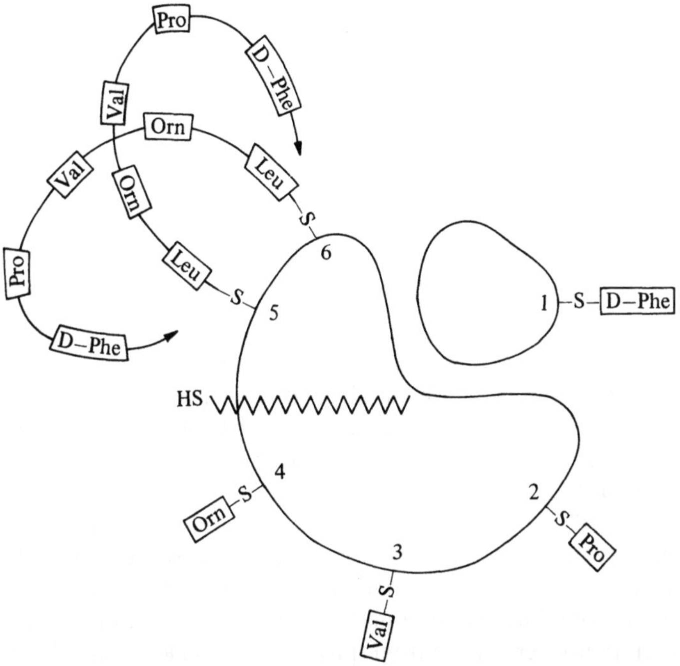

Fig. 5. Model for the intramolecular cyclization of two pentapeptides to form gramicidin S. Position 5, the thiol site for leucine; Position 6, the thiol waiting site. The zig-zag line represents the 4′-phosphopantetheine arm. (Reproduced with permission of S.G. LALAND)

In contrast to tyrocidine synthetase, trials to dissociate the HE of gramicidin S synthetase into subunits by various treatments have failed. KOISCHWITZ and KLEINKAUF (1976b) and FRØYSHOV et al. (1978) postulate that HE with a molecular weight of 280,000 may consist of subunits which are covalently linked. However, a proline-activating subunit and possibly an ornithine-activating subunit with a molecular weight of 80,000–100,000 were found in extracts of a gramicidin S-nonproducing mutant of *B. brevis* (KAMBE et al., 1974). The use of mutants may be appropriate for studies of the subunits of HE.

SAITO and his associates also obtained a number of mutants that could not produce gramicidin S (IWAKI et al., 1972). Recently KANDA et al. (1978) purified LE from one mutant strain. It possessed L- and D-phenylalanine-activating activity, but lacked the activity to bind them as thioesters. Racemization of phenylalanine was not catalyzed either. These results confirm the finding that racemization of phenylalanine takes place at the thioester-linked stage on LE (TAKAHASHI et al., 1971).

IV. Linear Gramicidins

Linear gramicidins, gramicidin A, B, and C (Fig. 6) are produced by *Bacillus brevis* ATCC 8185 which also elaborates tyrocidines. The feature of the structure

A

N–Formyl–Val → Gly → Ala → D–Leu → Ala → D–Val → Val → D–Val
(Ile) ↓
Ethanolamine ← Trp ← D–Leu ← Trp ← D–Leu ← Trp ← D–Leu ← Trp

B

← Phe ←

C

← Tyr ←

Fig. 6. Structure of gramicidin A, B, and C

is the presence of a formyl group at the N-terminal valine, an ethanolamine moiety at the C-terminus, and an alternative sequence of L- and D-amino acid residues. AKASHI and KURAHASHI (1977) and AKERS et al. (1977) partially resolved gramicidin A synthetase. The features of the enzyme fractions are summarized in Table 3.

BAUER et al. (1972) reported that a Sephadex G-200 fraction of crude extracts catalyzed the synthesis of a protein-bound unformylated pentadecapeptide. Upon chemical formylation and ethanolaminolysis of the enzyme-bound pentadecapeptide they obtained a compound which migrated with an authentic linear gramicidin in thin-layer chromatography. Later AKERS et al. (1977) partially purified two enzyme fractions (glycine enzyme and alanine enzyme) that were in combination presumably capable of synthesizing the N-terminal heptapeptide without a formyl group. AKASHI and KURAHASHI partially purified a valine- and glycine-activating enzyme (Component I) (AKASHI et al., 1977; AKASHI and KURAHASHI, 1977) and an alanine-, leucine-, and valine-activating enzyme (Component II) (AKASHI and KURAHASHI, 1977). The mechanism of activation of the substrate amino acids and thioesterification to the enzyme was found to

Table 3. Features of gramicidin A synthetase

Fraction number	Nomenclature	Amino acid activated	PPan[a] mole/mole of enzyme	Molecular weight	References
I	Glycine enzyme	Val (Ile)[b], Gly	1	180,000[c] 160,000[d]	AKASHI and KURAHASHI, 1977, 1978; AKERS et al., 1977
II	Alanine enzyme	Ala, L- and D-Leu, Val	1	300,000[e] 350,000[d]	AKASHI, 1977; AKASHI and KURAHASHI, 1977; AKERS et al., 1977
III		L- and D-Val	ND[f]	ND	AKASHI, 1977
IV		Leu, Trp	ND	ND	AKASHI, 1977

[a] 4′-Phosphopantetheine
[b] The amino acid in parentheses can be activated and incorporated into gramicidin A
[c] According to AKASHI and KURAHASHI, 1977
[d] According to AKERS et al., 1977
[e] According to AKASHI, 1977
[f] Not determined

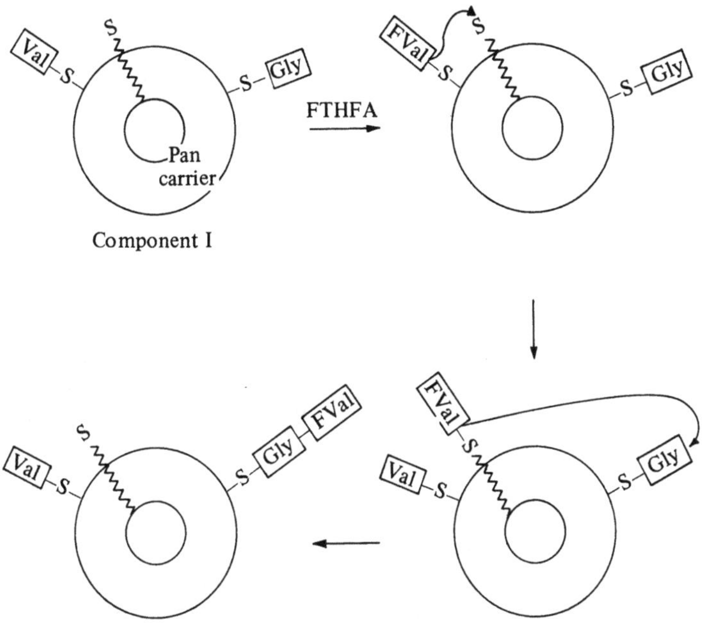

Fig. 7. Model for the initiation of gramicidin A synthesis. Pan Carrier, 4′-phosphopantetheine carrier protein

be similar to that in gramicidin S and tyrocidine synthesis. However, Component I was found to catalyze a novel reaction, the transfer of the formyl group from formyltetrahydrofolate (formyl-THFA) to the valine thioesterified to Component I, followed by peptidation to form formylvalylglycine bound to the enzyme as shown schematically in Figure 7 (AKASHI et al., 1977; AKASHI and KURAHASHI, 1978). The addition of Component II together with alanine, leucine, and ATP to the above system gave rise to a formyl-Val-Gly-Ala-Leu-Ala (even longer) intermediary peptide bound to the enzyme (AKASHI and KURAHASHI, 1977). They showed that the formyltransferase activity was intrinsic to Component I (AKASHI and KURAHASHI, 1977; AKASHI and KURAHASHI, 1978). Thus, they concluded that initiation of gramicidin A synthesis began with the activation and thioesterification of valine to Component I followed by formylation and peptidation with glycine bound to Component I. AKERS et al. (1977) found that 1 mole each of 4′-phosphopantetheine was present in glycine enzyme (Component I) and alanine enzyme (Component II).

AKASHI (1977) further isolated two other components of gramicidin A synthetase, Component III and IV, which activated L- and D-valine, and leucine and tryptophan, respectively. The incubation of the four components together with all constituent amino acids, formyl-THFA, and ATP produced a formylpentadecapeptide thioesterified to the enzyme, which gave rise to gramicidin A upon chemical ethanolaminolysis.

The mechanism of incorporation of the ethanolamine moiety has not been elucidated. There is a possibility that serine is incorporated next to the C-terminal tryptophan of the linear chain to form a formylhexadecapeptide. The decarboxylation of it would produce gramicidin A. However, the enzymatic ethanolaminolysis of the formylpentadecapeptide thioesterified to the enzyme is also plausible, because it was shown that D-phenylalanylamide was formed enzymatically from the D-phenylalanine thioesterified to the LE of gramicidin S synthetase in the presence of ammonium ions (TAKAHASHI et al., 1971; TOMINO et al., 1967b).

V. Edeine

Edeine is an antibiotic which consists mostly of unusual amino acids and the carboxyl terminus is masked by spermidine (edeine A) or guanylspermidine (edeine B) as shown in Figure 8. Edeine synthesis has been studied by KURYLO-BOROWSKA and TATUM and their associates (KURYLO-BOROWSKA, 1975; KURYLO-BOROWSKA and ABRAMSKY, 1972; KURYLO-BOROWSKA and SEDKOWSKA, 1974; KURYLO-BOROWSKA and TATUM, 1966).

Edeine synthetase is present in the edeine-producing organism, *Bacillus brevis* Vm4, in two forms, soluble and cytoplasmic membrane-DNA bound. KURYLO-BOROWSKA and her associates (KURYLO-BOROWSKA, 1975; KURYLO-BOROWSKA and SEDKOWSKA, 1974) resolved the synthetase of both soluble and particulate fractions into several fractions by DEAE-cellulose column chromatography and Sephadex G-200 gel filtration. The features of the representative fractions that are complementary in the total synthesis of the peptide are summarized in Table 4. The fact that edeine synthesis was inhibited by neither chloramphenicol nor RNase and the multienzyme nature of the synthetase indicate that the

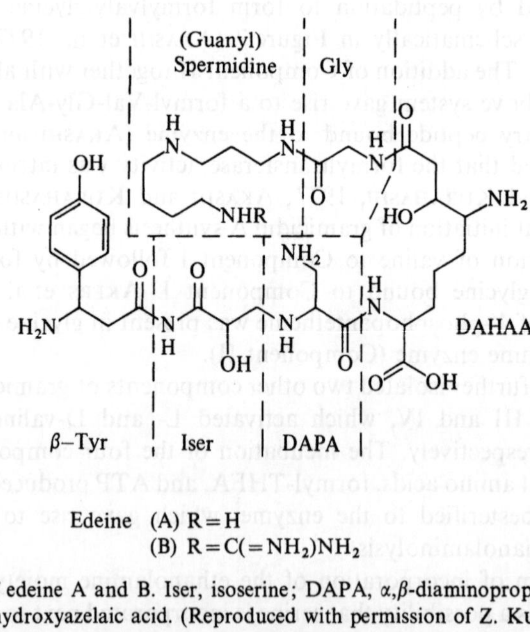

Edeine (A) R=H
(B) R=C(=NH_2)NH_2

Fig. 8. Structure of edeine A and B. Iser, isoserine; DAPA, α,β-diaminopropionic acid; DAHAA, 2,6-diamino-7-hydroxyazelaic acid. (Reproduced with permission of Z. KURYLO-BOROWSKA)

Table 4. Features of edeine synthetase

Fraction number	Amino acid activated	PPan[a]	Molecular weight	References
I (A)	β-Tyrosine	+[b]	210,000	KURYLO-BOROWSKA, 1975; KURYLO-BOROWSKA and SEDKOWSKA, 1974
II (B)	Isoserine, DAPA[c], DAHAA[d], Gly, α- and β-alanine[e]	+[b]	180,000	KURYLO-BOROWSKA, 1975; KURYLO-BOROWSKA and SEDKOWSKA, 1974

[a] 4′-Phosphopantetheine
[b] Not quantitatively determined
[c] α,β-Diaminopropionic acid
[d] 2,6-Diamino-7-hydroxyazelaic acid
[e] Not constituent amino acids of edeine

peptide formation must follow the nonribosomal mechanism. However, it is rather puzzling to find that Component A which activates and binds only β-tyrosine as a thioester has a molecular weight of 210,000 and contains 4′-phosphopantetheine. Component B was shown to thioesterify glycine. They also isolated another fraction, Component C, with a molecular weight of 100,000 (revised later to be 60,000 (KURYLO-BOROWSKA and KIERAS, 1976)) by Sephadex G-200 gel filtration. Component C activated α- and β-alanine and leucine in addition to isoserine and α, β-diaminopropionic acid and enhanced the synthesis of edeine by Component A and B. Further purification of the enzyme fractions and rigorous identification of their properties seem necessary to clarify fully the mechanism of edeine biosynthesis.

The mechanism of β-tyrosine formation from L-α-tyrosine was reported by the same group (KURYLO-BOROWSKA and ABRAMSKY, 1972) but the pathway of the synthesis of the other unusual amino acids in edeine is unknown. Like the introduction of the ethanolamine moiety into linear gramicidin, the incorporation of (guanyl)spermidine into the C-terminus presents problems to be solved in the future.

VI. Alamethicin

There are two proposed structures for alamethicin, a cyclic (PAYNE et al., 1970) and a linear, open-chain peptide (MARTIN and WILLIAMS, 1976; PANDEY et al., 1977). Both structures are shown in Figure 9. Based on the cyclic structure, KLEINKAUF and RINDFLEISCH (1975) proceeded to obtain a cell-free enzyme system that was able to synthesize alamethicin. They presented evidence to suggest that a labeled peptide which behaved like an authentic sample of alamethicin in thin-layer chromatography was formed in an incubation of crude extracts of *Trichoderma viride* together with the constituent eight amino acids and ATP. Neither puromycin nor RNase inhibited the synthesis, but rather enhanced it. They fractionated the synthetase into two complementary fractions by Sepha-

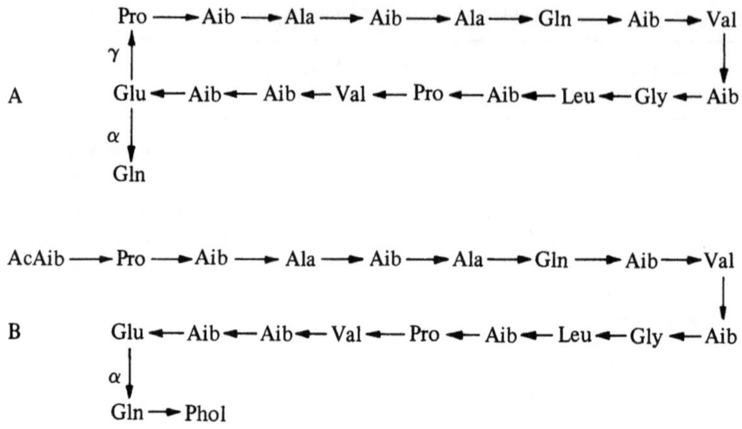

Fig. 9. Structure of alamethicin. **A** Cyclic structure (PAYNE et al., 1970); **B** Linear structure (MARTIN and WILLIAMS, 1976; PANDEY et al., 1977). Aib, aminoisobutyric acid; AcAib, N-acetylaminoisobutyric acid; Phol, phenylalaninol

dex G-200 gel filtration and hydroxylapatite column chromatography, which activated and thioesterified some of the constituent amino acids, though their exact roles in synthesis were not clear because of the contamination of the fractions with aminoacyl-tRNA synthetases (KLEINKAUF and RINDFLEISCH, 1975; RINDFLEISCH and KLEINKAUF, 1976). Since the recent structural analysis had proposed a linear nonadecapeptide structure with phenylalaninol as a component as shown in Figure 9B, they tested the influence of phenylalaninol on the in vitro synthesis of alamethicin (RINDFLEISCH and KLEINKAUF, 1976). They could not detect any effect. However, in a more recent paper, MOHR and KLEINKAUF (1978) reported the incorporation of ^{14}C-phenylalaninol into alamethicin in vivo. They also showed that enzyme-bound N-acetylaminoisobutyric acid was synthesized by incubating a partially purified enzyme with ATP, acetyl-CoA, and aminoisobutyric acid. This result agrees with the initial formylation of the enzyme-bound valine in gramicidin A synthesis. Still further fractionation and purification of enzymes are essential for elucidation of the biosynthetic mechanism of alamethicin.

VII. Bacitracins

Biosynthesis of bacitracin, a branched cyclic dodecapeptide produced by a strain of *Bacillus licheniformis*, has been extensively studied and shown to be carried out by a multienzyme thiotemplate system. The structure is shown in Figure 10 (RESSLER and KASHELIKAR, 1966). ISHIHARA et al. (1968) were the first to obtain a cell-free enzyme system that catalyzed bacitracin synthesis. The enzyme system was fractionated into two complementary components by ISHIHARA et al. (1974) and FRØYSHOV and LALAND (1974) and later one of the components was separated into two components (FRØYSHOV, 1974; ISHIHARA

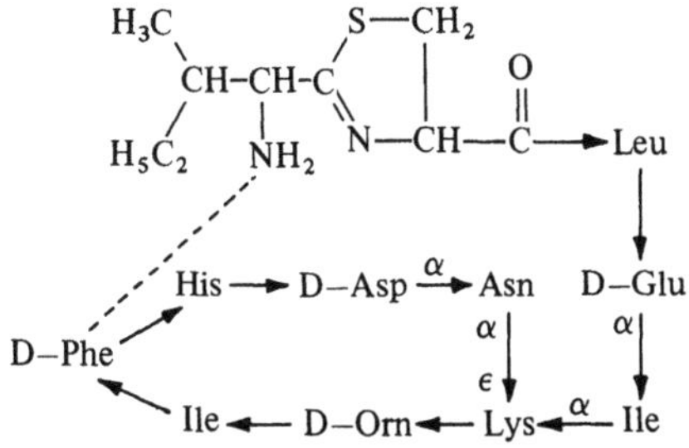

Fig. 10. Structure of bacitracin (RESSLER and KASHELIKAR, 1966).

et al., 1975). Table 5 shows the features of the synthetase. All three components activate multiple amino acids and contain 1 mole each of 4′-phosphopantetheine (ISHIHARA et al., 1975; ROLAND et al., 1975). By sequential additions of the constituent amino acids to the synthetic reaction FRØYSHOV (1975) demonstrated the presence of intermediary peptides attached to each component of the synthetase. PFAENDER et al. (1973) obtained a number of bacitracin synthetase fractions with a variety of molecular weights, but the nature of those fractions is not clear.

At what stage the N-terminal thiazoline ring is formed or how cyclization of the carboxyl terminal heptapeptide is directed has remained unanswered. Recently ISHIHARA and SHIMURA obtained evidence that the N-terminal dipeptide, Ile-Cys, thioesterified to Component I contained the thiazoline ring (K. SHIMURA, personal communication). It suggests that dipeptide synthesis followed by the thiozoline ring closure is prerequisite for further elongation of the chain.

Table 5. Features of bacitracin synthetase

Fraction number	Amino acid activated	PPan[a] mole/mole of enzyme	Molecular weight	References
I (A)	Ile, Cys, Leu, Glu	1	200,000	FRØYSHOV and LALAND, 1974; ISHIHARA et al., 1975; ISHIHARA and SHIMURA, 1974; ROLAND et al., 1975, 1977
II (B)	Lys, Orn	1	210,000	FRØYSHOV, 1974; ISHIHARA et al., 1975; ROLAND et al., 1975, 1977
III (C)	Ile, L- and D-Phe, His, Asp, Asn	1	380,000	FRØYSHOV, 1974; ISHIHARA et al., 1975; ROLAND et al., 1975, 1977

[a] 4′-Phosphopantetheine

VIII. Polymyxins

Polymyxins, colistins, and circulins are a group of antibiotic peptides with a cyclic structure and a linear side chain produced by *Bacillus polymyxa* and

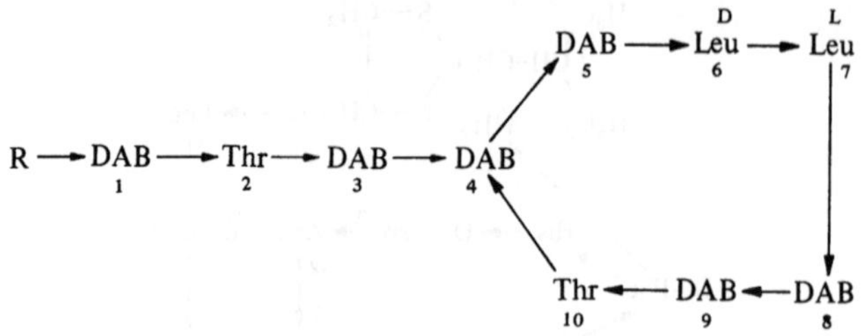

Polymyxin E_1 : R=6–Methyloctanoic acid (MOA)

Polymyxin E_2 : R=Isooctanoic acid (IOA)

DAB: 2,4–Diaminobutyric acid

Polymyxin B:	Residue 6	D–Phe
Polymyxin D:	Residue 3	L–Ser
Circulin A :	Residue 7	L–Ile

Fig. 11. Structure of polymyxins

some other microorganisms. The feature of the structure is the presence of a number of diaminobutyric acid residues and N^{α}-6-methyloctanoyl (or isooctanoyl)-α, γ-diaminobutyric acid (MOA-DAB or IOA-DAB) at the N-terminus of the peptides as shown in Figure 11. A number of studies on biogenesis of polymyxins (Daniels, 1968; Ito et al., 1970a; Monreal and Paulus, 1970; Paulus and Gray, 1964) have been carried out, but no cell-free enzyme system that can synthesize polymyxins or intermediary peptides has been found. Jayaraman et al. (1969) and Paulus (1975) partially purified a DAB-activating enzyme, present in both soluble and particulate-bound state in a polymyxin-producing organism, *B. polymyxa* strain Pfizer 2459. The enzyme was absent in mutants which lost the ability to produce polymyxin. Ito et al. (1970b) reported that the addition of MOA-DAB or IOA-DAB together with the unlabeled substrate amino acids enhanced about three-fold the incorporation of L-^{14}C-threonine into colistins (polymyxin E) by a soluble fraction obtained from *Bacillus colistinus* Koyama. However, no control in which only MOA-DAB or IOA-DAB was omitted from the complete reaction system was run; thus the role of the acyl-DAB in polymyxin synthesis is obscure.

Komura and Kurahashi (1973) partially purified a DAB-activating enzyme (about 23-fold) from crude extracts of *Aerobacillus polyaerogenes* which produces polymyxin E_1 and E_2. The enzyme protein binds DAB, leucine, and threonine as an acid stable form in a molar ratio of 3:1:1.4. They are released by a mild alkali or mercuric acetate treatment, indicating that they are bound to the enzyme as thioesters. The enzyme activity appears at the late logarithmic phase of growth, just prior to the accumulation of polymyxin and reaches the highest level at the beginning of the stationary phase. The activity disappears rapidly thereafter. They tried to synthesize polymyxin by incubating crude extracts, ATP, ^{14}C-DAB, and other unlabeled amino acids together with IOA-

DAB without success. From the finding that the formylation of valine takes place on the valine-activating subunit of gramicidin A synthetase, a mechanism of acylation of DAB on the DAB-activating enzyme should be taken into consideration for further studies on the total synthesis of polymyxin.

IX. Valinomycin

Valinomycin is a cyclododecadepsipeptide produced by certain strains of *Streptomyces* with thrice-repeating sequence of L-lactyl-valyl-D-α-hydroxyisovaleryl-D-valyl as shown in Figure 12. McDonald and Slater (1968) showed that D-α-hydroxyisovaleric acid (D-Hov) and valine were incorporated into valinomycin by whole cells. Ristow et al. (1974) reported that labeled valine, alanine, and threonine were incorporated into valinomycin by a growing culture of *S. fulvissimus*. They prepared an enzyme fraction by Sephadex G-200 gel filtration and DEAE-cellulose column chromatography that activated only L-valine and to a much lesser extent threonine. No activating activities of L- and D-Hov and L-lactic acid were detected. By incubating this enzyme preparation with ATP, L-^{14}C-valine, L-threonine, NAD, and pyridoxalphosphate they obtained a compound which had characteristic properties of valinomycin.

Anke and Lipmann (1977), however, obtained an enzyme fraction(s) that activated D-Hov and L-lactic acid from valinomycin-producing *Streptomyces* sp. (ATCC 23836). They failed to synthesize the antibiotic by cell lysates, but observed that L-lactic acid, rather than L-alanine, was a direct precursor of L-lactyl residues of valinomycin in resting cells. At present there is not enough information for predicting the mechanism of the total synthesis of valinomycin; where the chain initiates or how and what depsipeptide units join together to form the cyclic peptide.

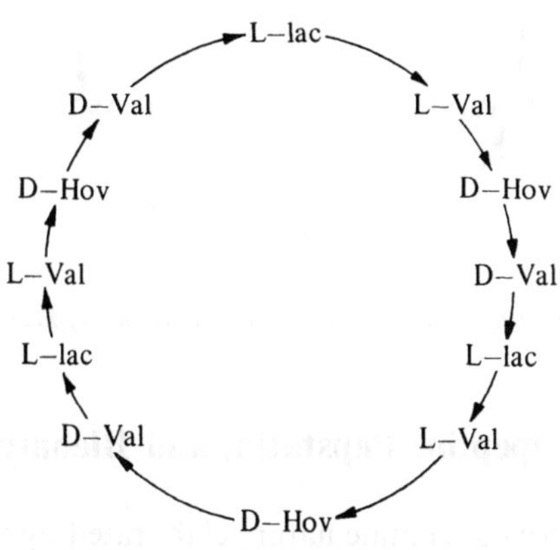

Fig. 12. Structure of valinomycin. Hov, α-hydroxyisovaleric acid; lac, lactic acid

X. Enniatin B

The results of work of ZOCHER and KLEINKAUF (1978) and ZOCHER et al. (1976) on the biosynthesis of enniatin B, a lower analog of valinomycin, are clearer than those on valinomycin. Enniatin B (Fig. 13) is produced by various strains of *Fusarium*. ZOCHER and KLEINKAUF (1978) purified about 50-fold enniatin B synthetase from crude extracts of *Fusarium oxysporum* ETC 1536/9. In contrast to valinomycin synthetase, this purified enzyme exhibited the activating activity of D-Hov in addition to that of L-valine. The enzyme binds valine and D-Hov in an acid stable form, that can be released by an alkali or performic acid treatment, indicating that they are thioesterified to the enzyme. As shown in Figure 13, the amino acid in enniatin B is not valine, but N-methyl-L-valine. They demonstrated that the addition of S-adenosylmethionine was essential for the synthesis of the peptide. N-Methylvaline could not serve as a precursor and the incubation of the enzyme with L-^{14}C-valine and ATP in the presence of S-adenosylmethionine produced exclusively N-methyl-^{14}C-valine thioesterified to the enzyme. From these results they suggest that the methylation occurs after activation of valine and before the subsequent peptide bond formation between the thioester-bound D-Hov and N-methylvaline takes place. The analogy between the formylation of the enzyme-bound valine in linear gramicidin synthesis as described in Section IV and the methylation step in enniatin B biosynthesis should be noted. Since the formation of the enzyme-bound formylvaline initiates the chain elongation in gramicidin A, I suggest that the ester rather than the peptide bond formation takes place after methylation of the enzyme-bound valine. Whether 4′-phosphopantetheine is involved in the ester and peptide bond formation has to be solved.

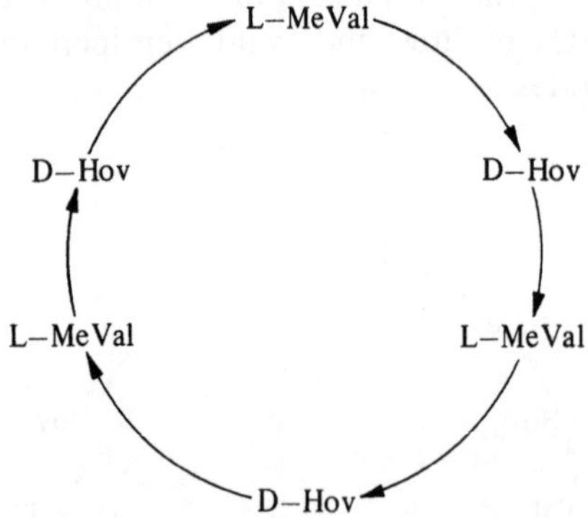

Fig. 13. Structure of enniatin B. Hov, α-hydroxyisovaleric acid; MeVal, N-methylvaline

XI. Leupeptin, Pepstatin, and Bleomycin

Many enzyme inhibitors of peptide nature elaborated by various microorganisms have been isolated and studied extensively by UMEZAWA and his associates

Acetyl or propionyl – L – Leu ⟶ L – Leu ⟶ Arginal

Fig. 14. Structure of leupeptins

(AOYAGI and UMEZAWA, 1975; UMEZAWA, 1977). Most of them have no antimicrobial activity, but they can be regarded as microbial secondary metabolites (UMEZAWA, 1977). The biosynthetic mechanism of leupeptin among them has been partially clarified by the use of a cell-free enzyme system. Leupeptin (Fig. 14) exhibits a strong inhibitory effect on plasmin, trypsin, papain, and cathepsin B. HORI et al. (1978) prepared crude extracts from the leupeptin-producing organism, *Streptomyces roseus* MA839-Al and studied the efficiency of the incorporation of labeled arginine into leupeptin acid in the presence of acetate and leucine, acetylleucine and leucine, and acetylleucylleucine. The incorporation of arginine was the highest in the presence of acetylleucylleucine, indicating that the acetyldipeptide was the direct precursor of leupeptin acid. It was also shown that free acetylleucylleucine was synthesized in a reaction mixture of acetylleucine, ^{3}H-leucine, ATP, and an 80-fold purified enzyme (SUZUKAKE et al., 1978). These results in principle agree with the biosynthetic mechanism of glutathione or ophthalmic acid, in which free dipeptides are synthesized as intermediates and serve as precursors of the tripeptides (MEISTER, 1974). In gramicidin S synthesis by the multienzyme thiotemplate mechanism, it was shown that the intermediary tripeptide, D-Phe-Pro-Val, released from the enzyme prematurely did not serve as a precursor for gramicidin S synthesis (TOMINO and KURAHASHI, 1964), indicating that it could not be reactivated and thioesterified to the synthetase.

In connection with the above findings, the synthesis of pepstatin A (Fig. 15) is interesting. It is an acylpentapeptide produced by *Streptomyces testaceus* Hamada et Okami A-536 and inhibits the action of pepsin, cathepsin D, and renin. No cell-free enzyme studies have been made. Biogenetic studies showed that L-leucine and malonate were incorporated into the 4-amino-3-hydroxy-6-methylheptanoic acid (AHMHA) residues of the peptide (MORISHIMA et al., 1974). Labeled AHMHA was not incorporated into pepstatin by whole cells. MORISHIMA et al. (1974) postulate that AHMHA may be formed from leucine and malonic acid in the process of peptide synthesis. However, the permeability barrier has to be circumvented in order to make the proposal conclusive.

IVA ⟶ L – Val ⟶ L – Val ⟶ AHMHA ⟶ L – Ala ⟶ AHMHA

Fig. 15. Structure of pepstatin A. IVA, isovaleric acid; AHMHA, (3S,4S)-4-amino-3-hydroxy-6-methylheptanoic acid

If pepstatin is found to be synthesized by the multienzyme thiotemplate mechanism, the minimum length of peptides to be synthesized by such a mechanism would be tetra- or pentapeptides. The synthesis of malformin, a cyclic pentapeptide (Fig. 16) (BODANSZKY and STAHL, 1974), by a cell-free enzyme system was reported by YUKIOKA and WINNICK (1966). However, whether the activation of the constituent amino acids involves aminoacyl adenylates or aminoacyl phosphates is not known.

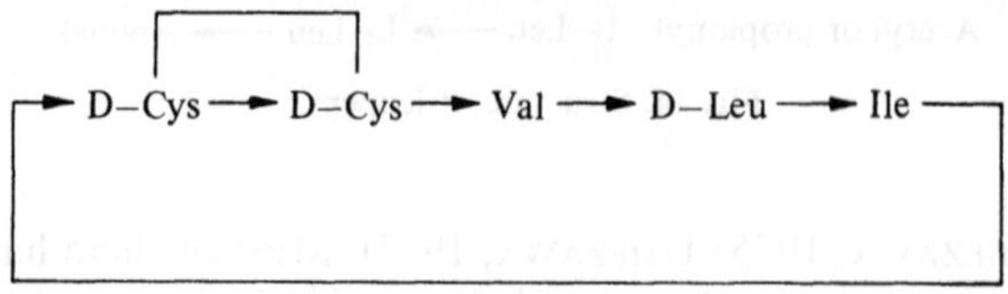

Fig. 16. Structure of malformin (BODANSZKY and STAHL, 1974)

Although biogenetic studies on bleomycin are very preliminary, the recent findings by UMEZAWA and his associates are briefly noted. Bleomycin, an antitumor agent, which causes a scission of single-stranded DNAs (UMEZAWA, 1977) is a glycopeptide antibiotic produced by *Streptomyces verticillus*. The recently revised structure (TAKITA et al., 1978) is shown in Figure 17.

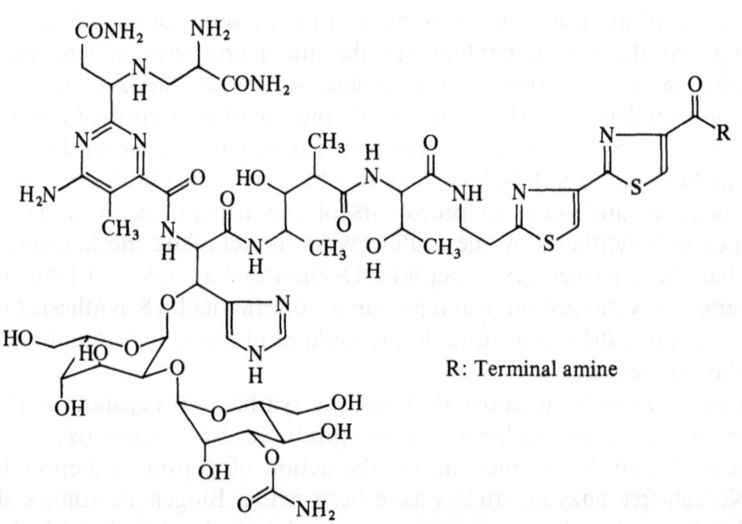

Fig. 17. Structure of bleomycin (TAKITA et al., 1978). (Reproduced with permission of H. UMEZAWA)

NAKATANI, FUJII, and UMEZAWA recently isolated intermediary peptides of various lengths with the N-terminal demethylblaminopyrimidyl residue and postulated that the synthesis of the peptide part of bleomycin might be catalyzed by a multienzyme complex (H. UMEZAWA, personal communication). They observed that the methylation of the demethylblaminopyrimidyl residue took place when the chain was elongated up to the stage of demethylblaminopyrimidyl-histidyl-(4-amino-3-hydroxy-2-methylpentanoyl)-threonine. They also noted that the β-hydroxyhistidine moiety of bleomycin was produced by oxidation of the histidine residue after completion of the peptide chain and prior to the addition of the C-terminal amines. Elucidation of the whole biosynthetic process of bleomycin with such a complicated structure that must involve not only the peptide bond formation catalyzed by multienzyme synthetase but also various modifications of intermediary peptides is a challenging problem. UMEZAWA considers that the production of many of the secondary metabolites is governed by genetic units of plasmid nature (UMEZAWA, 1977; UMEZAWA et al., 1978).

XII. Nisin and Subtilin

Nisin and subtilin are larger antibiotic peptides than those so far discussed. The former with 34 amino acid residues is produced by some strains of *Streptococcus lactis* and the latter with 32 amino acid residues by a particular strain of *Bacillus subtilis*. Despite the difference in taxonomy between the producing organisms, both antibiotics have a strikingly similar structure as revealed by GROSS et al. (1973) (Figs. 18 and 19). Both contain α,β-unsaturated amino acid residues, and lanthionine and β-methyllanthionine, which introduce cyclic structures to the molecules.

No attempts have been made to synthesize these peptides by a cell-free enzyme system, but HURST (1966) reported that nisin synthesis in growing cells was inhibited by chloramphenicol, puromycin, and actinomycin D, indicating the participation of the mRNA-ribosome system. INGRAM (1970) came to the same conclusion by incorporation studies of labeled cysteine into lanthionine moieties of nisin. The incorporation of cysteine by a *S. lactis* suspension was inhibited about 63% with 50 μg/ml chloramphenicol. HURST and PATERSON

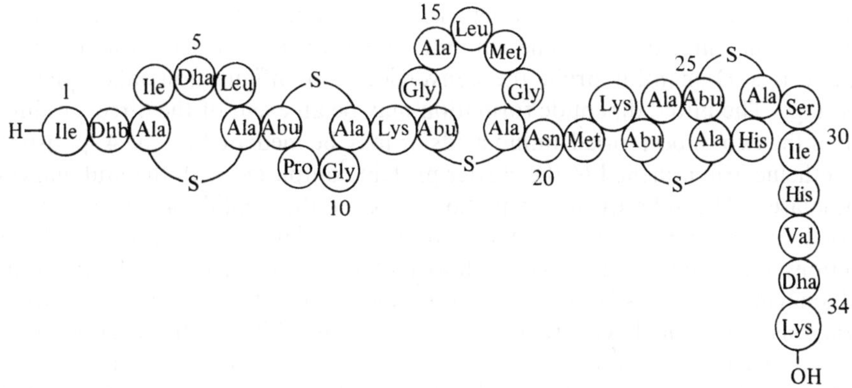

Fig. 18. Structure of nisin (GROSS et al., 1973). Abu, 2-aminobutyric acid; Dha, dehydroalanine; Dhb, dehydrobutyrine. (Reproduced with permission of E. GROSS)

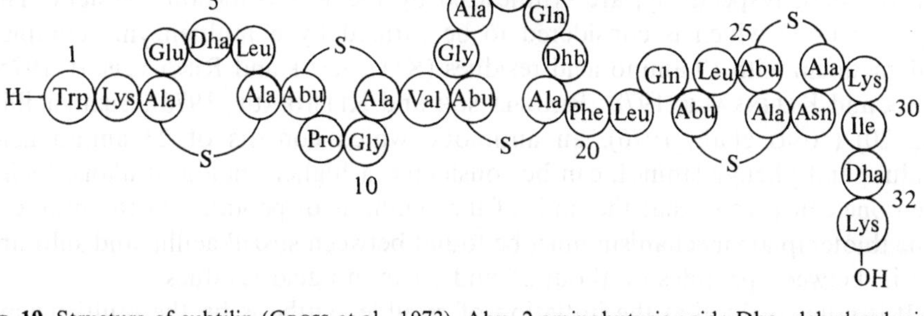

Fig. 19. Structure of subtilin (GROSS et al., 1973). Abu, 2-aminobutyric acid; Dha, dehydroalanine; Dhb, dehydrobutyrine. (Reproduced with permission of E. GROSS)

(1971) showed some evidence that there might be an inactive form of a precursor protein of nisin in a nisin-nonproducing mutant strain.

Biogenesis of subtilin by growing cells of *Bacillus subtilis* ATCC 6633 was found to be inhibited 80 to 90% by the addition of 10 µg/ml culture of chloramphenicol, puromycin and actinomycin D (C. NISHIO and K. KURAHASHI, unpublished results). The cell lysates contained basic proteins in which the presence of dehydroalanine was detected by its conversion to pyruvate in acid hydrolysis. Both nisin and subtilin, thus, seem to be derived from larger precursor peptides which are synthesized by the RNA-ribosome system. The formation of α,β-unsaturated amino acid residues, lanthionine, and methyllanthionine must be post-translational events.

XIII. Conclusions

It is now well established that medium-sized antibiotic peptides and depsipeptides are synthesized by the multienzyme thiotemplate mechanism. The substrate amino acids of antibiotic synthesis are activated as aminoacyl adenylates and bound to each subunit of the synthetases. Each aminoacyl group is then transferred to the thiol on the same subunit. When an amino acid residue in the peptide is a D-enantiomorph, the conversion of configuration takes place at this stage. The initial dipeptide formation may be an event of the direct conjugation of the two thioesterified amino acids or may be mediated by the 4′-phosphopantetheine arm attached to the carrier protein complexed with the multienzyme synthetases. The subsequent elongation steps of the peptide are shown to be carried out by repetition of alternative transthiolation and transpeptidation reactions mediated by the 4′-phosphopantetheine arm. The specificity of the multienzyme templates is not so strict as that of the RNA templates. Various analogous amino acids can replace each other, resulting in the production of a broad spectrum of antibiotic analogs by one organism under a variety of growth conditions. The sequence of amino acids in peptides is determined by the spatial arrangement of the active thiols on the multienzyme synthetases.

How prevalent this kind of mechanism is in nature is an interesting question, because there must be a limit in the size of multienzymes capable of carrying out such reactions. Nisin and subtilin, antibiotic peptides with 34 and 32 amino acid residues, respectively, are synthesized by the RNA-ribosome system. The largest peptide which is considered to be formed by a multienzyme complex is alamethicin with 19 amino acid residues (KLEINKAUF and RINDFLEISCH, 1975; MOHR and KLEINKAUF, 1978; RINDFLEISCH and KLEINKAUF, 1976). Suzukacillin (Fig. 20) (JUNG et al., 1976), an antibiotic which consists of 23 amino acid residues and phenylalaninol, can be considered a higher analog of alamethicin. Then one can predict that the limit of the synthesis of peptides by the multienzyme thiotemplate mechanism must be found between suszukacillin and subtilin, that is, between peptides of about 25 and 30 amino acid residues.

It is noteworthy that the initiation of peptide synthesis by the multienzyme thiotemplate mechanism starts with either unnatural amino acids such as D-

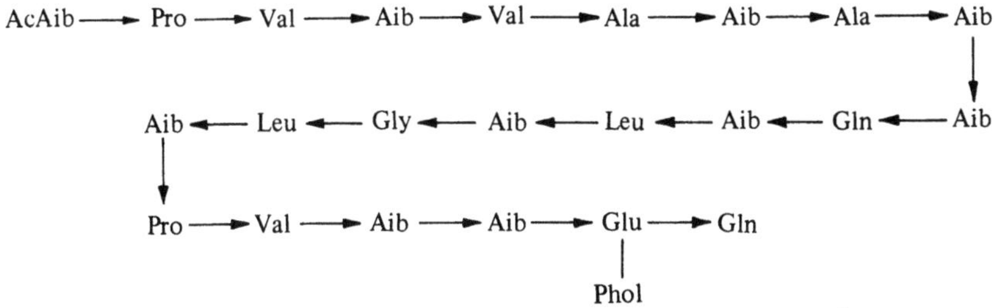

Fig. 20. Structure of suzukacillin (JUNG et al., 1976). Aib, aminoisobutyric acid; AcAib, N-acetylisobutyric acid; Phol, phenylalaninol

phenylalanine or β-tyrosine, acylated amino acids, or a dipeptide with a thiazoline ring.

A cyclic tridecapeptide, mycobacillin (Fig. 21), was proposed to be synthesized in a different manner than the multienzyme thiotemplate mechanism by SENGUPTA and BOSE (1972, 1974). An ammonium sulfate fraction obtained from the mycobacillin-producing organism, *Bacillus subtilis* B_3, contained ATP-P_i exchange activity dependent on proline. They isolated prolyl-peptides of various lengths which they considered as intermediates in the synthesis of the antibiotic. However, their enzyme preparation was also shown to catalyze a proline dependent ATP-PP_i exchange (BANERJEE and BOSE, 1968). We have to wait for the purification of the enzyme before coming to any conclusion on the mechanism of mycobacillin synthesis.

Biosynthesis of other peptide antibiotics such as serratamolide, sporidesmolide, pyridomycin, etamycin, and glyotoxin or other diketopiperazines are not discussed here, because little progress has been made in the pursuit of cell-free systems or in understanding their biosynthetic mechanisms since the subject was reviewed in 1974 (KURAHASHI, 1974).

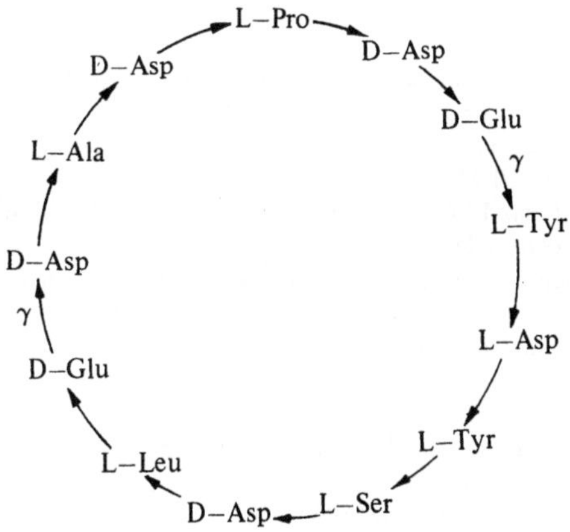

Fig. 21. Structure of mycobacillin

Acknowledgment. I am grateful to Drs. H. UMEZAWA, K. SHIMURA, S.G. LALAND, and H. KLEINKAUF who made unpublished manuscripts and results available.

References

Akashi K (1977) Biosynthesis of gramicidin A by a cell-free enzyme system of *Bacillus brevis* ATCC 8185. Thesis, Faculty of Science, Osaka University

Akashi K, Kurahashi K (1977) Formylation of enzyme-bound valine and stepwise elongation of intermediate peptides of gramicidin A by a cell-free enzyme system. Biochem Biophys Res Commun 77:259–267

Akashi K, Kurahashi K (1978) Enzyme-bound formylvaline and formylvalylglycine; an initiation complex for gramicidin A biosynthesis. J Biochem 83:1219–1229

Akashi K, Kubota K, Kurahashi K (1977) Biosynthesis of enzyme-bound formylvaline and formylvalylglycine. A possible initiation complex for gramicidin A biosynthesis. J Biochem 81:269–272

Akers HA, Lee SG, Lipmann F (1977) Identification of two enzymes responsible for the synthesis of the initial portion of linear gramicidin. Biochemistry 16:5722–5729

Altmann M, Koischwitz H, Salnikow J, Kleinkauf H (1978) (3,3′-Leu)-Gramicidin S formation by gramicidin S synthetase. FEBS Lett 93:247–250

Anke T, Lipmann F (1977) Studies on the biosynthesis of valinomycin. FEBS Lett 82:337–340

Aoyagi T, Umezawa H (1975) Structures and activities of protease inhibitors of microbial origin. In: Reich E, Rifkin DB, Shaw E (eds) Proteases and biological control, pp 429–454. Cold Spring Harbor Laboratory, Cold Spring Harbor

Asselineau J, Zalta J-P (1973) Les antibiotique, pp 103–173. Hermann, Paris

Banerjee AB, Bose SK (1968) Biosynthesis of mycobacillin, an antifungal peptide: Part III – Incorporation of constituent D-amino acids. Indian J Biochem 5:35–36

Bauer K, Roskoski R Jr, Kleinkauf H, Lipmann F (1972) Synthesis of a linear gramicidin by a combination of biosynthetic and organic methods. Biochemistry 11:3266–3271

Berg TL, Frøholm LO, Laland SG (1965) The biosynthesis of gramicidin S in a cell-free system. Biochem J 96:43–53

Bhagavan NV, Rao PM, Pollard LW, Rao RK, Winnick T, Hall JB (1966) The biosynthesis of gramicidin S. A restudy. Biochemistry 5:3844–3850

Bodanszky M, Stahl GL (1974) The structure and synthesis of malformin A. Proc Natl Acad Sci USA 71:2791–2794

Christiansen C, Aarstad K, Zimmer TL, Laland SG (1977) A rapid method for the preparation of pure heavy enzyme of gramicidin S synthetase. FEBS Lett 81:121–124

Daniels MJ (1968) Studies of the biosynthesis of polymyxin B. Biochim Biophys Acta 156:119–127

Frøyshov Ø (1974) Bacitracin biosynthesis by three complementary fractions from *Bacillus licheniformis*. FEBS Lett 44:75–78

Frøyshov Ø (1975) Enzyme-bound intermediates in the biosynthesis of bacitracin. Eur J Biochem 59:201–206

Frøyshov Ø, Laland SG (1974) On the biosynthesis of bacitracin by a soluble enzyme complex from *Bacillus licheniformis*. Eur J Biochem 46:235–242

Frøyshov Ø, Zimmer TL, Laland SG (1970) The nature of the enzyme bound intermediates in gramicidin S biosynthesis. FEBS Lett 7:68–71

Frøyshov Ø, Zimmer TL, Laland SG (1978) Biosynthesis of microbial peptides by the thiotemplate mechanism. Int Rev Biochem 18:49–78

Fujikawa K, Suzuki T, Kurahashi K (1966) Incorporation of L-leucine-C^{14} into tyrocidine by a cell-free preparation of *Bacillus brevis* Dubos strain. J Biochem 60:216–218

Fujikawa K, Sakamoto Y, Suzuki T, Kurahashi K (1968a) Biosynthesis of tyrocidine by a cell-free enzyme system of *Bacillus brevis* ATCC 8185. II. Amino acid substitution in tyrocidine. Biochim Biophys Acta 169:520–533

Fujikawa K, Suzuki T, Kurahashi K (1968b) Biosynthesis of tyrocidine by a cell-free enzyme system of *Bacillus brevis* ATCC 8185. I. Preparation of partially purified enzyme system and its properties. Biochim Biophys Acta 161:232–246

Fujikawa K, Sakamoto Y, Kurahashi K (1971) Biosynthesis of tyrocidine by a cell-free enzyme system of *Bacillus brevis* ATCC 8185. III. Further purification of Components I and II and their functions in tyrocidine synthesis. J Biochem 69:869–879

Gevers W, Kleinkauf H, Lipmann F (1968) The activation of amino acids for biosynthesis of gramicidin S. Proc Natl Acad Sci USA 60:269–276

Gevers W, Kleinkauf H, Lipmann F (1969) Peptidyl transfers in gramicidin S biosynthesis from enzyme-bound thioester intermediates. Proc Natl Acad Sci USA 63:1335–1342

Gilhuus-Moe CC, Kristensen T, Bredesen JE, Zimmer T-L, Laland SG (1970) The presence and possible role of phosphopantothenic acid in gramicidin S synthetase. FEBS Lett 7:287–290

Gross E, Kiltz HH, Nebelin E (1973) Subtilin, IV. Die Struktur des Subtilins. Hoppe-Seylers Z Physiol Chem 354:810–812

Holm H, Frøholm LO, Laland S (1966) Isolation of a peptide conjugate with the sequence Phe-Pro-Val-Orn from a cell-free system producing gramicidin S. Biochim Biophys Acta 115:361–370

Hori K, Kurotsu T, Kanda M, Miura S, Nozoe A, Saito Y (1978) Studies on gramicidin S synthetase. Purification of the heavy enzyme obtained from some mutants of *Bacillus brevis*. J Biochem 84:425–434

Hori M, Hemmi H, Suzukake K, Hayashi H, Uehara Y, Takeuchi T, Umezawa H (1978) Biosynthesis of leupeptin. J Antibiot 31:95–98

Hurst A (1966) Biosynthesis of the antibiotic nisin by whole *Streptococcus lactis* organisms. J Gen Microbiol 44:209–220

Hurst A, Paterson GM (1971) Observations on the conversion of an inactive precursor protein to the antibiotic nisin. Can J Microbiol 17:1379–1384

Ingram L (1970) A ribosomal mechanism for synthesis of peptides related to nisin. Biochim Biophys Acta 224:263–265

Ishihara H, Shimura K (1974) Biosynthesis of bacitracin. III. Partial purification of a bacitracin-synthesizing enzyme from *Bacillus licheniformis*. Biochim Biophys Acta 338:588–600

Ishihara H, Sasaki T, Shimura K (1968) Biosynthesis of bacitracin. II. Incorporation of ^{14}C-labeled amino acids into bacitracin by a cell-free preparation from *Bacillus licheniformis*. Biochim Biophys Acta 166:496–504

Ishihara H, Endo Y, Abe S, Shimura K (1975) The presence of 4′-phosphopantetheine in the bacitracin synthetase. FEBS Lett 50:43–46

Ito M, Aida K, Uemura T (1970a) Biosynthesis of colistin by *Bacillus colistinus* Koyama. Biochim Biophys Acta 213:244–247

Ito M, Koyama Y, Aida K, Uemura T (1970b) Biosynthesis of colistin by a cell-free system *Bacillus colistinus* Koyama. Biochim Biophys Acta 215:418–420

Itoh H, Yamada M, Tomino S, Kurahashi K (1968) The role of two complementary fractions of gramicidin S synthesizing enzyme system. J Biochem 64:259–261

Iwaki M, Shimura K, Kanda M, Kaji E, Saito Y (1972) Some mutants of *Bacillus brevis* deficient in gramicidin S formation. Biochem Biophys Res Commun 48:113–118

Jayaraman K, Monreal J, Paulus H (1969) L-α,γ-Diaminobutyrate-activating enzyme from *Bacillus polymyxa*. Properties and distribution. Biochim Biophys Acta 185:447–457

Johne S, Gröger D (1977) Naturstoffe mit Diketopiperazinstruktur. Pharmazie 32:1–16

Jung G, König WA, Leibfritz D, Ooka T, Janko K, Boheim G (1976) Structural and membrane modifying properties of suzukacillin, a peptide antibiotic related to alamethicin. Part A. Sequence and conformation. Biochim Biophys Acta 433:164–181

Kambe M, Sakamoto Y, Kurahashi K (1971) Biosynthesis of tyrocidine by a cell-free enzyme system of *Bacillus brevis* ATCC 8185. IV. Further separation of Component II into two fractions. J Biochem 69:1131–1133

Kambe M, Imae Y, Kurahashi K (1974) Biochemical studies on gramicidin S non-producing mutants of *Bacillus brevis* ATCC 9999. J Biochem 75:481–493

Kanda M, Hori K, Kurotsu T, Miura S, Nozoe A, Saito Y (1978) Studies on gramicidin S synthetase. Purification and properties of the light enzyme obtained from some mutants of *Bacillus brevis*. J Biochem 84:435–441

Katz E, Demain AL (1977) The peptide antibiotics of *Bacillus*: chemistry, biogenesis, and possible functions. Bacteriol Rev 41:449–474

Kleinkauf H (1979) Antibiotic polypeptides – biosynthesis on multifunctional protein templates. Planta Med 34:1–18

Kleinkauf H, Gevers W (1969) Nonribosomal polypeptide synthesis: the biosynthesis of a cyclic peptide antibiotic, gramicidin S. Cold Spring Harbor Symp Quant Biol 34:805–813

Kleinkauf H, Koischwitz H (1978) Peptide bond formation in non-ribosomal systems. Prog Mol Subcell Biol 6:59–112

Kleinkauf H, Koischwitz H (1980) Gramicidin S-synthetase. In: Bisswanger H, Schmincke-Ott E (eds) Multifunctional proteins. John Wiley & Sons, New York, pp 217–233
Kleinkauf H, Rindfleisch H (1975) Non-ribosomal biosynthesis of the cyclic octadecapeptide alamethicin. Acta Microbiol Acad Sci Hung 22:411–418
Kleinkauf H, Gevers W, Lipmann F (1969) Interrelation between activation and polymerization in gramicidin S biosynthesis. Proc Natl Acad Sci USA 62:226–233
Kleinkauf H, Gevers W, Roskoski R Jr, Lipmann F (1970) Enzyme-bound phosphopantetheine in tyrocidine biosynthesis. Biochem Biophys Res Commun 41:1218–1222
Kleinkauf H, Roskoski R Jr, Lipmann F (1971) Pantetheine-linked peptide intermediates in gramicidin S and tyrocidine biosynthesis. Proc Natl Acad Sci USA 68:2069–2072
Koischwitz H, Kleinkauf H (1976a) Gramicidin S-synthetase. Preparation of the multienzymic complex with a high specific activity. Biochim Biophys Acta 429:1041–1051
Koischwitz H, Kleinkauf H (1976b) Gramicidin S-synthetase. Electrophoretic characterization of the multienzyme. Biochim Biophys Acta 429:1052–1061
Komura S, Kurahashi K (1973) Biosynthesis of polymyxin E – L-2,4-diaminobutyric acid activating enzyme. Seikagaku 45:484
Kurahashi K (1961) Enzymatic combination of L-phenylalanine with L-proline. Abstr 5th Int Congr Biochem, Moscow, p 37
Kurahashi K (1974) Biosynthesis of small peptides. Annu Rev Biochem 43:445–459
Kurahashi K, Yamada M, Mori K, Fujikawa K, Kambe M, Imae Y, Sato E, Takahashi H, Sakamoto Y (1969) Biosynthesis of cyclic oligopeptide. Cold Spring Harbor Symp Quant Biol 34:815–826
Kurylo-Borowska Z (1975) Biosynthesis of edeine: II. Localization of edeine synthetase within *Bacillus brevis* Vm4. Biochim Biophys Acta 399:31–41
Kurylo-Borowska Z, Abramsky T (1972) Biosynthesis of β-tyrosine. Biochim Biophys Acta 264:1–10
Kurylo-Borowska Z, Kieras J (1976) On the structure of edeine synthetase. Abstr 10th Int Congr Biochem, Hamburg, p 181
Kurylo-Borowska Z, Sedkowska J (1974) Biosynthesis of edeine. Fractionation and characterization of enzymes responsible for biosynthesis of edeine A and B. Biochim Biophys Acta 351:42–56
Kurylo-Borowska Z, Tatum EL (1966) Biosynthesis of edeine by *Bacillus brevis* Vm4 in vivo and in vitro. Biochim Biophys Acta 114:206–209
Laland SG, Zimmer T-L (1973) The protein thiotemplate mechanism of synthesis for the peptide antibiotics produced by *Bacillus brevis*. In: Campbell PN, Greville GD (eds) Essays in biochemistry, vol IX, pp 31–57. Academic Press, London New York
Laland SG, Frøyshov Ø, Gilhuus-Moe C, Zimmer TL (1972) Gramicidin S synthetase, an enzyme with an unusually large number of catalytic functions. Nature New Biol 239:43–44
Lee SG (1976) On the mechanism of racemization of thioester-linked L-phenylalanine by an enzyme participating in tyrocidine biosynthesis. Abstr 10th Int Congr Biochem, Hamburg, p 181
Lee SG, Lipmann F (1974) Isolation of a peptidyl-pantetheine-protein from tyrocidine-synthesizing polyenzymes. Proc Natl Acad Sci USA 71:607–611
Lee SG, Lipmann F (1975) Tyrocidine synthetase system. In: Hash JH (ed) Methods in enzymology, vol 43, pp 585–602. Academic Press, London New York
Lee SG, Lipmann F (1977) Isolation of amino acid activating subunit – pantetheine protein complexes: their role in chain elongation in tyrocidine synthesis. Proc Natl Acad Sci USA 74:2343–2347
Lee SG, Roskoski R Jr, Bauer K, Lipmann F (1973) Purification of the polyenzymes responsible for tyrocidine synthesis and their dissociation into subunits. Biochemistry 12:398–405
Leung DC, Baxter RM (1972) Substrate-derived reversible and irreversible inhibitors of the multienzyme I of gramicidin S biosynthesis. Biochim Biophys Acta 279:34–47
Lipmann F (1971) Attempts to map a process evolution of peptide biosynthesis. Science 173:875–884
Lipmann F (1973) Nonribosomal polypeptide synthesis on polyenzyme templates. Acc Chem Res 6:361–367
Lipmann F, Gevers W, Kleinkauf H, Roskoski R Jr (1971) Polypeptide synthesis on protein templates: The enzymatic synthesis of gramicidin S and tyrocidine. Adv Enzymol 35:1–34
Ljones T, Vaage O, Zimmer TL, Frøholm LO, Laland SG (1968) The presence of protein bound intermediates in the biosynthesis of gramicidin S. FEBS Lett 1:339–342
MacDonald JC, Slater GP (1968) Biosynthesis of valinomycin. Can J Biochem 46:573–578
Mach B, Tatum EL (1964) Environmental control of amino acid substitutions in the biosynthesis of the antibiotic polypeptide tyrocidine. Proc Natl Acad Sci USA 52:876–884

Maier W, Gröger D (1972) Biosynthese der Peptidantibiotica. Pharmazie 27:491–505
Martin DR, Williams RJP (1976) Chemical nature and sequence of alamethicin. Biochem J 153:181–190
Meister A (1974) Glutathione synthesis. In: Boyer PD (ed) The enzymes, vol X, pp 671–697. Academic Press, London New York
Mohr H, Kleinkauf H (1978) Alamethicin biosynthesis. Acetylation of the amino terminus and attachment of phenylalaninol. Biochim Biophys Acta 526:375–386
Monreal J, Paulus H (1970) Nonparticipation of transfer RNA in the biosynthesis of polymyxin B. Biochim Biophys Acta 199:280–282
Morishima H, Sawa T, Takita T, Aoyagi T, Takeuchi T, Umezawa H (1974) Biosynthetic studies on pepstatin. Biosynthesis of (3S, 4S)-4-amino-3-hydroxy-6-methylheptanoic acid moiety. J Antibiot 27:267–273
Pandey RC, Cook JC Jr, Rinehart KL Jr (1977) High resolution and field desorption mass spectrometry studies and revised structure of alamethicin I and II. J Am Chem Soc 99:8469–8483
Pass L, Zimmer TL, Laland SG (1974) On the use of affinity chromatography in demonstrating the transfer of thioester-bound D-phenylalanine from the light enzyme of gramicidin S synthetase to an acceptor site for this amino acid on the heavy enzyme. Eur J Biochem 47:607–611
Paulus H (1975) Polymyxin synthetase: L-2,4-diaminobutyrate activating enzyme. In: Hash JH (ed) Methods in enzymology, vol 43, pp 579–584. Academic Press, London New York
Paulus H, Gray E (1964) The biosynthesis of polymyxin B by growing cultures of *Bacillus polymyxa*. J Biol Chem 239:865–871
Payne JW, Jakes R, Hartley BS (1970) The primary structure of alamethicin. Biochem J 117:757–766
Perlman D, Bodanszky M (1971) Biosynthesis of peptide antibiotics. Annu Rev Biochem 40:449–464
Pfaender P, Specht D, Heinrich G, Schwarz E, Kuhnle E, Simlot MM (1973) Enzymes of *Bacillus licheniformis* in the biosynthesis of bacitracin A. FEBS Lett 32:100–104
Rao RK, Bhagavan NV, Rao KR, Hall JB (1968) Peptide synthesis in cell-free extracts of *Bacillus brevis* 8185. Biochemistry 7:3072–3077
Ressler C, Kashelikar DV (1966) Identification of asparaginyl and glutaminyl residues in *endo* position in peptides by dehydration-reduction. J Am Chem Soc 88:2025–2035
Rindfleisch H, Kleinkauf H (1976) Biosynthesis of alamethicin. FEBS Lett 62:276–280
Ristow H, Salnikow J, Kleinkauf H (1974) Biosynthesis of valinomycin. FEBS Lett 42:127–130
Roland I, Frøyshov Ø, Laland SG (1975) On the presence of pantothenic acid in the three complementary enzymes of bacitracin synthetase. FEBS Lett 60:305–308
Roland I, Frøyshov Ø, Laland SG (1977) A rapid method for the preparation of the three enzymes of bacitracin synthetase essentially free from other proteins. FEBS Lett 84:22–24
Roskoski R, Jr, Gevers W, Kleinkauf H, Lipmann F (1970a) Tyrocidine biosynthesis by three complementary fractions from *Bacillus brevis* (ATCC 8185). Biochemistry 9:4839–4845
Roskoski R, Jr, Kleinkauf H, Gevers W, Lipmann F (1970b) Isolation of enzyme-bound peptide intermediates in tryocidine biosynthesis. Biochemistry 9:4846–4851
Roskoski R, Jr, Ryan G, Kleinkauf H, Gevers W, Lipmann F (1971) Polypeptide biosynthesis from thioesters of amino acids. Arch Biochem Biophys 143:485–492
Saito Y, Otani S, Otani S (1970) Biosynthesis of gramicidin S. Adv Enzymol 33:337–380
Saxholm H, Zimmer TL, Laland SG (1972) The mechanism of the inhibition of gramicidin-S synthesis by D-leucine. Eur J Biochem 30:138–144
Sengupta S, Bose SK (1972) Peptides from a mycobacillin-synthesizing cell-free system. Biochem J 128:47–52
Sengupta S, Bose SK (1974) A proline-dependent ATP-$^{32}P_i$ exchange in *Bacillus subtilis* B_3 producing mycobacillin. Indian J Biochem 11:335–336
Stoll E, Frøyshov Ø, Holm H, Zimmer TL, Laland SG (1970) On the mechanism of gramicidin S formation from intermediate peptides. FEBS Lett 11:348–352
Suzukake K, Fujiyama T, Hori M, Umezawa H (1978) Purification and properties of leupeptin synthetase. Seikagaku 50:668
Takahashi H, Sato E, Kurahashi K (1971) Racemization of phenylalanine by adenosine triphosphate-dependent phenylalanine racemase of *Bacillus brevis* Nagano. J Biochem 69:973–976
Takita T, Muraoka Y, Nakatani T, Fujii A, Umezawa Y, Naganawa H, Umezawa H (1978) Chemistry of bleomycin. XIX Revised structures of bleomycin and phleomycin. J Antibiot 31:801–804

Tomino S, Kurahashi K (1964) Enzymic synthesis of D-phenylalanyl-L-prolyl-L-valine, a peptide sequence present in gramicidin S. Biochem Biophys Res Commun 17:288–293
Tomino S, Yamada M, Fujikawa K, Itoh H, Kurahashi K, Suzuki T (1967a) Biosyntheses of gramicidin S and tyrocidines by cell free enzyme systems. Abstr 7th Int Congr Biochem, Tokyo, p 583
Tomino S, Yamada M, Itoh H, Kurahashi K (1967b) Cell-free synthesis of gramicidin S. Biochemistry 6:2552–2560
Umezawa H (1977) Recent advances in bioactive microbial secondary metabolites. Jpn J Antibiot 30:Suppl S-138-S-163
Umezawa H, Okami Y, Hotta K (1978) Transfer of the leupeptin-producing ability of the strain, *Streptomyces roseus* MA839-Al, by conjugation. J Antibiot 31:99–102
Vater J, Kleinkauf H (1976) Gramicidin S-synthetase. A further characterization of phenylalanine racemase, the light enzyme of gramicidin S-synthetase. Biochim Biophys Acta 429:1062–1072
Yamada M, Kurahashi K (1968) Adenosine triphosphate and pyrophosphate dependent phenylalanine racemase of *Bacillus brevis* Nagano. J Biochem 63:59–69
Yamada M, Kurahashi K (1969) Further purification and properties of adenosine triphosphate-dependent phenylalanine racemase of *Bacillus brevis* Nagano. J Biochem 66:529–540
Yamada M, Tomino S, Kurahashi K (1964) Conversion of L-phenylalanine to D-phenylalanine by cell-free extracts of *Bacillus brevis*. J Biochem 56:616–618
Yukioka M, Winnick T (1966) Synthesis of malformin by an enzyme preparation from *Aspergillus niger*. J Bacteriol 91:2237–2244
Yukioka M, Tsukamoto Y, Saito Y, Tsuji T, Otani S, Otani S (1965) Biosynthesis of gramicidin S by a cell-free system of *Bacillus brevis*. Biochem Biophys Res Commun 19:204–208
Zimmer TL, Laland SG (1975) Gramicidin S synthetase. In: Hash JH (ed) Methods in enzymology, vol 43, pp 567–579. Academic Press, London New York
Zocher R, Kleinkauf H (1978) Biosynthesis of enniatin B: Partial purification and characterization of the synthesizing enzyme and studies of the biosynthesis. Biochem Biophys Res Commun 84:1162–1167
Zocher R, Salnikow J, Kleinkauf H (1976) Biosynthesis of enniatin B. FEBS Lett 71:13–17

Addendum

KOMURA and KURAHASHI (1979, 1980a, b) recently reported that the DAB-activating enzyme partially purified from crude extracts of *A. polyaerogenes* (KOMURA and KURAHASHI, 1973) catalyzed the synthesis of octanoyl-DAB thioesterified to the enzyme and also the total synthesis of polymyxin E.

SUZUKAKE et al. (1979, 1980) and HAYASHI et al. (1980) have succeeded in the total synthesis of leupeptin. The enzymes involved are leucine acylase, leupeptin acid synthetase and leupeptin acid reductase, and the reaction requires ATP, NADPH and magnesium ions in addition to acetyl CoA, L-leucine and L-arginine as substrates.

Hayashi H, Suzukake K, Hori M, Umezawa H (1980) Purification and properties of leupeptin acid reductase. Seikagaku 52:859
Komura S, Kurahashi K (1979) Partial purification and properties of L-2,4-diaminobutyric acid activating enzyme from a polymyxin E producing organism. J. Biochem. 86:1013–1021
Komura S, Kurahashi K (1980a) Biosynthesis of polymyxin E by a cellfree enzyme system. II. Synthesis of enzyme-bound octanoyldiaminobutyric acid. J. Biochem. 88:285–288
Komura S, Kurahashi K (1980b) Biosynthesis of polymyxin E. III. Total synthesis of polymyxin E by a cell-free enzyme system. Biochem. Biophys. Res. Commun. 95:1145–1151
Suzukake K, Fujiyama T, Hayashi H, Hori M, Umezawa H (1979) Biosynthesis of leupeptin. II. Purification and properties of leupeptin acid synthetase. J Antibiot 32:523–530
Suzukake K, Hayashi H, Hori M, Umezawa H (1980) Biosynthesis of leupeptin. III. Isolation and properties of an enzyme synthesizing acetyl-L-leucine. J Antibiot 33:857–862

Biosynthesis of the Nucleoside Antibiotics

ROBERT J. SUHADOLNIK

I. Introduction

About seventy naturally occurring nucleoside analogs have been isolated to date. As with the numerous other analog types that have been isolated from microorganisms, these nucleoside analogs have also been useful biochemical probes in the elucidation of the complex steps of RNA, DNA, protein, and cell wall synthesis as well as cytoplasmic, mitochondrial, and nuclear processes. The structures of the nucleoside analogs can be classified into five groups. One group is structurally similar to the purine nucleosides or nucleotides; a second group is structurally similar to the pyrimidine nucleosides; a third group is the pyridine nucleosides; a fourth group is the diazepine nucleosides; and the fifth group is the maleimide nucleosides.

There are 34 purine-like naturally occurring nucleoside analogs. They are: agrocin 84, 3′-amino-3′-deoxyadenosine, 2′-aminoguanosine, amipurimycin, antibiotic A201A, angustmycin A (decoyinine), angustmycin C (psicofuranine), ara-A, aristeromycin, bredinin, the clindamycin purine ribonucleotides, cordycepin (3′-deoxyadenosine), crotonoside (isoguanosine), eritadenine, formycin, herbicidins A and B, homocitrullylaminoadenosine, lysylaminoadenosine, nebularine, nucleocidin, O-glycosyl ribonucleosides, puromycin, pyrazofurin, raphanatin, sangivamycin, septacidin, sinefungin (antibiotic A9145), spongoadenosine, spongosine, thraustomycin, thuringiensin, toyocamycin, and tubercidin.

There are 26 pyrimidine-like naturally occurring nucleoside antibiotics. They are: anthelmycin (hikizimycin), ara-T, ara-U, 5-azacytidine, bamicetin, blasticidin S, blasticidin H, clindamycin pyrimidine ribonucleotides, 5,6-dihydro-5-azathymidine, ezomycins, gougerotin, ileumycin, l-methylpseudouridine, mildiomycin, minimycin (oxazinomycin), norplicacetin, the octosyl acids, oxamicetin, pentopyranines, platenocidin, plicacetin, polyoxins, spongothymidine, spongouridine, streptovirudins, and tunicamycin.

There are two naturally occurring nucleoside analogs with the pyridine aglycon (clitidine and nikkomycin), two with the diazepine ring (coformycin and deoxycoformycin) and one with the maleimide aglycon (showdomycin). The production, isolation, physical and chemical properties, structures, and biochemical properties of the above nucleoside antibiotics have been recently reviewed (SUHADOLNIK, 1979).

The biosynthesis of 21 of the naturally occurring nucleoside analogs has been reported. Although the carbon-nitrogen skeleton of the purine and pyrimidine-like nucleoside antibiotics requires all or part of the purine or pyrimidine rings, the carbon-linked ribonucleosides, which are classified as purine-like (i.e., formycin and pyrazofurin), pyrimidine-like (i.e., minimycin), and the maleimide nucleoside (showdomycin) use either two carbons of acetate or three carbons of glutamate for the biosynthesis of the aglycon.

This review on the biosynthesis of the above naturally occurring nucleoside antibiotics is subdivided into three parts. The first (Section II) describes the biosynthesis of the nucleoside analogs that utilize either the preformed adenine or guanine ring. Section III describes the biosynthesis of the nucleoside analogs that utilize either the preformed uracil, cytosine, or thymine ring. Section IV describes the biosynthesis of purine and pyrimidine-like analogs that utilize acetate or glutamate but do not depend on preformed adenine, guanine, uracil, cytosine, or thymine.

II. The Biosynthesis of the Nucleoside Analogs that Utilize either Adenine or Guanine

A. 3′-Amino-3′-deoxyadenosine

3′-Amino-3′-deoxyadenosine is found in the culture filtrates of *Helminthosporium*, *C. militaris*, and *A. nidulans*. It has antitumor activity and inhibits *Candida albicans* (SUHADOLNIK, 1970). 3′-Amino-3′-deoxy-5′-ATP is a strong inhibitor of RNA and DNA synthesis when added to cell-free extracts of Ehrlich ascites tumor cells (TRUMAN and KLENOW, 1968).

The biosynthesis of 3′-amino-3′-deoxyadenosine has been described by CHASSY and SUHADOLNIK (1969). [U-^{14}C]Adenosine is a direct precursor for 3′-amino-3′-deoxyadenosine (Fig. 1).

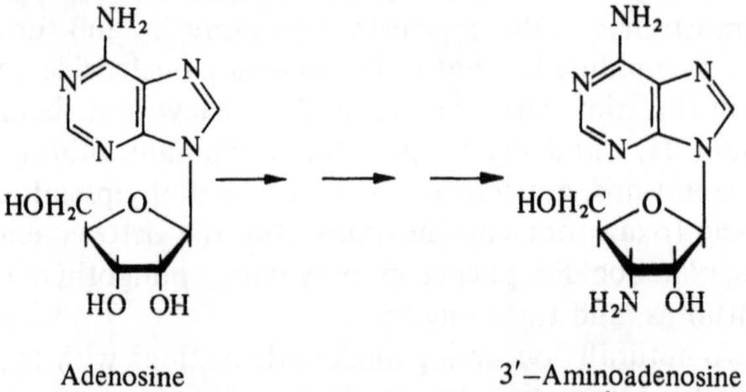

Fig. 1. Biosynthesis of 3′-aminoadenosine

B. Decoyinine and Psicofuranine

Decoyinine and psicofuranine are two naturally occurring ketohexose nucleoside antibiotics elaborated by *S. hygroscopicus* var. *decoyicus*. They inhibit bacte-

Glucose → Glucose-6-P → Fructose-P → Psicose-6-P

Hexose → Hexose-1-P → XDP-hexose → XDP-allose → Psicose-1-P

Fructose → Fructose-2-P → XDP-fructose → XDP-psicose → Psicose

Adenine + Psicose-6-P or Psicose-1-P or Psicose → Psicofuranine → Decoyinine

XDP = purine or pyrimidine nucleoside diphosphate

Fig. 2. Biosynthesis of psicofuranine and decoyinine

rial cells and Walker adenocarcinoma 256 in rats. Psicofuranine and decoyinine inhibit XMP aminase at the nucleoside level.

The biosynthesis of psicofuranine and decoyinine is shown in Figure 2. Adenine and glucose are the precursors for the adenine and D-psicose moieties of psicofuranine and decoyinine (SUGIMORI and SUHADOLNIK, 1965). [U-^{14}]-Psicofuranine is converted to [U-^{14}C]decoyinine by *S. hygroscopicus*; this reaction is also reversible. The biosynthesis of psicofuranine and decoyinine could conceivably occur as shown in Figure 2.

C. Ara-A

Ara-A (9-β-D-arabinofuranosyladenine) is isolated from the culture filtrates of *S. antibioticus* (Parke, Davis Laboratories, 1967). HUBERT-HABART and COHEN (1962) were the first to report on the effect of ara-A on bacteria. They reported that ara-A was very toxic to a purine-requiring strain of *E. coli.* DNA synthesis and, to a lesser extent, RNA synthesis were inhibited. Ara-A also has been used successfully in the treatment of herpes simplex encephalitis (WHITLEY et al., 1977). The reader is referred to reviews on ara-A by COHEN (1966, 1976), SUHADOLNIK (1970, 1979), and PAVAN-LANGSTON et al. (1975). Ara-A is incorporated into the internucleotide linkage (DOERING et al., 1966; MÜLLER et al., 1977; COZZARELLI et al., 1977; PLUNKETT and COHEN, 1975).

LIM and COHEN (1966) postulated that the biosynthesis of ara-A might proceed either by the condensation of D-arabinose-l-phosphate with adenine or D-arabinose-5-phosphate could form l-pyrophosphoryl-D-arabinose-5-phosphate and condense to form ara-AMP which would be dephosphorylated to form ara-A. Experimentally, FARMER and SUHADOLNIK (1972) and FARMER et al. (1973) reported that adenosine is directly converted to ara-A. These studies were accomplished in vivo with adenosine labeled with either ^{3}H, ^{14}C, or ^{15}N. More recently, WU and SUHADOLNIK (manuscript in preparation) have isolated and partially purified adenosine 2′-epimerase from *S. antibioticus*. In these in vitro studies, adenosine is the substrate for the enzymatic synthesis of ara-A. The loss of tritium from the 2′-carbon of adenosine (FARMER et al., 1973) suggested the formation of 2′-ketoadenosine as an intermediate. In the in vitro studies, the addition of $NaB^{3}H_4$ to the enzyme assays did not produce [^{3}H]ara-A. However, $^{3}H_2O$ was isolated when [2′-^{3}H]adenosine was the substrate and ara-A was the product. Although all of the ^{3}H on C-2′ of [2′-^{3}H]adenosine is lost

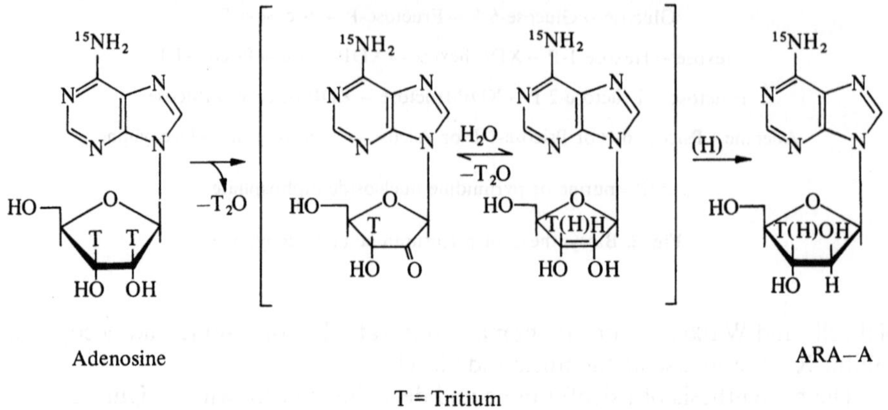

Fig. 3. Mechanism proposed for the biosynthesis of ara-A

and 85% of the ^3H is lost from C-3′ of [3′-^3H]adenosine, the lack of incorporation of ^3H from NaB^3H_4 suggests that the enzymic conversion of adenosine to ara-A may not proceed via a free form of 2′-ketoadenosine. The mechanism proposed for the biosynthesis of ara-A is shown in Figure 3. When the enzyme assays are done in tritium oxide, tritium is incorporated into the D-arabinose of ara-A. This type of epimerization is similar to UDP-N-acetylglucosamine 2′-epimerase described by SALO and FLETCHER (1970).

D. Clindamycin Purine Ribonucleotides

COATS and ARGOUDELIS (1971) and ARGOUDELIS et al. (1977) reported that clindamycin is readily converted to clindamycin 3-(5′-adenylate) and clindamycin 3-(5′-guanylate) (Fig. 4) following the addition of *S. coelicolor* to growing cultures. The biosynthesis of the adenylate and guanylate involves the addition of AMP or GMP to the hydroxyl group on carbon-3 of clindamycin. The clindamycin ribonucleotides are not inhibitory to *S. aureus*, but they do protect mice infected with *S. aureus* (ARGOUDELIS et al., 1977).

E. Cordycepin

Cordycepin is found in the culture filtrates of *Cordyceps militaris* and *Aspergillus nidulans* (CUNNINGHAM et al., 1951; KACZKA et al., 1964). Cordycepin 5′-triphosphate specifically inhibits the polyadenylating enzyme in the nucleus of the eukaryote. The formation of the poly(A) at the 3′-end of mRNA is blocked by cordycepin 5′-triphosphate.

The biosynthesis of cordycepin, like puromycin, 3′-amino-3′-deoxyadenosine, and 3′-acetamidoadenosine, proceeds directly from adenosine (SUHADOLNIK et al., 1964). LENNON and SUHADOLNIK (1976) have reported that the type reduction that occurs at C-3′ of adenosine to form cordycepin (Fig. 5) is similar to the biosynthesis of the deoxyribonucleotides by ribonucleotide reductase.

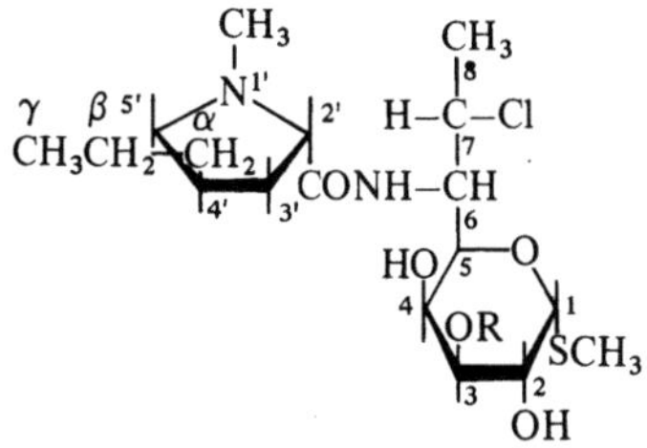

Clindamycin
R = H

Clindamycin 3–(5′–adenylate)
R = adenyl–5′–yl

Clindamycin 3–(5′–guanylate)
R = guanyl–5′–yl

Fig. 4. Structures of clindamycin, clindamycin 3-(5′-adenylate), and clindamycin 3-(5′-guanylate) (COATS and ARGOUDELIS, 1971)

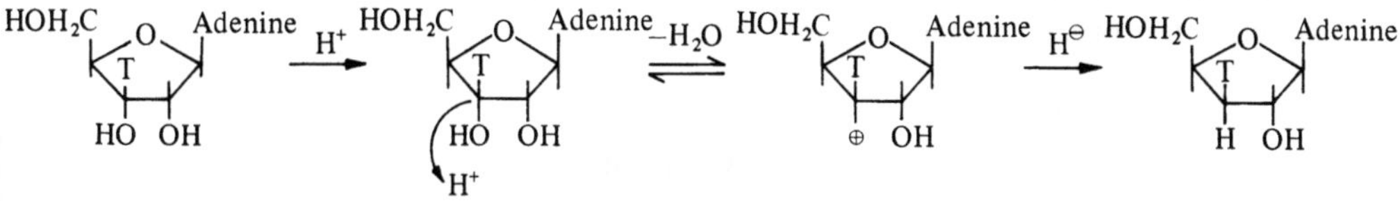

[3′–^{3}H]Adenosine

[3′–^{3}H]3′–Deoxyadenosine

T = Tritium

Fig. 5. Biosynthesis of cordycepin (3′-deoxyadenosine). (Reprinted with permission from LENNON and SUHADOLNIK, 1976)

F. Eritadenine

Eritadenine ((2′*R*, 3′*R*)-9-(4-carboxy-2,3-dihydroxybutyl)-adenine) has been isolated from *Lentinus edodes* Sing. Deoxyeritadenine and 9-(3-carboxylpropyl) adenine have also been isolated. Eritadenine has hypocholesterolemic activity. Because this is the first example of a naturally occurring adenine with a four-

Table 1. Distribution of C-14 from [8-^{14}C]Adenine into eritadenine and deoxyeritadenine. (Reprinted in modified form with permission from ITOH et al., 1973)

Peaks	Effluent (ml)	Radioactivity (cpm × 1000)	
		Time of culture after infusion	
		6 h	24 h
Eritadenine	178–185	39.8	64.6
Deoxyeritadenine	208–212	52.7	30.5
Adenine	361–375	33.7	18.8

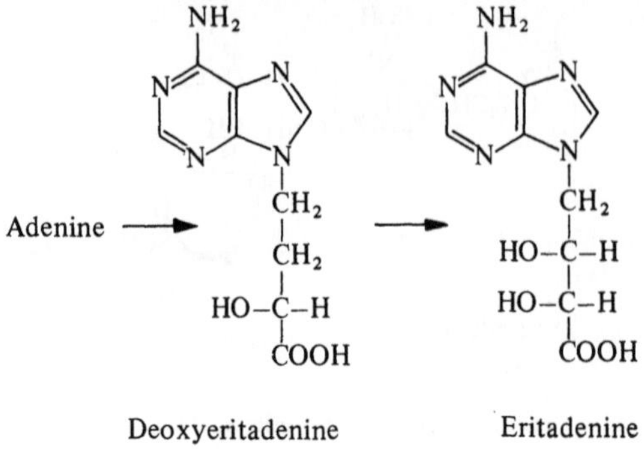

Fig. 6. Conversion of adenine to eritadenine by *Lentinus edodes*. (Reprinted in modified form with permission from ITOH et al., 1973)

carbon hydroxy acid attached to nitrogen-9, ITOH et al. (1973) studied the biosynthesis. They reported that [8-^{14}C]-adenine is the adenine precursor for deoxyeritadenine and eritadenine. The incorporation is shown in Table 1. From these data, ITOH et al. (1973) concluded that adenine is converted to deoxyeritadenine which is the precursor for eritadenine (Fig. 6).

G. Puromycin

Puromycin is isolated from the culture filtrates of *S. alboniger*. It acts as a codon-independent functional analog of aminoacyl-tRNA. Puromycin acts by catalyzing the release of incomplete peptide chains from the peptidyl-tRNA-

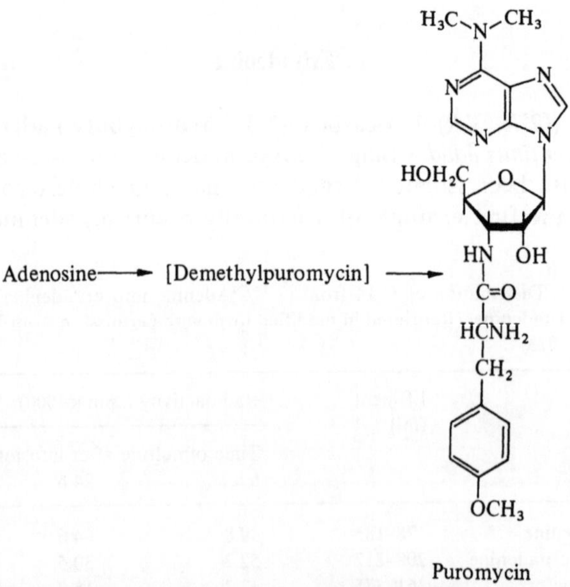

Fig. 7. Adenosine as the precursor for the biosynthesis of puromycin

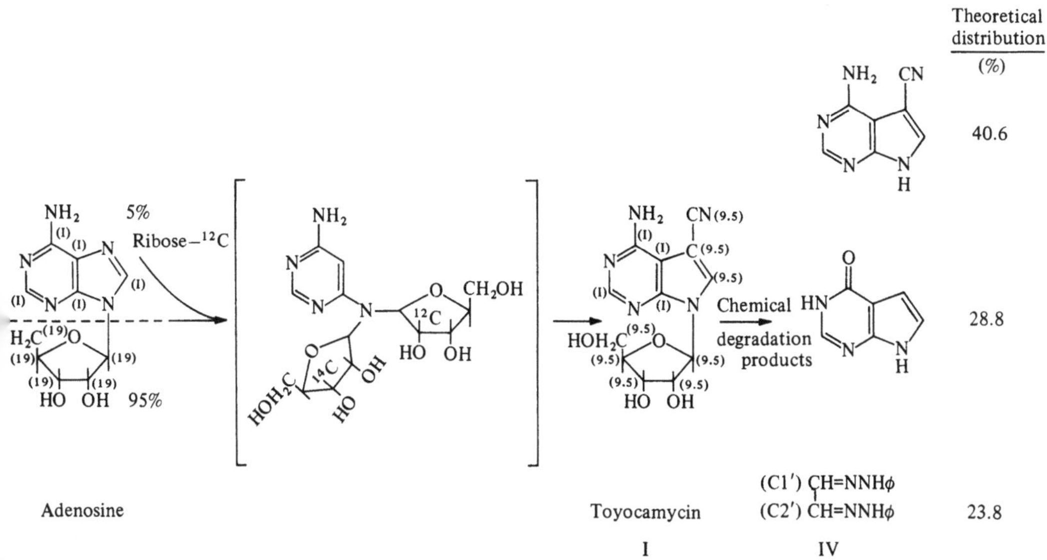

Fig. 8. Theoretical distribution of ^{14}C in toyocamycin from adenosine with a ^{14}C ratio of 5:95 for adenine to ribose (Reprinted with permission from SUHADOLNIK and UEMATSU, 1970)

mRNA. SUHADOLNIK et al. (unpublished results) have demonstrated that [U-^{14}C]adenosine is a direct precursor for the 3′-aminodemethyl-adenosine moiety of puromycin (Fig. 7). PATTABIRAMAN and POGELL (1969) have isolated O-demethylpuromycin which strongly suggests that the methylation of the tyrosine moiety of O-demethylpuromycin is the last step in the biosynthesis of puromycin.

H. Pyrrolopyrimidine Nucleoside Analogs (Tubercidin, Toyocamycin, and Sangivamycin)

The role of the pyrrolopyrimidine ring in natural products biochemistry has expanded from the *Streptomyces* to nucleoside Q which is widely distributed in the prokaryotes and the eukaryotes (KASAI et al., 1975; OKADA et al., 1978).

The biosynthesis of the pyrrolopyrimidine nucleosides utilizes the carbon-nitrogen skeleton of the purine ring and carbon atoms 1′-, 2′-, and 3′- of the ribosyl moiety (SMULSON and SUHADOLNIK, 1967; UEMATSU and SUHADOLNIK, 1970). The enzyme, GTP-8-formylhydrolase, that removes C-8 as formic acid from GTP in the biosynthesis of toyocamycin has been isolated and partially purified by ELSTNER and SUHADOLNIK (1971). The molecular weight of the enzyme is about 500,000. DEAE-chromatography splits the enzyme into two active proteins. Because carbons 1′, 2′, and 3′ of the ribosyl of GTP are used in the biosynthesis of the pteridine ring (BURG and BROWN, 1968), experiments were designed to determine 1. the biosynthetic origin of the pyrrole carbons and the cyano carbon of toyocamycin and 2. if a second ribose is added to N-8 of the purine ring following the elimination of C-8, but prior to pyrrole

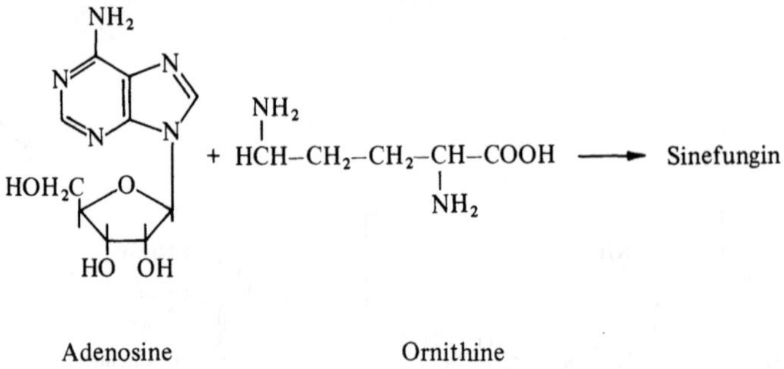

Fig. 9. Proposed biosynthetic mechanism for sinefungin. (Reprinted in modified form with permission from BERRY and ABBOTT, 1978)

ring formation (Fig. 8). By using adenosine, labeled in the aglycon and the ribosyl moieties, SUHADOLNIK and UEMATSU (1970) demonstrated that, following the removal of C-8, a second ribose is added to N-9. These two ribosyl units contribute equally to the three carbons needed for the pyrrole ring and the cyano group of toyocamycin (Fig. 8).

I. Sinefungin (Antibiotic A9145)

Sinefungin is one of several nucleosides produced by *S. griseolus* (HAMILL and HOEHN, 1973; GORDEE and BUTLER, 1973; BOECK et al., 1973; HAMILL et al., 1977; NAGARAJAN et al., 1977). Sinefungin is structurally similar to S-adenosylmethionine. Sinefungin inhibits fungi, Newcastle disease virus, and methyl transferase (PUGH et al., 1978). BERRY and ABBOTT (1978) have reported that ^{14}C from [8-^{14}C]adenine and [U-^{14}C]ornithine added to cultures of *S. griseolus* were incorporated into sinefungin. They proposed a biosynthetic mechanism as shown in Figure 9.

J. Thuringiensin

Thuringiensin (exotoxin) is an adenine nucleotide elaborated by *Bacillus thuringiensis*. The isolation, purification, structural elucidation, and chemical syntheses have been reviewed (SUHADOLNIK, 1979).

This unique nucleotide consists of adenine, ribose, glucose, and allaric acid. Phosphoric acid is attached to C-4 of allaric acid. The production of thuringiensin in the culture medium by *B. thuringiensis* reaches a maximum 16 h after inoculation (HORSKÁ et al., 1975). The role of adenine as a precursor for the biosynthesis of thuringiensin has been reported by MYSLOVATAYA (1974). 8-Azaguanine inhibits the growth of *B. thuringiensis*; adenine or guanine reverse this inhibition. Mutants resistant to 8-azaguanine had lowered amounts of thuringiensin.

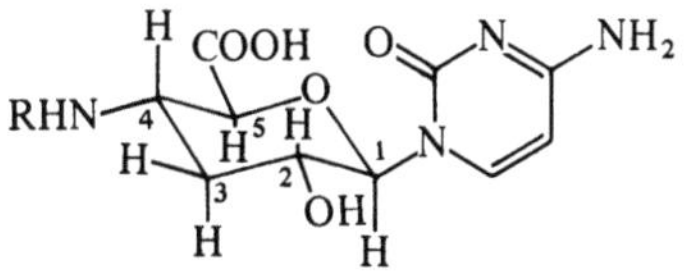

(I) Blasticidin H R = A
(II) Pentopyranamine D R = H
(III) Cytomycin H R = B

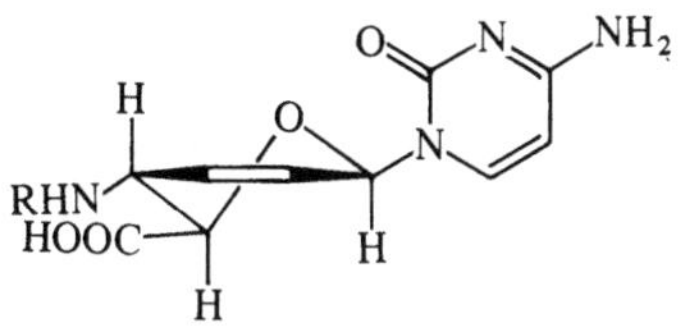

(IV) Blasticidin S R = A
(V) Cytomycin R = B

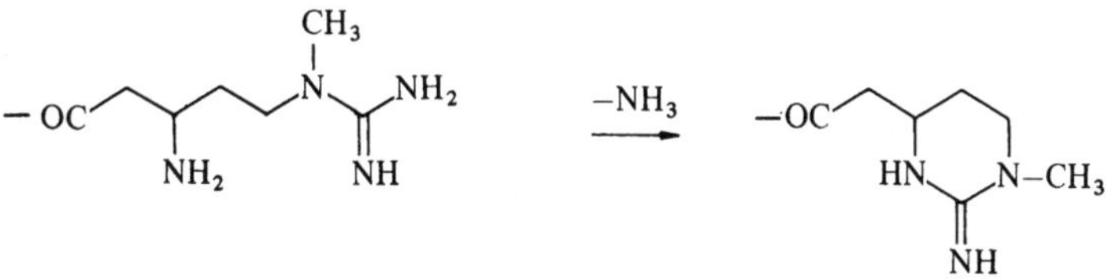

(A) Blastidyl (B) Pseudoblastidonyl

Fig. 10. Biosynthesis of blasticidin S from blasticidin H. (Reprinted with permission from SETO and YONEHARA, 1977)

III. The Biosynthesis of the Nucleoside Analogs that Utilize the Uracil, Cytosine, or Thymine Ring

A. Blasticidin H and S

The aminoacyl aminonucleoside antibiotics, blasticidin H and S, are isolated from the culture filtrates of *S. griseochromogenes* and *S. moro-okeansis* (TAKEUCHI et al., 1958; TSURUOKA and NIIDA, 1963). SETO et al. (1968) reported that ^{14}C from cytosine was incorporated into blasticidin S. Most recent studies by SETO and YONEHARA (1977) strongly suggest that blasticidin H (Fig. 10, I) loses a molecule of water which would make blasticidin H a direct precursor for blasticidin S (IV).

B. 5,6-Dihydro-5-azadeoxythymidine

The *s*-triazene naturally occurring nucleoside antibiotic is isolated from the fermentation culture of *S. platensis* var. *clarensis* (BANNISTER et al., 1976). 5,6-Dihydro-5-azadeoxythymidine (DHAdT) is a *s*-triazene nucleoside that is similar to the naturally occurring nucleoside antibiotic, 5-azacytidine.

DHAdT inhibits viruses in culture. It also has antibacterial activity against *E. coli.* The resistance of *E. coli* strains to this antibiotic is attributed to thymidine phosphorylase.

Although the biosynthesis of DHAdT does not depend on the uracil, cytosine, or thymine chromophore, it is included in this section. The biosynthesis of

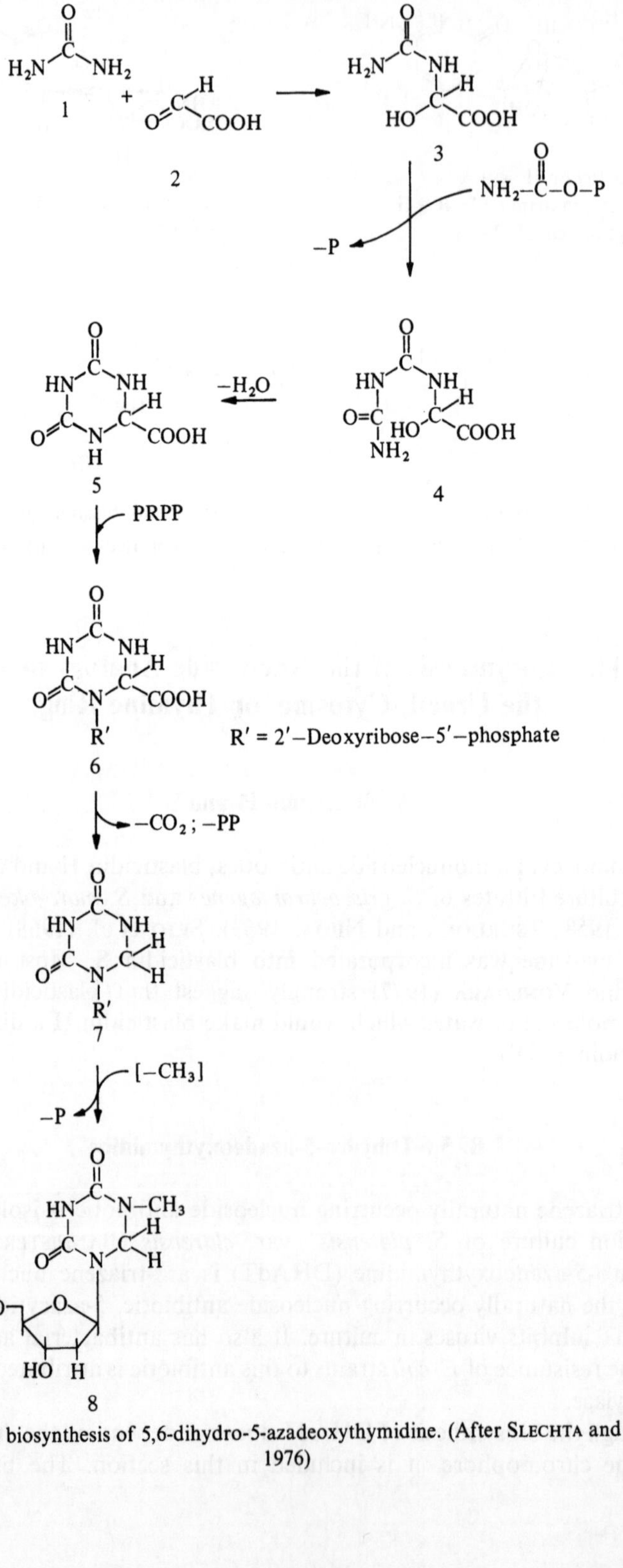

Fig. 11. Proposed biosynthesis of 5,6-dihydro-5-azadeoxythymidine. (After SLECHTA and CIALDELLA, 1976)

DHAdT has been studied by SLECHTA and CIALDELLA (1976). In their studies, they were able to show that [2-^{14}C]5-azaorotic acid was incorporated into DHAdT. The biosynthesis of DHAdT (*6*) is summarized in Figure 11. Urea (*1*) condenses with glyoxylic acid (*2*) to form glyoxyl urea (*3*). Condensation of *3* with carbamoyl phosphate forms glyoxyl biuret (*4*). The subsequent reactions (*4*→*6*) are analagous to normal purine nucleotide biosynthesis except that the N-methyl group of DHAdT is supplied by [^{14}C-methyl]methionine.

C. Clindamycin Pyrimidine Ribonucleotides

The biosynthesis of the uracil and cytosine-containing clindamycin ribonucleotides occurs as described in Section II, D.

D. Polyoxins and Octosyl Acids

The polyoxin complex (A-M) and the octosyl acids (A-C) are synthesized by *S. cacaoi*. The structure of polyoxin C and the general structure for the

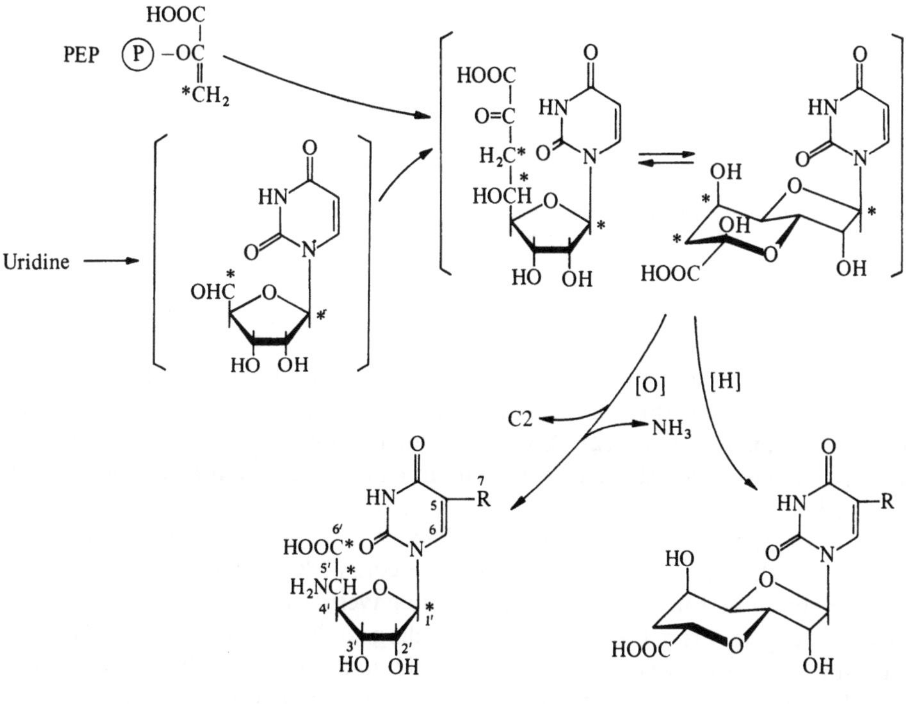

1 2

Fig. 12. Proposed biosynthetic pathway for the nucleoside skeleton of the polyoxins (*1*) and the octosyl acids (*2*) via an aldol condensation of uracil-5′-aldehyde with PEP. R = $-CH_3$, $-CH_2OH$, or $-COOH$; * = ^{13}C enrichment from D-[1-^{13}C]glucose (see text). (Reprinted with permission from ISONO et al., 1978)

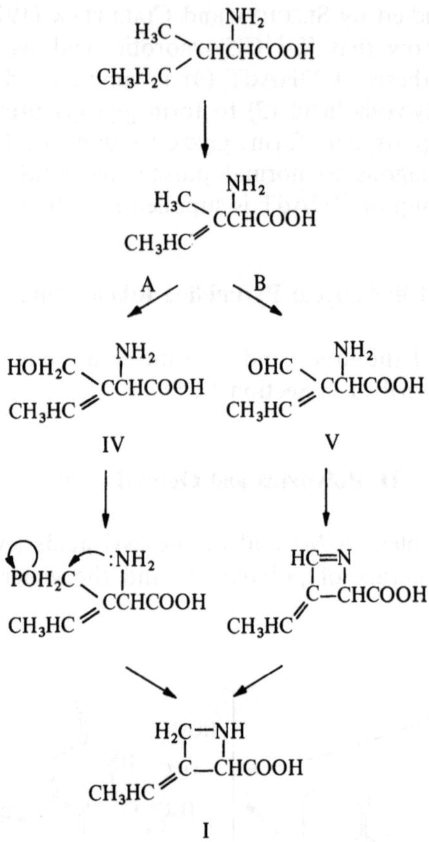

Fig. 13. Biosynthetic pathway of polyoximic acid (I) from L-isoleucine. (Reprinted with permission from ISONO et al., 1975)

octosyl acids are shown in Figure 12. The polyoxins are excellent inhibitors of phytopathogenic fungi (for review, see SUHADOLNIK, 1979).

The biosynthesis of polyoxin C (*1*) and the octosyl acids (*2*) by *S. cacaoi* proceeds via the oxidation of the hydroxymethyl group of uridine to the intermediate C-5′-aldehyde (Fig. 12). A C-8 keto-nucleoside is formed from PEP and uracil-5′-aldehyde which then forms the anhydro ring structure of the octosyl acids (*2*).

The six-carbon uronic acid in the polyoxins (*1*) is not formed directly from the carbon skeleton of glucose. Instead, the equal ^{13}C enrichment of C-1′ and C-5′ of ribose in *1* indicates that glucose is converted to ribose via the pentose phosphate cycle. From the ^{13}C and ^{14}C labeling studies, the most likely explanation for the biosynthesis of the aminouronic acid moiety of the polyoxins (*1*) and the octose carbon skeleton of the octosyl acids (*2*) involves the condensation of ribose and a three-carbon unit (Fig. 12).

The addition of the one-carbon unit (i.e., $-CH_3$, $-CH_2OH$, or $-COOH$) to C-5 of the uracil ring occurs at a step near the completion of the biosynthesis of polyoxins A–J (ISONO et al., 1978; ISONO and SUHADOLNIK, 1976; FUNAYAMA

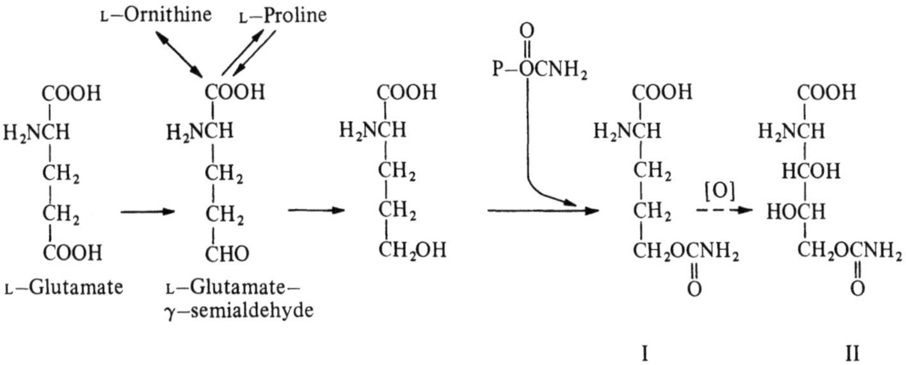

Fig. 14. Biosynthetic pathway for carbamoyl-polyoxamic acid (II). (Reprinted with permission from FUNAYAMA and ISONO, 1977)

and ISONO, 1977). The one-carbon donor for the five-substituted uracil ring in the polyoxins is C-3 of serine and not the methyl group of methionine. In addition, thymine can not serve as the thymine precursor for polyoxins H and J (ISONO and SUHADOLNIK, 1976). Therefore, the biosynthesis of the thymine chromophore in the polyoxins proceeds via a pathway independent of the dUMP thymidylate synthetase to TMP pathway that is needed for synthesis of dTTP for DNA synthesis.

The biosynthesis of 3-ethylidene-L-azetidine-2-carboxylic acid (polyoximic acid, I) occurs by the direct utilization of L-isoleucine (Fig. 13). The biosynthesis of 2-amino-2-deoxy-L-xylonic acid for the polyoxin complex utilizes glutamic acid (FUNAYAMA and ISONO, 1975). The δ-carboxyl group of glutamate is reduced to the hydroxymethyl group. The carbamoyl group is added to C-5 of α-amino-δ-carbamoyloxyvaleric acid (I) to form 5-*O*-carbamoyl-2-amino-2-deoxy-L-xylonic acid (carbamoyl-polyoxamic acid, II) (Fig. 14).

IV. Biosynthesis of the Carbon-linked Nucleoside Antibiotics

A portion or all of the carbon skeleton of showdomycin, oxazinomycin, formycin, and pyrazofurin is formed from either acetate or glutamate (Fig. 15). ELSTNER and SUHADOLNIK (1973) showed that ^{14}C from [1-^{14}C]acetate was found exclusively in C-5 of the maleimide ring of showdomycin. The asymmetric incorporation of ^{13}C from [1-^{13}C]acetate into C-5 of showdomycin and ^{13}C from [2-^{13}C]acetate into C-2, -3, and -4 of showdomycin was demonstrated by ^{13}Cnmr (ELSTNER et al., 1973). This distribution of ^{14}C from acetate provides an accurate picture of the biochemistry of acetate via the Krebs cycle in *S. showdoensis*. Further proof that the incorporation of the carboxyl group of acetate exclusively into C-5 of either glutamate or α-ketoglutarate and the subsequent formation of an asymmetric four-carbon intermediate was established by a double-labeled experiment with [5-^{14}C; 4-^{3}H]glutamate and [1-^{14}C; 2-^{3}H]acetate. All of the ^{14}C from [1-^{14}C]acetate and from [5-^{14}C]glutamate resides

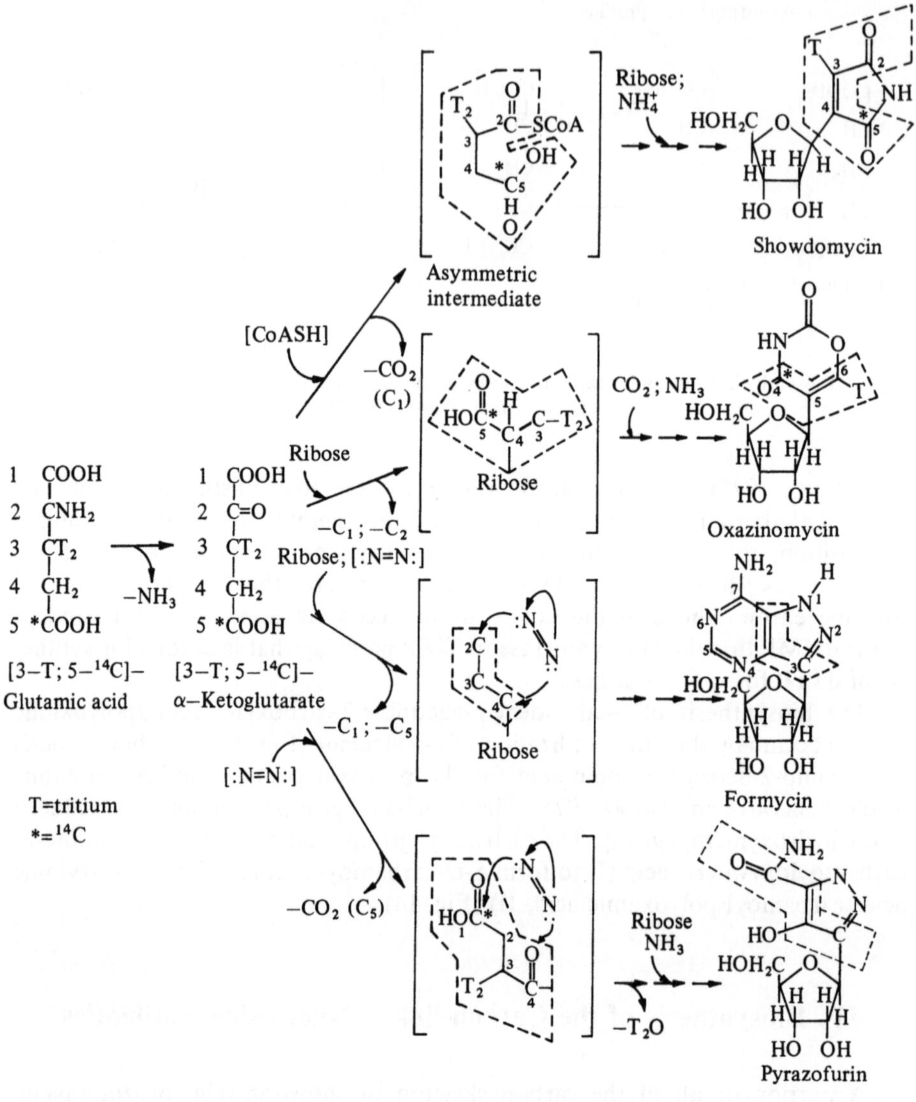

Fig. 15. Glutamic acid as the common precursor for the C-3 or C-4 carbon skeleton of the aglycon of showdomycin, oxazinomycin, formycin, and pyrazofurin

in C-4 of the maleimide ring of showdomycin. The tritium on C-4 is lost in this transformation. These findings are consistent with the conversion of glutamate to α-ketoglutarate from acetate, once acetate enters the Krebs cycle (ELSTNER and SUHADOLNIK, 1973). Although the aglycon of the C-nucleoside, oxazinomycin, is the 1,3-oxazine 2,4-dione ring, C-3, -4, and -5 of glutamate are incorporated into C-6, -5, and -4 of the aglycon of oxazinomycin (Fig. 15). In a more recent study, ISONO and UZAWA (1977) reported a sensitive and reliable method for studying the biosynthesis of the aglycon of oxazinomycin.

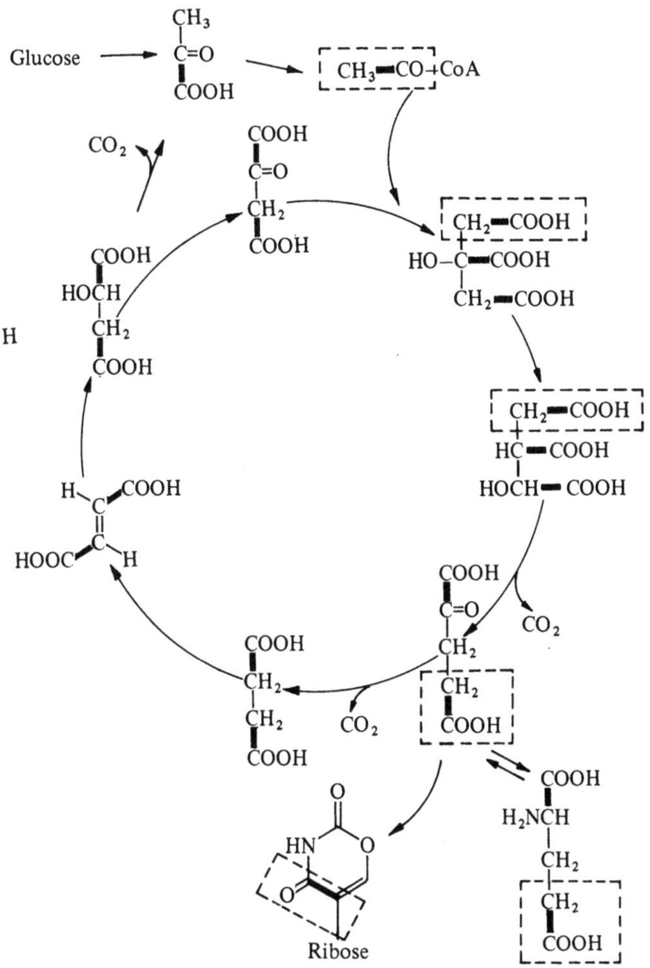

Fig. 16. The role of the Krebs cycle and malic enzyme in the distribution of acetate unit (C–C) and the biosynthesis of minimycin. The boxes show the primary site for an incorporated acetate unit. (Reprinted with permission from ISONO and UZAWA, 1977)

They demonstrated that [1,2-^{13}C]acetate is incorporated exclusively into C-4 and C-5 of the oxazine ring (Fig. 16).

KUNIMOTO et al. (1971) showed that the biosynthesis of formycin by *Nocardia interforma* does not appear to be closely related to either purine or pyrimidine metabolism. This was based on the observation that the incorporation of glycine into adenine was ten times greater than the ^{14}C incorporated into formycin and also the absence of incorporation of ^{14}C or ^{3}H from adenine and uridine into formycin. As with the biosynthesis of the aglycon of showdomycin, pyrazofurin, and oxazinomycin, [^{14}C]-glutamate is a good precursor for the biosynthesis of formycin (OCHI et al., 1974, 1975, 1976). The biosynthesis of formycin from formycin B has also been reported (OCHI et al., 1975).

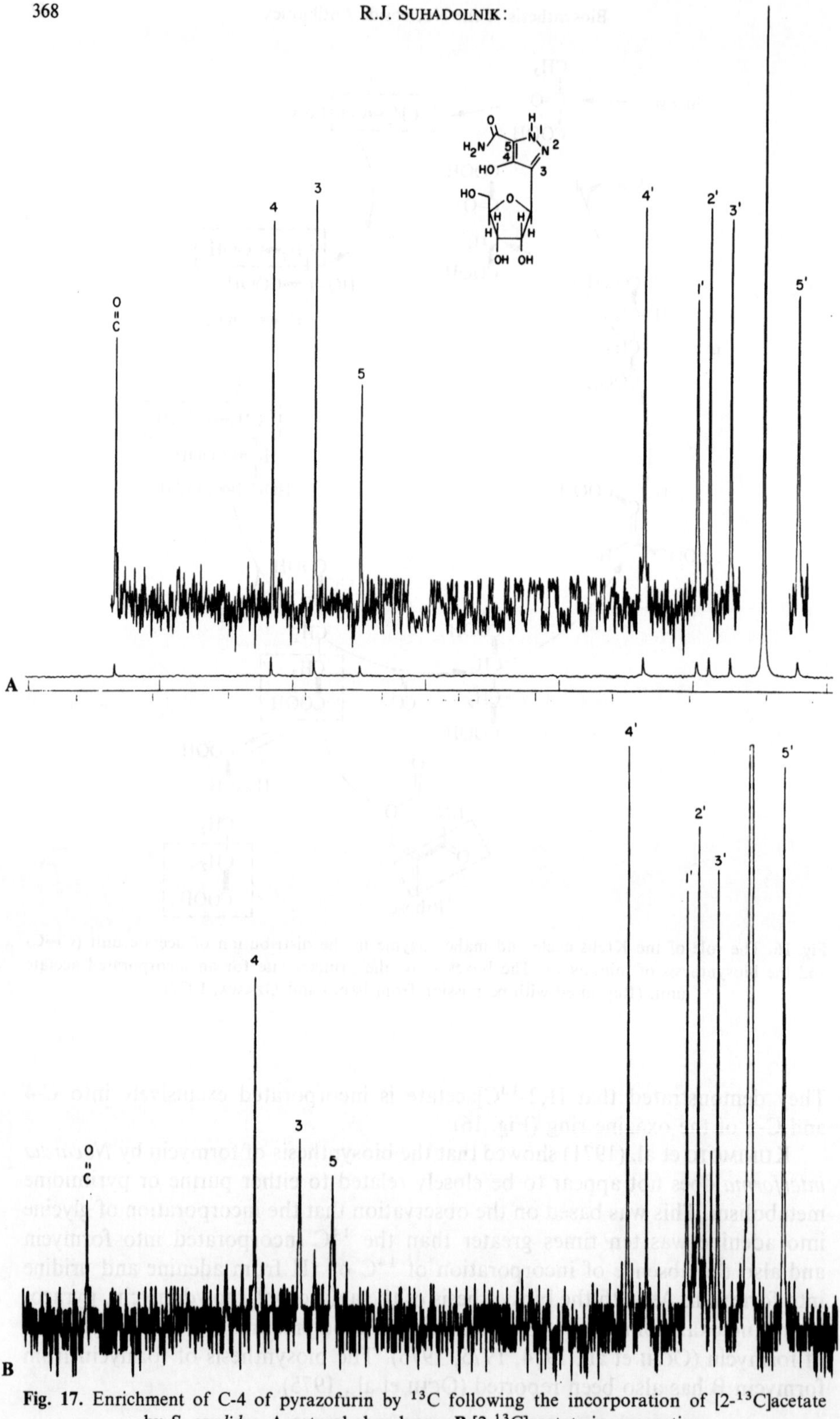

Fig. 17. Enrichment of C-4 of pyrazofurin by ^{13}C following the incorporation of [2-^{13}C]acetate by *S. candidus*. **A** natural abundance; **B** [2-^{13}C]acetate incorporation

Pyrazofurin, a pyrazolo nucleoside similar to formycin, is not a precursor of formycin (KUNIMOTO et al., 1971). The high incorporation of ^{14}C from [U-^{14}C]glutamic acid suggests that the biosynthesis of the aglycon of formycin utilizes several of the carbon atoms of this amino acid. From the acetate-glutamate precursor relationship for showdomycin, oxazinomycin, and pyrazofurin (Fig. 15), it is likely that a three-carbon fragment of glutamate may be incorporated into the pyrazolopyrimidine ring (OCHI, personal communication). Lysine also appears to be important in the biosynthesis of formycin (OCHI et al., 1974).

The ^{13}C-nmr spectra of the pyrazofurin isolated from [2-^{13}C]acetate displayed three enhanced resonances at 140.5, 134.0 and 128.2 ppm from dioxane which is 1.45, 1.45 and 1.8 times natural abundance (SUHADOLNIK, unpublished results). These are the signals for C-4, C-3 and C-5 (Fig. 17). ^{13}C from [1-^{13}C]acetate was not incorporated into pyrazofurin. BUCHANAN et al. (1980) reported that ^{14}C from [U-^{14}C]glutamate and [1-^{14}C]glutamate was incorporated into pyrazofurin; only a slight incorporation of [U-^{14}C]lysine was observed. The ^{14}C and ^{13}C incorporation data suggest that C-1, C-2, C-3 and C-4 of glutamate become the carboxamide carbon, C-5, C-4 and C-3 of pyrazofurin, respectively (Fig. 15).

References

Argoudelis AD, Coats JH, Mizsak SA (1977) Antibiot 30:474–487
Bannister B, Slechta L, Argoudelis AD (1976) 10th Int Symp Chem Nat Prod, Abstr C28
Berry DR, Abbott BJ (1978) J Antibiot 31:185–191
Boeck LD, Clem GM, Wilson MM, Westhead JE (1973) A9145, a new adeninecontaining antifungal antibiotic: Fermentation. Antimicrob Agents Chemother 3:49–56
Buchanan JG, Hamblin MR, Sood GR, Wightman RH (1980) J C S Chem Common 917–918
Burg AW, Brown GM (1968) J Biol Chem 243:2349–2358
Chassy BM, Suhadolnik RJ (1969) Biochim Biophys Acta 182:307–315
Coats JH, Argoudelis AD (1971) J Bacteriol 108:459–464
Cohen SS (1966) In: Davidson JN, Cohn WE (eds) Progress in nucleic acid research and molecular biology, vol V, pp 1–88. Academic Press, London New York
Cohen SS (1976) Med Biol 54:299–326
Cozzarelli NR (1977) Annu Rev Biochem 46:641–668
Cunningham KG, Hutchinson SA, Manson W, Spring FS (1951) J Chem Soc 2299–2300
Doering A, Keller J, Cohen SS (1966) Cancer Res 26:2444–2450
Elstner EF, Suhadolnik RJ (1971) J Biol Chem 246:6973–6981
Elstner EF, Suhadolnik RJ (1973) Biochemistry 11:2578–2584
Elstner EF, Suhadolnik RJ, Allerhand A (1973) J Biol Chem 248:5385–5388
Farmer PB, Suhadolnik RJ (1972) Biochemistry 11:911–916
Farmer PB, Uematsu T, Hogenkamp HPC, Suhadolnik RJ (1973) J Biol Chem 248:1844–1847
Funayama S, Isono K (1975) Biochemistry 14:5568–5572
Funayama S, Isono K (1977) Biochemistry 16:3121–3127
Gordee RS, Butler TF (1973) J Antibiot 26:466–470
Hamill RL, Hoehn MM (1973) J Antibiot 26:463–465
Hamill RL, Carrell CB, Nash SM, Nagarajan R (1977) 17th Annu ICAAC Meet Abstr No 48
Horskà K, Vanková J, Šebesta K (1975) Z Naturforsch 30C:120–123
Hubert-Habart M, Cohen SS (1962) Biochim Biophys Acta 59:468–471
Isono K, Suhadolnik RJ (1976) Arch Biochem Biophys 173:141–153
Isono K, Uzawa J (1977) FEBS Lett 80:53–56
Isono K, Funayama S, Suhadolnik RJ (1975) Biochemistry 14:2992–2996

Isono K, Sato T, Hirasawa K, Funayama S, Suzuki S (1978) J Am Chem Soc 100:3937–3939
Itoh H, Morimoto T, Kawashima K, Chibata I (1973) Experientia 29:271
Kaczka EA, Trenner NR, Arizon B, Walker RW, Folkers K (1964) Biochem Biophys Res Commun 14:456–458
Kasai H, Ohashi Z, Harada F, Nishimura S, Oppenheimer NJ, Crain PF, Liehr JG, von Minden DL, McCloskey JA (1975) Biochemistry 14:4198–4208
Kunimoto T, Sawa T, Wakashiro T, Hori M, Umezawa J (1971) J Antibiot 24:253–258
Lennon MB, Suhadolnik RJ (1976) Biochim Biophys Acta 425:532–536
Lim R, Cohen SS (1966) J Biol Chem 241:4304–4315
Müller WEG, Zahn RK, Beyer R, Falke D (1977) Virology 76:787–796
Myslovataya ML (1974) Genetika 10:151–153
Nagarajan R, Chao B, Dorman DE, Nash SM, Occolowitz JL, Schabel A (1977) 17th Annu ICAAC Meet Abstr No 50
Ochi K, Iwamoto S, Hayase E, Yashima S, Okami Y (1974) J Antibiot 27:909–916
Ochi K, Yashima S, Eguchi Y (1975) J Antibiot 28:965–973
Ochi K, Kikuchi S, Yashima S, Eguchi Y (1976) J Antibiot 29:638–645
Okada N, Shindo-Okada N, Sato S, Itoh YH, Oda KI, Nishimura S (1978) Proc Natl Acad Sci USA 75:4247–4251
Parke, Davis and Company (1967) Belg Patent 671, 557
Pattabiraman TN, Pogell BM (1969) Biochim Biophys Acta 182:245–247
Pavan-Langston D, Buchanan RA, Alford CA, Jr (eds) (1975) Adenine arabinoside: An antiviral agent. Raven Press, New York
Plunkett W, Cohen SS (1975) Cancer Res 35:1547–1554
Pugh C, Borchardt RT, Stone HO (1978) J Biol Chem 253:4075–4077
Salo WL, Fletcher HG Jr (1970) Biochemistry 9:882–885
Seto H, Yonehara H (1977) J Antibiot 30:1022–1024
Seto H, Yamaguchi I, Ōtake N, Yonehara H (1968) Agric Biol Chem 32:1292–1298
Slechta L, Cialdella J (1976) 10th Int Congr Biochem, Hamburg, Abstr No 01-8-012
Smulson M, Suhadolnik RJ (1967) J Biol Chem 242:2872–2876
Sugimori T, Suhadolnik RJ (1965) J Am Chem Soc 87:1136–1137
Suhadolnik RJ (1970) Nucleoside antibiotics. John Wiley and Sons, New York
Suhadolnik RJ (1979) Nucleosides as biological probes. John Wiley and Sons, New York
Suhadolnik RJ, Uematsu T (1970) J Biol Chem 245:4365–4371
Suhadolnik RJ, Weinbaum G, Meloche HP (1964) J Am Chem Soc 86:948–949
Takeuchi S, Hirayama K, Ueda K, Sakai H, Yonehara H (1958) J Antibiot Ser A 11:1–5
Truman JT, Klenow H (1968) Mol Pharmacol 4:77–86
Tsuruoka T, Niida T (1963) Meiji Seika Kenkyu Nempo p 23
Uematsu T, Suhadolnik RJ (1970) Biochemistry 9:1260–1266
Whitley RJ, Soong S, Dolin R, Galasso GJ, Ch'ien LT, Alford CA (1977) N Engl J Med 297:289–294
Wood WA (1972) In: Boyer PD (ed) The enzymes, vol VII, pp 281–302. Academic Press, London New York

Subject Index

f. = also following page; ff. = also following pages; *italics* = figure, scheme, table

Antibiotics

Volume I

Mechanism of Action

Editors: D. Gottlieb, P. D. Shaw
1967. 197 figures. XII, 785 pages
ISBN 3-540-03724-1

Volume II

Biosynthesis

Editors: D. Gottlieb, P. D. Shaw
1967. 115 figures. XII, 466 pages
ISBN 3-540-03725-X

Volume III

Mechanism of Action of Antimicrobial and Antitumor Agents

Editors: J. W. Corcoran, F. E. Hahn
1975. 193 figures. XII, 742 pages
ISBN 3-540-06653-5

"This review is to be commended. It is deliberately selective and concise, has little redundancy, is well edited, and quite complete... These books should provide excellent reference volumes and, in addition, pleasurable reading. They will be extremely useful to all investigators using the techniques of modern molecular biology, handy for graduate students, and will provide an important adjunct to the physicians' library." *Annals of Internal Medicine*

Volume V (in 2 parts)
Part 1

Mechanism of Action of Antibacterial Agents

Editor: F. E. Hahn
1979. 80 figures, 38 tables. XII, 376 pages
ISBN 3-540-09342-7

Contents: Bacitracin. – Bicyclomycin. – Chloramphenicol. – Ethambutol. – Ionophore Antibiotics. – Isonicotinic Acid Hydrazide. Kidamycin and Acetyl Kidamycin. – Lincomycin. – Moenomycin and Related Phosphorus-Containing Antibiotics. – Nalidixic Acid. – Nitrofurans. – Novobiocin and Coumermycin A_1. – Phenomycin and Enomycin. – Quinone Antibiotics. – Sparsomycin. – Streptomycin and Related Antibiotics. – Tetracycline. – Thiostrepton and Related Antibiotics. – Tiamulin and Pleuromutilin. – Tirandamycin. – Subject Index.

Part 2

Mechanism of Action of Antieukaryotic and Antiviral Compounds

Editor: F. E. Hahn
1979. 138 figures, 53 tables. XIII, 470 pages
ISBN 3-540-09396-6

Contents: Anisomycin and Related Antibiotics. – Antitumor Platinum Compounds. – 9-β-D-Arabinofuranosyladenine (Ara A). – 8-Azaguanine. – Bleomycin. – Diphtheria Toxin and Exotoxin A from Pseudomonas aeruginosa. – Echinomycin, Triostin, and Related Antibiotics. – Ellipticine. – 2-Hydroxy-3-Alkyl-1,4-Naphthoquinones. – Hydroxystilbamidine-5-Iodo-2'-Deoxyuridine. – Neocarzinostatin Nitracrine. – Phleomycin. – Polyene Antibiotics: Nystatin, Amphtericin B, and Filipin. – Protein and Glycoprotein Toxins That Inactivate the Eukaryotic Ribosome. – Quinine. – Showdomycin. – Streptonigrin. – Tilorone Hydrochloride. – The Vinca Alkaloids. – Virazole (Ribavirin). – Subject Index.

Springer-Verlag
Berlin
Heidelberg
New York

MIX
Papier aus verantwortungsvollen Quellen
Paper from responsible sources
FSC® C105338
FSC
www.fsc.org

If you have any concerns about our products,
you can contact us on
ProductSafety@springernature.com

In case Publisher is established outside the EU,
the EU authorized representative is:
Springer Nature Customer Service Center GmbH
Europaplatz 3, 69115 Heidelberg, Germany

Printed by Libri Plureos GmbH
in Hamburg, Germany